INFECTIONS
and
NURSING PRACTICE
prevention and control

161342

INFECTIONS
and
NURSING PRACTICE
p r e v e n t i o n   a n d   c o n t r o l

Barbara M. Soule, RN, MPA, CIC

Director, Epidemiology & Outcomes Research
St. Peter Hospital
Olympia, Washington
Coordinator, HIV/AIDS Services
Sisters of Providence Health System
Seattle, Washington

Elaine L. Larson, RN, PhD, FAAN, CIC

Dean and Professor
Georgetown University School of Nursing
Washington, D.C.

Gary A. Preston, MA, PhD, CIC

Epidemiologist
Healthcare Management Alternatives, Inc.
Vashon Island, Washington

with 24 illustrations

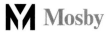 Mosby

St. Louis Baltimore Berlin Boston Carlsbad Chicago London Madrid
Naples New York Philadelphia Sydney Tokyo Toronto

161342

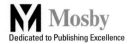
Mosby
Dedicated to Publishing Excellence

Editor: Timothy M. Griswold
Developmental Editor: Jolynn Gower
Project Manager: Karen Edwards
Production Editor: Gail Brower
Production: Graphic World Publishing Services
Designer: Elizabeth Fett
Manufacturing Supervisor: Betty Richmond
Cover Design: GW Graphics & Publishing

Copyright © 1995 by Mosby–Year Book, Inc.

All rights reserved. No part of this publication may be reproduced, stored in a retrieval system, or transmitted, in any form or by any means, electronic, mechanical, photocopying, recording, or otherwise, without prior written permission from the publisher.

Permission to photocopy or reproduce solely for internal or personal use is permitted for libraries or other users registered with the Copyright Clearance Center, provided that the base fee of $4.00 per chapter plus $.10 per page is paid directly to the Copyright Clearance Center, 27 Congress Street, Salem, MA 01970. This consent does not extend to other kinds of copying, such as copying for general distribution, for advertising or promotional purposes, for creating new collected works, or for resale.

Printed in the United States of America
Composition by Graphic World, Inc.
Printing/binding by R.R. Donnelley & Sons Company

Mosby–Year Book, Inc.
11830 Westline Industrial Drive
St. Louis, Missouri 63146

Library of Congress Cataloging in Publication Data

Soule, Barbara M.
  Infections and nursing practice: prevention and control/Barbara M. Soule, Elaine L. Larson, Gary A. Preston.
      p.   cm.
  Includes bibliographical references and index.
  ISBN 0-8016-6947-2
  1. Communicable diseases—Nursing.   2. Communicable diseases—Prevention.   3. Communicable disease—Case studies.   4. Communicable diseases—Etiology.   I. Larson, Elaine.   II. Preston, Gary A.
III. Title.
    [DNLM: 1. Communicable Diseases—nursing.   2. Communicable Disease Control—methods—nurses' instruction.   3. Communicable Diseases—nursing—case studies.   4. Cross Infection—prevention & control.
WC 18 S722i 1994]
  RC112.S63   1994
  616.9'045—dc20
  DNLM/DLC
  for Library of Congress   94-21881
                                                                                                CIP

95 96 97 98 99 / 9 8 7 6 5 4 3 2 1

Contributors

Kaye Bender, RN, MS
Chief of State Health Officer's Staff
Mississippi State Department of Health
Jackson, Mississippi

Rosemary Berg, M Ed, MBA
Director, Tucson Orthopedic Institute
Tucson Medical Center
Tucson, Arizona

Linda D. Bobo, PhD
Research Associate, Pediatric Infectious Diseases
Department of Medicine
Johns Hopkins University
Baltimore, Maryland

Arlene M. Butz, BSN, ScD, CPNP
Associate Professor, School of Nursing
Johns Hopkins University
Baltimore, Maryland

Patricia J. Checko, MPH
Chief of Epidemiology, AIDS Section
Connecticut Department of Public Health and
Addiction Services
Hartford, Connecticut

Brian W. Cooper
Director, Hospital Epidemiology
Division of Infectious Disease
Hartford Hospital, Hartford, Connecticut
Assistant Professor of Medicine
University of Connecticut School of Medicine
Farmington, Connecticut

Wendy A. Cronin, MT(ASCP), MS
Instructor, Consultant in International Infection
Control
School of Nursing, Johns Hopkins University
Baltimore, Maryland

Sue Crow, RN, MSN
Nurse Epidemiologist
Infection Control Department
Louisiana State University Medical Center
Shreveport, Louisiana

T. Grace Emori, RN, MS
Nurse Epidemiologist, Hospital Infections Program
National Center for Infectious Diseases
Centers for Disease Control and Prevention
Atlanta, Georgia

Hala Fawal, MT(ASCP), MPH, MBA, CIC
Program Manager
Department of Epidemiology
School of Public Health
University of Alabama at Birmingham
Birmingham, Alabama

Candace Friedman, MT(ASCP), MPH, CIC
Manager, Infection Control Services
University of Michigan Hospitals
Ann Arbor, Michigan

Barbara A. Goldrick, RN, PhD, CIC
Assistant Professor and Director
Center for Research and Scholarship
School of Nursing, Georgetown University
Washington, D.C.

Lorraine M. Harkavy, RN, MS, CIC
President, LMH Health Associates, Inc.
Potomac, Maryland

Gail A. Harkness, DrPH, RN, FAAN
Professor and Chair, Health Promotion Unit
School of Nursing
University of Connecticut
Storrs, Connecticut

Eddie R. Hedrick, BS, MT(ASCP), CIC
Manager, Infection Control/Staff Health Services
University Hospitals and Clinics
Columbia, Missouri

Teresa C. Horan, MPH, CIC
Surveillance Coordinator, Hospital Infections
Program
Centers for Disease Control and Prevention
Atlanta, Georgia

Elaine L. Larson, RN, PhD, FAAN, CIC
Dean and Professor
Georgetown School of Nursing
Georgetown University
Washington, DC

Marguerite McMillan Jackson, RN, MS, CIC, FAAN
Administrative Director
Medical Center Epidemiology Unit
University of California
San Diego Medical Center
San Diego, California;
Assistant Clinical Professor
Department of Family and Preventive Medicine
University of California
San Diego, California

Jeanne Leclair, MPH
Epidemiologist, Infectious Disease Department
The Johns Hopkins Bayview Medical Center
Baltimore, Maryland

Martha Long, RN, MSN, CIC
Infection Control Practitioner
University of Alabama Hospital
Birmingham, Alabama

Patricia Lynch, RN, MBA
Director, Epidemiology Associates
Seattle, Washington

Barbara R. Mooney, RN, BSN, CIC
Nurse Epidemiologist, Hospital Epidemiology
University of Utah Hospital
Salt Lake City, Utah

Norann Y. Planchock, PhD, RN
Professor and Associate Director of Graduate Studies in Nursing
Division of Nursing
Northwestern State University of Louisiana
Shreveport, Louisiana

Jean M. Pottinger, MA, RN, CIC
Nurse Epidemiologist
Veteran's Affairs
Lakeside Medical Center
Chicago, Illinois

Emily Rhinehart, BSN, RN, CIC
Director, CQI Services
AIG Consultants, Inc.
Boston, Massachusetts

Mary Schoenthal, RN, BSN, CCRN
Senior Clinical Nurse
Surgical Intensive Care
Perry Hall, Maryland

Barbara Soule, RN, MPA, CIC
Director, Epidemiology & Outcomes Research
St. Peter Hospital
Olympia, Washington
Coordinator, HIV/AIDS Services
Sisters of Providence Health System
Seattle, Washington

Marjorie J. Stenberg
Nurse Epidemiologist
Veterans Affairs Medical Center
West Palm Beach, Florida

Beth Hewitt Stover, RN, CIC
Infection Control Nurse, Alliant Health System
Kosair Children's Hospital
Louisville, Kentucky

Patricia A. Tabloski, PhD, RNC
Assistant Professor, School of Nursing
University of Connecticut
Storrs, Connecticut

Dorothy J. Thomas, BSN, CIC
Director, Infection Control
Miami Children's Hospital
Miami, Florida

Linda G. Tietjen, RN, BSN, MPH
Infection Prevention Consultant
Baltimore, Maryland

Marie Ciacco Tsivitis, MT(ASCP), MPH, CIC
Infection Control Coordinator
Long Island State Veterans Home
State University of New York
Stony Brook, New York

Joan G. Turner
Professor, University of Alabama
Birmingham, Alabama

Carol O'Boyle Williams, RN, MS, CIC
Clinical Nurse Specialist/Infection Control
Acute Disease Epidemiology Section
Minnesota Department of Health
Minneapolis, Minnesota

Reviewers

Chris L. Algren, RN, MSN, EdD
Associate Clinical Professor
University of Texas Health Sciences Center
Assistant Director
Education, Operating Room, PACU, & Same Day
Surgery
Texas Children's Hospital
Houston, Texas

Trisha Barrett, RN, BS, CIC
Manager, Infection Control Program
Alta Bates Medical Center
Berkeley, California

Rex Bolin, MD
Division of Pulmonary Medicine
Director, Critical Care Medicine
St. Peter Hospital
Olympia, Washington

Elizabeth Bolyard, RN, MPH
Chief, Prevention Activities
HIV Infections Branch
Hospital Infections Program
National Centers for Infectious Diseases
Centers for Disease Control and Prevention
Atlanta, Georgia

Jerry K. Bryant, RN, MPH, CIC
Clinical Epidemiologist
Cleveland Clinic Foundation
Adjunct Assistant Professor
Cleveland State University School of Nursing
Cleveland, Ohio

Linda A. Chiarello, RN, MS, CIC
Director, Infection Control/Occupational
Health Unit
New York State Department of Health
AIDS Institute
Albany, New York

Jackie Cohran, RN, BSN
Infection Control Coordinator
Prince Georges Hospital Center
Cheverly, Maryland

Michael F. Cole, PhD
Associate Professor
Microbiology and Immunology
Georgetown University School of Medicine
Washington, DC

Henry L. deGive, MD
Pediatric Department
St. Peter Hospital
Olympia, Washington

John Duncan III, MD
Department of Neurosurgery
Georgetown University Medical Center
Washington, DC

Dorrie Fontaine, RN, PhD
Coordinator, Critical Care Program
Georgetown University School of Nursing
Washington, DC

Sheila Fitzgerald, RN, PhD
Division of Occupational Health
School of Hygiene and Public Health
Johns Hopkins University
Baltimore, Maryland

Dorothy Gauthier, MSN, DSN
Associate Professor
School of Nursing
University of Alabama
Birmingham, Alabama

Robert P. Gruninger, MD
Associate Director
Clinical Microbiology Laboratory
Duke University Medical Center
Durham, North Carolina

Janice Harral, RN, BSN
Assistant Nurse Coordinator
Neurosurgical Intensive Care Unit
Georgetown University Hospital
Washington, DC

Susan J. Hockenberger, EdD, RN
Dean
Allan and Donna Lansing School of Nursing
Bellarmine College
Louisville, Kentucky

W. Charles Huskins, MD
Instructor in Pediatrics
Harvard Medical School
Assistant in Infectious Diseases
Children's Hospital
Boston, Massachusetts

Heidi Jenkins
Assistant Program Director
STD Control Program
Connecticut Department of Public Health
& Addiction Services
Hartford, Connecticut

LaVohn Josten, PhD, RN, FAAN
Associate Professor and Coordinator Public Health
Nursing
School of Nursing
University of Minnesota
Minneapolis, Minnesota

Princy Kumar, MD
Division of Infectious Diseases
Department of Medicine
Georgetown University Medical Center
Washington, DC

Cole Mason, MD
Pediatric Department
St. Peter Hospital
Olympia, Washington
Clinical Associate Professor
University of Washington School of Medicine
Seattle, Washington

R. Michael Massanari, MD, MS
Medical Director
Professional Practice Review Group
Hospital Epidemiologist
Henry Ford Hospital
Detroit, Michigan

Michael L. Matlock, MD
Division of Infectious Diseases
St. Peter Hospital
Olympia, Washington

William J. Mitchell, MD
Division of Gastroenterology
St. Peter Hospital
Olympia, Washington

Patricia A. Mshar
Epidemiologist
Epidemiology Section
Connecticut Department of Public Health
& Addiction Services
Hartford, Connecticut

Roger Mshar
Senior Environmental Sanitarian
Environmental Health/Food Protection Program
Connecticut Department of Public Health
& Addiction Services
Hartford, Connecticut

Gregory A. Poland, MD
Associate Professor of Medicine
Chief, Mayo Vaccine Research Group
Mayo Clinic and Foundation
Rochester, Minnesota

Gina Pugliese, RN, MN
Director, Infection Control
American Hospital Association
Chicago, Illinois

Helen Roach, RN, MSN
Clinical Educator
Georgetown University Hospital
Washington, DC

Karin K. Roberts, MN
Assistant Professor
Research College of Nursing
Kansas City, Missouri

William A. Rutala, PhD, MPH
Division of Infectious Diseases
Department of Medicine
University of North Carolina
Director, Hospital Epidemiology
University of North Carolina Hospitals
Chapel Hill, North Carolina

Bruce Silverman, MD
Division of Gastroenterology
St. Peter Hospital
Olympia, Washington

Carol Scott, RN, MSN
Clinical Instructor
Georgetown University School of Nursing
Washington, DC

Mariah Snyder, PhD, RN, FAAN
Professor
School of Nursing
University of Minnesota

Linda Thiel, RN, MS, CFMP
Assistant Professor of Nursing
Catholic University of America
Washington, DC

Donald Vesley, PhD
Professor
Environmental and Occupational Health
School of Public Health
University of Minnesota
Minneapolis, MN

Joan Weber, RN, CIC
Infection Control Nurse
Shriners Burns Institute
Boston, Massachusetts

We wish to acknowledge authors who also served
as reviewers:

Patricia J. Checko, MPH
T. Grace Emori, RN, MS
Teresa C. Horan, MPH, CIC
Marguerite M. Jackson, RN, MS, CIC, FAAN
Patricia Lynch, RN, MBA
Barbara R. Mooney, RN, BSN, CIC
Marjorie J. Stenberg, MS, RN, CIC
Beth H. Stover, RN, CIC
Carol O'Boyle Williams, RN, MS, CIC

To our families, especially Oscar, Steve, and Lyn
For their confidence and support

Preface

The health services planners of the Pew Health Profession Commission concluded in their 1991 report that, if we are to be prepared for the next century, educators of our health care practitioners must shift their emphasis from specialized "sickness" care in acute care institutions to community-based, preventive, primary care.[1] Nurses are the traditional caregivers who must be prepared to participate in health promotion, disease prevention, and community health care as well as technically complex acute care.

We intend this book to prepare nurses to prevent and manage infectious diseases typically encountered in these diverse settings. Section One discusses the host, microorganism, physical environment, and social influences on host-microorganism interactions which determine whether or not disease occurs. Each chapter describes one of these in detail and considers its interactions with the other three as determinants of the natural history of infectious disease. Section One provides the basis for the review of prevention and control methods in Section Two and for the application of these methods illustrated in the clinical studies of Section Three. Our emphasis is on the patient as the host. However, the role of family members, caregivers, and others as potential hosts is also considered. The efficacy of traditional infection control strategies is critically assessed and the implications of setting are considered throughout.

This book is designed to supplement course work in infectious disease or infection prevention and control. It may support study at several levels of preparation or serve as a reference for nurses practicing in diverse settings. It is not intended to be a comprehensive infectious disease, microbiology, or immunology text or a clinical procedure manual. Its use should be supported by references, articles, and texts from the health science literature consistent with the level of the reader's experience and instructor's focus.

We have tried to describe principles of human biology and practical infection prevention and control methods based on them. The importance of adapting these methods to the ecology of host-environment interactions[2] and the circumstances of the care setting are emphasized and integrated into the clinical study presentations. We hope this approach logically connects basic science to general methods and general methods to specific patient care practices in a way that assists you in responding to the variations and complexities of your practice of nursing.

THE EDITORS: *Barbara M. Soule*
Elaine L. Larson
Gary A. Preston

---

[1] Healthy America: Practitioners for 2005, Durham, N.C., 1991, Pew Health Professions Commission.

[2] Burnet M, White DO. *Natural History of Infectious Disease.* 4th ed. Cambridge, 1972, Cambridge University Press.

Acknowledgments

This book exists because of the hard work of many people. We thank the authors for their contributions and forbearance with our suggestions, the reviewers for their time and attention to important details, and the editors of Mosby–Year Book and Graphic World Publishing Services for seeing the book through to completion.

The production of numerous drafts, maintenance of complicated correspondence, and meeting of many deadlines would not have been possible without the extraordinary efforts of Bonnie Matson, Christina Orange, Laurent Dubois, and Marilyn Graham who managed every request with energy and good humor.

We are grateful for the assistance of librarians Edean Berglund, Kathy Wagner, and Lewis Daniel for literature research, and to our professional colleagues and friends who provided encouragement and counsel: Lou Hilken, Mike Matlock, Bev Masini, Marcia Kliban, Becky Cant, Gail Stewart, Judy Dubois, Diane Marinig, Cynthia Strauss, Charles Hawley, Marilyn Otoupal, Carol O'Boyle Williams, Gina Pugliese, Carla Alvarado, Patricia Lynch, Marguerite Jackson, Emily Rhinehart, and Camilla Stivers.

Finally, we thank our children Sarah and Adam Soule, Justine and Nathan Larson, and Morgan, Meridith, and Mallory Preston for their understanding and willingness to accommodate their lives to their parents' chaotic schedules.

Contents

Section One

The Host-Environment Interaction

There is no single determinant of health and disease. At one time, the microbiologic agent was considered the only and sufficient cause of infectious disease and the roles of the host's condition, the physical environment, and social factors were not well appreciated. We now understand that the infectious agent is but one important element of the host's environment and that a variety of factors work interactively to determine whether infection and clinical disease result. This perspective, the ecologic perspective, assesses the interaction of a host with its environment.

This section describes the interrelationships that influence risk of infection. These are depicted in Figure I-1. Each chapter is accompanied by a similar illustration that emphasizes the elements of cause discussed in that chapter. Chapter 1 assesses characteristics of the potential human host that may influence risk of infectious disease. Chapter 2 considers the mechanisms by which microorganisms establish themselves in or on the human host and reviews microbial characteristics that affect the host and result in disease. Chapter 3 describes how the physical environment can influence the host-microorganism interaction and Chapter 4 reviews the influence of human society on one's risk of infection. Successful nursing strategies for prevention and management of infectious disease can evolve only from an understanding of the forces that influence risk.

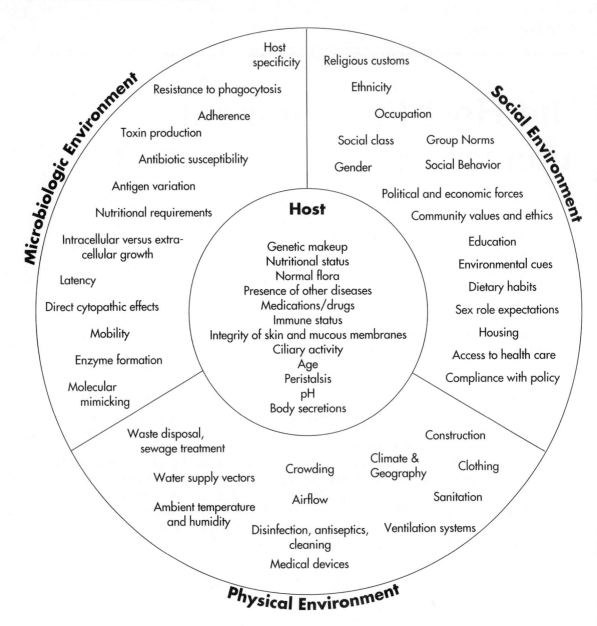

FIGURE I-1 Factors that influence the infectious process.

Chapter 1

The Host

ELAINE L. LARSON

he host plays a major role in determining the outcome of interactions involving the host, microbe, and environment. Humans are equipped with a myriad of natural and acquired defenses that usually prevent harmful consequences of an encounter with a microorganism. The body's armamentarium to resist or control the spread of microorganisms includes innate defenses and those acquired throughout life by interactions with microorganisms. It is essential for the health care professional to understand the immune system and other factors that influence immunity to assess the patient's risk of infection, to identify strategies to enhance the patient's resistance, and to protect the vulnerable patient.

It is not possible to predict unerringly whether a clinical infection will occur under specific conditions. An encounter between a human host and a microbe can result in any of several outcomes. The microbe may pass on or through the host without a trace or may establish itself in a comfortable niche (skin, gut, mouth) and persist without apparent ill effect. At other times, the body recognizes the organism as a foreign invader, mounts its immune defenses, and kills or rids itself of the invader. When this defense process becomes more than a mild skirmish, war breaks out in the body and is recognized by clinical signs and symptoms as infection. This chapter focuses on the attributes of the human host that influence the infectious process and presents an overview of the immune system and factors that affect immune function.

HOST IMMUNE SYSTEMS

The nature of the ecologic balance between the host and microorganisms is influenced by a variety of environmental and host factors. Some important host factors are listed in Figure 1-1. These host factors influence why some individuals become very ill and others have no symptoms after an encounter with the same microorganism. The immune system has many interacting parts and a variety of simultaneous activities that work in concert. Although components of the immune system are interdependent, this discussion classifies a host immune mechanism as nonspecific if it is active against a variety of potentially infective microorganisms or specific if it is targeted against a specific microorganism as a consequence of previous experience.

Nonspecific immune mechanisms

Each species is equipped with natural immune mechanisms that act against a range of infectious microorganisms to protect it from certain infectious diseases. Natural immunity can be specific to an individual host or to all hosts of a species. For example, humans are

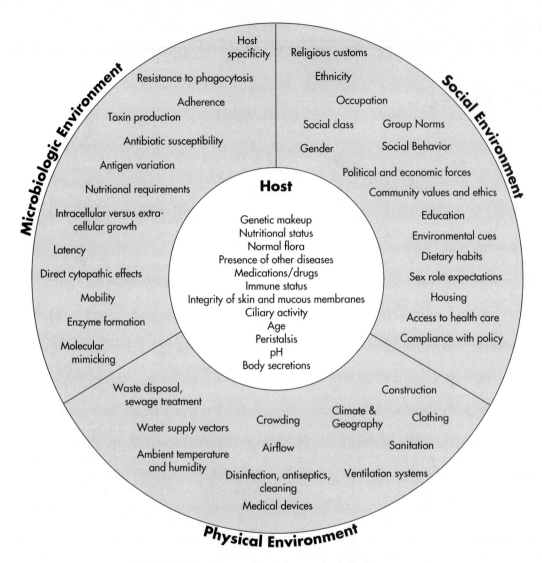

FIGURE 1-1. Host factors that influence the infectious process.

not susceptible to the distemper virus that affects cats and dogs. When a host encounters a microorganism to which the host is susceptible, a series of events must occur before an infection can result. The organism must: (1) successfully gain access to the host; (2) find a suitable site for growth; and (3) be able to survive the host's various defenses. Host-protective mechanisms affect each step of this process. Mechanisms that prevent entry or rid the host of microorganisms by the inflammatory response are nonspecific (Table 1-1).

Physical Barriers

Most infectious agents do not make it past the host's physical and chemical barriers. The human body is encased in its largest organ, the skin, which provides a relatively impermeable

TABLE 1-1. General defense mechanisms and protective effects against microorganisms

Organ	Defense mechanism	Protective effect
Intact skin	Physical barrier	Prevents penetration of organism into body
	Normal flora Low pH from fatty acids Dryness, dessication, desquamation	Inhibit growth of organisms
Respiratory tract	Mucociliary lining of upper and lower tracts	Sweeps inhaled organisms to throat to be swallowed
	Cough and sneeze reflex	Forces organisms out of respiratory tract
	Lysozymes in nasal secretions	Lyse cell wall of some bacteria
	Alveolar macrophages	Phagocytize of some organisms
Gastrointestinal tract: Small intestine	Peristalsis	Sweeps organisms to large intestine, minimizing attachment and multiplication
	Hydrochloric acid	Lowers pH; kills organisms
	Mucous gel on epithelial surface	Limit establishment of organisms in intestine
	Normal flora Secretory IGA Bile acids and enzymes	
Large intestine	Fatty acids	Inhibit growth of organisms
	Bacteriocin	Provides competition to exogenous organisms for nutrients and attachment
Urogenital tract	Flushing action and bacteriostatic pH of urine	Inhibits establishment and growth of organisms
	Normal flora (*lactobacilli*)	Produces lactic acid and low pH to inhibit organism
Conjunctiva	Flushing action of tears	Carries organisms away from eye
	Lysozymes	Lyse organisms

barrier to the outside world. The normal openings in this barrier—the ear, conjunctiva, and respiratory, gastrointestinal, and genitourinary tracts—are themselves protected from microbial invasion by various mechanisms (e.g., mucociliary activity, acidic pH, antibodies, enzymes) and an indigenous microbial population that make it difficult or impossible for newcomers to attach, compete successfully for nutrients, or overcome growth inhibitors produced by the resident microbes.

To cause infection, a microbe must penetrate or attach to intact skin or mucous membranes or take advantage of a break in some protective barrier that would normally exclude it. Some organisms have developed mechanisms and strategies to overcome these defenses. The influenza virus and rhinovirus, a cause of the common cold, attach to and reside in respiratory epithelial cells, precluding the need to enter further into the body. The adenovirus and chlamydia live in the conjunctiva, resulting in "pinkeye" and other eye infections. *Streptococcus pyogenes* can grow in the epithelium of the pharynx and can cause streptococcal throat infections ("strep throat"). Fungi can settle on intact skin to cause ringworm without ever having to enter the body. Certain strains of *Escherichia coli*, when ingested, can attach to intestinal surfaces and cause diarrhea.

Organisms' access to epithelial surfaces, their ability to replicate there, and their frequent exclusion from other body sites by host immune mechanisms explains why most infections among otherwise healthy individuals affect the integumentary, respiratory, genitourinary, and intestinal tracts. Generally, the body is protected from entry of microorganisms except when alterations occur in the usual host barriers. For example, some organisms that cannot normally enter intact skin must be delivered into the host by a vector such as a mosquito (e.g., malaria), a bite such as from a skunk (e.g., rabies), or even a contaminated needle (e.g., hepatitis B and C). Before infection can occur, there must be a suitable reservoir, portal of exit from the reservoir, mechanism of transmission to the host, portal of entry, and most important, a susceptible host. Infectious agents can be transmitted by one of four major routes: contact, air, vehicle, or vector. Table 1-2 gives examples of specific infectious diseases transmitted by these four major routes. In health care settings contact is by far the most important mode of transmission.

Microbe Inhibitors

If microorganisms penetrate the host's physical and chemical barriers and are recognized as invaders, the body marshals an inflammatory process that expedites delivery of two types of specialized phagocytic cells, macrophages and neutrophils, to the affected site. These cells engulf and digest microbes and other debris by a process called *phagocytosis* (ingesting cells), which consists of four phases: chemotaxis, attachment, ingestion, and killing.

Phagocytic cells are biochemically attracted to microorganisms by a process called *chemotaxis*. These cells migrate from the circulating bloodstream across the vessel wall to the site of infection. Chemicals that can serve as chemotactic agents and stimulate migration include components of the organism itself, damaged body cells, and components of lymphocytes and complement (see Humoral Immunity). When the phagocyte arrives on site, its plasma membrane adheres to the microorganism's surface. This process often requires the help of specific antibodies called *opsonins*, plasma proteins that coat the microbe and promote the attachment. When the microbe and the phagocyte are attached, the phagocyte surrounds the microbe in an intracellular vacuole, into which enzymes and other antimicrobial agents are released to kill the invader. Some phagocytes active at the infection site migrate to the lymphatic circulation to dispose of debris. Other phagocytes die and are removed from circulation via the lymphatic system or become part of a localized necrotic process such as an abscess.

The process of phagocytosis is considered to be a nonspecific host defense because it can be initiated in the presence of any substance recognized to be foreign without the need for specific priming by previous immune experience with the microorganism. The classic signs of the inflammatory process are a result of the body's phagocytic response to foreign invaders (Table 1-3). However, phagocytic activity is greatly enhanced by components and interactions of the specific immune response, including humoral and cellular immune functions (see Specific Immune Mechanisms). In some cases, organisms are not affected by phagocytosis and live successfully within cells. Some

TABLE 1-2. Examples of infections spread by four major routes

	Air	Contact	Vehicle	Vector
Infectious agent	Varicella zoster virus	*Salmonella*	Hepatitis B virus	Western equine encephalitis virus
Reservoir of agent	Humans only: respiratory tract, skin, mucous membranes	Intestinal tract of humans, domestic fowl, other animals	Humans; primary site of replication unknown	Birds, hibernating mosquitoes
Portal of exit	Respiratory secretions, skin vesicles	Intestinal tract, feces	Parenteral primarily; also urine, bile, semen, feces, nasopharyngeal secretions	Parenteral via mosquito blood meal
Portal of entry into host	Respiratory tract	Intestinal tract; mouth	Often parenteral (transfusion or needle stick); occasionally by mucous membrane	Mosquito bite
Susceptible host	Any human who has not had chickenpox or been immunized	Most humans if dose adequate; some strain-specific immunity develops after infection	Any human who has not been previously infected or immunized	Birds, snakes, frogs, rodents, horses; humans become accidental hosts

bacteria, including the organisms causing tuberculosis and chlamydial infection, as well as viruses, are therefore unaffected by phagocytosis. The human immunodeficiency virus (HIV), for example, survives ingestion by macrophages, which then serve as a reservoir for the HIV. Consequently, specific cellular immunity is vital against these intracellular parasites.

Specific immune mechanisms

The mechanisms of nonspecific resistance—physical and chemical barriers and the inflammatory response—respond against all foreign invaders and are not specific to any particular pathogen. Specific immune responses, on the other hand, are learned by the body as a result of exposure to a microbe and are targeted specifically to that one invader. Substances that are recognized as foreign and trigger specific and nonspecific immune responses are called *antigens* (Ag, *anti*body *gen*erating). Two types of immune reactions to specific antigens exist: *humoral* immunity, so named because the protective elements circulate in the bloodstream, and *cellular* immunity, which involves direct contact between the foreign invader and certain immune cells. The cells responsible for major immune function are white blood cells. All originate from the hematopoietic cell line in the bone marrow (Figure 1-2).

Humoral Immunity
Complement

The two components of the humoral defense system are complement and antibody. *Comple-*

TABLE 1-3. Relationship between signs/symptoms of inflammatory response and phagocytosis

Sign/symptom	Mechanism
Rubor (redness)	Vascular phase; increased permeability of endothelial functions induced by chemotaxis; dilatation of arterioles and capillaries
Dolor (pain)	Cellular phase; assimilation of phagocytes at site of infection; release of enzymes into surrounding tissue; irritation of nerve endings
Tumor (swelling)	Cellular phase; same as for dolor
Humor (exudate or pus)	Accumulation of large numbers of phagocytes and cellular debris
Color (heat)	Vasodilatation; irritation of nerve endings

TABLE 1-4. Functions of components of humoral immune response

Complement	Antibody
Enhancement of chemotaxis	Agglutination (clumping) of bacteria to enhance phagocytosis
Opsonization	Opsonization (enhancing) of phagocytosis
Microbial lysis	Activation of complement
	Prevention of antigen binding to target cells
	Recruitment of killer cells to lyse antigen
	Precipitation of antigen-presenting cell
	Inhibition of microbial motility
	Neutralization of toxins
	Interference with growth metabolism of extracellular microbes

ment is a series of about 25 proteins that circulate in the lymph and blood in an inactive form until they are triggered to activity. The system's name stems from its role: to complement the immune system by performing three major functions. Complement (1) enhances chemotaxis, attracting more phagocytes to a site of microbial invasion; (2) enhances the phagocyte's ability to ingest and destroy the microbe in a process called *opsonization;* and (3) causes the destruction (lysis) of bacteria by puncturing their cell walls (Table 1-4).

Complement activation occurs in two ways. The usual *classic pathway* is triggered by an antigen-antibody interaction. When the first component of complement is activated, it acts on the next, so that a series of reactions known as the *complement cascade* occurs. Complement components bind with antibody that has attached to the antigen on the microbe's surface. Attachment allows the complement to initiate the reactions that destroy the organism. In the *alternative pathway,* complement is activated directly, without the involvement of antibody, usually by polysaccharides of invaders' cell walls. Thus, complement, as with phagocytosis, can be available for immediate action.

Antibody

The second major component of humoral immunity consists of the *antibody* (Ab; also called immunoglobulin, Ig), which is produced by B lymphocytes. When a specific Ag is encountered, these B lymphocytes differentiate into plasma cells that serve as Ab-producing factories. Each plasma cell is able to manufacture a unique Ab that will react with only one of thousands of antigens. This specificity is attained because the plasma cell is capable of rearranging and splicing together hundreds of DNA (deoxyribonucleic acid) segments in order to develop the genetic code

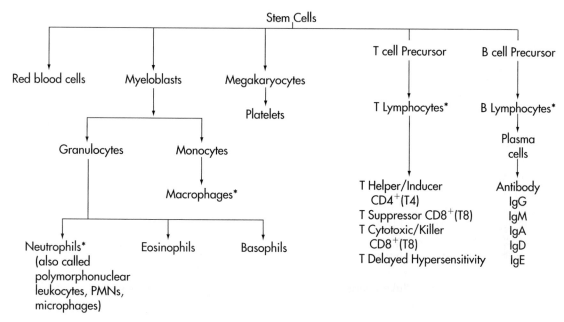

Bone Marrow

*Primary cells of the immune response

FIGURE 1-2. Origin of leukocytes.

necessary to produce an Ab that fits only one specific target antigen. As long as the foreign invader is present, B cells continue to mature into clones of plasma cells that make specific Ab. In addition, small numbers of memory B cells are produced and retained, usually for life, even after the infection is gone. If the body subsequently encounters the same Ag, these memory cells immediately replicate and respond by rapid mass production of specific Ab.

A time lag occurs between the first encounter of a B cell and an antigen and the formation of a new antibody. Thus the primary immune response is slower (1 to 2 weeks), weaker, and less efficient than the secondary or anamnestic (memory) response, which is almost immediate. In fact, once specific antibody is formed as a result of an encounter with a microbe, the host may be completely asymptomatic after a second encounter with the same microbial invader. For example, most adults have had chickenpox. When a child develops chickenpox, the parents who had the disease in their own childhood will not become ill, even when closely tending the sick child. Their memory cells have been activated, and a rapid secondary immune response ensues. This prevents disease in the parents.

Antibodies are acquired naturally by an individual who has an infection and mounts an immune response. This is called *natural active immunity.* Antibody can be acquired in several other ways as well. The immunity resulting from natural acquisition of antibody produced by another individual is called *natural passive immunity.* For example, infants are born with their mother's antibody, acquired through the placenta during the last trimester of pregnancy. Antibodies are also passed to the infant in breast milk and colostrum. This passively acquired antibody is vital during the first 4 to 5 months of life because neonates have not yet produced their own antibody. An infant's antibody levels do not reach those of an adult until about age 12 to 18 months.

Sometimes individuals need short-term protection from an infectious disease to which they are not immune. In such circumstances, *passive artificial immunity* is attained by administration of immune globulin or antitoxin that are antibodies prepared from an immune individual. Examples are hepatitis B immune globulin (HBIG) and tetanus antitoxin (preformed Ab). *Active artificial immunity* results when an individual produces antibody in response to a vaccine or toxoid that contains antigens of killed or reduced virulence (attenuated) microorganisms, toxins, or genetically engineered equivalents that are recognized by the immune system but do not produce disease (see Table 1-5). Thus the host mounts an immune response and produces antibody, but the danger of clinical infection is minimized. Vaccines are discussed in chapters 5 and 6.

The five types of Ab are IgG, IgM, IgA, IgD, and IgE. Each has unique characteristics and function. For example, IgG is the only antibody that passes across the placenta. IgM is the prominent antibody in the primary immune response, later replaced by a sustainable level of IgG. IgA is the major Ab in human secretions: tears, sweat, breast milk, and urine. IgD seems to be linked to IgM activity and complement activation. IgE is active in some allergic reactions, but its specific immune function remains unclear. Antibodies can act in a variety of ways to help protect the host from microbial devastation; these functions are summarized in Table 1-4. Antibodies can also produce adverse effects. For example, when the host misidentifies self antigens as foreign, components of the immune system may be activated and destructive autoimmune conditions result, as when the immune response to group A streptococcus damages renal or cardiac valve tissue.

Cellular Immunity

Cell-mediated immunity has its origins in the genetic ability of the host to differentiate between self and nonself. The immune system normally recognizes cells labeled "self" and will react only against molecules it does not recognize.

Cellular immunity is activated when the macrophage ingests and digests a foreign invader and then displays an antigen fragment of the foreign invader on its own surface. The T lymphocyte recognizes the antigen as foreign and initiates the cellular immune response.

TABLE 1-5. Origin of selected vaccines and toxoids

Origin	Vaccines
Killed or inactivated microorganisms	Influenza, pertussis, typhoid, polio (Salk), rabies
Live or attenuated microorganisms	Measles, mumps, rubella, polio (Sabin), yellow fever, BCG, *Varicella
Purified polysaccharides	Pneumococcal, meningococcal
Protein conjugated polysaccharide	Haemophilus influenzae type b
Genetically engineered	Hepatitis B

	Toxoids
Modified toxins	Diphtheria, tetanus

*Licensure is anticipated at this writing.

T lymphocytes comprise about 70% of the circulating lymphocytes and are differentiated by markers on their surface and by their function into several subsets. The two major functions of T lymphocytes are to coordinate the cellular and humoral immune responses and to attack infected or malignant cells directly.

T helper/inducer cells, which express the CD4+ or T4 surface antigen, initiate the cellular immune response by activating cytotoxic, or killer, cells, which directly attack and lyse target cells. The helper/inducer cells also stimulate the B cells to begin antibody production. T suppressor cells are at the other end of the regulatory spectrum. They express the CD8+ or T8 surface antigen, and slow the immune response when it is no longer needed. As with B cells, memory T cells recognize previous invaders and expedite response to repeat exposure. A fourth subset of T cells, which are responsible for delayed hypersensitivity, such as the tuberculin skin test reaction, are also activated by the T helper/inducer cells. The profound consequences of HIV infection are a result of the death of T helper/inducer cells, which have a central role in immune function, and the subsequent imbalance in T helper and T suppressor cells.

Whereas antibodies are the primary mediators of humoral immunity, *lymphokines* are the primary mediators of the cellular response. The T cell works by secreting a variety of these potent chemical messengers. Some lymphokines increase phagocytic activity. Others perforate cell membranes. The most familiar lymphokines are interferons, which have antiviral activity. Lymphokines and their activities are listed in Table 1-6. In addition to Ab, produced by the action of B cells, and lymphokines, secreted by T cells, natural killer (NK) cells are another type of lymphocyte that can kill infected or malignant cells. These do not require previous sensitization or contact with antigen, as do antibody and T cells.

The cells responsible for major immune function, including the B and T lymphocytes described previously, are white blood cells (leukocytes), and all originate from the hematopoietic cell line in the bone marrow (Figure 1-2).

Lymphocytes other than B and T lymphocytes that have important immune functions include granulocytes, named for the granular appearance of their intracellular vacuoles. Granulocyte subtypes include neutrophils, basophils, and eosinophils, each with specific functions. Neutrophils are the major phagocytic cells. Basophils are involved in acute allergic reactions. Their specific immune function is unknown. Eosinophils respond to parasitic invaders such as helminths (worms) and regulate immediate-type hypersensitivity. They play a minor role in phagocytosis and are

TABLE 1-6. Examples of lymphokines secreted by T cells

Lymphokine	Function
Interferons	Inhibit viral replication
Interleukin-2	Stimulates growth of killer T cells; activates B cells
Interleukin-3	Stimulates growth of bone marrow stem cells and mast cells
Lymphotoxin	Kills tumor cells
Macrophage chemotactic factor	Attracts macrophages to site of invasion
Macrophage-activating factor	Increases phagocytic activity of macrophages
Perforin	Perforates target cell membranes
Transfer factor	Sensitizes lymphocytes to become intensified cytotoxic T cells

TABLE 1-7. Differential white blood cell counts

Type of cell	Normal serum values/ mm^3 (% of total)	Examples of interpretation of abnormalities	
		Increase	Decrease
Granulocytes			
Neutrophils	3650 (60-70)	Infection, burns, stress, inflammation	Radiation therapy, chemotherapy, vitamin B$_{12}$ deficiency, lupus erythematosus
Eosinophils	150 (2-4)	Parasitic infection, allergy, autoimmune disease, adrenal insufficiency	Certain drugs, stress, Cushing's syndrome
Basophils	30 (0.2-0.5)	Allergy, cancer, hypothyroidism	Pregnancy, hyperthyroidism
Lymphocytes	2500 (25-30)	Acute infections, immune diseases, leukemia	Chronic infection, corticosteroids
Monocytes/macrophages	430 (5-7)	Infection	

of much less importance in the immune response than the neutrophils. The nomenclature for the various cells involved in the immune function are diagrammed in Figure 1-2. The differential white blood cell count from the clinical laboratory provides helpful information about a patient's infection status, as summarized in Table 1-7. All these components working together make up the host's response to microbiologic challenge. Figure 1-3 summarizes the immune response to an invading organism.

HOST FACTORS AFFECTING IMMUNE RESPONSE

Many host factors affect immune functions directly or indirectly and influence the outcome of the host-microbe encounter. These factors include nutrition, stress, age, hormonal status, and coincident diseases (see Chapter 5).

Nutrition

Nutritional status is a major determinant of host resistance to infection. Some increased risk of infection associated with aging may actually be caused by poor nutrition. Protein-energy malnutrition most dramatically influences immunity, particularly cell-mediated immunity, which has profound effects on all aspects of the immune response.[4]

Deficits in specific nutrients have been associated with particular immunologic effects (Table 1-8). In individual patients, however, it may be difficult to identify consequences resulting specifically from nutritional deficiencies when malnutrition is associated with poor hygiene, low socioeconomic status, or significant levels of environmental microbial contamination.

Breastfeeding increases the infant's resistance to gastrointestinal, respiratory, and middle ear infections. Breast milk contains high levels of IgA; lactoferrin, which limits microbial growth by competing for iron; enzymes that lyse bacteria; macrophages; fatty acids that have antiviral and antiparasitic activity; and complex carbohydrates that inhibit the binding of some pathogens in the gut. The protective effects of breastfeeding are most profound in developing countries, where high levels of contamination of water sources present a risk of infection from water-prepared alternatives to breast milk.[2,5]

Poor nutrition, unintentional weight loss, and low serum albumin levels are associated with risk of developing nosocomial infection.[7] Thus, nutritional support has been used to improve immune function and reduce risk of nosocomial infection. Ironically, some infec-

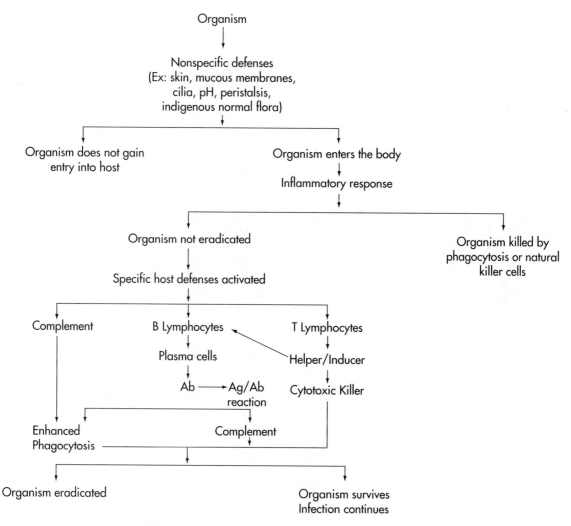

FIGURE 1-3. Host defenses against an invading microorganism.

TABLE 1-8. Specific nutritional deficits known to decrease functions

Type of deficiency	Neutrophil	Macrophage	Complement	B cell	T cell	Delayed hypersensitivity
Protein	↓	↓	↓	↓	↓	↓
Lipids				↓	↓	
Zinc	↓				↓	↓
Iron	↓	↓		↓	↓	↓
Iron	↓	↓		↓	↓	↓
Selenium	↓			↓		
Vitamin A				↓	↓	↓
Vitamin B$_6$ (pyridoxine)				↓	↓	↓
Vitamin B$_{12}$	↓				↓	↓
Vitamin C						↓

Adapted from Alexander JW. Nutritional management of the infected patient. In Kinney KN, et al, eds. Nutrition and Metabolism in Patient Care. Philadelphia: W.B. Saunders Co.; 1988; and Meydani SN: Micronutrients and immune function in the elderly. *Ann NY Acad Sci.* 1990; 587:196-207.

tions, such as typhus and malaria, are less severe in poorly nourished individuals.

Stress

The role of physiologic and emotional stress in stimulating or modulating the immune response has been recognized for decades. In the 1980s and 1990s, *psychoneuroimmunology,* which examines the reciprocal influence between the immune and nervous systems, emerged as a discipline.[3] This field has particular relevance to nursing because of the nurse's interest in mind-body interactions. Nursing care can incorporate physiologic and psychosocial interventions that might reduce the effects of stress and improve immune function. Depression, hope, and grief have been shown to be associated with biochemical changes that affect body systems. Death of a spouse, football games for players and spectators, test taking, psychotropic drugs, exercise, waiting for surgery, unemployment, divorce, and fear of an airplane flight may all be stressful enough to influence changes in immune function.[1,9] Childbirth, stress, anxiety, and depression have been associated with reduced amounts of secretory IgA in maternal breast milk.

The mechanisms by which stress affects immune function are not well understood. One explanation is that stress increases adrenal activity which results in increased levels of epinephrine and cortisol that act on lymphocytes to reduce competence. Although stress generally reduces immune reactivity, some reactions of the immune system may be increased, particularly the autoimmune response. The box below summarizes stress-related immunologic changes.

Solomon[9] proposed more than 30 mechanisms for specific interactions between the

---

POTENTIAL STRESS-RELATED IMMUNOLOGIC CHANGES

Numbers of circulating macrophages and lymphocytes
Natural killer cell activity
Ratio of B cells to T cells
Ratio of T cell suppressors to helpers
Autoimmune reactivity
Response to mitogens
Surface and steroid receptors

central nervous and immune systems. Some hypotheses relevant to nursing practice describe the relationships of the following:

- Coping styles and personality traits to immune system alterations
- Emotional distress to incidence, severity, and course of infectious diseases
- Mental dysfunction to immunologic abnormalities

Interventions such as support groups to enhance coping skills, exercise and conditioning, and biofeedback are being assessed to determine whether immune function can be improved by these interventions.

Age

Extremes of age are associated with increased risk of infection. Mechanisms for this increased risk are summarized in Table 1-9. Although the newborn receives immune protection from transplacental maternal IgG, generalized immunologic immaturity, lack of resident flora, and certain anatomic features (e.g., narrow airways) make the neonate highly susceptible to infection. Likewise, the waning immune responsiveness and physiologic changes such as increased skin fragility and decreased clearance of bacteria by the respiratory mucociliary system make the elderly individual highly susceptible to infection.[6,8,10] Some viral diseases, such as polio, mumps, measles, herpes, and varicella, are often less severe in early childhood than in adulthood. On the other hand, other viruses, such as cytomegalovirus and rubella, usually cause mild disease in healthy adults but can cause severe fetal malformations. Immune function generally peaks during childhood and begins to decline with sexual maturity.

Other factors

A variety of genetic or congenital disorders, categorized in Table 1-10, cause immunodeficiency syndrome. Certain hormones, can have a profound effect on the infectious process by inhibiting the inflammatory reaction and causing general depression of the immune response, which may exacerbate latent infections. Additionally, persons with hypoadrenalism (Addison's disease) who have low levels of corticosteroids are prone to severe consequences of infection. Some of the increased susceptibility to infection associated with physiologic and psychologic stress may be the result of persistent increases in corticosteroid production. The hormonal changes of pregnancy also are associated with increased risk of infection. The metabolic changes associated with diabetes and malignancies increase susceptibility to a variety of infections.

TABLE 1-9. Mechanisms associated with increased risk of infection at extremes of age

Neonates	
Immature splenic function	Thin, absorbent skin
Paucity of normal flora	Narrow airways
Lack of antibody response, including complement activation and phagocytic function	Reduced mechanical barriers (e.g., cilia)

Elderly	
Weakening of respiratory muscles, cough reflex, and alveolar elasticity	Thinning, drying skin
Urinary retention	Shift in T cell helper and suppressor regulatory functions
Impaired ability in cytoplasm to generate energy	Reduced stomach acidity
Greater prevalence of other diseases (diabetes, neoplasms, heart failure, dementia)	Urinary retention
	Increased anergy

TABLE 1-10. Congenital and genetic immune disorders

Functional abnormality	Example	Activity affected
Abnormal maturation	DiGeorge syndrome	T cell function (congenital thymic aplasia) Antibody formation
Abnormal proliferation and differentiation	X-linked hypogammaglobulinemia Ataxia, telangiectasia	Deficits in IgA and IgE; T cell deficits Antibody formation IgA antibody
Abnormal regulatory cell function	Selective IgA deficiency Common variable immunodeficiency	Antibody formation
Enzyme deficit	Severe combined immunodeficiency syndrome	Both humoral and cellular immunity
Abnormal cytokine response	Hyper-IgE syndrome	IgE function

Adapted from Hassner A, Adelman DC. Biologic response modifiers in primary immunodeficiency disorders. *Ann Intern Med.* 1991; 115:294-307.

Except as associated with pregnancy, gender seems to have much less influence on susceptibility to infection than age or physical condition. Certain social behaviors, particularly sexual promiscuity and self-injection with drugs, increase risk of exposure to infectious agents. Ingestion of alcohol impairs chemotaxis, and alcoholics are at increased risk for respiratory diseases. Smoking inhibits respiratory ciliary action and enhances attachment of certain pathogens to pharyngeal epithelium.

INFLUENCE OF SETTING ON HOST-SPECIFIC DETERMINANTS OF INFECTION

The physical, social, and microbial environments have considerable effect on the host. Several host factors contribute to increased risk of infection among residents of long-term care facilities, many of whom are elderly and undernourished and have impaired mobility and a variety of chronic diseases. Decreased resistance to new infection or activation of chronic infection, such as tuberculosis or varicella, may occur as immune function wanes with age. High endemicity and sometimes outbreaks of infections caused by multiply resistant strains of *Staphylococcus aureus*, *Clostridium difficile*, or other organisms may be facilitated by circumstances in institutions.

Day-care centers and other group living arrangements present specific problems. The proximity of many young children whose personal hygienic habits are less than optimal is ideal for the spread of microbes by the fecal-oral and droplet routes. Enteric infections caused by organisms such as hepatitis A, rotavirus, salmonella, and respiratory infections due to rhinovirus or influenza virus often occur (see Clinical Study 15, 18). Military barracks and boarding schools occasionally are sites of outbreaks of meningococcal disease and conjunctivitis from adenoviruses. Such infections are not so much a result of intrinsic host factors as they are a function of the opportunities for transmission presented by these physical and social environments.

Crowding and inadequate hygiene cause special infection control problems. The difficulty is compounded by other environmental factors, such as lack of clean drinking water, poverty, and inadequate immunization, as well as host factors such as malnutrition (see Clinical Study 25). High infant death rates may result from a combination of malnutrition and poor environmental conditions. Breast milk has a vital immune protective effect, and breastfeeding should be encouraged for at least the first 6 months of life.

The hospitalized patient is often immunologically compromised because of changes in endogenous flora (e.g., from antibiotic therapy), compromises in the skin and mucous membrane barriers (e.g., from IV therapy, surgery, bladder catheterization, invasive monitoring), chemotherapy, stress, and other diseases (e.g., malignancy, vascular insufficiency, diabetes). (See Chapters 5 and 8.)

SUMMARY

Humans have many defenses against microbial invasion. Nonspecific immune mechanisms include natural, species-specific immunity, physical and chemical barriers (e.g., skin, body secretions), phagocytosis, and inflammation. Specific immune responses are mediated by B cells, which produce antibodies, and T cells, which control the cellular response to infection. Nutritional status, stress, age, certain congenital abnormalities, steroids, and underlying disease are among the human host characteristics that affect the immune response and susceptibility to infection.

REFERENCES

1. Ader R, Felten D, Cohen N. Interactions between the brain and the immune system. *Ann Rev Pharmacol Toxicol.* 1990;30:561-602.
2. Arnold LDW, Larson E. Immunologic benefits of breast milk in relation to human milk banking. *Am J Infec Control.* 1993;21:235-242.
3. Biondi M, Kotzalidis GD. Human psychoneuroimmunology today. *J Clin Lab Anal.* 1990;4:22-38.
4. Chandra RK. Nutrition is an important determinant of immunity in old age. *Prog Clin Biol Res.* 1990;326: 321-334.
5. Edelman R. Infant nutrition and immunity. *Ann N Y Acad Sci.* 1990;587:232-235.
6. Geokas MC. The aging process. *Ann Intern Med* 1990;113:455-466.
7. Gorse GJ, Mesner RL, Stephens ND. Association of malnutrition with nosocomial infection. *Infect Control Hosp Epidemiol.* 1989;10:194-203.
8. Sinha AA, Lopez MT, McDevit HO. Autoimmune diseases: the failure of self-tolerance. *Science.* 1990;24: 1380-1386.
9. Solomon GF. Psychoneuroimmunology: interactions between central nervous system and immune system. *J Neurosci Res.* 1987;18:1-9.
10. Weigle WO. Effects of aging on the immune system. *Hosp Pract* 1989;24:88-95.

SUGGESTED READINGS
Immune system

Benjamin E, Leskowitz S. *Immunology: A Short Course.* New York: Wiley-Liss; 1991.

Goodenough UW. Deception by pathogens. *American Scientist.* 1991;79:344-355.

Hassner A, Adelman DC. Biologic response modifiers in primary immunodeficiency disorders. *Ann Intern Med.* 1991; 115:294-307.

Klein J. *Immunology.* Boston: Blackwell Scientific Publications; 1990.

Mims CA. *The Pathogenesis of Infectious Disease,* 3rd ed. San Diego: Academic Press; 1987.

Ram B, Harris MC, Tyle P. *Immunology: Clinical Fundamental and Therapeutic Aspects.* New York: VCH; 1990.

Schindler LW. *Understanding the Immune System.* Bethesda,

MD: U.S. Department of Health and Human Services; 1990. publication NIH 90-529.

Nutrition

Alexander JW. Nutritional management of the infected patient. In: Kinney KN, et al, eds. *Nutrition and Metabolism in Patient Care*. Philadelphia: W.B. Saunders Co.; 1988.

Chandra RK (1990 McCollum Award Lecture): Nutrition and immunity: lessons from the past and new insights into the future. *Am J Clin Nutr*. 1991;53:1087-1101.

Daly JM, et al: Effect of dietary protein and amino acids on immune function. *Crit Care Med*. 1990;18(2suppl): 586-593.

Gorse GJ, Messner RL, Stephens ND. Association of malnutrition with nosocomial infection. *Infec Control Hosp Epidemiol*. 1989;10:194-203.

Keusch GT. Micronutrients and susceptibility to infection. *Ann N Y Acad Sci*. 1990;587:181-188.

Meydani SN. Micronutrients and immune function in the elderly. *Ann N Y Acad Sci*. 1990;587:196-207.

Mims CA. *The Pathogenesis of Infectious Disease*, 3rd ed. San Diego: Academic Press; 1987:284-286.

Stress

Adair MN, et al: New behavior strategies for enhancing immune functioning. *AIDS Patient Care*. 1991;297-300.

Fawzy FI, et al: A structured psychiatric intervention for cancer patients. *Arch Gen Psychiatry*. 1990;47:729-735.

Groer M: Psychoneuroimmunology. *Am J Nurs*. 1991;91:33.

Levy SW, et al: Persistently low natural killer cell activity factors for infectious disease. *Life Sciences*. 1991;48: 107-116.

Solomon GF: Phsychoneuroimmunology: interactions between central nervous system and immune system. *J Neuroscience Res*. 1987;18:1-9.

Schleifer SJ, et al: Lymphocyte function in major depressive disorder. *Arch Gen Psychiatry*. 1984;41:484-486.

Waller KV: Effects of short-term exercise on immunologic tests. *Clin Lab Sci*. 1991;4:175-180.

Chapter 2

The Microbiologic Environment

LINDA D. BOBO

icroorganisms by definition play a central role in the infectious disease process. Their presence or absence, ability to live in harmony with the host, and their pathogenicity affect the outcome of a host-microbial interaction. This chapter describes microorganisms encountered in clinical practice: where they reside in the body, some of their mechanisms of disease production, and how they are detected by routine laboratory procedures. It is important for health care professionals to understand the microbe's preferred habitat, disease-causing mechanisms, and the mechanisms of transmission of infectious, potentially pathogenic microbes. This knowledge, in concert with clinical expertise and attention to the social environment will contribute to better nursing practice.

From the moment of conception, the developing embryo is affected by the mother's immune status, general health, and social behavior and by the physical environment, including the universe of microorganisms. As the individual matures, the complex interplay of environmental factors, the host's inherited attributes, and the microorganism's tenacity will determine the success or failure with which the individual combats infectious diseases (Figure 2-1).

One's earliest encounter with the microbial world occurs in utero as some organisms cross the placental barrier. Later, the newborn is colonized with organisms from the mother's genital tract during passage through the birth canal. Neonatal gonorrheal conjunctivitis is an example of an infection acquired during birth. The presence of certain microorganisms in the mother and the passage of protective maternal antibodies to the infant via the placenta influence the risk of disease in the neonatal and perinatal periods. As the individual matures, exposure to various microbes increases and organisms establish themselves in various body sites. Some encounters establish resident microbial flora; others do not result in permanent residence for the microbe or cause harm to the host. Growth of microorganisms in or on a host that does not lead to clinical manifestation or a detectable immune response is referred to as *colonization*. However, traumatic injury, environmental pollutants, inadequate nutrition, aging, unregulated cellular growth, metabolic changes, immune dysfunction, or alterations in the physical environment or social habits can provide opportunities for organisms to establish themselves in new niches. *Infection* is said to be present when microorganisms replicate in host tissues causing a detectable immune response. When signs or symptoms are absent, the infection is considered subclinical. When overt manifestations are apparent, the infection is commonly referred to as *disease*. Healthcare providers attempt to monitor the quality and clinical outcomes of care. One outcome is an infection

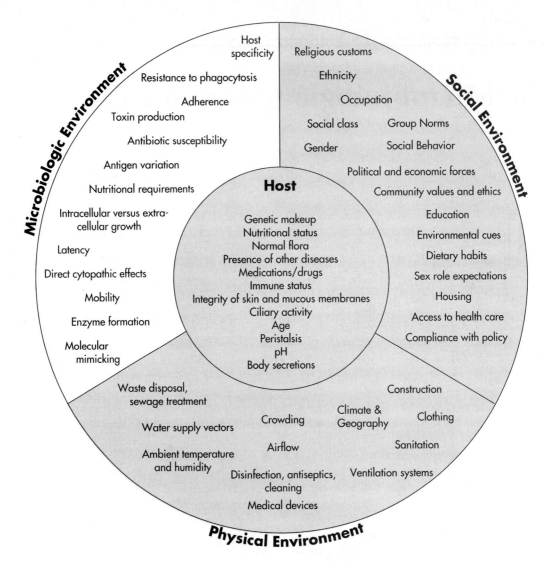

FIGURE 2-1. Factors of the microbiologic environment that influence the infectious process.

that was not incubating or present when a patient was admitted to a health care facility. These infections are referred to as *nosocomial,* a term derived from the Latin word *nosocomium,* meaning hospital. Infections present or incubating at the time of admission are typi-

cally referred to as *community acquired* infections.

The physical environment exposes persons to microorganisms. Soon after entering a hospital or other health facility, a patient may encounter microorganisms that have adapted to the hostile pressures of disinfectants and antibiotics. These nosocomial (hospital-acquired) organisms may colonize the patient and under suitable conditions initiate disease. In addition, these microbes may infect other patients or staff if a lapse occurs in infection control practices. In the community, infectious diseases are usually initiated in healthy but susceptible hosts who contact infected individuals or a contaminated physical environment. Living conditions, personal habits, leisure activities, sexual behaviors, occupation, and other social factors also affect the risk of infection. However, for both hospital-acquired and community-acquired infections, the occurrence of disease is not always predictable. Finally, if the host is compromised immunologically, functionally or structurally, *opportunistic* microorganisms may cause disease. Opportunists are considered harmless to most normal hosts when found at their usual anatomic locations.

THE MICROORGANISMS

Microbiology includes the study of a large variety of unicellular and multicellular organisms, only some of which typically cause human disease. These organisms have been sub-divided into prokaryotes and eukaryotes, based primarily on compartmentalization of genetic material within the cell. *Prokaryotes*, including bacteria, are unicellular organisms having nuclear material consisting of a single loop of double-stranded DNA chromosome distributed throughout the cell's cytoplasm, which is not contained within a nuclear membrane (Figure 2-2). Bacteria have a rigid cell wall, with the exception of the mycoplasma and chlamydiae. *Eukaryotes* have a well-defined nuclear membrane containing chromosomes (Figure 2-3). Fungi, protozoa, complex organisms such as the parasitic worms, and other multicellular members of the animal kingdom, even humans, are examples of eukaryotic organisms. Viruses are neither eukaryotic nor prokaryotic. The relationships of organisms and the distinctions used to group them are changed as submicroscopic life forms are discovered and sensitive genetic profiling techniques are developed.[6]

Bacteria

Classification and differentiation of bacteria has traditionally been based on microscopic morphology (shape), staining properties, atmospheric oxygen and nutritional requirements, and other metabolic capabilities.

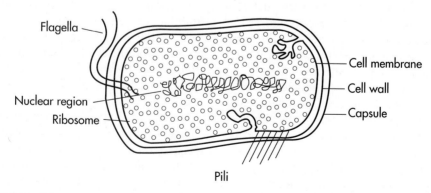

Flagella

Nuclear region

Ribosome

Cell membrane

Cell wall

Capsule

Pili

FIGURE 2-2. Schematic of a procaryotic cell. Adapted from Checko P. Microbiology. In: Soule BM, ed. *The APIC curriculum for Infection Control Practice.* 1983. Dubuque, Iowa; Kendall Hunt, 138.

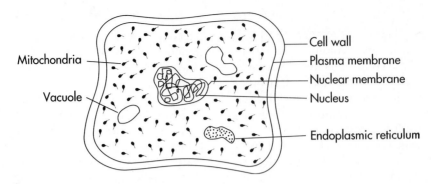

FIGURE 2-3. Schematic of a eucaryotic cell. Adapted from Checko P. Microbiology. In: Soule BM, ed. *The APIC Curriculum for Infection Control Practice.* 1983. Dubuque, Iowa; Kendall Hunt, 139.

Newer techniques of genetic characterization are proving to be valuable tools to assess relatedness of microorganisms and detect them in the clinical laboratory.[6] Nurses and other health care professionals should be familiar with basic determinants of microbe identification and diagnostic tools used by the clinical laboratory.

Although bacteria lack some internal structures, such as a nucleus, membrane-bound mitochondria, and endoplasmic reticulum, they have both DNA and RNA. DNA is present as a single chromosome with many genes. Extrachromosomal pieces of DNA, called *plasmids,* may also be present in some bacteria. Plasmids are important clinically because they can code for a variety of characteristics, such as resistance to antibiotics, and can be transferred between bacteria of the same or different species. Bacteria contain several types of RNA that function in protein synthesis.

The cell wall protects the bacteria and confers a characteristic shape. The characteristics of the organism's cell wall have significance for laboratory identification and host response. Some microorganisms are classified by the composition and shape of their cell wall. Many bacteria are classified according to their cell wall's reaction to purple (aniline) dyes, alcohol decolorization, and red (safranin)

counterstaining (Gram Stain). Gram-negative bacteria appear pink, and gram-positive organisms appear purple under the microscope after Gram staining. Microscopic identification of *Mycobacterium* (including *M. tuberculosis*) and *Nocardia* depends on their resistance to acid-alcohol decolorization after staining with phenolic dye. Acid-fast species and species without a cell wall stain poorly or not at all by Gram stain. Cell wall components also influence the host's immune response. The cell wall of some gram-negative bacteria contain lipopolysaccharides, which can induce septic shock in the host.

Some bacteria have one or more flagella, which propel the cells, giving them characteristic motility. Other bacteria have pili or fimbriae, which aid attachment of bacterial cells to the host target cell or serve as the bridge through which genetic material can be transferred between "male" and "female" bacterial cells. Flagella and pili are antigenic and can elicit the formation of antibody.[1,3]

Some rod-shaped bacteria, such as *Clostridium* species (sp.), which can cause tetanus, gas gangrene, or diarrhea, form spores. Spores are dormant forms of bacteria that are resistant to adverse environmental conditions such as heat, cold, drying, and various harsh chemicals. Other structures, such as polysaccharide capsules and slime layers, may surround bacterial cells and confer resistance to phagocytosis.

Bacteria have evolved to live in various atmospheric conditions, including anaerobic (no O_2), aerobic (room air), both anaerobic and aerobic (facultative) and microaerophilic (reduced O_2). Some organisms require other gases, such as carbon dioxide (CO_2) or methane, for survival. Adaptation to survive at select temperatures is another characteristic that influences the organism's relationship to a human host. Thermophilic bacteria inhabit high-temperature niches such as hot springs. Mesophiles, including the normal human microbiota, prefer the midrange or body temperature. Psychrophiles prefer cooler temperatures such as tap water or refrigerated blood products. Most pathogenic organisms are mesophiles that grow optimally at body temperature. Most bacteria can grow outside the host cell (extracellular) but may eventually invade an epithelial cell or be phagocytized by white blood cells. Other bacteria, such as the chlamydiae, must live inside a host cell because they do not possess cell walls and may lack their own metabolic systems.

Bacteria are always named by genus and species, which may be underlined or in italics, such as *Staphylococcus aureus*. Two organisms of the same genus are more closely related than two organisms belonging to different genera. Many genus and species names refer to the shape of the individual cell, arrangement of cells, pigmentation, or disease the organism is or was thought to cause. For example, the name *Staphylococcus aureus* indicates that coccal or round cells are present in *staphylo*, or cluster aggregates, and that the colonies are naturally an aureus, or golden, color. Purulence containing this organism may be yellow.

The characteristic shape, or morphology, of the cell can be used to group bacteria. Cells may be coccoid and arranged in pairs (diplococci), in clusters (staphylococci), or in chains (streptococci). Alternatively, cells may be bacillary, or rodlike, in shape. Rods may be straight, comma shaped, or spiral. Some cells have an irregular or amorphous appearance because they lack a cell wall. Bacterial cells may multiply to form characteristic masses or colonies on artificial laboratory media. Bacterial identification tests may be based on detection of specific microbial metabolic products, reactivity to specific chemicals, detection of bacterial-species-specific antigens, staining characteristics or genetic characterization. Most clinical laboratories also measure bacterial susceptibility to antimicrobial agents.[2]

Initial results of these assays are combined to give preliminary information to the nurse or physician concerning the presence of a bacterium in a clinical specimen. This preliminary information may be enough to guide antibiotic selection or determine the need for surgical intervention without waiting for the organism's precise identification. Table 2-1 lists disease-producing bacteria and their classification according to some of the characteristics just described.

Fungi

Fungi may produce localized or systemic infection in humans. Classic fungal identification is based on whether the species reproduces sexually or asexually. Table 2-2 lists groups of fungi most commonly associated with human disease.

Fungi are unicellular or multicellular, have cell walls, and are eukaryotic. Most fungi are stationary, although rarely some developmental forms are motile. Diagnosis of fungal infection can be made by observing characteristic forms in tissue sections, skin scrapings, exudates, or body fluids. In general, organisms may exhibit an oval, budding form known as a *yeast* or branchlike structures called *hyphae*. Preliminary information can be gained microscopically from clinical material using special stains (e.g., Giemsa). Fungal morphology can

TABLE 2-1. Bacteria: selected characteristics and disease

Genus/species	Stain/morphology[1]	Motility[2]	Atmosphere[3]	Disease[4]
Staphylococcus	+/cluster	−	aer, fac	
aureus				All, fp, TSS[5]
epidermidis				All
saprophyticus				u
species				all
Streptococcus	+/chain	−	fac	
pyogenes (group A)				c, o, t,[6]
agalactiae (group B)				b, g, m
Groups C, F, G				w
Enterococcus				
faecalis (group D)				b, g, i, u
Nonenterococcus				g, i, u
(group D)				
viridans group				n, SBE[7]
pneumoniae	+/diplococcus			b, m, o, p
morbillorum, etc.				a, b, g
Peptococcus sp.	+/cluster	−	ana	b, g, i, n
Peptostreptococcus sp.	+/chain	−	ana	a, b
Neisseria	−/diplococcus	−	aer[8]	
gonorrhoeae				g[9]
meningitidis				b, m, n
Other sp.				n
Moraxella (Branhamella)		−	aer	n, p
catarrhalis				
Kingella		−	aer	a, b, n
Veillonella		−	ana	a, g, n
Bacillus	+/bacillus (spores)	+/−	aer (some fac)	
anthracis		−		Anthrax
cereus		+		fp, n
species		+/−		n
Listeria monocytogenes		+	fac	b, m
Corynebacteriun	+/bacillus	−	aer	
diphtheriae				Diphtheria
"Diphtheroids"				n
jaikaiem				a, b
Erysipelothrix		+	ma	Erysipelas
Lactobacillus		−	ana	n
Nocardia	Partial AF/branching	−	aer	a, m, p

TABLE 2-1. Bacteria: selected characteristics and disease—cont'd

Genus/species	Stain/morphology[1]	Motility[2]	Atmosphere[3]	Disease[4]
Clostridium	+/bacillus (spores)	+/−	ana	
tetani				Tetanus
botulinum				Botulism
perfringens				Gangrene, fp
difficile sp.				i, PMC[10]
				Gangrene, n
Propionibacterium	+/bacillus	−	ana	n, rarely b
Actinomyces				
israelii	Branching	−	ana	Oral/brain/pelvic
species				Oral a
Mycobacterium	AF/bacillus	−	aer[8]	
tuberculosis				Tuberculosis
avium-intracellulare				Lung, disseminated
(MAI)				
kansasii				Lung
marinum				Skin, a
scrofulaceum				Scrofula
leprae				Leprosy
fortuitum				n
Eschericia coli	−/bacillus	−	fac	n, u, i, all
Klebsiella	−/bacillus	−		n, b, p, m
Enterobacter	−/bacillus	+/−		
Salmonella	−/bacillus	+		
typhi				Typhoid
Other sp.				b, i
Shigella	−/bacillus	−		
dysenteriae sp				Dysentery
Proteus	−/bacillus	+		n, u, all
Serratia	−/bacillus	+		All
Yersinia		+/−	aer, fac	
enterocolitica				Pseudoappendicitis
pestis				Bubonic plague
Pseudomonas	−/bacillus	+/−	aer	n, all
aeruginosa				
cepacia				
mallei				Glanders

Continued.

TABLE 2-1. Bacteria: selected characteristics and disease—cont'd

Genus/species	Stain/morphology[1]	Motility[2]	Atmosphere[3]	Disease[4]
Flavobacterium	−/bacillus	+	aer	w, b, n
Xanthomonas maltophilia	−/bacillus	+	aer	b, m, n
Achromobacter	−/bacillus	+	aer	w, b, n
Vibrio	−/bacillus	+	fac	
cholerae				Cholera
parahaemolyticus				i, w
species				i, w
Aeromonas	−/coccobacillus	−	fac	n, wound
Campylobacter	−/curved rod	+	ma	
fetus				Abortion
jejuni				i
Haemophilus	−/coccobacillus	−	fac	
influenzae				b, e, o, p, s
aegyptius				e
ducreyi				Soft chancroid
species				Abscess
Pasteurella multocida	−/coccobacillus	−	aer, fac	Cat/dog bite
Francisella tularensis	−/bacillus	−	aer	Tularemia
Bordetella pertussis	−/coccobacillus	−	aer	Pertussis
Brucella	−/coccobacillus	−	aer[8]	Brucellosis
Legionella	−/bacillus	+	aer	p
Gardnerella vaginalis	variable/bacillus	−	fac	n, vaginitis
Bacteroides	−/bacillus	−	ana	
fragilis				b, g, i, n
species				b, g, i, n, oral a, pulmonary
Fusobacterium	−/bacillus	+	ana	a, n
Mobiluncus	−/bacillus	+	ana	Vaginitis

BACTERIA LACKING CELL WALL[11]

Genus/species	Stain/morphology[1]	Motility[2]	Atmosphere[3]	Disease[4]
Chlamydia	NA	−	[11]	
trachomatis				Trachoma, g, p[12]
psittaci				p
pneumoniae				p
Mycoplasma				
pneumoniae	NA	−	[11]	"Atypical" p
hominis				g, n
Ureaplasma urealyticum	NA	−	[11]	g, u

TABLE 2-1. Bacteria: selected characteristics and disease—cont'd

Genus/species	Stain/morphology[1]	Motility[2]	Atmosphere[3]	Disease[4]
ORDER SPIROCHAETALES	−/spirals			
Borrelia	NA/spirals	+	ana	
vincentii				Vincent's angina
recurrentis				Relapsing fever
burgdorferi				Lyme disease
Treponema	NA/spirals	+	fac	
pallidum				Syphilis; yaws, pinta
denticola				Periodontal
Leptospira	NA/spirals	+	aer	
interrogans				Leptospirosis
biflexa				n
Spirillum minus	SS/spirals	+	aer or ma	Rat-bite fever
Rickettsia[11]	−/coccobacilli		[11]	
rickettsii		−		Rocky Mountain spotted fever
prowazekii				Epidemic typhus
typhi (mooseri)				Murine fever
tsutsugamushi				Scrub typhus
akari				Rickettsial pox
Coxiella burnetii				Q fever
MISCELLANEOUS				
Bartonella (Rochalimaea spp.)	−/bacillus	+	ma	b, Oroya fever, cat scratch fever
Streptobacillus moniliformis	−/pleomorphic	−		Rat-bite fever
Helicobacter pylori	−/spiral	+	ma	Gastritis, ulcers

[1]Gram positive (+) or negative (−), acid fast (AF), not applicable (NA), or special stains required (SS).
[2]+, motile; −, not motile.
[3]Atmospheric growth requirements: aer, aerobic; ana, anaerobic; ma, microaerophilic; fac, facultative.
[4]Codes for diseases listed alphabetically: a, abscess; all, all sites including normal flora; b, blood; c, cellulitis; e, eye; fp, food poisoning; g, genital; i, intestinal; m, meningitis; n, normal flora; o, otitis media; p, pneumonia; s, sinusitis; t, throat; u, urinary; w, wound.
[5]Toxic shock syndrome.
[6]Occasionally scarlet fever; occasional sequelae are rheumatic fever, heart valve damage, and glomerulonephritis.
[7]Subacute bacterial endocarditis.
[8]Special CO_2 requirements. Some *Neisseria* species capable of anaerobic growth.
[9]Postgonoccal arthritis.
[10]Pseudomembranous colitis.
[11]Obligate intracellular parasites.
[12]Inclusion conjunctivitis, pelvic inflammatory disease (PID); other sequelae include sterility, arthritis, and blindness.

TABLE 2-2. Fungi: yeast, filamentous, and dimorphic forms; features; and disease

Genus/species	Features	Disease*
YEAST FORMS		
Candida		
albicans sp.	Oval	g, n, thrush, all†
		n, all
Cryptococcus neoformans	Round, encapsulated	b, m, p, sk
Trichosporon	Rectangular	n, sk
Geotrichum	Rectangular	b, n, sk, u
Torulopsis	Oval, small	b, g, n, u
Pityrosporum orbiculare	Nonculturable, oval	Pityriasis, ? seborrheic dermatitis
FILAMENTOUS FORMS		
Aspergillus sp.	Septate hyphae	p, sk, bone‡
Fonsecaea, Phialophora, Rhinocladiella	Septate hyphae	sk (chromoblastomycosis)
Exophiala, Alternaria, Cladosporium, Curvularia	Septate hyphae	sk (phaeohyphomycosis)
Actinomadura, Madurella, Pseudoallescheria, Acremonium, Streptomyces/ Actinomyces§	Septate hyphae	sk (mycetoma)
Trichophyton, Microsporum	Septate hyphae	Ringworm of scalp, body; athlete's foot, jock itch
Phycomycetes	Aseptate hyphae	
Mucor, Rhizopus, Absidia		n, p, sk, bone, brain
Conidiobolus		Subcutaneous granuloma
Basidiobolus		p, sinusitis
DIMORPHIC FORMS		
Histoplasma capsulatum	Tissue—small, round yeast; filamentous, bumpy spores	p (histoplasmosis), bone marrow, sk, disseminated
Coccidioides immitis	Tissue—spherule with endospores; filamentous, barrel-shaped spores	p (San Joaquin Valley fever), sk, disseminated
Sporothrix schenckii	Tissue—yeast; filamentous, daisy-clustered spores	Lymphocutaneous, disseminated
Blastomyces dermatitidis	Tissue—large, broad-based yeast; filamentous	Pulmonary blastomycosis, sk, disseminated
Paracoccidioides brasiliensis	Tissue—double-walled yeast with multiple buds; filamentous	Mucocutaneous, pulmonary, disseminated
Malessezia furfur	Yeast form is *Pityrosporum*; nonculturable	Pityriasis; sepsis caused intralipid therapy

TABLE 2-2. Fungi: yeast, filamentous, and dimorphic forms; features; and disease—cont'd

Genus/species	Features	Disease*
OTHER		
Pneumocystis carini ‖	Methenamine-silver stain for cyst, Giemsa stain for trophozoite	p; disseminated
Prototheca wickerhamii	Alga-like unicellular fungus	Cutaneous/subcutaneous infection following trauma

*Codes for diseases listed alphabetically: all, all sites; b, blood; g, genital; m, meningitis; n, normal; p, pneumonia; sk, skin; u, urinary.
†Important in immunocompromised patients; also catheter infections.
‡Also allergic bronchiolitis; aflatoxin produced by some species contaminating food linked to liver carcinoma.
§Soil bacteria.
‖Uncertain classification of *Pneumocystis carinii* has placed it with the parasites in the past; presence of chitin in cell wall bears resemblance to the fungi. *Prototheca* resembles yeast on artificial laboratory media but is a member of the colorless algae.

also be observed by using potassium hydroxide (KOH) slide preparations, which dissolve host tissue material but preserve fungal structures, or negative staining using India ink. For example, it is important to note whether yeast forms are oval or round, have one or multiple buds, appear double walled, or are encapsulated. Most yeasts (e.g., *Candida* sp.) stain gram positive, although some (e.g., *Pneumocystis carinii*) may require special silver impregnation staining to be seen. A clear halo-appearing structure called a *capsule* may be observed surrounding some yeasts (e.g., *Cryptococcus neoformans*) in India ink preparations. Hyphae can appear as long strands or may have cross-walls called *septations*. Reproductive structures known as *fruiting bodies* are also associated with spores. Observation of whether spores are enclosed in walled structures (endospores) or borne externally aids in identification. In some cases, antibodies specific for a unique fungal antigen that have been tagged with fluorescein, a fluorescent dye, can provide rapid, definitive identification of a species.

Identification of fungi is often based on the appearance of the colony and reproductive structures in culture. Yeasts can be biochemically characterized according to nutrient utilization or production of specific cell wall components. The filamentous fungi, which have hyphae, usually produce characteristic fruiting bodies at some point in their life cycle. Some fungi (e.g., *Pityrosporum orbiculare*) cannot be grown in culture. Identification of these fungi must rely on the host's clinical presentation and the microscopic appearance of the organism in the specimen obtained from the host. A few fungal species are *dimorphic,* producing both a yeastlike form at 37° C or in tissue and a hyphal form at room temperature; however, most fungi have only one form at both temperatures.

Parasites and Arthropods

The term *parasite* can refer to an organism that maintains itself in or on a host at the expense of the host while contributing little in return. In this section the term refers to the eukaryotic, unicellular or multicellular subset of organisms that may associate with a human host. Traditional classification separates these organisms into protozoa, such as amebae, blood or tissue flagellates, and intestinal and tissue helminths (worms) (Table 2-3).

The amebae can exist as fragile, mobile configurations called *trophozoites* when condi-

TABLE 2-3. Parasites: protozoa, blood and tissue flagellates, helminths and disease

Genus/species	Disease
PROTOZOA	
Intestinal amebae	
Entamoeba	
histolytica	Intestinal; rarely: lung, liver, brain
coli, hartmanni, gingivalis,	Low or inconsistent pathogenicity
polecki	
Iodamoeba butschlii	Low or inconsistent pathogenicity
Endolimax nana	Low or inconsistent pathogenicity
Dientamoeba fragilis	Acute/chronic diarrhea
Free-living amebae (water)	
Naegleria gruberii	Fulminant meningitis
Acanthamoeba	More chronic meningitis; corneal infection with contact lens or corneal transplant
Intestinal ciliate	
Balantidium coli	Diarrhea (history of contact with pigs)
Intestinal flagellate	
Giardia lamblia	Diarrhea, intestinal malabsorption
Intestinal sporozoa	
Cryptosporidium	Diarrhea, invasion of intestinal organs (immunocompromised)
Isospora belli	Diarrhea
Blood sporozoa	
Plasmodium	Blood, liver
falciparum	Most life-threatening; severe systemic complications, coma, death
vivax	Relapse, splenic rupture
ovale	Same as with other species
malariae	Chronic, limited
Tissue sporozoa	
Toxoplasma gondii	Eye, lung, brain; congenital malformations
Blood piroplasmids	
Babesia microti, bovis,	Anemia
bigemina, divergens, major	Anemia
BLOOD AND TISSUE FLAGELLATES	
Leishmania	
donovani	Visceral leishmaniasis (kala-azar)
tropica, mexicana, viannia	Cutaneous and mucocutaneous (espundia, leishmaniasis)
Trypanosoma	
brucei (rhodesiense,	Sleeping sickness
gambiense)	
cruzi	Chagas' disease

TABLE 2-3. Parasites: protozoa, blood and tissue flagellates, helminths and disease—cont'd

Genus/species	Disease
HELMINTHS	
Nematodes	
Intestinal roundworms	
Trichuris trichiura (whipworm)	Colon: diarrhea, rectal prolapse
Enterobius vermicularis (pinworm)	Intense anal pruritus; rare vulvovaginitis
Ascaris lumbricoides	Löffler's syndrome (cough, pneumonitis), intestinal pain/obstruction
Capillaria philippinensis	Fatal diarrhea if untreated
Trichostrongylus	Mild diarrhea
Intestinal hookworms	
Ancylostoma duodenale	Rarely pneumonitis; severe anemia, hypoproteinemia
Necator americanus	Abdominal pain, anemia
Strongyloides stercoralis	Pneumonitis, abdominal pain
Tissue nematodes	
Wuchereria bancrofti, Brugia malayi	Lymphatic obstruction, elephantiasis
Tissue nematodes	
Trichinella spiralis	Trichinosis
Onchocerca volvulus	Onchocerciasis (skin, ocular)
Mansonella	Skin
Dirofilaria immitis	Pulmonary
Dracunculus medinensis	Skin ulcer
Angiostrongylus cantonensis	Eosinophilic meningitis
Gnathostoma sp.	Creeping eruptions; rarely eye and central nervous system (CNS) involvement
Trematodes	
Blood flukes: flatworms	
Schistosoma	
mansoni	Portal hypertension, splenomegaly
haematobioum	Hydronephrosis, carcinoma
japonicum	Seizures, splenomegaly, hepatic dysfunction
Tissue flukes	
Paragonimus sp.	Lung abscess, seizures (CNS), gastrointestinal ulceration
Intestinal flukes	
Heterophyes heterophyes	Diarrhea, abdominal pain, or asymptomatic
Fasciola buski	Diarrhea, abdominal pain, malabsorption, or asymptomatic
Metagonimus yokogawai	Diarrhea, abdominal pain, or asymptomatic
Liver flukes	
Clonorchis sinensis	Cholangitis, carcinoma, cirrhosis, or asymptomatic
Opisthorcis sp.	Asymptomatic, cholangitis
Fasciola sp.	Hepatomegaly, biliary obstruction

Continued.

TABLE 2-3. Parasites: protozoa, blood and tissue flagellates, helminths and disease—cont'd

Genus/species	Disease
Cestodes (Tapeworms)	
Taenia	
solium (pork)	Asymptomatic; weight loss, nausea, constipation; cysticercosis (CNS, skeletal muscles)
saginata (beef)	Vague
Hymenelopis nana	Vague; abdominal, diarrhea
Diphyllobothrium latum (fish)	Weight loss, pernicious anemia, abdominal pain
Echinococcus granulosus	Cystic hydatid disease: liver, brain, anaphylaxis

tions are optimal. Under adverse conditions the trophozoites encyst. Laboratory identification is based on size of cysts, arrangement of intracellular structures, and the type of trophozoite motility observed (directional, revolving, leaflike fluttering).

The blood and tissue flagellates, including *Plasmodium, Leishmania,* and *Trypanosoma* sp., produce characteristic forms depending on the stage of the life cycle at which the clinical specimen is taken. Accurate identification of the particular species, especially for malaria, is very important for selection of effective treatment (see Clinical Study 35). Microfilaria are observed in tissue and blood smears.

Helminths are subclassified as roundworms (nematodes), or flukes (trematodes), or flatworms (cestodes). Macroscopic observation of the worms in stool samples is often possible, but identification is usually confirmed microscopically, most often by examination of the specimen and identification of eggs (ova) with species-specific features. The distinctive appearance of the body segments (proglottids) or mouth parts (scolex) allows identification of some adult or juvenile forms.

The arthropods, especially the class *Insecta,* are tremendously important intermediate hosts for *Entamoeba, Plasmodium, Trypanosoma,* and select bacteria (enteric, rickettsia, borrelia) and viruses (enteric, hemorrhagic) (see Clinical Study 35). Arthropods may also spread disease directly by invasion, colonization at the site of entry, and production of local irritants or poisons. Classification is normally based on examination of mouth parts, body segmentation, wing or leg types, and coloration. Table 2-4 summarizes arthropod, microorganism, and disease relationships.

Viruses

All viruses and subviral agents (e.g., prions) must either live in the host cell cytoplasm (e.g., rabies virus) or integrate into the host cell's DNA (herpes, retroviruses). Unlike bacteria, fungi, and parasites, which contain both DNA and RNA, viruses contain *either* RNA or DNA, which may be single-stranded (ss) or double-stranded (ds). Generally, DNA viruses that integrate into the host cell DNA do so directly. Single-stranded RNA retroviruses such as the human immunodeficiency virus (HIV) must first *reverse transcribe* their RNA genetic code into DNA before the viral DNA can integrate into the host cell's DNA.

Viral nucleic acid is surrounded by a protein coat called a *nucleocapsid.* The capsid may be enclosed by a lipid-containing membrane susceptible to organic solvents. Rhinovirus, one cause of common colds, is not enveloped by such a membrane and is thus resistant to ether,

TABLE 2-4. Arthropods as vectors and primary disease agents

Arthropod (Host)	Disease (Microorganism)
MITES	
Sarcoptes scabiei	Scabies
Dermatophagoides sp.	Dust mite allergy
TICKS	
Ixodes dammini (deer)	Lyme disease (*Borrelia burgdorferi*)
Dermacentor sp. (dog)	Rocky Mountain Spotted fever tick paralysis (*Rickettsia rickettsii*)
Amblyomma americanum (Lone Star)	Cellulitis
Ornithodoros sp.	Relapsing fever (*Borrelia recurrentis*)
All ticks	Encephalitides (viruses)
LICE	
Pediculus humanus	Head and pubic (crabs) pediculoses; relapsing fever (*Borrelia*)
FLEAS	
Pulex irritans (human)	Dermatitis; Plague (Yersinia), Typhus, tapeworm
Ctenocephalides felis (cat)	Dermatitis
Tunga penetrans (chigoe, jigger)	Dermatitis
FLIES	
Screwworm, botfly	Myiasis (traumatic, furuncular, intestinal, creeping, ocular)
Glossina sp. (tsetse)	African trypanosomiasis or sleeping sickness (*Trypanosoma brucei*)
Phlebotomus sp. (sandfly)	Leishmaniasis (*Bartonella*, *Leishmania*)
Fluid and filth flies	Bacterial and viral intestinal diseases
MOSQUITOES	
Anopheles sp.	Malaria (*Plasmodium*)
Aedes sp.	Dengue fever (Dengue virus)
All mosquitoes	Encephalitides (viruses)
REDUVIID BUGS	
Triatoma sp.	Chagas' disease (*Trypanosoma cruzi*)
SPIDERS	
Latrodectus sp. (widow)	Venom-related neuromuscular transmitter blockade; shock; rarely death
Loxosceles sp. (recluse)	Severe necrosis at bite site; occasionally shock
BEES, WASPS, HORNETS	Severe edema; occasionally anaphylaxis

chloroform, ethanol, and weak phenol. The capsid may have external proteins, such as the *hemagglutinin* and *neuraminidase* molecules of influenza A, which aid in attachment to and penetration of host cells. Viruses may exhibit a distinctive, even crystalline shape, or they may be revealed as amorphous by electron microscopy. Viruses are classified according to their nucleic acid (DNA or RNA, single or double stranded), shape (e.g., spheric, icosahedral, bullet), and presence or absence of an envelope.

Viruses can gain access to the host cell by binding to or *adsorbing* specific receptor molecules on the host cell membrane. The viral particle is then engulfed by the host cell membrane and internalized. For example, HIV-1 binds to CD4$^+$ molecules on the surface of CD4$^+$ T lymphocytes. Once inside the host cell, the virus may replicate, producing progeny that exit the host cell by budding from or rupturing the cell membrane. This process frequently results in cell death. The host cell may also die as a result of viral subversion of its metabolism to production of viral proteins. Alternatively, viruses that integrate into host DNA, such as herpesviruses and HIV-1, may become *latent* for a time and later initiate replication after some stimulus.

Host cell pathology resulting from viral infection may be seen on cytologic preparations using light microscopy and special stains to visualize cytoplasmic or nuclear *inclusions* (herpesvirus). In addition, cytologic preparations may indicate that epithelial or white blood cells have undergone a transformation in appearance *(dysplasia)* or have increased in number *(hyperplasia)*, behaving as a carcinoma. This may be observed in some types of genital human papillomavirus (HPV) infection of epithelial cells. Retroviruses are responsible for feline and human T cell leukemia. Another retrovirus, HIV-1, causes a decrease in helper T lymphocytes (CD4$^+$ cells), leading to acquired immunodeficiency syndrome (AIDS). Interest-

ingly, host response to infection may be greatly affected by host genetic differences. For example, in most people the clinical manifestation of Epstein-Barr (EB) virus infection is a self-limited mononucleosis of atypical lymphocytes, but in some Africans it can produce a tumor known as Burkitt's lymphoma. Table 2-5 presents diseases and symptoms for selected human viruses.

Laboratory diagnosis of viral infection is complex. The virus may be identified by electron microscopy, grown in tissue cultured cells, detected by observing whether red blood cells will stick to the surface of infected tissue culture cells, or identified indirectly when antibodies against the virus are detected in the blood. Since many viruses do not survive very long outside the host, it is crucial to transport a viral specimen for culture to the laboratory *immediately*. Table 2-6 lists some appropriate specimens for viral detection. If swab scrapings are taken, they should be placed in a viral transport medium for immediate delivery. It is also possible to diagnose viral infection by looking directly for viral antigens (enzyme-linked immunosorbent assay, ELISA) or nucleic acids (hybridization, polymerase chain amplification) in clinical material. These tests are increasingly available and will likely replace traditional staining, culture, and other identification methods in the future.

MICROBIAL RESERVOIRS

Disease (pathology)-producing microbes are referred to as *pathogens*. They may originate outside the host *(exogenous)* or may normally reside within the host *(endogenous)*. Exogenous organisms may be free living in water, soil, or air or on environmental surfaces, or they may require a living host. For example, legionella lives freely in soil or air conditioner condensates. Exogenous organisms gain entry to the host through portals that include the mouth and respiratory system or through the skin or

TABLE 2-5. Selected viruses and syndromes

Virus	Syndromes
Adenovirus	Asymptomatic; coryza, pharyngitis, tracheitis, or pneumonia; epidemic keratoconjunctivitis; diarrhea; hemorrhagic cystitis
Arenavirus, other hemorrhagic viruses	Lassa fever; other hemorrhagic fevers; lymphocytic choriomeningitis
Coronavirus	Acute upper respiratory infection
Coxsackievirus, echovirus, other enteroviruses	Aseptic meningitis, "nonparalytic poliomeningitis"; herpangina; pleurodynia; rash; myocarditis, pericarditis; mild upper respiratory or gastrointestinal disease
Cytomegalovirus	Congenital defects; pneumonia, gastrointestinal disease
Dengue	Dengue (febrile exanthem); dengue hemorrhagic fever/dengue shock syndrome
Epstein-Barr	Infectious mononucleosis
Flavivirus, togavirus, Bunyaviridae	Encephalitis; hemorrhagic fever with renal syndrome (hantavirus)
Hepatitis A, B, C, D	Hepatitis
Herpes simplex	Gingivostomatitis, pharyngotonsillitis, herpes labialis (cold sore); whitlow, erythema multiforme; encephalitis, meningitis; esophagitis, genital infection
Influenza	Constitutional (fever, myalgia, chills, headache); respiratory (cough); cardiac complications (myocarditis, pericarditis); neurologic (Guillain-Barré syndrome); Reye syndrome
Mumps	Parotitis; meningitis; orchitis
Norwalk, calicivirus, astrovirus	Gastroenteritis
Papillomavirus	Skin warts; genital warts (condylomas); oral conjunctival and respiratory papillomas; association with cervical carcinoma
Parainfluenza	Upper respiratory infection; bronchiolitis, pneumonia
Parvovirus	Fifth disease; transient aplastic crisis; chronic bone marrow failure; hydrops fetalis
Poliovirus	Aseptic meningitis, polio; mild constitutional symptoms
Polyomavirus	Mild respiratory infection; progressive multifocal leukoencephalopathy
Rhabdovirus	Rabies
Respiratory syncytial	Bronchiolitis (infants), pneumonia, croup; otitis media
Retroviruses	Adult T cell leukemia (HTLV-1), hairy cell leukemia (HTLV-2); AIDS (HIV-1, HIV-2)
Rhinovirus	Common cold
Rotavirus	Diarrhea
Rubella	German measles; congenital birth defects
Rubeola	Measles; subacute sclerosing panencephalitis (SSPE)
"Slow" viruses	Subacute spongiform encephalopathies: Creutzfeldt-Jakob disease
Varicella-zoster	Chickenpox; shingles; pneumonia
Yellow fever	Yellow fever (total system involvement)

TABLE 2-6. Some appropriate specimens for viral isolation*

	Specimen					
Agent	Throat	Stool	Cerebrospinal fluid	Urine	Vesicle fluid	Other
Meningitis and encephalitis						
Mumps	++++	−	++	+	−	−
Enteroviruses	+++	++++	++	−	−	−
Herpes simplex	±	−	±	−	+	++++ (Brain biopsy)
Arboviruses†	−	−	+	−	−	++ (Brain) + (Blood)
Respiratory diseases						
Influenza and parainfluenza viruses	++++	−	−		−	−
Adenoviruses	++++	++++	−		−	−
Exanthems						
Measles	++++	−	−	+	−	
Rubella†	++++	−	−	+	−	
Varicella	−	−	−	−	++++	
Herpes simplex	++	−	−	−	++++	
Cytomegalovirus	++	−	−	++++	−	+ (Leukocyte tissue biopsy)

From Sherris JC, editor: *Medical microbiology: an introduction to infectious diseases,* Norwalk, Conn, 1990, Appleton & Lange.
−, No yield; ± to ++++, relative yield (low to high).
*In general, it should be remembered that virus shedding often diminishes rapidly after onset of acute illness; it is therefore important to attempt specimen collection as early as possible.
†Because it is frequently very difficult to isolate these agents from the disease in question, it is emphasized that serologic tests are particularly important to ensure a diagnosis.

mucous membranes by direct penetration or traumatic injury. The intestine, genitourinary system, and oral cavity normally contain many different endogenous microbial species. Enteric organisms, such as *Escherichia coli,* live in the human intestinal tract. Both exogenous and endogenous microorganisms may cause disease if they enter a normally sterile body site or body sites that they do not normally inhabit. Organisms may travel from an adjacent site or be transported via the bloodstream to other locations (hematogenous spread).

Surgical and other manipulative trauma (e.g., dental procedures, diagnostic tests), invasive tumors, or autoimmune diseases causing breaks in the skin or mucous membranes also facilitate transport of microbes.[3,5]

Once a microbe has entered the host, colonization of one or more body sites may occur. The relationship established between the microorganism and the human body depends on characteristics of both the microorganisms and the host. For example, some organisms attach to the cell via recognition of receptors on the host cell surfaces (see Chapter 1). These organisms may thus be said to have *tropism* for a cell type. However, microorganisms compete with each other for sites of attachment and nutrients. The commensal microbiota already present at the site may successfully prevent attachment and colonization or disease production by a microbial invader. In addition, some microorganisms produce substances with antimicrobial activity against other microbes. Microbial competition has been used as a treatment strategy by giving lactobacilli in the form of capsules or yogurt for diarrheal diseases and vaginal yeast infections. There have been conflicting results in the literature regarding the efficacy of this treatment.

Symptomatology gives a clue as to *where* the focus of infection is and *what* organisms can be found at the site. In many cases the patient is treated empirically, before final identification of the pathogen, with an antimicrobial agent active against microbes most likely to be found at the site. Once the laboratory diagnosis has been made and susceptibility of the organism to antimicrobial agents determined, antibiotic coverage may be changed accordingly. Surgical intervention (removal or drainage) may be used alone or in addition to antimicrobials when infection occurs at sites where penetration of antimicrobial agents is poor or when the infection is causing pressure on adjacent structures. Table 2-7 lists body sites, symptomatology, and the microorganisms most likely to be encountered at each site. It is very helpful to be familiar with the normal commensal microbiota likely to be found at various body sites. This knowledge can guide interpretation of laboratory reports, collection of specimens, and infection prevention strategies.

MICROBIAL FACTORS IMPORTANT IN DISEASE PRODUCTION

Many known microbes have been associated with disease production at one time or another.

The initiation of disease is known as *pathogenesis* and is influenced by the organism's *virulence*. Virulence is determined by the microbe's ability to evade local and specific immune factors and to adapt rapidly to changes in the external environment or host behavior and by the degree, location, and duration of disruption of host systems.

One characteristic of microbes is the dose needed to initiate infection in a typical host. For example, ingestion of as many as 100,000 (10^5) *Vibrio cholerae*/ml may be required to cause cholera, whereas ingestion of only a few *Salmonella typhi* bacilli may be necessary to initiate typhoid fever. However, once disease occurs, cholera may be immediately more devastating for the host, causing death within a few hours, whereas typhoid less frequently results in death. Thus a lower infectious dose does not necessarily imply that the organism causes more severe, immediate disease.

The type and location of infection have significant implications for the consequences of infection. For example, many enteroviruses cause diarrhea and mild, self-limited aseptic meningitis. However, poliovirus (an enterovirus) can also produce flaccid asymmetric paralysis and is thus regarded as more virulent. *Neisseria meningitidis,* which may be carried in the nasophargnyx, may cause fulminant meningitis and adrenal collapse and death within 1 day of onset if it enters the bloodstream. On the other hand, the viral agents of kuru and Creutzfeldt-Jakob disease may live in the host with minimal symptoms for decades but eventually may cause fatal neurologic disease. Thus, manifestations of organism virulence may also vary with time.

Microorganisms use various attachment factors, enzymes, toxins, and evasion mechanisms to avoid or inactivate nonspecific immune clearance and promote invasiveness. Invasiveness may be mediated by specialized surface structures called *pili* or *fimbriae,* which help *Neisseria gonorrhoeae* and uropathic and

TABLE 2-7. Normal flora and typical infections by body site

System/body site	Flora	Disease state
CENTRAL NERVOUS		
Brain and spaces	None	Abscess
Meninges	None	Meningitis
Nerves	None	Neuritis
CARDIOVASCULAR AND LYMPHATIC		
Blood	None	Bacteremia, sepsis, shock, intravascular coagulation, death; anemia, hemolysis
Bone marrow	None	Anemia, aplasia; leukemia; same as for blood
Vessels	None	Endothelial inflammation, hemorrhagic thrombophlebitis
Heart	None	Endocarditis, myocarditis
Pericardium	None	Pericarditis
Lymph nodes, lymphatics	None	Abscess, granuloma, blockage (elephantiasis)
MUSCULOSKELETAL		
Muscles	None	Gangrene, myositis, paralysis
Bone	None	Osteomyelitis
HEAD AND NECK		
Oral	Normal†	Thrush, ulcer, periodontal/endodontal abscess, sinus tract disease, angina, pharyngitis/tonsillitis
Nares, lower	Transient†,§	Abscess, rhinitis
Sinuses	Transient†,§	Sinusitis
Ears		
External	Normal§	Otitis externa
Middle	None	Otitis media
Inner	None	Vestibular inflammation
Eyes		
External	Transient§	Blepharitis, conjunctivitis, trachoma, blindness, keratitis
Humors	None	Cloudiness, blindness
Retina	None	Retinitis
RESPIRATORY		
Trachea	Mouth flora†	Tracheitis
Bronchi	Transient†	Bronchitis, bronchiolitis
Lungs	None	Pneumonia, abscess
Pleura	None	Pleuritis
GASTROINTESTINAL AND ABDOMINAL		
Peritoneum	None	Peritonitis, ascites
Liver	None	Hepatitis, abscess, cirrhosis; hepatomegaly

TABLE 2-7. Normal flora and typical infections by body site—cont'd

System/body site	Flora	Disease state
Gallbladder	Transient intestinal microbes*	Cholecystitis, cholangitis
Spleen	None	Abscess; rupture
Stomach	Transient mouth flora†	Gastritis, ulcer
Small and large intestine	Normal flora‡	Diarrhea, dysentery, malabsorption, pseudomembranous colitis, obstruction, abscess, gangrene, fistula, appendicitis; small intestine: bacterial overgrowth
Rectum	Normal*,§	Abscess, prolapse, ulcer
GENITOURINARY AND REPRODUCTIVE		
Kidney	None	Pyelonephritis, abscess, glomerulonephritis
Bladder	None	Cystitis
Urethra	Normal*,†,§	Urethritis, fistula
Penis	Normal§	Abscess, chancre, ulcer
Vulva, labia	Normal	Abscess, ulcer
Vaginal	Normal*,†,§	Vaginitis, Bartholin gland abscess
Cervix	None (transient)†,§	Cervicitis, ulcer
Reproductive (e.g., uterus, prostate)	None	Abscess, sterility
Fetus	None	Congenital defects; any infection
Membranes, placenta, cord	None	Any infection
INTEGUMENT		
Skin	Normal§	Abscess, ulcer, cellulitis, sinus tract, petechiae, exanthem, bullae, granuloma; trauma, wound; surgical hypo- or hyperpigmentation; epidermal thickening
Nails	Normal§	Erosion, loss
Hair	Normal§	Breakage, loss

*Intestinal flora includes Enterobacteriaceae, anaerobic gram-negative and gram-positive rods, anaerobic cocci, enterococci, some other streptococcal/staphylococcal species, lactobacilli, *Candida* and *Torulopsis* sp.
†Mouth and genitourinary flora includes viridans streptococcus, *Branhamella* and *Neisseria* sp., staphylococci, anaerobic gram-positive cocci and rods, anaerobic gram-negative cocci and rods, and lactobacilli.
‡Large intestine is most highly colonized.
§Skin flora includes diphtheroids, staphylococci, streptococci, *Bacillus* and *Propionibacterium* sp., and peptococci.

enteropathogenic *Escherichia coli* to attach to their target cells and outcompete nonpiliated species. Other organisms, such as *Staphylococcus aureus, Streptococcus pyogenes, Treponema pallidum,* and *Entamoeba histolytica,* have surface molecules that allow them to attach to specific sites on cell surfaces such as fibronectin or laminin in tissues' basement membranes. *Candida albicans*'s attachment to epithelial cells and plastics is assisted by a protein in the yeast cell wall.

Enzymes produced by microbes may damage the host cell and tissue. For example, hyaluronidase produced by some *S. pyogenes* dissolves intercellular hyaluronic acid and allows the spread of streptococci to adjacent sites. Some enzymes (proteases, e.g., hemoglobinase of *Plasmodium,* elastase of *Schistosoma,* and nucleases, e.g., neuraminidase) are associated with virulence.

Some bacteria produce toxins that have specific, significant effects. Toxins fall into two major categories. *Endotoxins* are components of the lipopolysaccharide of the outer membrane of gram-negative bacteria and have profound systemic effects on host circulatory and complement systems. Shock, disseminated intravascular coagulation, and death may result from overwhelming endotoxemia. *Exotoxins* are produced and released extracellularly by a variety of primarily gram-positive bacteria. These toxins can (1) damage the host cell membrane, (2) cross the host cell membrane and catalyze lethal intracellular metabolic events, or (3) remain attached to the external cell membrane and affect second messengers. Examples of exotoxins include α- and δ-toxins of *S. aureus,* streptolysin O and S of pyogenic streptococci, and phospholipases of *Clostridium perfringens.* Damage to the host cell membrane disturbs osmosis and ion flow, causing cell death.

Exotoxins include some of the most potent bacterial toxins known. Tetanus toxin and diphtheria toxin act by blocking neurotransmitters and cell protein synthesis, respectively. Cholera toxin increases adenosine diphosphate–ribosyl Gs, causing formation of cyclic adenosine monophosphate and concomitant loss of fluid from the small intestine (see Clinical Study 25). The heat-stable toxins of *E. coli* cause severe diarrhea. Toxic shock syndrome toxin of *S. aureus* induces interleukin-1 and tumor necrosis factor with T lymphocyte stimulation.

Microorganisms' ability to evade nonspecific and specific immune killing is definitely advantageous to promoting both symptomatic and asymptomatic infection. Evasion of nonspecific immune agents is aided by polysaccharide capsules, which prevent phagocytes from engulfing organisms in the absence of opsonic antibodies or complement. Some organisms may evade intracellular killing by lysosomal enzymes or toxic oxygen-free radicals. *Legionella pneumophila, Chlamydia psittaci,* and *Mycobacterium tuberculosis* inhibit fusion of the phagosome, which contains the phagocytized microbe with the digestive enzyme containing lysosome. *Leishmania* sp. and *Salmonella typhimurium* possess lysozyme resistance necessary to survive and replicate within the lysosome.

Microbes may evade specific antibodies. The structure of surface-exposed epitopes (antibody-binding molecules) of some microbes change over time. Host antibodies that may have been produced initially will not recognize the new epitopes. Genetic mutation or reassortment of gene fragments allows HIV-1 and influenza A viruses, respectively, to evade immune components specific for its previous configuration. Rapid rearrangement of the pilin genes of *Neisseria gonorrhoeae* allows it to evade antibodies that would block cell surface attachment. This change in genetic structure can be minor (antigenic drift) or major (antigenic shift) and make development of effective vaccines very difficult.

Some bacterial components may activate or block activity of cytokines and lymphokines, causing increased cell damage or downregulation of antibody production. Finally, antigenic cross-reactivity between microbial components and the host cell results in the host not seeing the components as foreign (immune tolerance). Conversely, microbe-host antigenic similarity may result in formation of antibodies that react with both the microbe and the host cell, resulting in formation of host antibodies against the host's own cells (autoantibodies). Autoantibodies produced in response to *Streptococcus pyogenes* infection may react with the heart and valves, resulting in acute rheumatic fever within several weeks. Antibodies formed against certain peptides in the streptococcal M protein may also react against cardiac tissue.

INFLUENCE OF SETTING ON MICROBE-SPECIFIC DETERMINANTS OF INFECTION

Characteristics of the external environment and behavioral practices of the host have a considerable effect on microorganisms and thus on one's state of health. Microorganisms persist in the hospital setting despite adverse conditions imposed by use of antibiotics and disinfectants. Microbes may acquire resistance to chemical insults through change in existing genetic information (mutation) or by acquisition of new genetic material from other organisms. Selection in favor of resistant microorganisms can occur rapidly. For example, a genetic change may allow the production of extracellular enzymes (e.g., penicillinase), resistance of the cell membrane to antimicrobials, or alteration of previously susceptible components of DNA replication or protein synthesis. Extrachromosomal DNA, *plasmids,* have become associated with resistance to aminoglycoside and beta-lactam antibiotics. Plasmids not only confer resistance to the bacterium but may be transferred to sensitive microbes of the same or other species. Subplasmid genetic components, *transposons,* can excise themselves and be transferred from plasmid to plasmid. Some pieces of DNA from the chromosome, such as that encoding macrolide antibiotic (e.g., erythromycin) resistance, can be transferred among different bacterial species.[4] Widespread use of antimicrobial agents results in increased occurrence of antibiotic resistance, such as the penicillin-resistant *N. gonorrhoeae.*

Care practices of health providers in the acute or chronic care setting are important in providing the backdrop for microbial adaptation. For example, increased use of multidrug "shotgun" antibiotic therapy, prophylactic drugs, and new drugs with a broad antimicrobial spectrum provide pressure that selects for survival of drug-resistant organisms. In some cases when drug resistance is a problem, temporary suspension of use of certain antibiotics may allow reemergence of drug-sensitive organisms. Failure to practice handwashing, gloving, and other precautions provides the opportunity for transfer of infectious and antibiotic-resistant organisms between patients and health care providers.

SUMMARY

Microorganisms are fundamental to the infectious process. Their inherent capabilities influence their role as do the specific attributes of the host and the physical and social environments with which they interact. Implicit in the study of the pathogenesis and infectious capability of microorganisms is the concept that they must first breach host defenses to enter the body and establish themselves, and

---

SELECTED CLINICAL STUDIES EMPHASIZING MICROBIOLOGIC ENVIRONMENT
(see Section Three)

NO.	TITLE
2.	Nursing Home Resident with Post-Antibiotic Oral Candidiasis
3.	Staphylococcal Food Poisoning in a University Cafeteria
5.	Methicillin-Resistant *Staphylococcus aureus* (MRSA) in a Sternal Wound Infection
34.	Group B Streptococcal Disease in an Infant
35.	School Teacher with Malaria

subsequently multiply and cause some damage to the host. The extent to which that damage (infection) can be avoided or moderated in patients relies in part on the techniques and methods used for nursing care. In Section 2, the microorganism is discussed in the context of infection prevention and control methods such as patient care practices, barrier precautions, disinfection and sterilization, antimicrobial therapy, health education and health policy. Each of the clinical studies in Section 3 presents a typical infection and describes the etiologic microorganism as it relates to the disease process and the care and outcome of the patient.

REFERENCES

1. Gorbach SL, Bartlett JG, Blacklow NR. *Infectious Diseases.* Philadelphia: W.B. Saunders Co.; 1992.
2. Koneman EW, et al. *Color Atlas and Textbook of Diagnostic Microbiology.* Philadelphia: J.B. Lippincott Co.; 1988.
3. Mims CA. *The Pathogenesis of Infectious Disease.* San Diego: Academic Press; 1987.
4. O'Brien TF, et al. Intercontinental spread of a new antibiotic resistance gene on an epidemic plasmid. *Lancet.* 1985;2:87.
5. Schaechter M, Medoff G, Schlessinger D. *Mechanisms of Microbial Disease.* Baltimore: Williams and Wilkins; 1989.
6. Thompkins LS. The use of molecular methods in infectious diseases. *N Engl J Med.* 1992;18:1290-1297.

SUGGESTED READINGS

Ewald PW. The evolution of virulence. *Sci Am.* 1993;268:86.

Hughes JM, Peters CJ, Cohen ML, Mahy BWJ. Hantavirus pulmonary syndrome: an emerging infectious disease. *Science.* 1993;262:850.

Muraca PW, Stout JE, Yu VL, et al. Legionnaire's disease in the work environment: implications for environmental health. *Ind Hyg.* 1988;584:590.

Stanier RY, et al, editors. *The Microbial World,* ed 5. Englewood Cliffs, NJ: Prentice-Hall; 1986.

Chapter 3

The Physical Environment

JEANNE LECLAIR

The physical environment is external to the microbial agent and the host. Air, water, sanitation, living conditions, and medical equipment all may influence the development of infection in community settings and health care institutions. This chapter explores environmental factors that play a role in the etiology of infection (Figure 3-1).

ENVIRONMENTAL COMPONENTS

Air

Air currents serve as conduits for only a limited number of bacterial, viral, and fungal agents. Before the identification of microorganisms, infections were thought to arise from "miasms," invisible particles of putrid material that circulated through the air. Vestiges of the miasm theory linger in some medical and nursing circles, leading to a general overemphasis on the role of air in the transmission of infection. When microorganisms were first viewed under a microscope, they were termed *animalcules* because of their resemblance to small animals. This term has some veracity. Bacteria share several traits of animals; they are living beings, have natural habitats, need nutrition and hydration, and have mass and weight. The relatively large mass and weight of most bacteria account for the fact that few remain airborne, at least in large enough numbers to cause infection.

Microorganisms present in the respiratory tract can be propelled into the environment on moist respiratory secretions by the cough or sneeze of an infected individual. Even talking results in the release of a large number of respiratory droplets. Most of the time, exposure to droplets laden with infectious agents is limited to a host who is close to where these droplets were expelled. This is termed *droplet spread* and is considered a form of contact spread. The droplets travel a few feet at most, then either settle to a surface or dry out while airborne, leaving behind the airborne droplet nuclei.[48] Relatively few organisms remain viable and suspended in infective doses in droplet nuclei. Those able to do so have the potential for being transmitted in the air.

The most common infections known to be transmitted via the airborne route are tuberculosis, varicella, influenza, rubeola (measles), and aspergillosis. *Aspergillus* is the only one of these agents originating from the environment and not spread person to person.

Mycobacterium tuberculosis is an acid-fast–staining bacteria transmitted almost exclusively by the airborne route. The size of the tubercle bacillus (1 to 5 µ) makes it an ideal candidate to bypass the upper respiratory defense system and be inhaled directly into the lung's alveoli, where primary infection begins. Persons who have active pulmonary disease and are coughing are contagious to others. Infectivity drops rapidly after *effective* treatment is begun, as symptoms (including coughing) subside, and numbers of organisms in respiratory secretions are reduced. If the organism is resistant to the drugs the patient is given, contagion persists. *M. tuberculosis* can infect organs other than the lungs, particularly bone and the urinary tract; patients with extrapulmonary disease are not contagious to others if the site of infection does not allow for dissemination of organisms. *M. tuberculosis* has occasionally been transmitted by biomedical devices in the health care setting (see Clinical Study 7).

The infectiousness of tuberculosis by the

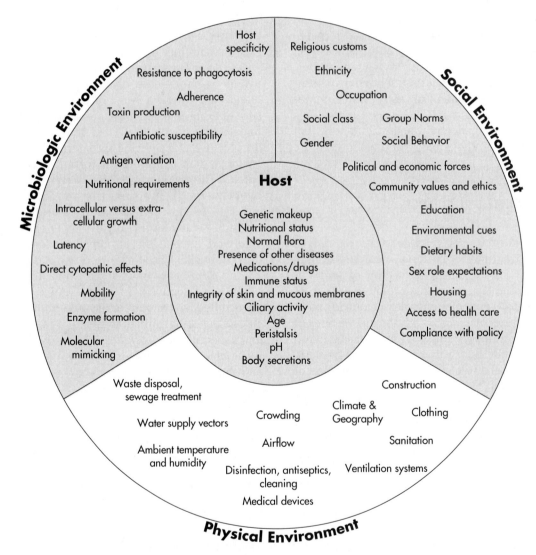

FIGURE 3-1. Factors in the physical environment that influence the infectious process.

airborne route was established in a 1962 study, when a tuberculosis ward was vented to a distant room containing a population of guinea pigs.[47] Most guinea pigs acquired the disease, confirming the significance of airborne droplet nuclei in the transmission of tuberculosis.

Before 1946, no drugs were available to treat tuberculosis, and control depended on prevention. In the 1990s we are faced with strains of *M. tuberculosis* that have become resistant to some or all available drugs, making prevention of transmission once again an urgent priority.

Viruses possess less mass and weight than bacteria and thus more easily remain airborne. The varicella-zoster virus causes two major clinical syndromes in immunocompetent persons: varicella (chickenpox) (see Clinical Study 6) and herpes zoster (shingles). A person who develops varicella carries a small quantity of virus in the respiratory tract and a large quantity of virus in vesicular fluid. Virus is shed into the environment, where it becomes airborne and is highly infectious when inhaled by susceptible persons.[55]

Varicella-zoster virus may infect and remain dormant in the cell body of the host's dorsal root ganglion. Later the virus may reactivate, usually as a response to stress or disease. The reactivated virus migrates down the nerve fiber to the skin served by that nerve system and produces localized vesicles known as herpes zoster, or shingles. Exposure to herpes zoster may lead to development of varicella in the nonimmune host. Children occasionally get chickenpox from a grandparent who has shingles.[34] Patients who have herpes zoster shed relatively small amounts of virus because of the small numbers of vesicles, and attack rates of varicella after exposure to herpes zoster are correspondingly lower.[34]

Influenza is a worldwide cause of virus res-

piratory infection every year (see Clinical Study 18). Because the virus mutates, the antibodies of individuals immune to previous strains of the virus may not be protective. The high attack rate among contacts and explosive onset of epidemics suggest that the air is an important means of transmission. Survival of influenza in droplet nuclei is enhanced when relative humidity is low.[48]

Many physical environments contain fungal spores. *Mycelia* produce a great number of spores that can remain dormant for many years and under certain conditions can become airborne. Under favorable conditions the spores can germinate and produce more mycelia. If these favorable conditions are in or on a human host, colonization or infection producing symptoms may result.

Aspergillus is ubiquitous in nature. It is found in soil, household dust, and many other environments. Spores are very small (2 to 5 μ) and can easily be inhaled. Individuals with normal immune systems are not affected by inhalation of even relatively large numbers of spores. However, persons with very specific types of immune deficiencies are at risk for serious fungal disease if they inhale large quantities of *Aspergillus* spores. The leukemias; lymphomas; immunosuppression associated with organ transplant protocols (bone marrow, cardiac, liver, renal); and burns all are associated with increased risk of aspergillosis (see Clinical Study 20).

Large quantities, or bursts, of spores can be released into the air when the environment is disturbed, such as when an old building is renovated or demolished. Spores from the air can stick to wet plaster during construction, where they can remain for years, protected by their resilient outer coat until they germinate to produce mycelia, which in turn produce more spores. High humidity or water leakage into walls can favor germination of spores. The demolition or renovation of a building or disturbance of poorly maintained air conditioning equipment can cause the release of clouds of spores, which can travel on air currents for some distance.[46] Outbreaks of nosocomial aspergillosis have occurred (see Clinical Study 10).

Water

The association of water with disease was recognized even before the discovery and acceptance of the germ theory. In 1853 a cholera epidemic occurred in London when a major source of drinking water became contaminated with sewage. Dr. John Snow, a surgeon, observed that people who obtained water from the Broad Street pump were most likely to develop cholera. He persuaded authorities to remove the pump's handle, and this was associated with an end to new cases.[6] Snow discovered that the diaper of a baby who had died of cholera had been rinsed in a cesspool found to be seeping into the well that supplied the Broad Street pump. He hypothesized that some disease-causing agent was present in the excreta of cholera victims and that drinking water containing the agent would produce the disease. Sporadic and epidemic cholera continues today in countries where water sanitation is inadequate (see Clinical Study 34).

In the United States, infectious agents associated with gastroenteritis traced to ingestion of contaminated water include *Giardia lamblia* (protozoan), *Shigella* (bacteria), hepatitis A (virus), Norwalk agent (virus), *Cryptosporidium* (protozoan), and certain strains of *Escherichia coli* (bacteria). Of these, *G. lamblia* is the most common cause of outbreaks associated with drinking water.[36]

Safety of public water systems depends on appropriate sewage treatment, protection of water reservoirs from contamination, and use of two or more preconsumption treatment processes. Treatments used to render water potable (safe for consumption) include filtration and disinfection, usually with chlorine.

Exposure to a minimum of 0.2 mg/L of free residual chlorine for 30 minutes at a pH less than 8 is considered adequate to kill coliform bacteria. *Giardia* cysts are relatively resistant to disinfection with chlorine. Narrow ranges of pH, turbidity, water temperature, contact time, and free chlorine concentration are necessary for chlorine treatment to kill *Giardia*. An ancillary process, usually filtration capable of removing 99.9% of *Giardia* cysts, is required to meet the U.S. Environmental Protection Agency (EPA) standard for potable water.[20]

Failure of one or more components of municipal water treatment processes can result in the survival of illness-producing levels of organisms in drinking water. Disinfection systems for public water supplies should have redundant components and an alarm system to detect disinfectant failure.[20]

Some enteric pathogens cause disease only after ingestion of a relatively large dose. Others, such as *Shigella*, a virulent gastrointestinal pathogen, require only small doses to infect. Cases of shigellosis have been traced to swimming in public pools in which the chlorine levels have been allowed to fall.

The most common organisms known to proliferate in water are *Pseudomonas aeruginosa*, *P. picketteii*, *P. cepacia*, and *Acinetobacter*, *Enterobacter*, *Aeromonas*, *Flavobacterium*, and *Legionella* species. One or more of these organisms is almost certainly present in all nonsterile water, especially standing water. Hot tubs and whirlpool baths have been implicated in cases of pseudomonas folliculitis.[14] Growth of pseudomonas in these recreational water sources can be controlled by maintaining the water at a pH of 7.2 to 7.8, with free residual chlorine levels of 1 mg/L.[13]

Legionella sp. are common microbial inhabitants of water. Tap water and distilled water provide a favorable environment for the growth of all strains of this bacteria. *Legionella* was discovered in 1977 after a 1976 outbreak of pneumonia and febrile respiratory illness in 221 people who attended an American Legion convention in Philadelphia; 34 people died of the illness. The fastidious gram-negative rod was grown from postmortem lung tissue.[31]

Legionella is the cause of two distinct syndromes: Legionnaires' disease and Pontiac fever. Legionnaires' disease is a multisystem disease characterized by pneumonia and has a 15% to 20% mortality rate. Pontiac fever, a milder form of febrile respiratory disease without pneumonia, is not fatal. *Legionella* can cause wound infections if sufficient numbers of organisms are introduced into the wound.

Transmission is primarily via contaminated environmental droplets. Person-to-person transmission occurs rarely if at all. Disease caused by *Legionella* occurs in both epidemic and sporadic form. Sporadic cases may be unidentified or source undetermined (see Clinical Study 33). The organism does not grow on ordinary laboratory culture media and is not found on routine sputum culture.

Air-conditioning equipment, shower heads, and faucets supplying potable water have been the sources of *Legionella* in several epidemics.[18] Cooling towers and evaporative condensers are widely used components of commercial and industrial air-cooling equipment. These devices are used to cool circulating water by dissipating excess heat into the atmosphere. In the process, water in droplet form escapes into the environment. When the water supplying these devices contains *Legionella*, the organism is propelled into the air to be inhaled by individuals in the vicinity.

Control measures have included prevention of accumulation of precipitates, known as *scale*, that may block the system. Heating to 70° C, hyperchlorination, and ultraviolet light have been successful in eliminating *Legionella* from water sources incriminated in epidemics.[31]

When a cluster of legionellosis is found in an institution, water sources should be tested for presence of the organism. Cultures should be taken from the bottom of hot water tanks and any areas in the water distribution system where sediment may accumulate, as well as faucets and shower heads.[31] This requires a coordinated effort and involvement of the microbiologist, engineer, and epidemiologist. In the absence of identified cases of *Legionella* infection, routine assays of water for *Legionella* are not warranted.

Sanitation

Since most diarrhea-causing pathogens are excreted in the feces of infected persons, sanitary disposal of human waste is important to prevent transmission of these pathogens. Studies have consistently shown an association between improved sanitation and reduced incidence of enteric disease.

The effectiveness of sanitation and other public health measures may be greatly influenced by the social environment. For example, improvements in physical facilities must be accompanied by education on how to use the facilities. Cultural influences must be acknowledged and incorporated into changes. For example, in many parts of the world, including Asia, the typical latrine is floor height and requires the user to assume a squatting position. Only the soles of the user's shoes come into direct contact with the latrine's hardware. Many refugees from Southeast Asia were confronted with the Western toilet for the first time on airplanes en route to their countries of destination. Unfamiliar with the device, the travelers attempted to use it while standing on the toilet seat. This resulted in environmental contamination of bathrooms and injuries sustained during bumpy flights. Educational efforts in refugee camps to familiarize residents with Western toilets helped improve sanitation (see Chapters 4 and 9).

Enteric disease may occur when water systems are significantly contaminated or the water from them is inadequately treated.

Domestic water systems are susceptible to contamination if sanitation is poor. Proximity of septic systems to wells can lead to leaching of fecal material into well water. Spring water is vulnerable to fecal and chemical contamination from above ground. Outbreaks of hepatitis A and other enteric diseases have occurred from drinking spring water into which an infected person has defecated.[42] Sporadic cases and outbreaks of hepatitis A have also been associated with eating raw or improperly steamed clams, oysters, and mussels harvested from fecally contaminated waters. Enteric infections associated with inadequate treatment of potable water occur in both endemic and epidemic form when sanitation is poor. These include typhoid fever, cholera, and amebic dysentery (see Clinical Study 25).

Turista, or traveler's diarrhea, is a common and temporarily debilitating ailment among persons traveling in foreign countries. Sometimes a pathogenic agent is involved. Most often the cause is ingestion of strains of enteric organisms with which the traveler is unfamiliar. In some countries there are very high numbers of enteric bacteria in drinking water because of inadequate or nonexistent water treatment. Travelers should avoid drinking tap water in countries with insufficiently managed water supplies. Bottled water should be purchased for drinking, brushing teeth, and preparing food that is not actually boiled. In restaurants and hotels, bottled water with the top already removed should be rejected; such bottles may contain tap water or their contents may be mixed with water from melted contaminated ice.

HOST-ENVIRONMENT INTERACTIONS

The encounter between microbial agent and host takes place in the physical environment. Social factors sometimes influence the course and outcome of the encounter. It is the interaction of these four elements—microbial agent, host, environment, and social factors—that together determine whether infection occurs. With the development and acceptance of the germ theory, an understanding of the complex interaction among biologic agent, environmental and social factors, and the host in the etiology of infection began to evolve. That evolution continues today.

Climate and geography

Climate is an environmental factor that can influence infectious disease patterns. Temperature and humidity not only determine which biologic agents survive and multiply outside a host but also influence human and vector behavior patterns, which in turn promote or inhibit microorganism transmission.

The complex relationship between ecological balance and human disease is illustrated by the epidemiology of a Hantavirus outbreak.[39] The deer mouse serves as the primary reservoir host of Hantavirus, which is shed in rodent droppings. In the spring of 1992 the southwestern United States received heavy rain following 6 years of severe drought. The sudden change in the ecologic balance brought about by the rain resulted in a large supply of piñon nuts and grasshoppers, foods eaten by rodents. With an increased food supply and since predators were eradicated by the preceding drought, the deer mouse population thrived and increased tenfold. This led to a sharp increase in the incidence of Hantavirus illness in humans. Efforts to eliminate the deer mouse seem reasonable but could result in other ecologic and health consequences. Deer mice also serve as hosts for fleas that transmit *Yersinia pestis*, the bacterium that causes plague. Eradication of deer mice would force fleas to seek new hosts, possibly leading to an increased risk of human plague.[11]

Social factors can exert a powerful influence on the physical environment. The practice of sharing needles has been integrated into the drug-using subculture, but since society generally disapproves of intravenous (IV) drug use and may view needle exchange programs as supportive of illegal use, drug users often have difficulty obtaining clean hypodermic equipment. When many hosts encounter the biologic agent of a bloodborne infection (such as HIV) in a social milieu where clean needles are not used, infection transmission of epidemic proportions may result.

Epidemiologic methods are used to identify the factors contributing to infection risk that may be influenced by specific interventions. Using the example of IV drug use, if society's attitudes toward drug addiction changed so that clean needles could be freely obtained, elimination of needle-sharing behavior in such a milieu would isolate the biologic agent (HIV) from the host (drug user), and no disease would occur.

Living conditions

Crowded living conditions favor the spread of microorganisms by contact and air. Organisms may be transmitted by three types of contact: direct, indirect, and droplet. *Droplets,* produced when an infected person coughs, sneezes, laughs, or talks, may deposit microorganisms directly on the nasal or conjunctival mucous membranes of another person. Airborne transmission is accomplished by particles carried in droplet nuclei.

Although crowding amplifies transmission of infection spread by contact and air, it may play a less important role in transmission of other infections such as those requiring exposure to blood or other body substances. Most HIV-infected persons remain asymptomatic for many years and mingle with family members and associates in the community, schools, and the workplace. Studies have established that the risk of HIV transmission to nonsexual family contacts even when crowding, sharing of eating utensils, and poor hygiene are present[21,49] is so low as to be unmeasurable.

Rhinovirus is a frequent cause of the most prevalent infectious human malady, the common cold. Infected individuals shed large amounts of virus during the first week of illness, when the severity of symptoms correlates with the amount of virus shed. Contrary to popular belief, colds are only moderately contagious, with infection resulting in 50% of susceptible household contacts after a week of exposure.[16] An epidemiologic study done in an isolated community in Antarctica focused on the role of the environment in the spread of colds.[54] When people with colds were introduced into the dormitory, the incidence of transmission was twice as high in the smaller, crowded living units than in the larger dormitory.

In another experiment, volunteers with rhinovirus colds and well volunteers occupied the same room for 72 hours. A double-wire mesh barrier separated the two groups and prevented contact between them but allowed free airflow. No transmission of infection occurred.[28] Another investigator staged a series of carefully controlled poker games to determine which types of contact transmit rhinovirus colds among adults.[17] Infected and uninfected people played cards around a table for 12 hours. Some uninfected individuals wore arm restraints, making it impossible for them to touch their faces. More than half the susceptible individuals caught the cold, suggesting large-droplet spread to be significant in the natural transmission of colds among adults. In another phase of the experiment, unrestrained, uninfected individuals played poker for 12 hours with cards that were heavily contaminated with rhinovirus. Participants were asked to rub eyes and noses frequently and were monitored for compliance. Every hour, freshly contaminated cards were introduced into the game. Despite this intensive exposure to contaminated fomites, no players became ill, suggesting that among adults, fomite transmission of rhinovirus colds occurs infrequently.

In a follow-up experiment, respiratory secretions from an infected person were traced and measured as they were deposited on fomites, then transferred to the hands and nasal or conjunctival mucosa of others.[33] The amount of virus diminished with each transfer, reaching negligible quantities by the time it reached the portal of entry of a potential host. Thus, the available evidence suggests that among adults most colds are transmitted when droplets expelled by an infected individual reach the mucous membranes of a nearby susceptible person. Transfer of abundant secretions that remain wet seems to be required for transmission of most colds. Droplets satisfy this requirement in most adult settings. Crowding favors this type of spread. Self-inoculation after direct or indirect contact with contaminated secretions is probably most significant among children, where hygiene is poor and transfer of infective still-wet secretions to nasal mucosa is most likely to occur.

Respiratory syncytial virus (RSV) is another common cause of upper respiratory infection. Colds caused by RSV tend to be more severe in infants and young children during their first experience with the virus. Studies have shown that the primary way RSV spreads among hospitalized infants is by contact, most likely on caregivers' hands[37] (see Clinical Study 29). The virus can be recovered for up to 6 hours from toys and environmental surfaces contaminated with secretions of RSV-infected persons, and transmission from fomites has been documented.[30] Droplets also play a role in RSV transmission. In one study, transmission was significantly lower in caregivers who wore eye/nose shields when having contact with infected patients.[23]

Sarcoptes scabiei infection, also known as scabies, is a parasitic infestation transmitted by direct contact and associated with crowding. Scabies is caused by mites that burrow into the uppermost layer of the skin, usually in skin folds. The eight-legged adult mite is most active at night, producing extreme nocturnal itching. The mites lay two to three eggs per day, which hatch and mature in 10 days. Once they have burrowed a niche in the stratum corneum, the mites are reluctant to leave and thus are not often encountered on fomites or in the environment. Scabies is usually transmitted after prolonged skin-to-skin contact.

There is one notable exception to the usual mode of scabies transmission. Mite-infested pigeons occasionally roost on window air conditioners. Bird mites can be sucked in through the air conditioner fan and heavily populate adjacent environmental surfaces.[51] Brigades of barely visible mites, each about the size of a grain of sand, march across window sills and other surfaces searching for a suitable host in which to burrow and lay their eggs. The only way to eradicate the problem is to relocate the pigeons, thoroughly clean and replace filters on air conditioners, and treat the affected individuals.

Vectors

Some microorganisms are spread by vectors. A *vector* refers to an insect or animal in whose body an infectious agent resides or multiplies before being directly or indirectly transmitted to a host by a bite or other means. Mosquitoes, ticks, and bloodsucking flies and fleas are all important vectors. Usually only a specific species of insect is capable of serving as the vector of a particular pathogen. For example, only the female *Anopheles* mosquito is capable of transmitting malaria. Therefore, malaria transmission occurs only in geographic regions where this variety of mosquito lives (see Clinical Study 35).

Some microorganisms are not transmitted by arthropod vectors despite an apparent theoretical possibility. A high incidence of HIV in a community in Florida led to speculation that HIV might be transmitted by insects. Mosquitoes and bedbugs were fed blood containing high titers of HIV. Virus could be cultured from the digestive tract of bedbugs but not mosquitoes. The insects then fed on uninfected blood; no transfer of virus to the uninfected blood could be detected.[40] Failure of insects to transmit HIV was subsequently confirmed by epidemiologic studies showing no HIV-seropositive persons younger than 10 years or older than 60 who resided in insect-infested areas.

Lyme disease is the most frequently reported tickborne infection in the United States. It is caused by a spirochete, *Borrelia burgdorferi*, carried by ticks of the genus *Ixodes* and is transmitted to humans through a tick's bite. *Ixodes* ticks are prevalent in nine states: New Jersey, Massachusetts, New York, Connecticut, Rhode Island, Pennsylvania, Wisconsin, Minnesota, and California. Ninety percent of cases of Lyme disease in the United States have been reported from these states. Surveys of tick populations in these states have shown that up to 20% of the ticks carry *Borrelia burgdorferi*.[5] The major reservoir of the organism is small rodents. Ticks acquire the organism while feeding on infected rodents, which are the major reservoir.

Preventing tick bites protects against Lyme disease. The tick is most active during May and June. Infested areas such as woods and tall grass should be avoided at these times. When in these areas, long pants with cuffs tucked into socks, long-sleeved shirts, and closed shoes should be worn to limit access of ticks to skin. Insect repellents known to be effective against ticks may also lower risk. Ticks that attach to the skin should be promptly removed using mechanical means. The likelihood of Lyme disease transmission is proportional to the amount of time the tick remains attached to the skin. Transmission is unlikely when the tick feeds for less than 24 hours[5] (see Clinical Study 1).

INFLUENCE OF SETTING ON ENVIRONMENTAL-SPECIFIC DETERMINANTS OF INFECTION
The home

Family members share air space, have direct contact, and handle common fomites for long periods on a regular basis. Experience with infection transmission within the family can be extrapolated to other settings in which the same type of interactions occur. For example, it is well established that HIV is not transmitted from infected children to their household contacts, despite hugging, kissing, and sharing of eating utensils.[21,49] These findings have been useful in predicting that the virus will not spread by similar or less intense forms of contact in schools and in the community.

In general, airborne infections such as tuberculosis, varicella, and influenza spread readily to susceptible hosts within households. Infections transmitted by contact or fecal-oral transmission also frequently spread within households because of the duration and nature of contact among family members.

Devices used in the home may present risk of infection. Home use of nebulizers filled with tap water can disseminate gram-negative organisms into the environment along with the nebulized water droplets. These devices should be emptied and all inside surfaces scrubbed daily while the machine is in use.

Day care

A shift toward single-parent families and reliance on dual wages in two-parent families in the United States have established day-care centers as integral to the livelihood of millions of Americans.

The day-care environment intermingles susceptible hosts who may have poor hygiene with potential sources of organisms in a crowded space. Most day-care centers attempt to exclude children known to be ill. However, some infections can be transmitted from asymptomatic carriers (*Haemophilus influenzae*, hepatitis B) or from individuals in the incubation stage of the infection (measles, varicella, influenza, hepatitis A).

One epidemiologic study in a day-care center found biting to be relatively common, especially among toddlers.[24] Male toddlers enrolled full time sustained an average of 9.4 bites per year. Although transmission of hepatitis B virus (HBV) by an infected biter has been documented[7] and the minimal infective dose for this virus is small, the HBV level in the saliva is low and risk of HBV transmission by this route is therefore also low. HIV transmission by biting is theoretically possible, but the level of virus carried in the saliva is thought to be orders of magnitude lower than the dose needed to produce infection. There is no documentation of HIV transmission by biting.[19]

Children under 5 years of age are at greatest risk for invasive *H. influenzae* infection. Seventy percent of cases occur in children less than 2 years of age. *H. influenzae* is a gram-negative bacterium that can reside harmlessly in the upper respiratory tract, a condition known as *asymptomatic carriage*. This organism is the most common cause of bacterial meningitis and may also cause epiglottitis, pneumonia, and septic arthritis in young children. *H. influenzae* is believed to be transmitted via respiratory droplets or direct contact with secretions from a person who harbors the organism. Usually the initial (index) case is an asymptomatic carrier, but transmission from individuals who have the disease also occurs. The risk of invasive *H. influenzae* disease in children who attend day care is approximately twice that of those who remain at home. Studies in day-care centers suggest that the risk increases with the size of the facility.[32] Presumably, larger numbers of potential carriers and susceptible hosts lead to a greater risk of infection (see Clinical Study 9).

Day-care centers may also provide opportunity for hepatitis A virus (HAV) transmission.[29] HAV is excreted in the feces and is transmitted via the fecal-oral route. HAV generally causes only mild or asymptomatic infection in preschool-age children. These children may be sources of infection for day-care staff and adult household members, who are much more likely to develop symptomatic disease with jaundice. Day-care centers have also been implicated in transmission of other organisms known to spread via the fecal-oral route, including *Salmonella, Shigella, Giardia,* and viruses causing gastroenteritis.

Several variables have been found to influence the risk of enteric disease transmission in day-care centers.[38] Presence of children under 2 years of age is associated with increased risk. Appropriate handwashing by staff approximately halves the incidence of diarrheal disease. Centers where one or more staff members diapered children and prepared or served a meal had a greater than threefold incidence of diarrhea than centers where these duties were performed by different individuals.[4]

Cytomegalovirus (CMV) is common in day-care settings, usually causing asymptomatic primary infection in healthy individuals. It is of concern because primary infection in pregnant women, regardless of trimester, may result in congenital CMV infection of the fetus in 5% to 10% of cases. Possible sequelae for these infants include hearing loss, visual impairment, seizures, cerebral palsy, and mental retardation.

Studies examining CMV excretion have demonstrated that up to 80% of toddlers in day-care centers excrete virus.[45] CMV is excreted in urine and saliva of infected individuals for 12 months or longer. Drooling and urine incontinence among diapered day-care children provide ample opportunities for CMV transmission from children who are asymptomatic shedders of the virus. The prevalence of CMV among children who attend day-care centers exceeds that of children who remain at home. Children who acquire CMV in the day-care setting usually remain asymptomatic and may serve as a reservoir of infection for family members and day-care workers who are pregnant. Seronegative mothers of children who attend day care and day-care workers have a documented increased risk of acquiring

CMV.[43] This contrasts with hospital pediatric nursing personnel, in whom the incidence of CMV acquisition is not discernibly higher than that in the general population.

Environmental and hygienic controls can reduce but not eliminate the risk of infection transmission in day-care centers. Since diaper changing carries the highest risk for environmental contamination with enteric pathogens, separation of age groups can reduce transmission of enteric pathogens from diapered toddlers. A separate area equipped with closed disposal containers and easily accessible handwashing facilities should be reserved for diaper changing. The diaper-changing surface should be cleaned and disinfected after each use with a disinfectant known to kill *Giardia* cysts. This area should be off-limits for eating and drinking. Staff should be trained in the proper method of cleaning body fluid spills such as urine and stool and proper methods used to avoid spreading contamination. Disposable gloves should be available for diaper changing and other activities when risk of contamination of hands is greatest.

The value of training and monitoring day-care staff in the proper methods of handwashing cannot be overemphasized. Hands should be washed after diaper changing and before preparing or serving food. Handwashing supplies must be easily accessible, and staff should recognize the importance of replenishing soap or paper towel dispensers that have been emptied during the work day. Waterless hand degerming agents are useful for quick decontamination of hands when handwashing facilities are unavailable. These products are supplied in small pocket-sized bottles that can be carried out to the playground and other areas where hands may become contaminated but handwashing is impractical.

The outpatient environment

The combination of high traffic volumes, crowding, and long waiting periods makes the waiting rooms of outpatient health care facilities a favorable environment for the transmission of some infections.[25] This risk is amplified in pediatric facilities, where waiting patients with poor hygiene may mingle.

Transmission of the childhood viral diseases, particularly varicella but also measles and rubella, may occur in this setting. Whenever possible, pediatric patients should be visually screened for symptoms of these infections on arrival to the outpatient setting. A negative-pressure room should be identified in advance for placement of patients who arrive with rash and fever or if preliminary findings suggest pulmonary tuberculosis. These patients should not mingle with other patients in the waiting room. If no negative-pressure room is available, a fan placed facing an open window may achieve this effect. However, it must first be determined that no air intake or other open window is situated near the exhaust window.

If the patient is subsequently diagnosed as having varicella, measles, or rubella, environmental surfaces and objects that the patient actually touched should be wiped with a disinfectant agent. If possible, susceptible patients should not be placed in the room for several hours after a patient with active infection has left.[50]

Long-Term Care

The long-term care environment bears similarities to both the home and the hospital. As in the home, residents share air space and engage in activities that bring them into daily contact with a relatively stable group of individuals. As in the hospital, the pool of potential contacts is large and includes patients who have received extended antibiotic therapy. These patients have an increased likelihood of becoming colonized with antimicrobial-resistant organisms or infected with *Clostridium difficile* (see Clinical Study 22). In addition, long-term care patients are at risk of reactivation of tuberculosis. Symptoms of active tuberculosis in the elderly may be masked by symptoms of other chronic conditions and therefore may go unrecognized. The infected person may be highly mobile within the long-term care institution and expose many patients, staff, and visitors.

The hospital

A 1982 study by Maki and Alvarado[41] clearly demonstrated that moving from an old hospital to a new, spacious facility having lower levels of contamination had no effect on the incidence of nosocomial infection. The study contributed to the increasing evidence that the vast majority of nosocomial infections are not caused by pathogens originating from inanimate reservoirs, such as floors, walls, doorknobs, window sills, and carpets. Nonetheless, some organisms shed from humans may remain viable in the environment for long periods. Though not often effectively transported to a susceptible host in numbers sufficient to establish themselves, the chance that microorganisms will reach vulnerable sites in susceptible hosts increases as environmental contamination accumulates. Consequently, maintaining a clean environment can be important. For example, if bacteria-laden skin squames carried in dust particles are allowed to accumulate on the lamp directly over the operating room table, some will eventually begin to drop off the lamp during surgery, directly into open wounds. In addition, visibly dirty surroundings create a perception of undue risk of infection in the minds of patients and staff. Certain environmental niches supply the nutrition and living requirements for microorganisms. Excess environmental contamination increases the chance that organisms will gain access to one of these niches and proliferate to high levels, creating a reservoir. Any area where moisture or nonsterile water collects or stands should be considered likely to harbor proliferating gram-negative organisms.

Transmission of organisms from environmental surfaces is of limited importance except for a few specific pathogens in certain hospital settings. *Clostridium difficile*, a gram-negative anaerobic bacterium, can cause severe gastrointestinal infection in patients who receive antibiotics. Spores produced by *C. difficile* may heavily contaminate the immediate environment of patients who have *C. difficile* diarrhea. Spores may persist in the environment for weeks or months because of their relative resistance to many disinfectants and cleaning agents.[35] Portable commodes, bedpans, electronic thermometers, and staff members' hands have all been shown to be a potential reservoir for *C. difficile*. A 1:10 dilution of household bleach may eliminate *C. difficile* spores from environmental surfaces. There is a trend in new construction to place unenclosed modular toilets in intensive care unit rooms several feet from the patient's bed. It is not advisable to equip these toilets with spray-type bedpan washes, as these devices generate considerable aerosols (see Figure 3-2). Such aerosols can lead to fecal contamination of the environment.

Hydrotherapy tanks used for single patient treatments bring water into direct contact with hosts who have sites vulnerable to bacterial invasion, such as open wounds and decubitus ulcers. Some patients, including those with burns, infected wounds, or decubitus ulcers, shed large quantities of organisms into the water of hydrotherapy tanks. These organisms may lodge and multiply in crevices in the agitator and contaminate subsequent treatment water.

The Centers for Disease Control and Prevention (CDC) recommends that the water in these tanks should be maintained at a constant pH of 7.2 to 7.6, with a free chlorine residual of 15 mg/L.[13] Other chemical disinfectant agents and protocols are also used. The tanks should be drained and all surfaces scrubbed with disinfectant after each use. The agitator, which can become a reservoir of debris and organ-

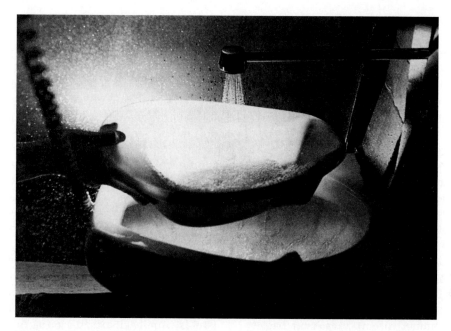

FIGURE 3-2. Spray-type bedpan washers generate considerable aerosols that may heavily contaminate the environment.

isms, should be disinfected at the end of each treatment day to flush out contamination from inner surfaces. The agitator may need to be disassembled periodically to remove debris.

Hydrotherapy pools can accommodate more than one patient at a time and are used to treat patients without open wounds or identified transmissible infection. These pools are generally not drained after each use. The CDC recommends continuous filtration with chlorination that maintains a free residual chlorine level of 0.4 to 0.6 mg/L. In pools without continuous filtration, a combination of iodine (which is not inactivated by organic material) and chloramine should be added to the water.[13]

Water used in hemodialysis is usually subjected to deionization or reverse osmosis processes that do not render it sterile. The water is then combined with concentrated salt solution, and the resulting solution leaches waste products from the patient's blood during hemodialysis.

Intact bacteria are too large to pass through the dialysis membrane, but remnants of the cell wall of gram-negative organisms called *endotoxins* can pass through the membrane and cause febrile reactions in the patient. With a damaged or otherwise nonintact membrane, bacteria contaminating the dialysate can directly invade the patient's bloodstream.

Prevention of bacteremia and endotoxic reactions during hemodialysis requires that the numbers of microbes in the dialysate be low. This involves proper cleaning of the machines' reusable components and monitoring levels of organisms in water used to prepare dialysate.[26] The acceptable count is 200 organisms/ml or fewer for water and 2000 organisms/ml or fewer for dialysate.[1]

Equipment used in patient care may pose infection risk unique to the device. Consequently, each piece of equipment should be carefully assessed and procedures developed for use.

Certain invasive medical devices create a conduit between the outside environment and areas of the human body that are normally inaccessible to microorganisms. The conduit is intended either as a delivery or drainage system, but inherent to all these systems is the risk of introducing microorganisms into a sterile body space (see Chapter 5).

Most urinary catheter–associated urinary tract infections (UTIs) are endogenous; the infecting organism comes from the patient's perineal flora.[22] Sometimes environmental organisms are carried to the system, usually on the hands of caregivers when they insert, empty, flush, or care for the drainage system. Clusters of UTIs among catheterized patients have been traced to the practice of using a common container to empty catheter bags.[27] The container may become contaminated with urine from an infected patient or from environmental sources between uses.

Most infections associated with intravascular devices occur when the patient's own flora travels through the skin wound and up the catheter track. Careful preparation of the insertion site with an appropriate antiseptic is essential to reduce the level of skin microbes through which the catheter must travel during insertion. Some organisms, especially *Staphylococcus epidermidis,* produce a slimy substance that helps the organism adhere to the catheter material and avoid both phagocytosis and antibiotics. Considerable research is now focused on developing materials that resist bacterial attachment[52] (see Chapter 5).

Environmental sources of intravascular system contamination include contaminated fluids and flushing solutions; hand, mouth, or skin bacteria shed by the caregiver during insertion or dressing changes; and cracked or leaking connections.[8]

Junctions on delivery systems occasionally leak because of manufacturing defects, use of incompatible components, or cracked plastic connectors. Taping directly over poorly fitting or leaking critical junctions can introduce bacteria into the system. (Leclair, J. Unpublished data, 1983). It is a common practice to tear tape with the fingers. This causes inoculation of hand flora onto the tape's sticky side. If tape is subsequently used to secure a loose or leaking connection, bacteria on the tape may wash into the delivery system. All efforts should be made to discover and remedy the cause of leaking or poorly fitting connections. If it is necessary to tape directly over critical connections temporarily, the tape should be cut with clean scissors and never torn with the fingers.

Pressure transducers are routinely used for cardiovascular monitoring of critically ill patients. The transducer setup consists of a reusable transducer head and a separate dome that is usually disposable or a complete disposable system. Epidemics of bacteremia have been traced to inadequate disinfection of the transducer head between patients.[3] The organisms have been gram negative and associated with environmental water sources: *Serratia marcescens, Pseudomonas cepacia, Klebsiella oxytoca,* and *Acinetobacter* sp. Presumably, these organisms contaminated transducer heads during some phase of the cleaning or rinsing process, which was followed by inadequate disinfection. It is well documented that contamination on the transducer head can reach the fluid column that communicates directly with the patient's circulation despite the presence of the dome diaphragm.[3] This can occur when personnel handle the components of the transducer system for tubing changes, calibration, or collection of blood specimens.

To understand the infection risk posed by respiratory therapy equipment, it is helpful to understand the difference between nebulizers and humidifiers.[15] Evaporative-type *humidifiers* produce humidity in the form of a gas from a reservoir of water. Bacteria contaminating the reservoir stay in the reservoir, since bacteria are solid and cannot travel in a gas. On the other hand, *nebulizers* lift tiny water droplets and propel them out of the reservoir. If the reservoir is contaminated, bacteria will be carried directly to vulnerable areas of the patient's respiratory tract. Ventilators are typically equipped with humidifiers that bubble gas through water, eliminating the hazard of microaerosols.

Water used to fill reservoirs may become contaminated or contain low levels of gram-negative organisms. Also, the reservoir may become contaminated when handled or changed. Once the reservoir water becomes even slightly contaminated, rapid proliferation of organisms may occur. Whether or not they are swept out of the reservoir and delivered into the patient's respiratory tract depends on whether the equipment uses a nebulizer (yes) or a humidifier (no). Cold-air room nebulizers are generally avoided by hospitals because of the ease with which the reservoirs may become contaminated and subsequently disseminate contaminated aerosols into the environment.

The source of infection associated with peritoneal dialysis is usually the patient's skin.[44] Organisms gain access by migration down the catheter from the skin entry site. External sources of infection include contaminated dialysis fluid, improperly disinfected peritoneal dialysis machines, water baths used to warm dialysate, and cracked or leaking intravascular line connections. Waste peritoneal dialysis fluid is one of the fluids believed capable of transmitting bloodborne pathogens such as hepatitis B and HIV. It must be disposed of carefully and splashing and the generation of aerosols avoided.

ENVIRONMENTAL ASSESSMENT AND MANAGEMENT
Environmental culturing

Routine microbiologic sampling was for many years considered an important infection control routine. However, it is expensive, can be time-consuming for the laboratory, and can provide potentially misleading information that rarely leads to meaningful action. Consequently, routine culturing of the environment is not recommended.[10] Exceptions are monthly cultures of hemodialysis solutions and the water used to prepare dialysate hemodialysis and cultures that may support educational efforts.

Environmental culturing may also be indicated when a cluster of infections suggests an environmental source of organisms. These cultures should be done as part of an organized investigation in collaboration with infection control and microbiology staff, who can advise regarding collection of specimens and interpretation of results.

Containment of airborne microorganisms

Patients in health care facilities who are in the contagious phase of infection from which airborne organisms may be shed should be in rooms that are maintained at a negative air pressure relative to the surrounding rooms and spaces and which prevent the patient's room air from flowing into other areas. Each room should have six or more air changes per hour, with exhausted air delivered directly to the outside at an appropriate distance (>20 feet) from any adjacent intake and not recirculated. This may be a particular challenge in newer buildings that recirculate air to conserve energy, in facilities where rooms originally designed for some other purpose are adapted for patient care, where private rooms are limited, and where ventilation is nonexistent or disrupted by the opening of windows or doors. Institutional engineering departments should determine which rooms, if any, have sufficient negative pressure and appropriate exhaust necessary to manage patients having airborne disease. The rooms should be designed for use by patients with suspected airborne disease in both inpatient and outpatient settings. Preventive maintenance should be frequently and routinely performed to

Aultman Hospital
Health Sciences Library
161342

ensure that airflow is appropriate. These engineering controls, airflow, and monitoring requirements have been included in recommendations from the CDC[12] and drafts of federal occupational safety regulations (see Chapter 6).

Infant isolettes maintain at positive air pressure relative to the surrounding environment in order to allow temperature control. Consequently, they expel air out of their openings and should not be used for infants who have an infection transmitted by air. Likewise, ventilators, even those equipped with exhalation filters, are capable of disseminating airborne pathogens into the environment from patients infected with airborne diseases. It is especially important for ventilated patients who are in the contagious phase of an airborne disease to be maintained in a negative-pressure room with the door closed.

The potential for airborne disease transmission should be addressed in the design phase of new facilities or renovation and should incorporate a sufficient number of negative-pressure rooms to accommodate patients with airborne disease. Nursing staff members often become involved in decisions regarding design of new or renovated patient care facilities. They should be aware of design considerations that are relevant to the prevention of infection in the hospital setting, and be prepared to manage patient room assignments to ensure that negative pressure rooms are used to manage patients with diagnosed or suspected airborne infectious diseases.

The use of positive-pressure rooms for patients who are immunosuppressed is unnecessary.[53] Except for *Aspergillus*, few organisms likely to cause infection are carried into the room on air currents. Furthermore, these patients are usually not confined to their rooms. However, immunosuppressed patients should be protected from environments containing large quantities of fungal spores. In the institution, this means that when major nearby demolition projects are planned, the air supply to these patients' rooms should be shut off or appropriately filtered and the windows closed until the dust has dissipated, usually several hours after implosion or demolition has occurred.[46] (See Clinical Study 10).

Since the major routes by which environmental *Aspergillus* usually enters patients' rooms are unfiltered supply air, open windows, and dusty room air conditioners, positive pressure in the patient's room has little or no effect on acquisition of nosocomial *Aspergillus*. Filters in wall-mounted room air conditioners in rooms housing vulnerable patients should be replaced or cleaned at least yearly, preferably just before first use of the season.

Organisms causing wound infections usually enter the wound at the time of the operation.[9] These organisms may be endogenous (originating from the patient) or exogenous (originating from someone or something external to the patient). Chapters 1 and 2, The Host and The Microbiologic Environment, discuss the role of endogenous organisms in infection. Exogenous sources of infection are discussed in this section in regard to surgical wounds and associated environments.

The physical environment of the operating room (OR) is far less important as a factor in exogenous wound infections than the people who inhabit it.[2] The surgical team shed skin squames that contain surface bacteria. Shedding of skin squames is intensified when dermatitis is present. If these squames fall or waft into the open wound in sufficient numbers over the course of surgery, a wound infection can occur. Environmental factors that influence the quantity and movement of skin squames shed in the OR also influence the risk of exogenous wound infection. This includes the number of people in the room, where they are standing, whether hair (including beards) is properly covered, the direction and velocity of airflow, and the amount of movement in the room, including movement of swinging doors.

ORs should have a minimum of 20 air changes per hour, of which at least four should be fresh air. The OR air pressure is maintained positive to adjacent spaces such as external hallways. All incoming air should be filtered.[9] Occasionally, clusters of wound infections can be traced to an individual who is a particularly efficient shedder of *Staphylococcus aureus* or group A streptococcus. Most often, the person has an area of dermatitis from which he or she is shedding large quantities of the organism into the environment. Less commonly, the shedder is someone who unknowingly carries the organism in the perineum, anus, or vagina. A search for these carriers should be limited to investigation of an apparent outbreak and requires culture screening of all who are epidemiologically linked to a series of wound infections.

SUMMARY

Forces in the physical environment may significantly influence the risk of infection. The effects of these environmental forces may be moderated by host, microorganism, and social factors. Prevention and management of infection have historically placed great emphasis on control of the physical environment. This has resulted, paradoxically, in an overemphasis on control of some environmental components and neglect of others.

Chapters 5 through 10 identify specific steps clinicians can take to minimize risk of infection by managing the physical environment. The clinical studies in Section Three demonstrate the interaction of the physical environment with host, microorganism, and social factors and illustrate how clinicians assessed and influenced these interactions to manage and prevent infections.

SELECTED CLINICAL STUDIES EMPHASIZING THE PHYSICAL ENVIRONMENT
(see Section Three)

NO.	TITLE
4.	*Pseudomonas* Bloodstream Infection from an Arterial Line
10.	Nosocomial Aspergillosis during Hospital Remodel
22.	*Clostridium Difficile* in a Nursing Home Resident
25.	Cholera in a 3-Year-Old Child in Bangladesh
33.	Legionnaires' Disease: Possible Acquisition on a Cruise Ship

---

REFERENCES

1. Association for the Advancement of Medical Instrumentation. *American National Standard for Hemodialysis Systems.* Arlington, VA: 1981.
2. Ayliffe GA. Role of the environment of the operating suite in surgical wound infection. *Rev Inf Dis.* 1991;13:S800-804.
3. Beck-Sague CM, Jarvis WR. Epidemic bloodstream infections associated with pressure transducers: a persistent problem. *Infect Control Hosp Epidemiol.* 1989;10:54-59.
4. Black RE. Handwashing to prevent diarrhea in daycare centers. *Am J Epidemiol.* 1981;113:445-451.
5. Buchstein SR, Gardner R. Lyme disease. *Infect Dis Clin North Am.* March 1991;5:103-116.
6. Cameron D, Jones I. John Snow, the Broad Street pump and modern epidemiology. *Int J Epidemiol.* 1983;12: 393-396.
7. Cancio-Bello TP. An institutional outbreak of hepatitis B related to a human biting carrier. *J Infect Dis.* 1982;146:652-656.
8. Centers for Disease Control. Guidelines for prevention of intravascular infection. *Infect Control.* 1982;3:61-72.
9. Centers for Disease Control. *Guidelines for Prevention of Surgical Wound Infections.* Atlanta, 1985.
10. Centers for Disease Control. *Guidelines for Handwashing and Hospital Environmental Control.* Atlanta, 1985.
11. Centers for Disease Control and Prevention. Hantavirus infection—southwestern United States: interim recommendations for risk reduction. *MMWR* July 30, 1993;42:1-13.
12. Centers for Disease Control and Prevention. *Draft Guidelines for Preventing the Transmission of Tuberculosis in Health Care Facilities.* Federal Register. Oct 12, 1993;58:52834.

13. Centers for Disease Control. *Disinfection of Hydrotherapy Pools and Tanks, Hospital Infections Program Center for Infectious Disease,* CDC, Atlanta, 1974.

14. Centers for Disease Control. Outbreak of *Pseudomonas aeruginosa* serotype 0:9 associated with a whirlpool. *MMWR.* 1981;30:329-331.

15. Craven DE, Steger KA. Nosocomial pneumonia in the intubated patient. *Infect Dis Clin North Am.* 1989;3:843-866.

16. D'Allessio DJ, et al. Short-duration exposure and the transmission of rhinoviral colds. *J Infect Dis.* 1984;150:189-194.

17. Dick EC et al. Aerosol transmission of rhinovirus colds. *J Infect Dis.* 1987;156:442-448.

18. Dondero TJ. An outbreak of legionnaire's disease associated with a contaminated air-conditioning cooling tower. *N Engl J Med.* 1980;301:365-370.

19. Drummond JA. Seronegative 18 months after being bitten by a patient with AIDS. *JAMA.* 1986;256:2342-2343.

20. Environmental Protection Agency. *Surface Water Treatment Requirements. Federal Register.* June 29, 1989;54:27486-514.

21. Friedland GH, et al. Lack of transmission of HTLV-III/LAV infection to household contacts of patients with AIDS or AIDS-related complex with oral candidiasis. *N Engl J Med.* 1986;14:344-349.

22. Garibaldi RA, et al. Meatal colonization and catheter-associated bacteriuria. *N Engl J Med.* 1980;303:316-318.

23. Gala CL, et al. The use of eye-nose goggles to control nosocomial respiratory syncytial virus infection. *JAMA.* 1986;256:2706-2708.

24. Garrard J, Leland N, Smith D. Epidemiology of human bites to children in a day-care center. *Am J Dis Child.* 1988;142:643-650.

25. Goodman RA, Solomon SL. Transmission of infectious diseases in outpatient health care settings. *JAMA.* 1991;265:2377-2381.

26. Gurevich I, Williams F, Cunha BA. Excessive levels of gram negative bacteria in hemodialysis machines because of inadequate cleaning guidelines. *Infect Contr.* 1981;2:373-376.

27. Gustafson M, Fuchs P. Unpublished study. St. Vincent Hospital, Portland, OR, 1976.

28. Gwaltney JM, Moskalski PB, Hendley JO. Hand-to-hand transmission of rhinovirus colds. *Ann Int Med.* 1978;88:463-467.

29. Hadler SC, et al. Risk factors for hepatitis A in day care centers. *J Infect Dis.* 1982;145:255-261.

30. Hall CB, Douglas RG. Modes of transmission of respiratory syncytial virus. *J Pediatr.* 1981;99:100-103.

31. Hguyen DMH, Stout JE. Legionellosis. *Infect Dis Clin North Am.* Sept 1991;5:561-577.

32. Istre GR. Risk factors for primary invasive *Haemophilus influenzae* disease: increased risk from day care attendance and school age household members. *J Pediatr.* 1985;106:190-195.

33. Jennings LC, et al. Near disappearance of rhinovirus along a fomite transmission chain. *J Infect Dis.* 1988;158:888-892.

34. Josephson A, Gombert ME. Airborne transmission of nosocomial varicella from localized zoster. *J Infect Dis.* 1988;158:238-241.

35. Kaatz GW. Acquisition of clostridium difficile from the hospital environment. *Am J Epidemiol.* 1988;127:1289-1294.

36. Kent GP, et al. Epidemic giardiasis caused by a contaminated public water supply. *Am J Public Health.* 1988;78:139-143.

37. Leclair JM, et al. Prevention of nosocomial respiratory syncytial virus infections through compliance with glove and gown isolation precautions. *N Engl J Med.* 1987;317:329-334.

38. Lemp GF, et al. The relationship of staff to the incidence of diarrhea in day-care centers. *Am J Epidemiol.* 1984;120:750-758.

39. Levins R, et al. The emergence of new diseases. *American Scientist.* 1994;82:52-60.

40. Lifson AR. Do alternate modes for transmission of human immunodeficiency virus exist? *JAMA.* 1988;259:1353-1356.

41. Maki DG, Alvarado CJ. Relation of the inanimate hospital environment to endemic nosocomial infection. *N Engl J Med.* 1982;307:1562-1566.

42. Morse LJ, et al. The Holy Cross College football team hepatitis outbreak. *JAMA.* 1972;219:706-708.

43. Pass, RF. Young children as a probable source of maternal and congenital cytomegalovirus infection. *N Engl J Med.* 1986;316:1414-1417.

44. Peterson PK, Matzke G, Keane WF. Current concepts in the management of peritonitis in patients undergoing continuous ambulatory peritoneal dialysis. *Rev Inf Dis.* 1987;9:604-612.

45. Pomeroy C, Englund JA. Cytomegalovirus: Epidemiology and infection control. *Am J Infect Contr.* 1987;15:107-119.

46. Rhame FS, et al. Extrinsic risk factors for pneumonia in the patient at high risk of infection. *Am J Med.* 1984;76:42-52.

47. Riley RL, et al. Infectiousness of air from a tuberculosis ward. *Am Rev Respir Dis.* 1962;84:511.

48. Riley RL. Airborne infection. *Am J Med.* 1974;57:466-475.

49. Rogers MF. Lack of transmission of human immunodeficiency virus from infected children to their household contacts. *Pediatr.* 1990;85:210-214.

50. Sawyer MH, Chamberlin CJ, Wu YN. Detection of varicella-zoster virus DNA in air samples from hospital rooms. *J Infect Dis.* 1994;169:91-94.
51. Sexton D, Haynes B. Bird-mite infestation in a university hospital. *Lancet,* page 445, Feb. 22, 1975.
52. Sheth NK, et al. Colonization of bacteria on polyvinyl chloride and Teflon intravascular catheters in hospitalized patients. *J Clin Microbiol.* 1983;1:1061-1063.
53. Wade JC, Schimpff SSC. Epidemiology and prevention of infection in the compromised host. In Rubin RH, Young IS, eds. Plenum Publishing Corp, New York, 1988.
54. Warshauer DM, et al. Rhinovirus infections in an isolated Antarctic station. *Am J Epidemiol.* 1989;129:319-340.
55. Weller TH. Varicella and herpes zoster (Part 2), changing concepts of the natural history, control and importance of a not-so-benign virus. *N Engl J Med.* 309:1434-1439.

SUGGESTED READINGS

Rhame FS. The inanimate environment. In Bennett JV, Brachman PS, eds. *Hospital Infections*, ed 3, 1992, 299-334.
Weber DJ, Rutala WA. Environmental Issues and Nosocomial Infections. In Wenzel RP, ed. Prevention and Control of Nosocomial Infections, ed 2, 1993, 420-449.

Chapter 4

The Social Environment

CAROL O'BOYLE WILLIAMS

Social support provides a sense of belonging. Being needed or valued by the group conveys a feeling of worth that contributes to the individual's self-esteem. A social network is the web of social ties that surrounds the individual and provides information, activities, and emotional, physical, and financial support. The social network influences an individual's health choices, since persons frequently feel pressure to model behaviors similar to those of other persons in their environment.

The social environment is composed of a wide range of variables and choices, including ethnic and cultural background, religious belief and custom, occupation, socioeconomic class and lifestyle. These circumstances raise specific questions about social health issues. Why and how do people stay healthy? What are the effects of lifestyle, cultural rituals, peer group support, and economic and social factors on health behavior and the risk of infection?

In the past, infections were often perceived as caused primarily by exogenous sources generally outside the individual's control. Health behavior is now recognized as one of the many determinants of disease and is influenced by the psychologic, emotional, and social factors woven into the cultural fabric that surrounds an individual or group. Contemporary health care providers strive to identify and understand the dynamics of the interaction between the social environment and health. The relationship among individuals, their lifestyles, and diseases has only recently been explored systematically.[10]

The challenge for those working in health care is to identify and support behaviors that enhance health and initiate interventions that lead to wide acceptance of those behaviors. Knowledge about the interaction between the person and the social environment is critical for nurses who work to promote, establish, or maintain human health and prevent infections (Figure 4-1). This chapter provides an overview of the components of the social environment that influence risk of infection, theories related to health behavior, and examples of their application.

The public health movement in developed nations has reduced the morbidity and mortality from many infectious diseases as basic human needs are met. Individuals can support health with adequate nutrition, protection from environmental hazards, and personal health behaviors that minimize risk (e.g., avoiding exposure to infectious disease agents, obesity, sedentary living).

Public health decisions may decrease exposure to microorganisms; however, personal beliefs and attitudes influence health behavior. For example, the decision to use resources to provide a safe water supply or sanitary sewer system is generally made by public health officials or political leaders. However, unless

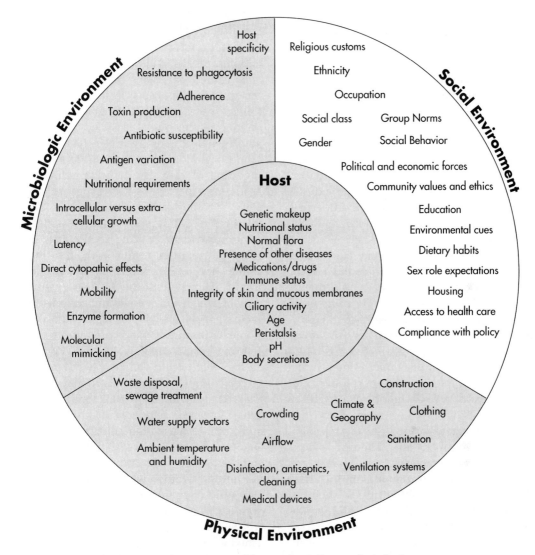

FIGURE 4-1. Social environmental factors that influence the infectious process.

the community values sanction the use of a piped water supply or toilets, the incidence of disease may remain unchanged because the individuals refuse to use these facilities. In the homes of many of the hill tribe villages in northern Thailand, villagers in some areas continued to defecate in the forests surrounding the villages despite installation of water-seal toilets. This practice contributes to continued transmission of waterborne and flyborne diarrheal diseases and to infestation with parasites such as the hookworm.[16] Personal choices about condom use or participation in an immunization program are examples of how persons reduce the risk of exposure to microorganisms or strengthen the host defense mechanisms against microorganisms. Although the individual's personal behaviors are important in determining exposure to microorganisms, the host's ability to cope and adapt to biologic stressors, once exposure occurs, is influenced by genetic factors, age, physiologic state (e.g., fatigue, pregnancy), and prior immunologic experiences, whether from maternal antibodies, immunizations, or previous infections (see Chapter 1).

Socially driven environmental cues often influence health behavior. Radio and television commercials; posters and advertisements in public buildings, buses, and magazines; labeling on food and drug packaging; comic books; movies; and newspapers all affect personal choices. Availability and accessibility of equipment and supplies may influence the epidemiology of infection. Support for certain health behavior occurs when bleach solution for rinsing intravenous (IV) needles and syringes is available to groups sharing injection drugs and equipment in gathering places called "shooting galleries," condoms are available in public bathrooms, immunization clinics are held in public places such as shopping centers and churches, and hand-washing soap is placed in bathrooms. The physical environment can also encourage or impede healthy behavior. The need to travel great distances for medical treatment and lack of access to safe drinking water are common examples of impediments in some countries. The decision to provide an immunization program to the infants of a community or to furnish a safe water supply and an adequate sanitary sewer system to a village in a developing nation illustrates the interaction of the social environment with the host, microbiologic agents and physical environments.

SOCIAL ENVIRONMENT AND THE INFECTIOUS PROCESS

Health is affected by behaviors that may be adopted because they are perceived as desired and valued by one's social group. Social factors that influence a person's risk for infectious diseases include ethnicity, religion, occupation, gender, social class, economic status, and the political environment. As an example, ethnic or national dietary customs such as the ingestion of raw fish or other undercooked foods may increase risk of exposure to parasites or other pathogens. The Far Eastern practices of eating crab soaked in vinegar or wine, instead of cooking to the appropriate temperature, often results in the transmission of the Oriental lung fluke *Paragonimus westermani*. Infection with the *Trichinella* nematode may be associated with ethnic customs, which include preparation and consumption of homemade pork sausage prepared according to some German, Italian, Polish, or Portuguese recipes that exclude adequate cooking.[22]

Perceptions of social class may influence risk. Many women in developing countries have increased the use of substitutes for breast milk and decreased the practice of breastfeeding because of the association of the breast milk substitute with affluence. In one study, the affluent women who elected to bottle-feed generally were literate, understood directions for mixing, and had access to refrigeration and a safe water supply. However, the impoverished women often lacked a safe water supply, refrigeration, and the skills to read and/or understand the directions. Consequently, the movement toward infant bottle-feeding by poor women often resulted in an increase in infant diarrheal disease and mortality.[22,23]

Religious beliefs can influence risk of infection. In countries without modern toilet facilities the Hindu rule that defecation should occur as soon as possible after rising and chanting the first prayer of the day may expose the bare feet of the devout Hindu to contact with the hookworm larvae, which frequently are still present on the damp early-morning soil. However, the Hindu is also expected to purify (or wash) his or her body immediately after defecation, and this practice may decrease the number of larvae present on the feet.[22] If religious prohibition of contraceptives decreases the use of condoms but does not successfully limit sexual activity to a single lifetime partner, the risk of exposure to microorganisms that cause sexually transmitted diseases may increase.

The degree to which a specific social group such as a religious community or sect is integrated into or segregated from the larger community will influence the extent to which the health behaviors of the larger population are emulated. In the United States, for example, certain religious communities or sects have proscriptions against immunization for diseases such as measles. When these proscriptions are respected, there can be periodic outbreaks of vaccine-preventable diseases in these communities.

Cultural norms affecting health also vary with one's sex and age. Adolescents responding to a survey in New York City reported that negotiating with one's sexual partner to use condoms was difficult for the person who wanted to establish a dating relationship, who wanted to increase his or her popularity, or who was simultaneously having sexual encounters and using alcohol or marijuana.[12] In Africa, where 90% of the new human immunodeficiency virus (HIV) infections in adolescents or adults occurs through heterosexual contact, Zimbabwean adolescent women claimed that the critical factor in determining the likelihood of condom use was the presence or lack of social support. The male adolescents in this study were less influenced by social support than by reminders or cues in the environment to use condoms.[31]

Treatment for infectious diseases may also be influenced by sex role expectations. If seeking treatment is perceived as dependent, weak, or unmanly, early symptoms may be ignored because the negative connotations associated with help-seeking behavior may outweigh the potential benefits of treatment.

Increased risk of exposure to disease agents may also be influenced by occupation. For example, meat-processing workers may be exposed to pathogens that cause brucellosis and health care workers may have an increased risk of exposure to bloodborne pathogens such as the hepatitis B virus.

Political, social, and economic factors can be barriers to health care. Consider the dilemma of a parent who will lose a day's wage if he or she takes the child to an immunization clinic to receive polio vaccine. In countries where polio is not widely perceived as an immediate danger, the parent may decide that the risk of polio is too small to justify the financial loss. In a similar risk-benefit analysis related to socioenvironmental factors, families in two Latino communities in New York City cited fear of the drug dealers as one of the impediments to an acquired immunodeficiency syndrome (AIDS) prevention program that would address the issue of IV drug abuse in their neighborhoods.[8]

Larger socioeconomic issues, such as access to adequate housing, health care, and employment, have a substantial impact on the health of communities, families, and the individual. Small, seemingly self-contained communities are interconnected with the larger units of the social structure, and their problems mirror the social problems of the larger communities. Community programs must address the multiple causes of poor health. For example, village women in Honduras determined that their children's health problems resulting from intestinal parasite infections were related to poverty, unemployment, and lack of education. By addressing these larger issues, they were able to improve their children's health.[21]

HEALTH BEHAVIOR THEORIES

Several theoretic models describe the interrelationships and interactions of variables that influence human health behavior. Four of these major theoretic models are the salutogenic theory, reasoned action theory, social learning theory, and health belief model. Each theory is applied to nursing practice in the following discussion.

Salutogenic theory

The salutogenic model identifies the themes common to health and those factors that maintain or improve health. In this model, health is a continuum with illness and death at one end and optimum well-being and health at the other (Figure 4-2). The individual's location on the continuum is the consequence of that person's response to stimuli. The charac-

terization of a stimulus as a stressor is a function of its meaning in the society or culture. The culture provides the person with an orientation to his or her place in the world, language, and a set of behavioral norms, including expected responses to stressors.[2]

Psychosocial stressors are inherent in human existence and include the tensions and positive or negative effects of new roles or new personal encounters. Societies have customs and rituals that provide methods for coping with stressors that produce anxiety. Ceremonies of birth and death and systems to select political leaders are examples of these customs and rituals. Stress is increased when a stimulus is encountered for which the culture has not

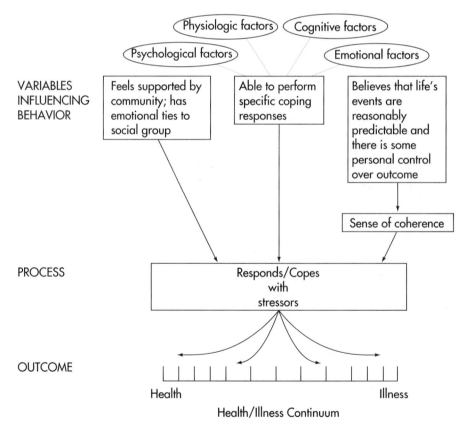

FIGURE 4-2. Salutogenic model.

modeled a response. In the 1980s, most cultures had not developed a response to accommodate AIDS, a terminal, chronic, transmissible infectious disease. Prevention of the transmission of the virus that causes AIDS has required changes in personal sexual practices and the culture's portrayal of sexual behavior. Discussions of sexual matters have been integrated into mainstream culture, influenced the way sex education occurs, and produced open debate concerning accommodation of various lifestyles (see Chapter 9).

In addition to the learned cultured responses to stressors, the individual's specific coping resources are important in the salutogenic model. These resources include physiologic, psychologic, cognitive (e.g., ability to understand and/or literacy), and emotional abilities. Social factors, such as role, group membership, intimacy, strong ties to others, commitment, and ties to the community, help individuals cope with stressors. Community support can include adequate living arrangements during an illness, health care, assistance in the activities of daily living, and maintaining a positive opinion of the ill person.

In the salutogenic model the concept of coherence incorporates the individual's belief that he or she has some control over the outcome of events and that things will turn out as well as can be expected. This sense of coherence is considered important for a person to cope with stress successfully. According to this model, when coping responses that support the individual's resistance to disease are overcome by nutritional deprivation, inadequate sanitation, and other similar factors, illness can result. Thus the salutogenic model suggests that when there is a reasonably adequate standard of living, differences in health status are determined by differences in psychosocial coping mechanisms.[2]

The salutogenic model proposes that health is enhanced or maintained if persons are confident that life's events are reasonably predict-able and that they will be able to mobilize sufficient resources to cope successfully with stressors[2] (Table 4-1).

Application of theory to practice

Clinical practice that incorporates the salutogenic model blends community and cultural elements into care. One example of a social support system found in some cultures is a female mothering figure called a *doula*.[23] The doula helps the postpartum woman cope with the stresses of lactating and managing a newborn infant by providing practical information and a nurturing environment for the infant and the mother. This support reinforces the practice of breastfeeding and reduces infant morbidity and mortality from diarrheal disease associated with nutritional substitutes for breastfeeding.[23] The doula helps the new mother meet the society's expectations, obtain social approval, and establish a sense of success in coping with her new role as mother. In the United States, nurses who are lactation specialists fulfill a similar role.

In some nations, social support for breastfeeding has begun to erode because bottle-feeding is marketed as being associated with affluence. Consequently, breastfeeding may become a symbol of inferior child care and associated with being underprivileged. The cultural expectation that a doula will be present to support the new mother has also decreased. To stabilize the internal social support for the practice of breastfeeding, nurses and health educators may need to incorporate methods to reward or support the doulas for their continuing work with lactating women and to portray breastfeeding as progressive and scientific.[23]

A social stigma attached to a disease may threaten group membership and contribute to delays in seeking diagnoses or adhering to the treatment. During the 1950s, reports from an African Zulu community stated that the diagnosis of pulmonary tuberculosis (TB) generally

TABLE 4-1 Health behavior theories

Theory	Main concepts	Predicting behavior	Modifiers
Salutogenic	A strong sense of coherence helps to mobilize resources to cope with stressors and maintain or enhance health.	• Able to cope successfully with stressors • A sense that life's events are somewhat predictable • Participates in decisions	• Ability to understand • Literacy • Social role • Social supports • Intimacy • Religion • Philosophy • Genetic • Biologic
Reasoned action	Health decisions are rational choices based upon desired outcome and expectations of social group.	• Attitudes and subjective norms influence the intentions to perform a behavior.	• Beliefs that behavior leads to specific outcomes • Value of the specific outcomes • Beliefs that certain individuals or groups do (or do not) expect specific behaviors • Motivation to comply with expectations of these individuals
Social learning theory	The link between knowledge and behavior is regulated by the self-image and one's sense of self-efficacy.	Observing others (models) being rewarded or punished for specific health behaviors. Recommended behavior more likely if observer can identify with the model and/or model is influential. Sense of *self-efficacy* (self-confidence) specific to the recommended behavior.	Behavior rehearsed mentally Positive outcome expected from performance of the behavior Successful performance of the behavior in practice situations.
Health belief model	Behavior related to the prevention treatment and cure of a disease, or health promotion is influenced by the *person's* perceptions more than by objective, scientific environment.	• Belief that one is susceptible to the disease • Belief that the disease is serious • Perception of the benefits associated with the recommended behavior • Perception of the risks associated with the behavior	The perceived risks and benefits balanced Environmental cues to action

Compiled from Ajzen (1), Antonovsky (2), Bandura (3), Rosenstock (24).

resulted in the patient terminating treatment because of the community belief that TB was associated with witchcraft.[25] Similarly, a study in India found that TB patients discontinued treatment if they thought they were ostracized by the community, whereas those who remained in treatment believed they were supported by family and community.[25] Many individuals in the United States at risk for infection with HIV have delayed being tested for the HIV antibody not only because of their fear of the diagnosis, but also because of the potential for social stigmatization and loss of support from the community.

Chlamydia trachomatis causes trachoma, a bacterial eye infection that is the world's leading cause of preventable blindness. Prevention of trachoma requires management of social, environmental, and cultural factors. The microorganism is transmitted by contact with the discharge from the eyes of infected persons. Transmission of pathogens from the eye can occur when the same cloths used to wipe the eyes of infected adults or children are subsequently used by others in the household. A South African prevention program was culturally tailored to the population by including villagers as primary health volunteers. Their efforts reduced the incidence of trachoma and improved the personal and environmental hygiene of the villagers.[20] One community in northern India found a method to provide treatment for trachoma that was efficacious and acceptable to the local culture when tetracycline was mixed with a traditional eye cosmetic that was believed to have healing properties.[20]

Social support was helpful in producing compliance with TB treatment during an outbreak of pulmonary TB on a Navajo Indian reservation when traditional healers who had received TB-specific training delivered TB treatment and education directly into patients' homes. This program incorporated medical interventions into the traditional health beliefs

and values of the community.[25] These examples illustrate how community support can influence health-enhancing behavior consistent with the salutogenic model.

Reasoned action theory

The theory of reasoned action is based on the premise that people make rational decisions based on the information available to them (Figure 4-3). This model proposes that people decide to engage in a behavior based on their belief that the behavior will lead to an outcome they desire, which may fulfill expectations of their social group.[1] Thus the strength of the intent to perform a behavior and the likelihood of action are determined by the desirability of the consequences of the behavior and the perceived social pressure (see Table 4-1).

The reasoned action theory suggests a person forms his or her beliefs regarding a behavior by considering, "What are the advantages and disadvantages of this specific behavior?" and "What else is associated with this behavior?" For example, if condoms are associated with negative consequences, such as a personal loss of pleasure or displeasing a desired sexual partner, an adolescent may have an unfavorable attitude toward using condoms. If condoms are associated with sophistication and erotic pleasure, adolescents may have a more accepting attitude. The reasoned action theory proposes that a person's perception of social pressure and expectations of friends or family also contribute to his or her intentions.[1]

Application of theory to practice

Application of reasoned action theory to clinical practice requires education and active participation of the client or patient. Persons who want to achieve a specific health behavior goal must have positive intentions and attitudes toward all the component behaviors that are steps to the overall goal or behavior. The health behavior goal of engaging only in

VARIABLES INFLUENCING BEHAVIOR   PROCESS   OUTCOME

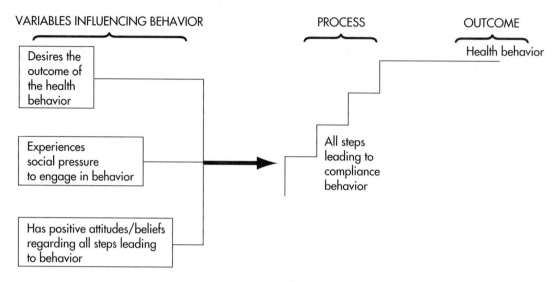

FIGURE 4-3. Reasoned action model.

"safe" sexual practices must be broken down into steps. For example, before persons use condoms as a component of engaging in safer sex behavior, they must believe that condoms reduce the risk of disease and that the social group expects and values condom use. Positive attitudes regarding each step that leads to the goal behavior are also required. These steps include purchasing condoms, negotiating with sexual partners, and learning techniques for condom use.

A person probably has more than one belief about a specific behavior such as condom use, for example, "condoms prevent pregnancy" or "are only used by immoral persons . . . will result in trouble for me if my parents find one in my billfold or purse . . . spoil sex, inhibit sex . . . turn off my partner . . . protect from AIDS." Since these assumptions are responsible for attitudes toward specific behaviors, changing behavior requires that the beliefs about the outcome of a behavior and about the expectations of others in the group regarding a specific behavior be changed. The reasoned action theory suggests that attempts to influence behavior that are based only on cognitive information about the behavior are unlikely to result in change unless the other important determinants such as attitudes and social norms are also altered.

The theory of reasoned action was applied to a study of condom use by college women in New Jersey.[11] Women who believed that sex was more enjoyable when a condom was used were more likely to use condoms. In addition, the perceived attitudes of their parents and sexual partners toward condom use were influential in determining the likelihood of use. A similar study of condom use by men and women was conducted in Zaire, Africa, where 6% to 8% of the population of the capital city, Kinshasa, were infected with HIV as reported in 1991.[4] Despite widespread knowledge of the transmission mechanisms for HIV, negative attitudes toward condom use (e.g., belief that condoms reduce sexual pleasure) were associated with a low rate of condom use.

Other reports from Tanzania identified concern that negative consequences resulted from condom use. Men there believed that imported condoms were contaminated with HIV. These men were also opposed to accepting free condoms from the government but were willing to pay for reasonably priced condoms.[26]

Cultural factors inhibiting condom use are present in many countries. For example, the importance of motherhood or the prestige of fatherhood can influence decisions regarding condom use. In a study of injection drug users, many women stated their belief that their partner would suspect a person who negotiated for condom use of having sex outside of the primary relationship and would consider that person untrustworthy.[15]

According to the reasoned action theory, behavior change requires education. For example, one approach to behavior change may be to promote positive attitudes toward condoms and change beliefs about the outcome of condom use. If condoms are believed to be erotic and are used by sophisticated, trustworthy persons, various beliefs resulting in negative attitudes may be overcome. Likewise, social pressure influences behavior when sexually active young people perceive that parents and sex partners value and respect persons who have the foresight to use condoms.

Factors important in preventing trachoma include beliefs about the cause of the disease and the efficacy of recommended actions. A study in Egypt found that many villagers did not associate the eye infection with blindness. In South Africa, trachoma was believed to occur as a normal part of life. It was essential to change the beliefs regarding trachoma before behavior could be changed.[20]

Thus, according to the theory of reasoned action, one can increase the understanding of a health behavior by identifying the beliefs underlying specific attitudes and the perceived social prescriptions for or against certain behaviors. Community interventions and publicity campaigns can be directed not only at the beliefs of the target population, but also at the beliefs of their social group.[1]

Social learning theory

In the social learning theory, persons are driven neither solely by internal forces nor solely by conditioned responses to environmental stimuli. Rather, behavior is a result of the continuous interaction between personal and environmental factors that support or penalize specific behaviors (Figure 4-4). Learning occurs through observing other persons who are either rewarded or punished for specific behaviors. People are more likely to emulate the behavior of those who are perceived to be influential or who share characteristics with the observer, such as age, sex, or lifestyle. People are more likely to initiate another's behavior if they observe the model receive a highly valued reward, if the model is perceived to be likable, or if the model is influential within the culture, such as a sports figure or television personality.

Social learning theory suggests that the use of a model is helpful when behaviors are complex and require a combination of motor and cognitive skills. Teaching family members how to irrigate and dress a large infected wound is an example of using a model to demonstrate the expected or desired behavior.

Motor processes are important in learning skills. The premise that behavior is a result of a continuous interaction between the person and the environment is depicted when persons attempt to learn complex skills. Because persons cannot generally observe their own actions, they depend upon onlookers for cues or verbal reactions. Based on the feedback from others about their behavior, persons are able to refine their performance.

It is also helpful for the person to know what specific behavior is expected and how and when to perform the behavior. Mental rehearsal in which the individual visualizes performing a behavior supports the memory of the desired behavior.

The behaviors of the persons with whom one regularly associates will be the behaviors most often observed and therefore most often learned. The need to belong may be met when the individual practices behaviors used by his or her social group. Observing others receive rewards or punishments for behaviors estab-

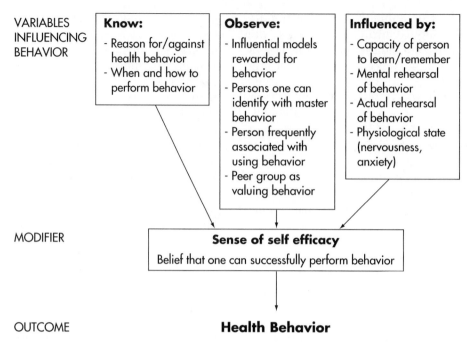

FIGURE 4-4. Social learning theory.

lishes a link in the person's mind between the observed behavior and the outcome. Thus, the decision to use a behavior is influenced by the anticipation that a valued outcome will be produced or a negative one averted.[3]

Persons do not enact all behavior that they observe. Modeled behavior is more likely to be adopted if the outcomes of the observed behavior are valued by the learner. Verbal persuasion, in which the negative and positive consequences of an action are described, also influences health decisions. As an example, adolescents may consider experimenting with drugs to demonstrate their independence from parents or other authority figures. They may also consider the use of drugs exciting, evidence of maturity, and an affirmation of their membership in a specific group. Peer group discussions about the negative consequences of drug use and demonstrations of acceptable methods for refusing drugs and for handling pressure to try drugs are an important stra-

tegy important strategy in adolescent drug prevention programs. The peer group approach may change the adolescent's expectations about the outcome of drug use and the effect the refusal may have on the relationship with peers.

Important sources of modeled behavior are television, films, and other types of visual media. Both adults and children acquire attitudes, emotional responses, and new types of behavior through these media. Exposure to modeled behavior can strengthen or weaken previous inhibitions regarding specific behaviors. For example, previously learned behavior is inhibited when one sees models punished. However, watching models participate in prohibited activities without suffering negative consequences can reduce inhibitions toward these same behaviors in the learner. It is more effective for learners to see models rewarded for specific health-related behaviors than to observe the models experiencing the negative results of not adopting the recommended practices. By focusing on the negative consequences of *not* practicing a behavior, observers may inadvertently associate the punishment with the recommended behavior.

In social learning theory, a critical prerequisite for behavior change is the sense of self-efficacy or confidence a person has about his or her ability to perform a specific behavior. The self-efficacy or confidence is specific to the task. That is, an adolescent may feel very confident about his or her basketball skills or reading capabilities but feel uncomfortable and awkward about discussing the use of condoms with a possible sexual partner.

Self-efficacy can be enhanced by rehearsing intended behaviors in a practice situation similar to the actual situation. Self-efficacy is derived from four sources: (1) successful performances of a behavior, (2) vicarious experiences in which models similar to the learner are observed mastering the behavior, (3) verbal persuasion in which the reasons to acquire or avoid the behavior and the expected positive outcomes are presented, and (4) the physiologic state that, when sufficiently aroused to include a feeling of anxiety, can impair self-efficacy expectations (e.g., rapid heart rate, extremely sweaty palms) (see Table 4-1).

If the person does not feel confident about performing a specific behavior, he or she may not attempt the behavior or may experience a substantial amount of stress when the behavior is attempted. Rehearsing specific social situations and responses allows an individual to build a sense of self-efficacy regarding the recommended behavior.

Application of theory to practice

In a study of gay men from San Francisco, a low sense of self-efficacy was the major predictor of participation in high-risk sexual behavior.[27] In an effort to influence the behavior of an entire gay community in a small city in Mississippi, the leaders of the community were involved in a training program. The trend setters within groups were identified and asked to serve as discussion leaders and to participate in role playing. These leaders provided information to their peers on specific strategies for avoiding HIV transmission, such as avoiding intoxicants before sex and having condoms readily available for use during sexual activity. During role playing the leaders demonstrated how to discuss the value of safer sex practices with sexual partners and how to resist pressure to engage in high-risk activities. The participants were provided multiple opportunities to role-play and receive feedback about their performance. Opportunities were available to discuss and plan strategies for problem situations. A 25% reduction in high-risk sexual activities was reported in a 2-month period.[14] The participants' sense of self-efficacy was enhanced as they were provided with specific strategies for implementing the recommended behaviors and opportunities to practice new behaviors in a low-stress environment. In addition, the use of peer group leaders as models illustrated the effect of appropriate models on the group's behavior.

In another example that demonstrates how self-efficacy can be strengthened by practicing new behaviors in a low-stress supportive environment, women at a methadone clinic in New York City were provided opportunities to develop skills for negotiating for safer sex practices with their partners. These former injection drug users often had contact with multiple male sexual partners at high risk for HIV and other sexually transmitted diseases. The group of women included African Americans and Latinas who, because of social group attitudes, were more likely to encounter resistance to condom use from their partners. The women who attended five skill-building sessions felt more comfortable talking about safer sex practices and were more likely to use condoms.[7]

Health belief model

A model that has had a major influence on health education is the health belief model. The health belief model proposes that four predictors of health behavior exist: (1) one's perception of personal susceptibility to disease, (2) perceived seriousness of the disease, (3) perception of the benefits of changing one's behavior, and (4) obstacles to compliance with the recommendations (Figure 4-5).

Susceptibility is related to the individual's belief or fear that he or she is personally vulnerable to a disease. Judgment of personal susceptibility is subjective and may range from denial of any possibility of contracting a disease to a perception of real danger.

Perceived seriousness is related to the emotional response that the thought of the disease arouses and includes the perceived effects on

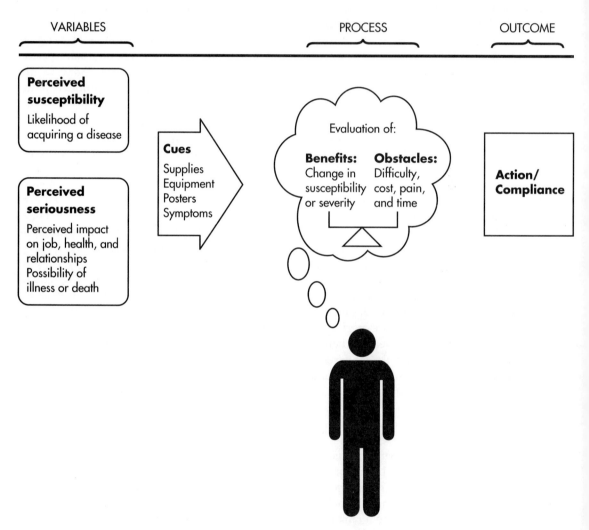

FIGURE 4-5. Health belief model.

job, social relations, and health (e.g., disability, death). The amount of harm the thought of the disease evokes in a person is related not only to the physical harm it may produce, but also to the harm it may cause economically, psychologically, and emotionally. Knowledge about a disease influences a person's perception of susceptibility and seriousness of that disease.

Benefits or obstacles to compliance with health recommendations include the person's perception of the physical, financial, and psychologic consequences of compliance. Persons weigh the obstacles or negative outcomes against the benefits of the action (e.g., reducing the severity of the disease), altering the person's susceptibility or totally preventing the disease. The person's beliefs about the effectiveness of the recommended action and the availability of a course of action influence the person's decision more than objective information. In a health belief model individuals who believe they are at risk for acquiring a disease are more likely to practice those preventive behaviors perceived as feasible and effective[24] (see Table 4-1).

If a person believes that an action will be effective in reducing the threat of disease but also perceives the action as costly, cumbersome, embarrassing, painful, or in any way problematic, conflict or stress will occur. The person will weigh the benefits (effectiveness in preventing or reducing the threat of disease) against the perceived negative aspects, then move toward the action believed to result in the greatest benefit with the smallest negative outcome. An important concept of the health belief model is that the person's *beliefs* about the effectiveness of treatment, not objective scientific data, determine the behavior the person will exhibit. In addition, if a person has a strong belief that he or she is susceptible to a serious disease but believes that no effective treatments exist, the person may avoid the issue because it seems to be unresolvable. This understanding of health behavior may be helpful to nurses interacting with persons whose behavior places them at increased risk for infection with HIV. These persons may know their behaviors have placed them at an increased risk for infection, but if they also believe no treatment exists for the disease, they may delay seeking diagnosis and treatment.

Cues to action, whether external stimuli (e.g., media campaigns, posters) or internal stimuli (e.g., awareness of disease symptoms), must occur for individuals to perform the recommended behavior. The level of intensity of the cue that will result in action varies with the individual. Persons who have a very low sense of susceptibility to a disease or believe a disease is of low severity need an intense cue from the environment to trigger action. However, those who believe they are susceptible to a serious disease are more likely to take action when a low-intensity cue is present. For example, if the person who works in a shelter for the homeless where outbreaks of multidrug-resistant tuberculosis have occurred believes that he or she is susceptible to a serious disease and is aware that treatment is effective, he or she will be likely to respond to a low-intensity cue to undergo tuberculin skin testing (see Clinical Study 7).

Application of theory to practice

In a study designed to test the health belief model in a Seattle clinic, postcards were used as environmental cues to prompt behavior for a group of patients at high risk for serious complications from influenza infection. Those patients who received postcards were more likely to receive the vaccine than those who did not. A belief that influenza was a potentially serious threat to their health and that the vaccine was effective in preventing influenza was also reported more often by patients who received influenza vaccine than by those who did not. Those who did not receive vaccine listed the vaccine's cost and dissatisfaction with their medical care as barriers to receiving vaccine.[17]

The health belief model premise that persons weigh the obstacles to compliance, such as pain or discomfort, against the perceived benefits was exemplified in a study of health care workers who did not take influenza vaccine. In this survey, those who elected not to receive vaccine cited "bad side effects" and misconceptions about the effectiveness of the immunization as important barriers to compliance with the recommendation.[28]

In a study of variables that influenced persons' behavior regarding Lyme disease, respondents who knew someone with Lyme disease or believed they were personally at a high risk for acquiring the disease were more likely to take precautions against ticks.[5] Knowing someone with the disease often supports the perception that one is personally vulnerable or susceptible to the disease. Lyme disease is discussed in Clinical Study 1.

The possible occupational transmission of HIV has stimulated interest in developing interventions to protect health professionals. *Universal precautions* were developed by the CDC to reduce risk of occupational transmission by protecting nurses and other health care workers from contact with blood and other body fluids that may transmit HIV or hepatitis B[6] (see Chapter 6).

It is likely that nurses perform analyses regarding the obstacles and benefits associated with compliance to health protection strategies in the work place. For example, although nurses might be motivated to avoid infection, the characteristics of the nurse-patient relationship may hinder compliance with universal precautions. In trauma or emergency situations, patients in crisis may be vulnerable and at risk for adverse clinical outcomes if treatment is delayed. If nurses believe the outcome of a patient's care depends on immediate action, they may not take the time necessary to use personal protective equipment. Taking this time in crises may indicate discordance between actions and beliefs. Thus, nurses' awareness of the time-sensitive, critical nature of the work may discourage the use of personal protective equipment in these circumstances. Nurses most frequently cite "lack of time" as a barrier to using personal protective equipment.[13,29]

In a national survey of 1127 registered nurse midwives, those who complied with universal precautions reported behavior consistent with the health behavior model, as they were more likely to believe they were personally susceptible to occupational acquisition of HIV or the hepatitis B virus. These midwives also received frequent reminders of the disease's seriousness in that more of their patients were infected with HIV.[30] One obstacle to compliance for the nurse midwives was the concern about loss of dexterity from using some barriers.

Contact with a greater number of AIDS patients provides reminders of the disease's seriousness and better compliance by nurses in adhering to universal precautions. Nurses and other health care workers have reported that they would be more likely to comply with universal precautions if they knew the patient was HIV infected.[9]

The health belief model can also be used to understand a patient's behavior related to treatment plans. For example, compliance with the medication regimen for TB is critical to treatment of the infection, however, difficulty with the patient's adherence to clinic appointments is an obstacle to effective treatment. The staff at a San Francisco clinic were able to reduce missed appointments from 26% to 4% by identifying and addressing obstacles to clinic appointments and incorporating patients' needs into the clinic plan. For example, the problem of lost work time for the patients was addressed by having the staff members available in some neighborhoods at times compatible with patients' work schedules.[25]

Injection drug users are at risk for HIV infection from the practice of sharing contaminated drug injection paraphernalia (see Clinical Study 26). A hospital-based methadone treatment center in New York City incorporated a voluntary AIDS education program and the opportunity to obtain HIV testing and counseling into the treatment program. Of those undergoing treatment, 27% attended AIDS educational sessions and 12% availed themselves of the opportunity for HIV testing. The obstacles to participating in the classes included a lack of time and a perceived lack of personal susceptibility to HIV because participants had discontinued their drug use. Other obstacles identified by those who refused testing included the fear of the emotional effects of discovering they were HIV positive and fear of the discovery and reaction by others should they be HIV positive.[18]

In Lima, Peru, dysenteric diarrheal disease in children under 1 year of age is often caused by the microorganism *Campylobacter jejuni*, which is commonly found in chickens. In the poor shantytown section of Lima, chickens often run freely in the homes and defecate frequently on the dirt floors. The hands of the infants and toddlers crawling or playing on the floor are often contaminated with the microorganisms carried by the chickens. Lack of running water impedes handwashing and contributes to transmission of the pathogens from the chickens to the toddlers and infants through hand-to-mouth contact. In this situation the obstacles to compliance with the recommendation that the children not have hand contact with chicken manure included the mothers' perceptions that free-roaming chickens are healthier and that the chicken manure is not related to illness. The presence of dirt or unfinished concrete floors and lack of water for washing also prevent adequate cleaning.[19] The strategy for addressing this health risk might include communicating the risk of disease for toddlers to the mothers, involving community leaders in strategies to create support for chicken pens, and since most inhabitants had access to mass media, using the media to educate the people about the risk of disease (susceptibility, seriousness) associated with these chickens.

INFLUENCE OF SETTING ON SOCIAL DETERMINANTS OF INFECTION

Human behavior related to health promotion or illness prevention is a complex phenomenon in which the person, the environment, and the behavior are continually interacting. The social environment provides the social and physical arenas in which the person must function. Health motivators are derived from the social environment. They influence behavior, which in turn influences both the person performing the behavior and the social environment. Regardless of the health care setting, support for persons learning and establishing new health behaviors should include information on the importance or value of certain behaviors and opportunities to practice the behavior. Finally, the physical and social environments must be structured so that the desired behavior is promoted, supported, and valued.

Viewing health behavior as the result of complex interactions among the various dimensions of human existence means disease prevention and health promotion efforts must occur in the context of the total human experience. Successful, sustained control of a disease cannot be accomplished with the use of a single approach related to diagnosis and treatment. It requires an integrated, multifaceted approach in which disease prevention is seen not as a vertical process where microorganisms are controlled or eliminated by medications but as a horizontal process in which disease prevention occurs within the person who initiates it and is supported (or not) by the surrounding physical and social environments.

SUMMARY

Four theoretic models related to health behavior in social environments have been described. In the salutogenic model, a sense of coherence, described as the belief that things will work out as well as can be expected and that the person has some control over the outcome, is considered important for a person to cope successfully with stressors. When a person's biologic resources are not overwhelmed by exposure to a critical threshold of microorganisms or an inadequate standard of living, the salutogenic model attributes differences in health to differences in dealing with psychosocial stressors. Successful coping is influenced by the social support systems.

The theory of reasoned action presents humans as rational beings who make decisions based on the information available to them and make decisions to engage in a behavior based on their belief that the behavior will lead to an outcome that they desire or that is expected by their social group. According to this theory, a health behavior is attributed to the beliefs underlying the specific attitudes and the perceived social pressures for or against certain behaviors.

The social learning theory stresses the importance of the influence of models on behavior. According to this theory, individuals observe models who are rewarded or punished for specific behaviors and thus observe not only how a behavior should occur, but also the link between the behavior and the outcome. A sense of confidence in one's ability to perform the behavior, referred to as self-efficacy, is essential to attempting new behaviors. Self-efficacy is achieved or strengthened by practicing the behaviors, observing models similar to the learner mastering the behavior, expecting positive outcomes from the behavior, and understanding the rationale for the recommended behavior.

The health belief model suggests that health-related behavior is the result of personal

---

SELECTED CLINICAL STUDIES EMPHASIZING THE SOCIAL ENVIRONMENT (see Section Three)

1. Lyme Disease at a Boy Scout Camp
7. Pulmonary Tuberculosis in a Homeless Person
14. Adolescent Female with *Chlamydia* infection
26. Human Immunodeficiency Virus (HIV) Infection in an Injection Drug User
31. Occupationally Acquired Hepatitis B in a Health Care Worker

---

perceptions regarding susceptibility to disease, seriousness of the disease, benefits of changing one's behavior, and obstacles to behavior change. In this model, the individual is thought to weigh obstacles to compliance against the benefits of the action. Beliefs about the effectiveness of the recommended action and the availability of the course of action influence the person's decision more than objective information.

These theories are ways of systematically describing the complexities of human behavior related to health decisions. In all the health behavior theories presented, decisions are influenced by the individual and the social group. Also, the expectations of the social groups regarding health behavior are in turn influenced by political and economic forces that determine how health resources are allocated within a community.

REFERENCES

1. Ajzen I, Fishbein M. Understanding Attitudes and Predicting Social Behavior. Englewood Cliffs, NJ: Prentice-Hall; 1980.
2. Antonovsky A. Health, Stress, and Coping. San Francisco: Jossey-Bass; 1980.
3. Bandura A. Social Foundations of Thought and Actions. Englewood Cliffs, NJ: Prentice-Hall; 1986.
4. Bertrand JT, et al. AIDS-related knowledge, sexual behavior, and condom use among men and women in Kinshasa, Zaire. *Am J Public Health.* 1991;81(1):53-58.

5. Centers for Disease Control. Lyme disease knowledge, attitudes and behaviors—Connecticut, 1992. *MMWR* 1992;41(28)505-507.

6. Centers for Disease Control. Update: universal precautions for prevention of transmission of human immunodeficiency virus, hepatitis B virus, and other bloodborne pathogens in health-care setting. *MMWR* 1988;37(24):378-388.

7. El-Bassel N, Schilling RF. 15-month follow-up of women methadone patients taught skills to reduce heterosexual HIV transmission. *Public Health Rep.* 1992;107(5):500-504.

8. Freudenberg N, Trinidad U. The role of community organizations in AIDS prevention in two Latino communities in New York City. *Health Edu Q.* 1992;19(2):219-232.

9. Gerberding JL, et al. Risk of exposure of surgical personnel to patients' blood during surgery at San Francisco General Hospital. *N Engl J Med.* 1990;332:1788-1793.

10. Janes CR, Stall R, Gifford SM, eds. *Anthropology and Epidemiology.* Dordrecht: D. Reidel; 1986.

11. Jemmott LS, Jemmott JB. Applying the theory of reasoned action to AIDS risk behavior: condom use among black women. *Nurs Res.* 1991;40(4):228-233.

12. Kasen S, Vaughan RD, Walter HJ. Self-efficacy for AIDS preventive behaviors among tenth grade students. *Health Edu Q.* 1992;19(2):187-202.

13. Kelen GD, et al. Adherence to universal (barrier) precautions during interventions on critically ill and injured emergency department patients. *J Acquir Immune Defic Syndr.* 1990;3:987-994.

14. Kelly JA, et al. HIV risk behavior reduction following intervention with key opinion leaders of population: an experimental analysis. *Am J Public Health.* 1991;81(2):168-171.

15. Kenen RH, Armstrong K. The why, when and whether of condom use among female and male drug users. *J Community Health.* 1992;17(5):303-317.

16. Kunstadter P. Ethnicity, ecology and mortality in northwestern Thailand. In Janes CR, Stall R, Gifford SM, eds. *Anthropology and Epidemiology.* Dordrecht: D. Reidel; 1986.

17. Larson EB, et al. The relationship of health beliefs and a postcard reminder to influenza vaccination. *J Fam Pract.* 1979;8(6):1207-1211.

18. Magura S, et al. Correlates of participation in AIDS education and HIV antibody testing by methadone patients. *Public Health Rep.* 1989;104(3):231-240.

19. Marquis GS, et al. Fecal contamination of shanty town toddlers in households with non-coralled poultry, Lima, Peru. *Am J Public Health* 1990;80(2):146-149.

20. Marx R. Social factors and trachoma: a review of the literature. *Soc Sci Med.* 1989;29(1):23-34.

21. Minkler M. Improving health through community organizations. In Glanz K, Lewis FM, Rimer BK, eds. *Health Behavior and Health Education.* San Francisco: Jossey-Bass; 1990.

22. Nations MK. Epidemiological research on infectious disease: quantitative rigor or rigor mortis: insights from ethnomedicine. In Janes CR, Stall R, Gifford SM, eds. *Anthropology and Epidemiology.* Dordrecht: Reidel; 1986.

23. Raphael D. Warning: the milk in this package may be lethal for your infant. In Grollig FX, Haley HB, eds. *Medical Anthropology.* Chicago: Aldine; 1976:135.

24. Rosenstock IM. Historical origins of the health belief model. *Health Education Monographs.* 1974;2(4):328-335.

25. Rubel AJ, Garro LC. Social and cultural factors in the successful control of tuberculosis. *Public Health Rep.* 1992;107(6):626-636.

26. Sandman J. AIDS, the World Health Organization, and Central Africa. *Journal Association of Nurses in AIDS Care.* Oct-Dec 1992;3(4):33-41.

27. Stall RD, Coates TJ, Hoff C. Behavioral risk reduction for HIV infection among gay and bisexual men. *Am Psychol.* 1988;43(11):878-885.

28. Watanakunakorn C, Ellis G, Gemmel D. Attitude of health care personnel regarding influenza immunization. *Infect Control Hosp Epidemiol.* 1993;14(1):17-20.

29. Williams CO, et al. Variables influencing health care worker compliance with universal precautions in the emergency room, *Am J Infect Control.* in press.

30. Willy ME, et al. Adverse exposures and universal precaution practices among a group of highly exposed health professionals. *Infect Control Hosp Epidemiol.* 1990;11(7):351-356.

31. Wilson D, Lavelle S. Psychosocial predictors of intended condom use among Zimbabwean adolescents. *Health Education Research.* 1992;7(1):55-68.

Section Two

Infection Prevention and Control Methods

Infection prevention and control methods must be designed and implemented with an understanding of host-environment interactions in order to be effective. Much effort and money has been expended without effect on control measures not based on a solid understanding of these interactions. Opportunities to improve quality of care by efficiently preventing or managing infection will be missed if these relationships are not considered by individuals guiding and participating in patient care. When prevention and control measures are based on knowledge of these components, they can achieve important results.

This section describes infection prevention and control strategies, their scientific basis, and practical considerations for their use. The efficacy of traditional infection control practices is critically assessed. Chapter 5 reviews specific patient care practices that influence risk of infection. The role of medical devices is emphasized. Chapter 6 describes barrier precautions and methods of personal protection that have become important, visible tools to prevent transmission of infectious microorganisms to patients and care providers. Chapter 7 presents the theoretical and practical aspects of antisepsis, disinfection, and sterilization and their application to a range of patient care settings. Chapter 8 discusses the basis for antimicrobial therapy. Chapter 9 analyzes the importance of education and behavior modification tools that affect success of infection prevention strategies. Chapter 10 assesses the influence of the policy process on infection prevention and control efforts. The information in this section, together with understanding of host-environment interactions presented in Section One, provides a scientific and practical foundation on which to base nursing care.

Chapter 5

Patient Care Practices and Medical Devices

BARBARA R. MOONEY

ealth care practices influence the interactions and dynamic balance among the microbial agent, the host, and the physical, social, and cultural environments. Because each patient is unique and responds differently to preventive and therapeutic interventions, patient care practices must be individualized for each person or population to achieve maximum beneficial effect. Since nurses provide frequent, intimate, direct patient care, they are the ideal caregivers to adapt the prescribed care to the patient's distinctive characteristics and circumstances to produce a positive outcome.

The first part of this chapter is an overview of selected practices that can optimize the patient's resistance to infection. Since invasive devices contribute significantly to the risk of nosocomial infection, the second section reviews how these devices can be managed to minimize this risk. The need to validate patient care practices is discussed throughout this chapter; current practices are described and data provided when available. However, additional validation of many practices is needed, since much practice continues to be based on tradition and ritual. The final section of the chapter reviews various patient care settings that may require alterations in infection prevention methods to achieve the maximum benefit.

MAXIMIZING HOST DEFENSES

Infectious disease develops when a host's resistance to the microorganism and its effects is overcome. Risk can be reduced when the host's immune defenses are maximized. These defenses are supported when patient care practices are designed to maintain nutrition, manage stress, preserve skin integrity, support the respiratory tract, and enhance immunity.

Nutritional support

Nutrition is a combination of ingestion and digestion of food, absorption and metabolism of nutrients, and metabolic processes necessary for the organism's growth and function. Individual nutritional needs vary greatly with age, sex, energy expenditure, pregnancy, lactation, and general state of health.

Malnutrition is a condition of impaired growth or function resulting from inadequate or excessive intake of nutrients that leads to a deficiency of one or more essential nutrients. Malnutrition impairs a person's resistance to infection, wound healing, and ability to withstand stress[58] (see Chapter 1). In addition, children with malnutrition can have retarded growth and mental development. Infection and illness alter nutritional needs of the patient. Even in the presence of appropriate antimicrobial therapy, a patient with an infection may develop a nutritional deficiency and be unable to clear the infection without nutritional intervention or support. [23] In addition, noninfectious diseases may cause nutritional deficiency that can greatly increase the risk of an infectious complication.

Prevention of nutritional deficiencies is preferable to treatment of deficiencies after they occur. The nurse can assist in early recognition of a patient's nutritional problems and a registered dietician can determine the patient's nutritional needs based on an individualized assessment. A nutritional assessment includes a history (weight change, dietary intake changes, gastric disorders, functional capacity) and physical (loss of subcutaneous fat, muscle wasting, ankle or sacral edema, or ascites). [15] The dietitian can assist the nurse in planning a diet to prevent deficiencies and aid healing. Oral feedings are usually preferred to intravascular nutritional support because nutrients are more completely absorbed by the gastrointestinal tract. Oral feedings are also less expensive and present less risk of infectious complications. [58]

Stress reduction

Stress can adversely affect (1) immune function, (2) intake of nutrients, and (3) sleep patterns. Effective strategies to alleviate stress are extremely difficult to develop without identifying its source. Therefore a thorough nursing assessment for each patient should include identification of circumstances or forces that increase the patient's perceived stress and what helps alleviate it. Intervention by professionals with specialized training in stress reduction techniques may be necessary.

Sleep and exercise are important stress reduction tools. Adequate sleep is important to maintain disease resistance. The physiologic chores of cleansing, surveillance, and rebuilding the immune system are most efficient during sleep. It may be difficult to rest in a hospital or long-term care facility because of various factors, including pain, stress, noise, an uncomfortable mattress, and sleep interruptions

for nighttime care. The most common intervention to increase sleep is to give sleep-inducing medication. However, such medications may not induce a restful sleep. Nursing assessment and care can help identify problems with rest and sleep, support a strategy for decreasing identified stressors, and teach relaxation techniques that may reduce the need for medication. Nurses can determine when the patient is ready to walk or perform other exercise. Regular exercise helps to maintain adequate immune function and lung inflation. When active exercise is not feasible, regular passive exercise of the extremities assists in maintaining blood circulation and muscle function.

Skin preservation

The skin, the body's largest organ, defends the body against invading infectious organisms. Therefore, maintenance of intact skin is a vital part of maximizing the patient's normal defenses. Nurses can provide skin care that helps to maintain healthy, intact skin. Routine inspection will detect potential areas of concern and guide early intervention. Many therapeutic and diagnostic procedures result in penetration of, or damage to, the skin, creating the opportunity for entry of organisms. Poor healing of nonintact skin may increase the risk of infection, and conversely, infection may result in poor healing. Mattress overlays to relieve pressure, special fluidized or air beds, special dressings, and creams and lotions are used to prevent skin breakdown or promote healing, although the effectiveness of many of these techniques has not been methodically evaluated.

Respiratory support

The respiratory tract is equipped with various defense mechanisms against invading infectious organisms. Mucus production, cilia, coughing, and sneezing all serve as mechanical safeguards, trapping and expelling organisms. Unfortunately, many procedures and devices used to support patients (e.g., endotracheal suctioning, mechanical ventilators) also disrupt these mechanical barriers. Nurses play a major role in monitoring and maintaining respiratory function by encouraging the patient to turn, cough, and deep breathe. Turning helps maintain circulation and minimizes skin breakdown. Turning also assists normal respiratory defenses by preventing secretions from pooling and becoming potential growth media for organisms. An upright position, coughing and deep breathing help to inflate the lungs, expel secretions, and minimize risk of aspiration, as do walking and exercise. If a patient is being mechanically ventilated or has a tracheostomy, respiratory secretions may need to be removed by suctioning using aseptic, gentle technique to avoid trauma to, or contamination of, the mucociliary tree.

Enhancement of the immune system

Immunotherapy enhances immune system function to increase protection against infections (see Chapter 1). Therapies include immune stimulators, such as lymphokines or cytokines (e.g., interferon); preformed antibodies, (e.g., immune globulin); and antigens in the form of microorganism-specific vaccine to stimulate antibody production. There are effective vaccines against only a few of the many human infections.

Nurses can be instrumental in ensuring that patients have been appropriately immunized against measles, mumps, rubella, tetanus, diphtheria, hemophilus serotype B, polio, influenza, pneumococcus, and hepatitis B virus (HBV) by obtaining a complete immunization history from the patient and ensuring that needed immunizations are administered. Several of the clinical studies in Section Three illustrate the importance of immunizations (see Clinical Studies 9 and 16).

Many immunizations are offered to persons in specific age groups, those anticipating for-eign travel or military service, or those working in select professions. Nurses and other health care professionals should be immunized to protect themselves and their patients. Perhaps the most important immunizations for health care professionals in the United States are those against measles (rubeola), influenza, rubella, and HBV.[19] All these diseases can be transmitted from patients to care providers and directly or indirectly to other patients in health care settings. If the care provider becomes infected, there is potential for spread to patients, with possible life-threatening consequences. Additional discussion of immunizations for health care providers is presented in Chapter 6.

Currently recommended immunizations for adults, children, and health care professionals in the United States are found in Table 5-1. These recommendations are adjusted periodically as new vaccines and combinations become available and as additional information suggests the need for boosters. Updated recommendations are published regularly by the American Academy of Pediatrics, American College of Physicians, The Centers for Disease Control and Prevention, and others.

Health promotion

Health promotion and maintenance programs are based on the premise that it is easier to prevent than treat. Many programs promote smoking cessation and termination of drug and alcohol dependencies, since these addictions may increase the risk of health problems, including infections.

Educational promotion of health and wellness provides information to people who often already have firmly ingrained lifestyles and concepts, some of which may be incompatible with the new information. Therefore the challenge to these programs is to change behavior. Educational programs must be keyed to individuals, cultures, age groups, and other characteristics as necessary. Although many adult

TABLE 5-1 Routine immunization requirements and recommendations for use in the United States

Immunization	Children	Adults	Health care workers (HCW)
Polio	Complete series of 4 doses of oral (OPV) vaccine by 6 years old	In outbreak or if travel to endemic areas. Oral vaccine available (live virus) enhanced potency vaccine (e-IPV) inactive virus preferred	See "Adults"
Tetanus/diphtheria	Complete series of 5 doses by 6 years old	Every 10 years; if no childhood series, initiate series of three doses within one year[a]	See "Adults"
Pertussis[b]	Combined with tetanus/diphtheria, same schedule	None at this time (see "Health Care Providers")	None at this time. Possible use of acellular vaccine for adults in high-risk areas during outbreaks
Haemophilus[b] *influenzae* b (Hib)	Complete series by 15 months old (dosing depends on manufacturer)	Recommended for persons who have had splenectomy or who are HIV positive	See "Adults"
Measles[b]/mumps/rubella (MMR)	Two doses by 6 years old; first dose given between 12-15 months of age[c]	"Children" requirements; or two doses given at least 1 month apart	Documented immunity or 2 doses of vaccine at least 1 month apart
Varicella[d] (chickenpox)	Manufacturer's recommendations when available	See "Children"	See "Children"; will likely be recommended for all susceptible health care workers
Hepatitis B	Complete series of 3 doses within 6 months in infancy	Encouraged for all adolescents and young adults, especially those engaging in high-risk behaviors (3 doses within 6 months)	Complete series of 3 doses within 6 months for all health care students and workers who have contact with body substances

Continued.

TABLE 5-1 Routine immunization requirements and recommendations for use in the United States—cont'd

Immunization	Children	Adults	Health care providers (HCP)
Influenza[a]	Annually for children with pulmonary or cardiac problems, etc.; split virus vaccine if < 13 years old; if first dose ever and if < 9 years old, second dose needed in 4 weeks	Annually for persons with pulmonary or cardiac problems, etc., and for persons ≥ 65 years old	Annually
Streptococcus[b] *pneumoniae* (Pneumococcal)	For children ≥ 2 years old with serious chronic diseases, immuno-compromising diseases, and HIV; repeat doses as recommended	For adults ≥ 65 years old, and all adults with serious chronic diseases, immuno-compromising diseases, and HIV; repeat doses as recommended[e]	See "Adults"

Compiled from: 1. American Academy of Pediatrics. *Report of the Committee on Infectious Diseases* (the Redbook), 22nd ed. Elk Grove Village, IL: The American Academy of Pediatrics; 1991. 2. American College of Physicians. *The Guide for Adult Immunizations,* 3rd ed. Philadelphia: The American College of Physicians; 1994. 3. Benenson AS, ed. *Control of Communicable Diseases in Man,* 15th ed. Washington D.C.: American Public Health Association; 1990. 4. Centers for Disease Control and Prevention. Measles prevention: recommendations of the Immunization Practices Advisory Committee. *MMWR.* 1989;38(S-9):1-18.

[a]The American College of Physicians Task Force on Adult Immunizations states that an acceptable alternative after completion of appropriate childhood series is a single midlife tetanus/diphtheria booster.[2]

[b]For additional immunization information see Clinical Studies 6, 9, 16, 18, 28, 30, 31.

[c]The American Academy of Pediatrics recommends the second dose be given at 11-12 years.[1] The Advisory Committee on Immunization Practices recommends the second dose be given at age 4-6 years.[4]

[d]Not yet released.

[e]These recommendations also permit a pneumococcal immunization at age 50 with a booster at age 65.

health promotion programs emphasize basic needs and incorporate principles of adult learning intended to motivate change, they often are only minimally successful. (See Chapters 4 and 9 for a discussion of social and cultural issues and educational techniques for changing behavior.)

MINIMIZING RISK TO THE PATIENT

One author has commented about the role of medical devices in patient care and the associated risk[72]:

With yards of entrails, miles of vascular network, dozens of extravascular spaces, and several organ systems, any patient is a candidate for a staggering array of diagnostic and therapeutic procedures. Although many of these procedures provide information that is essential for sophisticated patient care or to supplant more traumatic intervention or are critical for life support, most procedures also bypass natural host defenses and place patients at increased risk of nosocomial infection.

Technology has made available many invasive, indwelling, and implantable devices that now play a vital role in patient care and treatment. One or more devices (e.g., intravenous lines, indwelling urethral catheters) are used for most patients during their care in a health facility and can contribute significantly to the patient's risk for nosocomial infection.

The risks attributable to medical devices and the methods that can decrease these risks must be understood if safe patient care is to be provided. Although many devices may be tested for effectiveness and safety in clinical trials before being released commercially, information obtained from these studies is often inadequate to evaluate all infection risks. For example, problems with cleaning or maintaining sterility may be identified only after marketing. The device may be used in the care of patients who are more severely ill than those studied in clinical trials.

Risk of infectious complications related to devices is minimized when three important principles are followed:

1. Devices must be used only as clinically required and never solely for the health care provider's convenience. The risks of using a device should always be considered, and the benefits should outweigh the risks.
2. Medical devices should be used only for the duration of the clinical need. Nurses should assist in continual evaluation of the patient's need for the device.
3. A device that is intended to be disposable or is labeled for single-patient use should not be reprocessed for use on another

patient unless processing and packaging and tested routines have been carefully developed to ensure sterility or disinfection, reliable function, and safety. Often this effort is coordinated with the manufacturer. The facility or person reprocessing such items may be liable for injury resulting from use.

Vascular access devices

Most nonepidemic infusion-related infections are caused during or after insertion by contamination of the catheter with organisms from the patient's own skin. Gram-positive bacteria such as *Staphylococcus aureus*, coagulase-negative staphylococci (including *Staphylococcus epidermidis*), enterococci, and *Candida* species account for a large and increasing proportion of infusion-related infections.[22,48]

Peripheral intravascular therapy

Most patients admitted to an acute-care facility receive intravenous (IV) therapy for at least some period, most often through a peripherally placed cannula (catheter). IV therapy devices provide organisms capable of causing infection with access to disrupted tissue that may become infected and a direct pathway to the bloodstream, either through the catheter lumen or underneath the skin on the outside of the catheter. Organisms that reach the bloodstream may produce sepsis or spread hematogenously to other sites in the body (Figure 5-1). (See Clinical Study 4).

Many factors affect the risk of nosocomial infection during IV therapy.[39] Probably the most important factor is the length of time the catheter remains in the insertion site. The risk of site infection, and subsequent bloodstream infection, dramatically increases if the catheter remains in the same site longer than 72 hours.[42] Therefore, the current standard of practice is to rotate the IV routinely to another

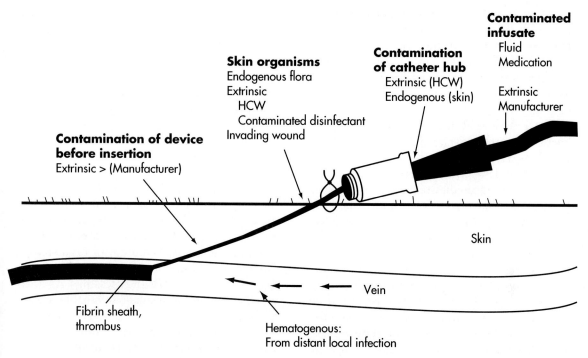

Contaminated infusate
Fluid
Medication

Extrinsic
Manufacturer

Contamination of catheter hub
Extrinsic (HCW)
Endogenous (skin)

Skin organisms
Endogenous flora
Extrinsic
HCW
Contaminated disinfectant
Invading wound

Contamination of device before insertion
Extrinsic > (Manufacturer)

Skin

Vein

Fibrin sheath,
thrombus

Hematogenous:
From distant local infection

FIGURE 5-1. Sources of intravascular cannula–related infection. Major sources are skin flora, contamination of catheter hub, contamination of infusate, and hematogenous colonization of intravascular device and its fibronectin-fibrin sheath. HCW-Healthcare worker. (From Maki DG, Infections due to infusion therapy, In: Bennett IV, *Hospital Infections*, ed 3, Boston: Little Brown; 1992.) Used with permission.

site within 72 hours, or sooner if signs and symptoms of infection develop. If limited sites are available and if the current site appears free from complications, catheters are sometimes left in place longer, although this may increase the risk of infection. Some facilities require a written physician's order for a peripheral IV cannula that is left in the same site longer than 72 hours.

The choice of cannula material may affect risk of infection. Foreign bodies introduced into the vascular system induce an immune reaction; a fibrin sheath is usually deposited on the IV cannula within several days. This sheath becomes a deposition and propagation site for organisms. Studies have demonstrated that cannulae made of steel were more bio-

logically inert and resulted in lower infection risks than cannulae made from early-generation plastic materials.[10] Steel needles are used frequently outside the U.S. However, steel cannulae are not the standard for use in the U.S. because of their susceptibility to infiltration, need for more frequent site rotation, and patient discomfort.

Catheters are made of a variety of materials. Since these cannulae must be inserted with a steel introducer or guide-wire needle, it is necessary that the material on the outside of the introducer be very smooth and not shred or split during insertion or removal of the cannula from the steel guide. A cannula that is not smooth will increase the possibility of vessel damage, potentially increasing the risk of infection. In addition, the material's composition should be as physiologically inert as possible to minimize immune response. Initially, materials such as polyvinyl chloride and Teflon were frequently used for cannulae but were not ideal because of rigidity and a tendency to split. Newer materials, such as Vialon®, resist splitting and soften with body heat to conform better within the vessel. Many materials have been and are being developed. Some of these materials incorporate antimicrobials or substances that release antimicrobial agents such as silver ions, antibiotics, or disinfectants. This is an area of continuing research and development.[22]

The preparation of the skin at the insertion site also plays a role in preventing infectious complications. Careful skin preparation decreases the risk that many organisms will be introduced into the vascular system when the IV cannula is inserted. Studies of skin antisepsis indicate that a broad-spectrum skin antiseptic or combination of antiseptics should be used before IV insertion.[10,22] To be effective, the antiseptic must be allowed to dry, usually at least 30 seconds. If two antiseptics are used, both should be allowed to dry.

Once a cannula is inserted, the type of dressing placed over the site may also affect the risk of infection. For many years the dressing placed on peripheral IV sites was a simple adhesive bandage or gauze. At least daily, this was removed, the site observed and cleaned as necessary, and the dressing replaced. An antimicrobial ointment was often applied at the insertion site. The advent of transparent, moisture-permeable dressings has changed this practice in many facilities. Since the site can be observed for visible signs of complications through the dressing, transparent dressings are usually left on until the catheter is removed or the dressing is not intact. Many facilities have stopped using an antimicrobial ointment because it may increase the likelihood of the transparent dressing falling off. Although evidence is conflicting, certain antimicrobial ointments may decrease the risk of infectious complications.[22,46] Some ointments predispose to the emergence of antimicrobial-resistant organisms. Some facilities continue to use ointment and place a folded gauze pad between the ointment and the transparent dressing, balancing the perceived need for ointment against the convenience of site observation through the dressing.

Transparent dressings have also been implicated as a risk factor for site infections.[39] Although these dressings are moisture permeable, fluids may accumulate beneath them, providing a growth medium for organisms.[16] There is a diversity of opinion regarding standards of practice for IV site dressings. An analysis combining the results of available studies identified significantly increased risk of central and peripheral catheter tip infection associated with transparent versus gauze dressings. Risk of bacteremia and catheter sepsis was greater when transparent rather than gauze dressings were used on central venous catheter sites.[27] Improved materials, combined with additional research into catheter design and care, should help to resolve some of these issues. Some facility guidelines allow nurses to individualize the dressing material and techniques based on the patient's circumstances, including the degree of diaphoresis and experience with dressing adherence.

The importance of site inspection, regardless of the dressing type or technique, cannot be underestimated. Complications discovered early may be more easily treated than those allowed to progress. A peripheral IV catheter should be removed at the first sign of potential infection (e.g., pain, redness, swelling). The standard for peripheral IV site selection and rotation is to use arms rather than legs, to start at distal veins and work to proximal sites and to alternate arms, if possible. Insertion sites with heavier contamination, for example, the groin or the neck of a patient with a tracheostomy, have higher risk of infection.[22] Nurses must individualize the application of these standards to specific patient requirements.

Many believe lines placed during an emergency while the patient is being stabilized and prepared for transport to a facility are associated with higher risk of infection as a result of lack of aseptic skin preparation and trauma to the vessel. Consequently, many facilities have policies that these field lines be discontinued and the site changed as soon as possible after the patient is admitted and stable.

Central intravascular access

Lines placed in large central vessels such as the subclavian or jugular vein, are often used for venous or arterial access and measurement purposes. In contrast to peripheral IV access catheters, these cannulae usually have a larger bore, are longer, enter a major vessel, may have multiple lumens, and may require surgical implantation. Although the risk factors for infection are similar to those of peripheral IV lines because a foreign body is placed into the vascular system, the outcome may be more severe.

Central catheters are used when peripheral sites are limited, when IV therapy will be required for a longer period, and when toxic medications such as hyperalimentation require rapid dilution in a large vessel. Multilumen cannulae are often used to replace several catheters at different sites.

No studies indicate precisely how long subclavian, jugular, and femoral cannulae may remain in place before infection risks outweigh the benefits of central vascular access. Although one study suggests that the sites be rotated every 96 hours,[45] some practitioners believe that these lines can stay in place longer. More research is required before a standard of practice can be established.

Catheters requiring surgical insertion or subcutaneous tunneling are used when vascular access is required for weeks to many months. A catheter that has cannula ports exiting into a major vein in the upper chest and that is inserted into an antecubital vein is also considered a long-term central line. These catheters may be used for chemotherapy, nutritional support, and antimicrobial administration. Given the extended duration of their use at a single site, infections associated with these lines may occur.[55] Lines are most often removed when intravascular access is no longer needed, the cannula ceases to work or is associated with infection. When central line–associated infection does occur, an attempt is often made to treat the infection while leaving the cannula in place. This strategy is inconsistent with peripheral line management techniques, which call for removal of the line when an infection occurs. This attempt to preserve the line and treat line-associated sepsis with antimicrobials balances the risk of infection against that of another trip to the operating room. These efforts are often successful.

Several risk factors for infection associated with peripheral IV access are also present when central cannulae are used. Skin preparation before catheter insertion is important for central catheters.[22] A more stringent technique than that used for peripheral catheters is recommended.[16] Sterile drapes often are placed around the insertion site and the health care worker inserting the line wears sterile gloves and possibly other sterile garb.

Large-bore, multilumen lines, used with increasing frequency, offer many advantages. Some studies suggest that the incidence of central venous catheter–related sepsis may be identical for single and triple lumen catheters.[17] However, the risks of all complications, including infections, may be higher for multilumen lines than for single-lumen catheters because their large size allows them to be frequently accessed for multiple uses, including collection of blood specimens.[16] The benefits of these large multilumen lines must be weighed against the potential risks to each patient.

Dressing material and technique may affect risk for infection in patients with central lines. Before the advent of transparent moisture-permeable dressings, standard care included an occlusive gauze dressing that was changed approximately every 48 hours. Often the adhesive tape used to anchor the dressing would separate before 48 hours and had to be reinforced. Site inspection was not possible except when the dressing was being changed. Though transparent dressings allow frequent inspection of sites and minimize manipulation of the line during dressing changes, there is evidence that transparent dressings, most particularly those having a low moisture vapor transmission rate, are associated with increased risk of infection.[22,27,40] These dressings should be changed at intervals of 72 hours to 7 days.[16]

Intravascular pressure monitoring

Measurement of intravascular pressures requires devices, such as the pressure transducer, or gauge, and stopcocks, that increase the risk of infection. Many nosocomial infections and outbreaks have been associated with transducers and their domes[3] (see Clinical Study 4). Outbreaks have also occurred when transducers were used to measure pressures of other body fluids (e.g., intrauterine, cerebrospinal).

When transducers were introduced, they were not accompanied by specific instructions for cleaning or sterilization. It was believed that a pressure gradient protected the patient from any contamination of the dome or transducer. This was quickly shown to be incorrect when outbreaks of bacteremia occurred as a consequence of transducer contamination. A disposable dome designed to prevent this problem included a thin membrane that separated the disposable dome from the transducer

(Figure 5-2). However, even these were associated with infections as a result of microscopic breaks in the dome membrane.[3] Disposable one-piece transducers and domes have since been introduced (Figure 5-2). When disposable transducers are not used, sterilization of the reusable transducer between patients can decrease infection risk. Other outbreaks occurred when some facilities preassembled and prefilled the transducer and dome, which would then sit for a variable period until use. These outbreaks ceased when the practice of preassembly and filling was discontinued.[3] Infections have also been attributed to contaminated stopcocks and flush solutions. These problems may be minimized when bottles or bags of fluid are changed every 24 hours, stopcocks are maintained aseptically, the entire pressure-monitoring system is changed every 48 to 96 hours, and the site of a peripheral arterial cannula is changed every 96 hours.[72]

Intravascular solutions

Contaminated solutions instilled through intravascular access devices have been the source of rare but dramatic outbreaks of bacteremia.[22] Most infusates typically used can support bacterial or fungal growth. In some instances, fluids can be heavily contaminated with bacteria yet appear clear on visual inspection. Infusates were initially recognized as a source of infection when a nationwide epidemic of bacteremia occurred in the early 1970s.[41] One manufacturer's product was contaminated at the factory and not identified as the source of the outbreak until the Centers for Disease Control received from many U.S. hospitals reports of outbreaks of bacteremia without an identified source. When the implicated product was recalled by the manufacturer, the epidemic ended.

This outbreak prompted the use of more stringent regulations for quality control by manufacturers and more rigorous preventive measures within facilities. Recommendations

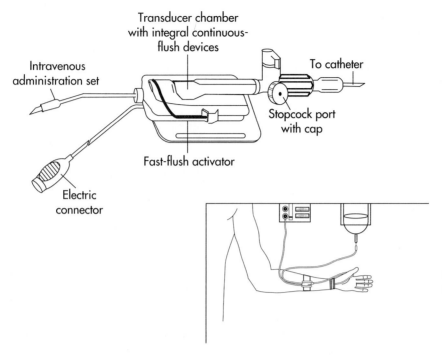

FIGURE 5-2. Disposable pressure transducer with intregal flow-through continuous-flush device. Insert shows body mounting of radial artery transducer. (From Luskin RL et al: Extended use of disposable pressure transducers, *JAMA* 255:916, 1986.) Used with permission.

were made to change the IV fluid, administration set and tubing every 24 hours.[10] Subsequent studies[69] have demonstrated that the fluid path (e.g., the tubing) is an unlikely source of infection. Consequently, these recommendations were modified to allow tubing to be changed every 3 days. Future studies may justify extension of this interval. Since the bottle or bag of fluid may become a potential source of infecting organisms once it is opened and sufficient time for microbial growth elapses, changing the bottle or bag every 24 hours continues to be the standard. Other methods that can decrease the risk of infusate-related bacteremia include use of strict aseptic technique while preparing or mixing fluids and meticulous preparation technique when entering and hanging fluid containers and

changing tubing. If an infusate-related infection is suspected, the bag or bottle and the tubing should be discontinued, disconnected from the patient immediately, and sent to the laboratory for culture and possibly for pyrogen testing. Adequate volumes of blood to be cultured should be drawn as part of the patient's evaluation for sepsis. Culture of the catheter tip may be helpful.[22,40]

Organizations such as The Centers for Disease Control and Prevention (CDC)[10] and the Intravenous Nurses Society (INS)[28] publish referenced guidelines for care of IV lines. While certain aspects of IV care, such as frequency of site rotation and tubing change, have been validated by research[44,61] data are equivocal regarding other aspects of care such as frequency of dressing changes, site cleansing techniques and products, types of dressings and use of filters during preparation or administration.[11,60] In the absence of convincing findings from studies of these practices, it is not surprising that considerable variation exists and that some costly practices are discontinued in the absence of data validating their use.

Urinary drainage devices

Catheter-associated urinary tract infections (UTIc) are the most common nosocomial infection and the most frequent device-related infection.[65,67] Data from the National Nosocomial Infections Study (NNIS) at the CDC indicate that between 1986 and 1991 36% of all nosocomial infections were catheter-associated.[7] Studies have consistently identified four major risk factors for UTIc. These include female gender, duration of catheterization, breaks in catheter care techniques, and the absence of systemic antimicrobials.[65] During the past decade, studies have demonstrated that 1% to 4% of patients with UTIc develop bacteremia and of these 13% to 40% die.[54,65] For those who are catheterized for more than 30 days, such as nursing home residents and persons with chronic bladder dysfunction, the incidence of bacteriuria is eventually 100%, and the bacteriuria often becomes chronic.[70,71] Thus, UTIc are significant infections (see Clinical Study 24.)

Indwelling urinary drainage was initially accomplished by a catheter that emptied into an open container. Virtually all patients with these open catheters had bacteria in their urine after 4 days.[33] Closed drainage systems having no interruption between the catheter and the urine receptacle were introduced to reduce this high infection risk. However, even with the closed system, bacteriuria occurs in 10% to 20% of those catheterized.[20]

Preventing UTIc is a challenge. The indwelling urethral catheter interrupts normal host defenses. Microorganisms causing UTIc can originate from the patient's endogenous flora, the hands of caregivers, and contaminated equipment. The portal of entry of bacteria into the urinary system of a catheterized patient differs by gender. In women, 70% of bacteriuria episodes occur via the periurethral route.[14,65] Organisms originating primarily from the rectum and found at the meatal and perineal areas may be pushed into the bladder at the time of catheterization or can migrate along the outside of the catheter into the bladder.[20,66] In men with catheter associated bacteriuria, the majority of organisms come from exogenous sources rather than the patient's own perineum. Organisms introduced into the drainage bag or tubing can reach the bladder via the inner lumen of the catheter in about 24 to 48 hours,[14] particularly in patients who are not receiving antibiotics.[65] Once organisms find their way into the bladder through any of these routes, small numbers increase to large numbers in under 24 hours.[68]

Perhaps the most important UTIc prevention technique is to use a urinary drainage device only when clinically indicated, such as to drain the bladder when the patient is unable to do so, to obtain critical measurements, and to drain the bladder while the patient is in the operating room. The catheter should be removed when it is no longer needed for this support. Nurses can be instrumental in making these clinical determinations by monitoring patients' need for catheterization, restricting catheterization to patients who require this procedure, and removing indwelling catheters when they are no longer essential. Incontinence is rarely an indication for a catheter. It can be best managed by diapers, timed urination, and fluid management.

Aseptic insertion of an indwelling catheter can reduce the risk of infection. The meatus and perineal area should be carefully prepared with an antiseptic solution and the sterility of the catheter rigorously maintained. Once inserted, the drainage tubing should be secured to avoid tension on the catheter and kept below the level of the bladder to facilitate drainage and prevent backflow of urine into the bladder. The system must be kept closed, specimens obtained through specimen ports, and the drainage bag emptied through a tube at the bottom of the bag. There is no standard time frame for changing the catheter or the drainage tubing and bag. If the system is functioning appropriately and its need persists, it may be left in place.

Clinicians, researchers and manufacturers of indwelling urinary drainage devices have developed a number of product or procedural options intended to decrease risk of infection. These include routine cleansing regimens in women and girls to block entry of bacteria from the meatal area; incorporating antimicrobial substances into the catheter structure such as impregnating the catheter with silver ions; disinfecting the catheter bag with agents such as hydrogen peroxide, iodophors, and chlorhexidine; selective decontamination of the gut flora in immunosuppressed women; and the use of systemic antimicrobials. Some of these measures have met with moderate success; others have been of questionable or no value.[5,20,64] Modifications will continue to be marketed with and without appropriate studies demonstrating efficacy. Nurses can be a valuable resource in the evaluation of their efficacy and insistence that product choices are based on demonstrated efficacy.

Opening the catheter system by disconnecting the junction between the catheter and tubing and other breaks in technique are significant factors for UTIc. Changes in product design have attempted to discourage or prevent opening of the drainage system with sampling ports and sealed catheter-to-tubing junctions. In one study using a sealed junction that minimized opening the system, there were fewer UTIc in patients who were not receiving antimicrobials.[53] The sampling port allows removal of urine for specimens with a needle and syringe without opening the drainage system and is generally acknowledged to help control infection risk. The antireflux valve

is designed to prevent the urine in the drainage bag from reentering the tubing and flowing back into the bladder. While studies have not proven efficacy, this device may be beneficial if the drainage bag is held above the level of the bladder or placed on the patient's abdomen during transport. Since these practices are firmly discouraged, the valve may simply be an unneeded and expensive addition.

There are several alternatives to indwelling catheter drainage of urine. One is the straight catheter, or in-and-out catheterization. This procedure consists of inserting the catheter, draining the urine and removing the catheter immediately after the urine is drained. A single catheterization using this technique has an associated risk for UTI of 0.5% to 8%.[32] Repeated intermittent catheterization with clean, not sterile, catheters is used for patients with spinal cord injury and has been demonstrated to be fairly safe.[35] Aseptic preparation of the meatus and sterile catheterization are still important to decrease infection risks.

Another alternative is the condom catheter used for men and boys. The condom, with the attached catheter drainage tube, is placed on the penis to collect urine from incontinent patients who can empty their bladder but cannot control urination. Although the entire system is external, patients with condom catheters can develop bacteriuria, urinary tract infection, local penile infections, and obstructed flow of urine.[26,30,52] In addition, the devices may be difficult to maintain, depending on placement technique and cooperation of the patient. A third alternative is a regimen of timed urination. Assisting the patient to empty the bladder regularly allows some patients who would otherwise be incontinent to avoid catheterization.

Dialysis

Hemodialysis-associated infections include bloodstream infection, infections of the vascular access site, and infections related to contamination of dialysis fluid.[18] If bacteremia is ruled out, pyrogenic reactions manifested by such symptoms as fever, rigors, low blood pressure, and muscle aches are presumed to be caused by endotoxins produced by gram-negative bacteria in the water system.[4] Although sterile disposable dialyzers intended for single use are available, they are frequently disinfected and reused.[1] Several outbreaks have been associated with this practice.[38] Permanent dialyzers are of two types: single pass (which are preferred) and recirculating. Whether a permanent dialyzer is used or a disposable dialyzer is reused, appropriate disinfection procedures are vital. Most commonly used agents include formaldehyde and peracetic acid with hydrogen peroxide.[4]

Complications of peritoneal dialysis include local skin infections, peritonitis, and bloodstream infections. Most infections are related to touch contamination; prevention is aimed at reducing this risk. For both hemodialysis and peritoneal dialysis, the most common infecting organisms are from the skin of the patient or the health care provider.

Ventilation assist devices

Nosocomial infections of the lower respiratory tract are associated with a high risk of mortality and are a common complication in hospitalized patients. Nosocomial pneumonias affect nearly a quarter of a million acute-care patients annually and account for approximately 13% to 18% of all nosocomial infections in the United States.[13] A number of factors are associated with colonization and infection of the respiratory tract (Figure 5-3). Patients who are over 70 years of age or who have chronic lung disease, depressed consciousness, or chest surgery or who take histamine type 2 (H_2) blockers with or without

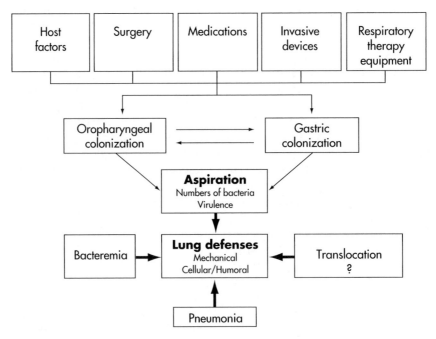

FIGURE 5-3. Summary of factors influencing colonization and infection of respiratory tract. (From Craven DE et al: *Semin Respir Infect* 5: 157-192, 1990.) Nosocomial pneumonia in the 90's: update of epidemiology and risk factors. Used with permission.

antacids have a greater risk of acquiring nosocomial pneumonia than patients without these characteristics.[12,13] Although devices such as nebulizers and humidifiers, feeding tubes, resuscitation bags, and spirometers have been associated with increased risk of respiratory infection, mechanical ventilators in particular substantially increase a patient's risk of nosocomial pneumonia.[21] Patients who are intubated have 7 to 21 times the pneumonia risk of patients not using a respiratory therapy device.[13]

Ventilators interrupt normal host defenses of the upper respiratory tract. The numbers and virulence of microorganisms that enter the lungs are one determinant of risk of infection. The ventilator equipment itself or poor management may contribute to large inocula. In some instances the endotracheal tube cuff may trap contaminated respiratory or gastric secretions and force them into the lungs.[56]

The risk of infection is proportional to the duration of mechanical ventilation. Therefore, limiting the time that a patient is mechanically ventilated is of utmost importance. The risk of early or premature weaning, with subsequent reintubation, must be balanced against the risks of prolonged ventilator use. The nurse can provide valuable input concerning the patient's respiratory status.

The route of intubation may also affect the risk of infection. Patients with nasal intubation have been shown to be at higher risk for sinus infections caused by blockage of sinus drainage passages.[6] Those with oral intubation may be at increased risk for aspirating oral secretions. Patients expected to have long-term intubation often undergo a tracheostomy in an attempt to bypass these risks. However, this procedure also has concomitant risks of insertion site infection. Nurses perform aseptic tracheostomy care to help decrease infectious complications for this route of ventilator access.

Regular clearing of secretions from the upper respiratory tract, oral cavity, and ventilator tubing is another important procedure for the patient on a ventilator. These secretions can provide a growth medium for organisms and block normal function of the lungs. Gentle manipulations and aseptic suctioning will minimize trauma and infection risk from the procedure. Nurses should use appropriate barrier precautions such as gloves on both hands to protect the patient and themselves from infection (see Chapter 6 and Clinical Study 13). Aspiration of gastric contents is a common problem in patients on mechanical ventilation. Although aspiration is not generally preventable, suctioning and positioning may decrease the inoculum of organisms or frequency of aspiration.

Appropriate management of equipment and medications is important. Ventilator tubing can be safely changed every 72 hours and perhaps at longer intervals without increasing risk of infection.[12] The condensate that collects in ventilator tubing may pose a risk to the patient if allowed to collect and incubate microorganisms and flow back into the patient's airway (Figure 5-4). Several products have been introduced to assist in evacuating or evaporating these secretions to protect the patient's airway.[13] As with all devices, one important component of care is to have ongoing, planned quality control programs in place.[31] Other respiratory devices, for example nebulizers and humidifiers, are discussed in Chapter 3.

Endoscopic Devices

Endoscopes are fiberoptic instruments that allow the practitioner to visualize internal organs, obtain specimens, and perform procedures. Endoscopes that are rigid are used for surgical procedures such as arthroscopy and laparoscopy. Flexible endoscopes have revolutionized some diagnostic tests and many surgical procedures in medical practice, particularly gastroenterology and pulmonology

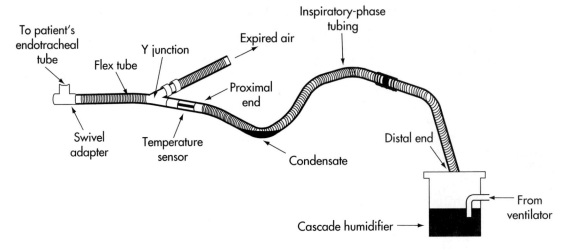

FIGURE 5-4. Schematic diagram of ventilator circuit demonstrating water condensate in dependent loop of ventilator tubing. (From Wenzel RP, ed. *Prevention and Control of Hospital Infection* ed 2. Baltimore: Williams & Wilkins; 1993:108.) Used with permission.

(Figure 5-5). However, endoscopes can also pose a risk of infection if inadequately cleaned and processed.

Thousands of patients in the United States undergo gastrointestinal and pulmonary endoscopic procedures every year. Although infections are not a frequently reported complication of endoscopy, there have been a number of infection-related deaths, and many infections may be difficult to recognize.[46] Two primary mechanisms are responsible for infections associated with flexible fiberoptic endoscopes. First, the patient's normal endogenous flora from the gastrointestinal or respiratory tracts can enter the bloodstream as a result of procedural manipulations. Transient bacteremia, endocarditis, cholangitis, and aspiration pneumonia in a sedated patient have been documented.[36,37,47,63] Second, exogenous microorganisms, primarily gram-negative bacilli, gain entry when endoscopic equipment, including the scopes and accessories, are contaminated.[46] Therefore, meticulous cleaning and adequate sterilization and disinfection procedures are critical to preventing infections from these devices.

Though sterilization is the preferred method of processing, endoscopes cannot be steam-sterilized because their fiberoptic lenses cannot withstand high temperatures. Facilities seldom have these costly endoscopes available in a sufficient quantity to use ethylene oxide (ETO) gas sterilization, which requires long aeration for removal of residual gas before the instrument can be used. ETO is also expensive. As technology continues to advance, a fast, safe, and cost-effective method for sterilization may become available. When this occurs, the standard for processing endoscopes should become sterilization. The minimal recommended practice for endoscope processing is high-level disinfection with an Environmental Protection Agency (EPA) registered disinfectant/sterilant.[46] These products assure that all viruses and vegetative bacteria (i.e., not in spore form) are killed along with a majority of bacterial and fungal spores. This process is one step less rigorous than sterilization, in which spores are eliminated (see Chapter 7). High-level disinfection can be achieved by using chemical agents, such as glutaraldehyde, stabilized hydrogen peroxide, or pericetic acid.

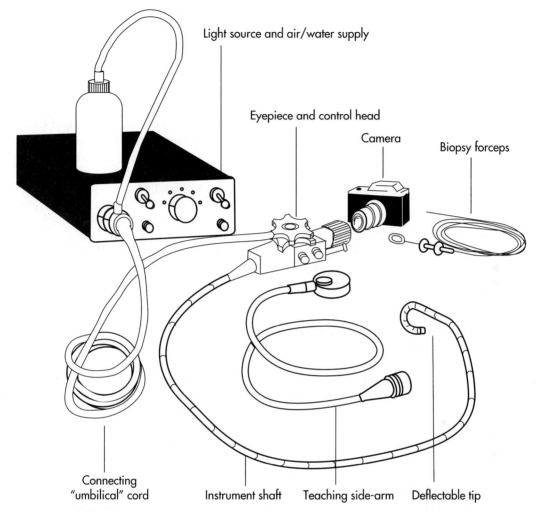

Light source and air/water supply

Eyepiece and control head

Camera

Biopsy forceps

Connecting
"umbilical" cord

Instrument shaft

Teaching side-arm

Deflectable tip

FIGURE 5-5. Gastrointestinal fiberoptic endoscope consists of control head with eyepiece and flexible shaft (insertion tube) with maneuverable tip. Head is connected to light source and air/water supply via connecting cord. (From Cotton PB: *Practical gastrointestinal endoscopy,* ed 2, St Louis, 1982, Blackwell.) Used with permission.

The endoscope must first be thoroughly cleaned, then soaked in the high-level disinfectant for at least the minimum time specified by the disinfectant manufacturer. The times range from 20 to 45 minutes. It is essential that all surfaces, internal and external, and all channels have contact with the disinfectant for the entire period. The scope is then rinsed in sterile water (often followed by alcohol) and dried and stored in a manner that avoids external contamination. Accessories are usually discarded after use or sterilized. Nurses can assure that consistent, appropriate processing is accomplished between uses with all patients.

Outbreaks have occurred as a consequence of inappropriate cleaning or disinfection.[2] One outbreak was associated with older-model endoscopes that had channels with no outlet, which made cleaning very difficult. When these blind channels became contaminated with organisms, the high-level disinfectant could not penetrate and disinfect, consequently, the organisms were transmitted to subsequent patients. Even if these endoscopes had been sterilized with ethylene oxide gas, organisms could have survived because residual organic matter would likely have been too dense to be penetrated by the gas. The outbreaks were terminated when channels were cleaned adequately. Manufacturers have ceased to produce endoscopes with blind channels.

Other outbreaks have been associated with inadequate cleaning, poorly designed automatic cleaning machines that became contaminated, and inappropriate use of the high-level disinfectant.[46] When appropriate procedures for endoscope cleaning, disinfection, and handling are carefully followed, risk of organism transmission occurs rarely.

Although endoscopes often undergo high-level disinfection, accessories that penetrate normally sterile tissues and that can withstand high-temperature processing (e.g., forceps) should be sterilized. Inadequate sterilization of forceps has been associated with transmission of organisms and infection.[34]

Permanently implantable devices

Many devices, such as cardiac pacemakers and valves, orthopedic prostheses, pins and rods, drainage devices, and vascular access devices, are permanently implanted into patients. These devices are made of materials that are as physiologically inert as possible to minimize the patient's immune response to the device. However, the long-term risks associated with many of these devices, including infections, are still being evaluated.

The infection risks associated with implantable devices continue for as long as the device is in place.[49,57] Practices to decrease infection risk associated with device insertion have had varied success. Strict sterile and aseptic technique during surgery is critical. Careful handling and sterilization of the implantable object, including placement of a biologic monitoring device in each sterilizer load containing implantables, is standard practice.[8] Holding the devices until test results are known is recommended but rarely done. Operating rooms with laminar air ventilation have been advocated as important for orthopedic prosthetic surgery, but studies have failed to show a consistent benefit.[49] Attention to equipment and instrument selection and processing can minimize risk of infections following procedures. Careful monitoring by nurses of signs and symptoms among individuals with permanently implanted devices can expedite early recognition and treatment of infections that might ultimately seed and infect an implanted device. This can occur within a few weeks or months after an implant.

Health care environment
Validation of patient care practices

The evaluation of efficacy of infection prevention strategies and safety of medical devices is incomplete. Some strategies have been repeatedly evaluated with conflicting results; others are used despite the absence of any rigorous testing. Infection precautions implemented to prevent organism transmission from the infected patient to others formed the rationale for isolation techniques. This strategy began as a public health measure to quarantine infectious persons from others and was adopted by hospitals and other health care settings. However, a major shift in strategy has occurred over the past decade. The new strategy advocates the use of barrier techniques when handling all body substances of all patients, regardless of diagnosis (see Chapter 6). Several examples below illustrate the importance of validating patient care practices—protective isolation, wound care, urinary catheter care, and visitor restrictions.

Protective isolation

Protective or reverse isolation was introduced in 1970 by the Center for Disease Control in the manual *Isolation Techniques for Use in Hospitals*. Unlike other barrier precaution strategies, protective isolation was developed to protect the very susceptible patient from exogenous organisms, both from other people and from the environment.

However, some research[50] has shown that such protective isolation does not prevent nosocomial acquisition of microorganisms or infections and that a majority of infections in immunocompromised patients originate from their own flora. Though many facilities have discontinued use of protective isolation as a result of these findings, modifications of protective precautions are still practiced. Except for the situation of the highly immunosuppressed bone marrow transplant recipient, few of these modifications have been validated by well-controlled research studies.[50]

Urinary catheter care

The high frequency of UTIc has prompted use of many procedures intended to prevent these infections. Meatal care using an antiseptic when an indwelling urethral catheter is in place has been investigated. Standard care of the patient with an indwelling urinary catheter used to include rigorous cleansing of the meatus with an antiseptic solution several times each day, but this practice was found to be unwarranted.[5] In fact, this rigorous routine actually increased the risk of infection for some patients. Daily cleansing with soap and water and cleansing after fecal soiling was found to be preferable to more intensive antiseptic care and manipulation.

Visitors

The relationship between restricted visiting and risk of infection is controversial and varies according to the circumstances. Visitors can be colonized or infected with microorganisms that can be transmitted within the care setting. However, this risk may be more perceived than real, since visitors have rarely been implicated in significant spread of disease. Visitors are not likely to present a greater risk to the patient than do the health care staff, provided clinically ill individuals and those who know they have been exposed to communicable infections refrain from visiting and any visitors who participate in care maintain appropriate hygiene. Visitors are vital to the patient's recovery, providing psychologic and often physical support. Nurses can teach visitors about handwashing and use of protective barrier techniques and can assess visitors for active infection. Most visitors do not want to cause harm to any patient and are cooperative.

Patients may pose risk of infection to visitors as well as to health care staff. When the patient's infection is communicable, particularly by the airborne route, visitors must be carefully managed. This will include consideration of the nature of the visitor's previous exposure, immune status, duration of the patient's communicability, and necessity for the visitor to see the patient.

Pets

Pets can provide valuable psychologic support to some patients. However, pet visitation is controversial. Patients who are hospitalized for an extended period may request a visit by their pet. Some facilities maintain shared pets or have formal pet visitation programs. The risk to other patients from these visits appears to be very low if reasonable precautions are taken, and there may be a definite psychologic benefit to the patient. Methodical, clear policies and procedures that assign care and responsibilities, define specific hygiene and management steps, and outline visitation guidelines can assist in safe management of these pets on an individual patient, unit, or facility basis. Support groups can assist health care providers with pet management issues.

Patient care practices are continually evaluated and changed to increase efficacy and improve the quality of care. Appendix A provides addresses of various professional and governmental organizations that publish infection prevention and control recommendations.

INFLUENCE OF SETTING ON PATIENT CARE PRACTICES

Patient care practices and management of devices in hospitals, extended care facilities, day-care and home health settings, ambulatory care clinics, and facilities in the midst of social disruption or severe economic deprivation present challenges unique to each setting. These challenges include limited staffing, limited budgets, and shortages of health care products. Patient care practice must balance patient and staff safety and effectiveness against the practical need to expedite care. Day-care and extended-care facilities should educate staff regarding essential infection control practices, such as handwashing, barrier use, and food service. Alternative methods may be developed to maintain appropriate standards of care depending on the setting. For example, though personnel are to wash their hands after diapering each child, many facilities do not have adequate sinks and cannot afford to have one installed in the diapering area. In these instances, a waterless hand degermer can be used as a substitute for handwashing.

The long-term care setting presents unique requirements. For example, linens are often heavily soiled with body substances such as urine and feces. Prerinsing linens by hand should be avoided to prevent exposure of staff to body substances. If funds to purchase large industrial washing machines that will prerinse linens are not available, prerinsing practices that incorporate use of protective equipment such as gloves, gowns, and face protection are necessary to prevent exposure of workers to body substances.

Management of urinary drainage can be a challenge in rehabilitation and extended-care facilities. Many patients in these facilities must have indwelling urine drainage catheters. For aesthetic reasons, many patients do not wish to use the usual drainage bags during the day because they cannot be concealed beneath clothing. Despite the risk of infection inherent in disrupting the closed system, a leg bag, which can be concealed, is often used during the day. Though not based on controlled studies demonstrating prevention of infection, routine care in some settings includes routine replacement of down-drain and leg bags. When economics requires, these bags can be decontaminated and reused rather than replaced.[15a,25] Thus, safe care may be provided and costs managed.

Transmission of microorganisms between patients is usually not a problem in home care as long as basic infection control practices, such as handwashing, and appropriate equipment cleaning and waste disposal are used by home care providers. Most home care–associated infections are related to devices and involve the patient's endogenous flora.[73] Consequently, practices and procedures designed to decrease device-related risks and inoculation of endogenous flora into sterile sites are important. Use of personal protective equipment and practices that protect the care provider from exposure to blood or body substances, such as gloves and appropriate sharps management, should be carefully integrated into care routines.

Various home care practices are applied widely but have not been studied to validate safety. For example, intermittent urinary catheterization has been performed with a reusable catheter and clean rather than sterile technique.[62] The catheter can be cleaned and dried thoroughly (e.g., in a microwave oven) between uses rather than sterilized. Frequent wound care with clean technique has been used in the home to prevent infection.

IV catheter care practices should vary little among inpatient, outpatient, and home care.[62] Peripheral, central, and peripherally placed central venous catheters have all been studied in the home setting.[24] However, the frequency of flushing of long-term cannulae may be decreased because the line is accessed less frequently in the home setting. There is a need for additional research into practices and outcomes in the home and comparison with those in the hospital if safe cost-effective practices are to be identified and standardized.

Social, political, and economic instabilities present significant challenges to safe patient care. Shortages of basic items, such as sterile needles, syringes, and gloves, require methodically implemented alternative strategies. For example, cleaning and reuse of the needle and syringe by the same patient, may decrease the risk of cross-infection and minimize supply requirements. Some persons with diabetes reuse their needles and syringes for a period. These are examples of problem solving that balances risk and benefit under stress.

SUMMARY

The risk of infection can be minimized if a patient's normal defenses are maximized and external compromises avoided. The infectious agent may be controlled or eliminated by proper management of the physical environment, including appropriate cleaning, disinfection, or sterilization of devices and instruments. The host's natural defenses are preserved when invasive devices are only used when absolutely necessary.

Not all practices and devices intended to decrease the risk of infection are effective. Many of these practices were instituted during outbreaks, were associated with termination of the outbreak, and consequently integrated into standard practice. Validation of each practice and device is important if patient care is to be efficient and effective. Nurses have a major role to play in studies that will guide changes in patient care practice standards. They are key participants in the investigations and decisions that refine and implement methods to decrease infection risks to patients and themselves. Patient care must be individualized so that the patient's characteristics are accommodated by health care practices that balance risks and benefits and incorporate standards intended to protect the patient (e.g., Medicare requirements) and health care providers (e.g., OSHA regulations).

REFERENCES

1. Alter MJ, et al. Reuse of hemodialyzers: results of nationwide surveillance for adverse reactions. *JAMA.* 1988;260:2073-2076.
2. Alvarado CJ, et al. Nosocomial infection and pseudo-infection from contaminated endoscopes and bronchoscopes. *MMWR.* 1991; 40(39):675-678.
3. Beck-Sague CM, Jarvis WR. Epidemic bloodstream infections associated with pressure transducers: a persistent problem. *Infect Control Hosp Epidemiol.* 1989;10(2):54-49.
4. Beck-Sague C, et al. Outbreak of gram-negative bacteremia and pyrogenic reactions in a hemodialysis center. *Am J Nephrol.* 1990;10:397-403.
5. Burke JP, et al. Prevention of catheter-associated urinary tract infections: efficacy of daily meatal care regimens. *Am J Med.* 1981;70:655-658.
6. Caplan ES, Hoyt NJ. Nosocomial sinusitis. *JAMA.* 1982;247:639-641.
7. Centers for Disease Control. Nosocomial infection rates for inter-hospital comparison: limitations and possible solutions: a report from the National Nosocomial Infections Surveillance System. *Infect Control Hosp Epidemiol.* 1991;12:609-621.
8. Centers for Disease Control. *Cleaning, Disinfection and Sterilization of Hospital Equipment: Guidelines for Hospital Environmental Control.* US Department of Health and Human Services, Public Health Department, 1982;1-6.
9. Centers for Disease Control. *Guideline for Prevention of Nosocomial Pneumonia.* US Department of Health and Human Services, Public Health Department; 1982;1-9.
10. Centers for Disease Control. *Guideline for Prevention of Intravascular Infections.* US Department of Health and Human Services, Public Health Department 1981;1-6.

11. Conly JM, Grieves K, Peters B. A prospective randomized study comparing transparent and dry gauze dressings for central venous catheters. *J Infect Dis.* 1989;159:310-319.

12. Craven DE, Steger KA. Nosocomial pneumonia in the intubated patient: new concepts on pathogenesis and prevention. *Infect Dis Clin N Amer.* 1989;3(4):843-866.

13. Craven DE, Steger KA, Duncan RA. Prevention and control of nosocomial pneumonia. In: Wenzl Rp, ed. *Prevention and Control of Hospital Infections*, ed 2. Baltimore: Williams & Wilkins; 1993;556-579.

14. Daifuku R, Stamm WE. Association of rectal and urethral colonization with urinary tract infection in patients with indwelling catheters. *JAMA.* 1984;252:2028-2030.

15. Detsky AS, Smalley PS, Chang J. Is this patient malnourished? *JAMA.* 1994;271:54-58.

15a. Dille CM, Kirchhoff KT. Decontamination of Vinyl Urinary Drainage Bags with Bleach. *Rehabilitation Nursing.* 1993;18:292-295.

16. Farber BF. The multi-lumen catheter: proposed guidelines for its use. *Infect Control Hosp Epidemiol.* 1988;9(5):206-208.

17. Farkas JC, et al. Single-versus triple-lumen central catheter-hyphen related sepsis: a prospective, randomized study in a critically ill population. *Am J Med.* 1992;93:277-282.

18. Favero MS, Alter JM, Bland LA. Dialysis-associated infections and their control. In Bennett JV, Brachman PS, eds: *Hospital Infections*, ed 3. Boston: Little, Brown; 1992;375-404.

19. Fedson D. Immunization for health-care workers and patients in hospitals. In Wenzel RP, ed. *Prevention and Control of Hospital Infections*, ed 2. Baltimore: Williams & Wilkins; 1993;214-294.

20. Garibaldi RA. Hospital-acquired urinary tract infections. In: Wenzel RP, ed. *Prevention and Control of Hospital Infections*, ed 2. Baltimore: Williams & Wilkins; 1993:600-613.

21. George DL. Epidemiology of nosocomial ventilator-associated pneumonia. *Infect Control Hosp Epidemiol.* 1993;14:163-169.

22. Goldmann DA, Pier GB: Pathogenesis of infections related to intravascular catheterization. *Clin Microbiol Rev.* 1993;6(2):176-192.

23. Gorse GJ, Messner RL, Stephens ND. Association of malnutrition with nosocomial infection. *Infect Control Hosp Epidemiol.* 1989;10(5):194-203.

24. Graham DR, et al. Infectious complications among patients receiving home intravenous therapy with peripheral, central, or peripherally placed central venous catheter. *Am J Med* 1991;91(suppl3B):95-100.

25. Hashisaki PA, et al. Decontamination of urinary bags for rehabilitation patients. *Arch Phys Med Rehabil.* 1984;65:474-476.

26. Hirsch DD, Fainstein V, Musher DM. Do condom catheter collecting systems cause urinary tract infections? *JAMA.* 1979;242:340-341.

27. Hoffman KK, et al. Transparent polyurethane film as an intravenous catheter dression: a meta-analysis of the infection risks. *JAMA.* 1992;267(15):2072-2076.

28. Intravenous Nurses Society. Intravenous Nursing Standards of Practice. *Journal of Intravenous Nursing.* Supplement 1990;S1-S95.

29. Irvine R, Johnson Jr L, Amstutz HC. The relationship of genitourinary tract procedures and deep sepsis after total hip replacement. *Surg Gynecol Obstet.* 1974;139:701-706.

30. Johnson ET. The condom catheter: urinary tract infection and other complications. *South J Med.* 1983;76:579-582.

31. Kellegham SI, et al. An effective continuous quality improvement approach to the prevention of ventilator-associated pneumonia. *Am J Infect Control.* 1993;21:322-330.

32. Kunin CM. Care of the urinary catheter. In: Kunin CM, ed. *Detection, Prevention and Management of Urinary Tract Infections.* Philadelphia: Lea & Febiger; 1987;245-287.

33. Kunin CM, McCormack RC. Prevention of catheter-induced urinary-tract infections by closed drainage. *N Engl J Med.* 1966;274:1155-1161.

34. Langenberg W, et al. Patient to patient transmission of *Campylobacter pylori* infection by fiberoptic gastroduodenoscopy and biopsy. *J Infect Dis.* 1990;161:507-511.

35. Lapides J, et al. Follow-up on unsterile intermittent self-catheterization. *J Urol.* 1974;111:184-187.

36. Le Frock J, et al. Transient bacteremia associated with sigmoidoscopy. *N Engl J Med.* 1973;289:467-469.

37. Logan RM, Hastings JGM. Bacterial endocarditis: a complication of gastroscopy. *BMJ.* 1988;296:1107.

38. Lowrey PW, et al. Mycobacterium chelonei infection among patients receiving high-flux dialysis in a hemodialysis clinic in California. *J Infect Dis.* 1990;161:85-90.

39. Maki DG. Infection due to infusion therapy. In: Bennett JV, Brachman PS, editors: *Hospital infections*, ed 3. Boston, 1992, Little, Brown. 849-898.

40. Maki DG, Band JD. Comparative study of polyantibiotic and iodophor ointments in prevention of vascular catheter-related infection. *Am J Med.* 1981;70:739-744.

41. Maki DG, et al. Nationwide epidemic of septicemia caused by contaminated intravenous products. *Am J Med.* 1976;60:471.

42. Maki DG, Ringer M. Risk factors for infusion-related phlebitis with small peripheral venous catheters. *Ann Intern Med.* 1991;14(10):845-848.

43. Maki DG, Ringer M. Evaluation of dressing regimes

for prevention of infection with peripheral intravenous catheters. *JAMA*. 1987;258(17):2396-2403.

44. Maki DG, Ringer M, Alvarado CJ. Prospective randomized trial of povidone iodine, alcohol, and chlorhexidine gluconate for prevention of infection associated with central venous and arterial catheters. *Lancet* 338:339-343, 1991.

45. Maki DG, Will L. Risk factors for central venous catheter-related infection in the ICU: a prospective study of 345 catheters. Abstract presented at the Third International Conference on Nosocomial Infections; August 2, 1991; Atlanta, GA.

46. Martin MA, Reichelderfer M. Apic guideline for infection prevention and control in flexible endoscopy. *Am J Infect Control*. 1994; 22:19-38.

47. Mellow MH, Lewis RJ. Endoscopy-related bacteremia: incidence of positive blood cultures after endoscopy of the upper gastrointestinal tract. *Arch Intern Med* 1976;136:667-669

48. Mermel LA, et al. The pathogenesis and epidemiology of catheter-related infection with pulmonary artery swan-ganz: a prospective study using molecular subtyping. *Am J Med* 1991;91(suppl 3B): 197-205.

49. Moggio M, Goldner L, McCollum D, Deissinger S. Wound infections in patients undergoing total hip arthroplasty. *Arch Surg*. 1979;114:815-823.

50. Nauseef WM, Maki DG. Study of the value of simple protective isolation in patients with granulocytopenia. *N Engl J Med*. 1981;304(8):448-453.

51. Occupational Safety and Health Administration. Occupational Exposure to Bloodborne Pathogens; Final Rule. *Federal Register*. 1991;56(235):64004-182.

51a. Raad II, et al. Prevention of central venous catheter-related infections by using maximal sterile barrier precautions during insertion. *Infect Control Hosp Epidemiol*. 1994;15(4 part 1):231-38.

52. Ouslander JG, Greengold B, Chen S. External catheter use and urinary tract infections among incontinent male nursing home patients. *J Am Ger Soc* 1987; 35:1063-1070.

53. Platt R, et al. Reduction of mortality associated with nosocomial urinary tract infection. *Lancet* 1983;1: 1893-7.

54. Platt R, et al. Mortality associated with nosocomial urinary tract infection. *N Engl J Med* 1982;307:637-642.

55. Richet M, et al. Prospective multicenter study of vascular-catheter related complications and risk factors for positive central catheter cultures in intensive care patients. *J Clin Microbiol*. 1990;28(11):2520-2525.

56. Sanderson PJ. The sources of pneumonia in ITU patients. *Infect Control*. 1986;7(2):104.

57. Saravolatz LD. Infection in implantable prosthetic devices. In: Wenzel RP, ed. *Prevention and control of nosocomial infections*, 2nd ed. Baltimore: Williams & Wilkins, 1993:683-707.

58. Scrimshaw NS. Malnutrition and nosocomial infection. *Infect Control Hosp Epidemiol*. 1989;10(5):192-193.

59. Shapiro M, et. al. A multivariate analysis of risk factors for acquiring bacteriuria in patients with indwelling urinary catheters for longer than 24 hours. *Infect Control* 1984;5(11):525-532.

60. Shivnan JC, et al. A comparison of transparent adherent and dry sterile gauze dressings for long-term central catheters in patients undergoing bone marrow transplant. *Oncol Nurs Forum* Nov-Dec;18:1349-56, 1991.

61. Simmons B. Guideline for prevention of intravascular infections. Atlanta, GA: Centers for Disease Control, 1981.

62. Simmons B, et al. Infection Control for Home Health. *Infect Control Hosp Epidemiol*. 1990;11:362.

63. Spach DH, Silverstein FE, Stamm WE. Transmission of infection by gastrointestinal endoscopy. *Ann Intern Med* 1993;118:117-128.

64. Stamm WE. Nosocomial urinary tract infections. In: Bennett JV, Brachman PS, eds. *Hospital Infections*, ed 3. Boston: Little, Brown; 1992;597-610.

65. Stamm WE. Catheter-associated urinary tract infection: epidemiology, pathogenesis, and prevention. *Am J Med*. 1991;91(suppl3B):65-71.

66. Stamm WE, et al. Urinary tract infections from pathogenesis to treatment. *J Infect Dis*. 1989;159:400-406.

67. Stamm WE. Infections due to medical devices. *Ann Intern Med*. 1978;89(pt2):764.

68. Stark RP, Maki DG. Bacteriuria in the catheterized patient: what level of bacteriuria is quantitatively relevant? *N Engl J Med*. 1984;311:560-564.

69. Syndman DR, et al. Intravenous tubing containing burettes can be safely changed at 72-hour intervals. *Infect Control*. 1987;8(3):113-116.

70. Warren JW. Catheter-associated urinary tract infections. *Infect Dis Clin North Am*. 1987;1:823-855.

71. Warren JW, et al. A prospective microbiologic study of bacteriuria in patients with chronic indwelling urethral catheters. *J Infect Dis*. 1982;146:719-723.

72. Weinstein RA. Other procedure-related infections. In Bennett JV, Brachman PS, eds. *Hospital Infections*, 3rd ed. Boston: Little, Brown; 1992;923-946.

73. White MC. Infections and infection risks in home care settings. *Infect Control Hosp Epidemiol*. 1992;13:535-539.

Chapter 6

Barrier Precautions and Personal Protection

PATRICIA LYNCH

The practices . . . represent an effort to make man's laws approximate the laws of nature, and when nature's laws are not well understood, man's rules are likely to be more or less irrational and their observance vacillating and ritualistic.[37]

Julius Roth, a sociologist, made this observation in the 1950s after experiencing the variation in caregivers' attitudes about the isolation practices used for him and other tuberculosis patients in a sanitarium where he received care. The role of rituals in the isolation practices used to "prevent" transmission of tuberculosis was obvious to him. Personnel did not understand how *Mycobacterium tuberculosis* was transmitted or how to prevent transmission to themselves, visitors, or other patients. As a result they frequently used ineffective practices and failed to use effective ones.

Ritualistic behavior has been used in an attempt to prevent the transmission of infectious organisms since the contagious nature of some diseases was recognized. It exists today to some extent in every community, family, and health care facility. Ritualistic behavior persists when we do not understand the laws of nature, that is, how disease transmission occurs.

Well-designed studies to evaluate specific elements of infection prevention practices have been performed only recently. The common use of certain practices despite the lack of studies to support their use is puzzling. Isolation precautions are expensive and play a major role in infection prevention and control programs in health care. However, the efficacy of many of these strategies has not been evaluated or is not supported by a reasonable theoretic framework.

For example, hospital personnel typically wear special gowns, masks, and gloves when caring for patients who have measles or chickenpox. In reality, people who have had these diseases or have been vaccinated are immune and have no need for additional protection. Furthermore, gowns, surgical masks, and gloves do not prevent transmission of airborne microorganisms to susceptible care providers and serve no useful purpose. Ineffective use of special clothing frequently occurs when the patient's infection is caused by a potentially airborne organism or when the patient has a particularly frightening or fatal disease. For example, when patients with human immunodeficiency virus (HIV) disease or acquired immunodeficiency syndrome (AIDS) are hospitalized, some facilities not only require staff to dress up but also require the patient's visiting friends, partner, and family to do so despite evidence that special clothing has no effect on organism transmission.

Some infection prevention practices are valuable but inadequately used. For example, when patients leave the hospital with open wounds, dressings, or indwelling drains or devices, the staff may not instruct family members to use aseptic technique and wear gloves for dressing changes because the staff believe these infection prevention methods are not necessary in the home setting or because the site is already infected. Thus the patient is at risk for acquiring new organisms at the site, and the person manipulating the wound is at risk for exposure to any microorganism present.

In the past, most barrier precautions were used only when patients' infections were diagnosed. These precautions made up the isolation system. That narrow focus has changed as it has become clear that precaution strategies must address these facts: (1) most infectious agents are transmitted by contact with the body substances that contain them and (2) most infections are communicable for some period when symptoms are absent and the infection is undetected. This chapter discusses personal protection, including the supplies and barrier precautions used to reduce infection risk for all patients and personnel, and the occupational health practices to protect health care staff from infection.

BARRIER PRECAUTIONS AND HOST-ENVIRONMENT INTERACTIONS

Barrier precautions are intended to modify the physical environment and affect the social and microbiologic environments for the benefit of potential hosts and caregivers.

The host

Depending on perspective, the host may be an individual, several people, or an entire community. A parent might focus on his or her child's risk of infection, a surgeon on his or her patients, an infection control professional on all the patients and personnel in the hospital or long-term care facility, or the public health officer on the entire county's population. The host's susceptibility to a particular infectious agent may be increased by such factors as lack of immunologic experience with the microbiologic agents, the number and severity of nonspecific compromises of the immune system (e.g., malnutrition, neutropenia), and the presence of indwelling medical devices (see Chapters 1 and 5). Some hosts have diseases that affect specific immune responses, which increase their risk for other infectious diseases. For example, persons with HIV infection are more likely to develop *Pneumocystis carinii* pneumonia than HIV-negative people.

In general, biologic alteration of host immunity with vaccine and immune globulin is very successful. With time, malnutrition and other host conditions may be overcome, but the strategies are cumbersome and complex and must be supplemented by manipulation of the physical environment to reduce infection risk.

The microbiologic environment

The number and type of organisms available to the host influence infection risk. The risk increases when a large dose of organisms can be delivered, when the dose of organisms required to establish infection is small, when the duration of contact between the host and the organisms is sufficient, and when the organism reaches a favorable site.

Microorganisms are abundant at all moist body sites and in moist body substances. The organisms live on or in the host, usually causing no harm and possibly even performing a useful function. These organisms are collectively called the *normal flora* and are remarkably similar, although not necessarily identical, from person to person.

If conditions at a particular body site change, resulting in an ecologic shift, organisms that are part of the normal flora may produce disease. For example, the normal flora of about one third of all people includes *Staphylococcus aureus*. Many more persons occasionally have this organism in their nasal and upper airway secretions without symptomatic infection. However, some develop staphylococcal pneumonia after viral respiratory infection, aspiration, or other disruption. Although antimicrobial therapy may successfully treat the pneumonia, the organism is likely to remain or return as part of the normal flora.

Organisms that are relatively avirulent and constitute the normal flora for one individual may produce serious infection when introduced into another person. For example, if the normal upper airway flora of methicillin-sensitive or methicillin-resistant *S. aureus* is transferred from one person to another, infection may result. The range of organisms that may successfully infect an individual is related to the individual's immune competence. Among severely compromised patients, virtually any organism can produce infection when introduced in sufficient numbers to susceptible sites. Consequently, no organism should be considered uniformly noninfectious or nonpathogenic.

It is difficult to determine whether an organism newly isolated from a given patient has been transferred from other patients or care providers or whether the organism has merely emerged, having been present but undetected. Moist body sites (e.g., mucous membranes, nonintact skin) and moist substances (e.g., airway secretions, lesion drainage, feces, urine from catheterized patients) should always be assumed to contain organisms. Many of these organisms may be the same species. Thus, sensitive and sophisticated laboratory tests, such as molecular biotyping methods, must be used to identify related subspecies (strains) within microbial populations particularly in an attempt to establish that two or more organisms have originated from a common source.

Transfer of organisms between patients and personnel may be common and clinically significant. One investigator found that almost 25% of all patients on a hospital medical unit acquired *Clostridium difficile* during their hospital stay. In this study, the organism was cultured from the hands of most caregivers after one episode of care, even after handwashing.[31] These findings suggest that contamination of caregivers' hands may transmit the organism and, by extension, that use of barriers (i.e., gloves) during direct patient care, and their timely removal, may prevent disease.

The physical environment

Barrier precautions change the effect of the physical environment on infection risk. Placing a clean layer of plastic or fabric between a susceptible site and a potential source of organisms reduces the likelihood that the organisms will reach the site in sufficient numbers to cause infection. In contrast to the difficulty of changing a host's immunity, barrier precautions can be implemented rapidly and can target specific sites. When used correctly, this makes them effective tools for reducing infection risk.

The social environment

All places where people receive health care are social settings, including acute and long-term care facilities, medical and dental offices, public health agencies, free-standing surgical centers, and homes. Care providers use techniques and strategies that were modeled for them by their families, teachers, and other influential figures and that have often been practiced long enough to become ingrained habits. Habitual behavior leads to consistency but also to inflexibility, since most people do not like to change their behavior, particularly when they are convinced that it is correct.

Consistent use of barrier techniques in health care has been complicated by different training of practitioners in diverse health care settings and their tendency to practice as they always have unless the incentive to change is profound. This affects handwashing, wearing gloves, and other elements of barrier precautions and ultimately determines whether organisms are likely to be transferred among patients and personnel. For instance, an accepted behavior or social norm in a particular setting may be to put on clean gloves just before contact with mucous membranes or nonintact skin. If the institutional leaders support this technique and there is socially imposed pressure that this is the "right" action, that practice is more likely to occur. If it is acceptable to wear gloves from one patient to another and not to put on clean gloves just before contacts, that becomes the norm and increases risk for the patient.

PATIENT CARE PRACTICES AND PRECAUTION STRATEGIES

Handwashing

Handwashing is so important and so much a part of infection prevention efforts that no discussion would be complete without it. Many researchers have demonstrated that hands become soiled during patient care, especially when caregivers have contact with moist body sites and substances. Further, soiled hands have played a major role in transferring organisms to new patient hosts. Many outbreaks of nosocomial infections among patients in health care facilities[24] and babies in day-care centers,[39] have demonstrated the important role of hands in transferring organisms.

Studies have demonstrated that caregivers do not wash their hands frequently or thoroughly enough to remove surface organisms completely.[1] In fact, it may not be possible for caregivers in some settings to wash often enough; facilities may not be available, or their hands may become irritated and chapped. Also, some people resist handwashing, claiming they do not like to do it because it is too time-consuming, irritating to their skin, inconvenient, or they forget to do it.

Handwashing is primarily a mechanical activity. The hands are moistened, cleanser is applied, hands washed for 10 to 15 seconds, then rinsed and dried with a clean towel or air.

Extended wash times are used in special settings such as surgery. The process is best done with running water.

At a minimum, hands should be washed whenever they are likely to have been soiled and before beginning care for a new person. Handwashing preparations that contain antibacterial chemicals may reduce the number of organisms residing on the skin (normal flora) as well as transient contaminants. These products are often recommended for people who work in surgical settings, intensive care units (ICUs), and other places where indwelling medical devices are typically used. Handwashing preparations without antibacterial chemicals are as effective in removing soil and transient organisms from the skin, but they may not reduce the number of organisms residing on the skin.[12,25,29]

Waterless hand cleansers that contain an antibacterial agent (e.g., alcohol) and an emollient do not effectively remove soil (stains, mucous, etc.). Consequently, if the hands look soiled, they need to be washed using running water and friction. However, the waterless hand cleaners are excellent for use when personnel do not need to wash soil from their hands but do need to ensure that they are not transferring organisms from one place to another. Examples include taking blood pressures on a series of patients and turning them in bed.

Waterless hand cleansers also work well for caregivers who do not have access to running water, especially in crowded places with poor sanitation. Clinics in poverty areas, immunization programs in rural areas, and caregivers in older facilities that have rooms without running water all benefit from these products. They are commercially manufactured and packaged in some places but are produced and bottled in the care facility in other areas. For example, an alcohol and glycerin solution is inexpensive and easy to prepare. Hospital studies have not demonstrated that caregivers who resist handwashing will use the waterless products, but the convenience is certainly greater.

Mechanical handwashing devices use antibacterial preparations and water to produce a comfortable 10- to 15-second handwash. They increase convenience and cost but have not been demonstrated to increase handwashing frequency.

Personal protective barriers
Purpose of barriers

The risk of symptomatic infection results from the interplay of host factors, the dose of organisms delivered, infectivity of the organism, the microorganism's virulence, and the social and physical environmental factors that determine the duration and intimacy of the contact between host and organism. Infection risk is greatest when (1) the host is compromised; (2) the dose, infectivity, and virulence are high; and (3) the organism is in prolonged, intimate contact with the host. These interactions are graphically displayed in Figure 6-1.

Susceptibility to infection increases as a function of the severity of the host's underlying illness or immune compromise and the number and nature of invasive procedures and indwelling devices used in care. Although patients are receiving care more frequently in outpatient or long-term care settings, few studies have evaluated risk in these settings, and those that do often include too few patients to be representative. Therefore, most recommendations for infection prevention and control are based on studies of hospitalized patients. Deemphasis on hospital-based care will require methodical study of infection practices in all of the non–hospital care settings and focused study of the most ill patients.

Transmission is related to the amount and type of organisms present and to the circumstances of contact. Punctures or lacerations with sharp instruments (e.g., needles and scalpel blades) and open skin contacts are very efficient methods of delivering organisms. Mucous membrane and minor nonintact skin contacts are less efficient. When moist body substances (including blood) touch intact skin, the skin acts as a barrier, and there is less risk of transmission. Since the presence and concentration of microorganisms in any given patient's body substances can never be known, caregivers should always assume that every patient's moist body substances contain potentially infectious, transmissible organisms. For example, hepatitis B virus (HBV) may be present in the body substances of chronically infected individuals whose infection never produced symptoms and was never diagnosed. HIV may be present when evidence of infection is absent. Cytomegalovirus (CMV) can be shed in urine of asymptomatic individuals.

Barriers are intended to affect these relationships by preventing transfer of an infective dose of organisms to a susceptible site. The prevented transmission can be from patient to caregiver or caregiver to patient. Risk increases for patients when the caregivers have contact with the patients' mucous membranes and nonintact skin, including insertion sites for indwelling devices. Risk increases for caregivers whenever they are in contact with moist body substances.

Types and uses of barriers
Gloves

One infection control researcher described gloves as "The most wonderful invention! You can choose a sterile or clean layer of skin that can be peeled off and reapplied...."[2]

Gloves are made of various materials, including latex, vinyl, and hypoallergenic materials. Many are easily punctured by sharp devices such as needles and fingernails. Latex gloves generally are stronger and less likely to develop pinholes or tears than vinyl gloves and are less likely to have pinholes before use.[33]

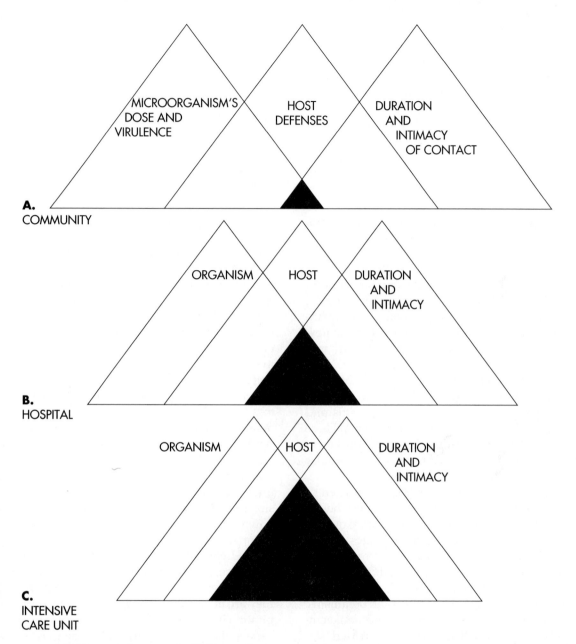

FIGURE 6-1. Infection risk *(black areas)* is greatest (1) when a person's host defenses are compromised, (2) when the microorganism's dose and virulence are increased, and (3) when the duration and intimacy of contact between host and organism is prolonged, a function of the physical and social environments. The risk of infection increases as the intersecting areas in each triangle increase. **A,** In the community, as illustrated by the darkened area, the overlap between the risk factors is small, indicating that infection risk is small. **B,** In the hospital, infection risk is increased as illness or injuries and indwelling devices compromise host defenses. **C,** In an intensive care unit, a person's host defenses are constantly compromised by illness and indwelling devices, making prolonged contact with microorganisms a typical occurrence.

Both latex and vinyl gloves deteriorate rapidly when exposed to chemicals such as those found in hand lotions, lubricants, detergents, disinfectants, and many laboratory reagents. These chemicals may cause the material to degrade and become permeable. Rewashing or disinfecting gloves for reuse is not recommended, except when the glove materials are particularly sturdy and adequate testing has confirmed that the gloves will withstand the reprocessing. In some settings, economics dictates that undamaged gloves be reused. They are washed, inspected for leaks, packaged, and sterilized by steam autoclave. Vinyl gloves are usually too flimsy to tolerate washing. Whether small glove leaks increase the risk of microorganism transmission to patients or caregivers outside the surgical setting is unclear.[33] Less contact with organisms should provide less risk of acquiring new flora, but whether that translates directly into lower infection risk is not known.

Well-designed studies have demonstrated that appropriate glove use can reduce the frequency of transmission of organisms and the incidence of infection in patients. These studies were performed in a variety of hospitals. It seems reasonable to expect similar results in other settings as well.

In one study, personnel were instructed to put on clean examination gloves just before touching patient's mucous membranes or nonintact skin, including insertion sites for indwelling devices.[29] Observers were hired to record compliance. As compliance with this gloving requirement increased, patient infection or colonization with marker organisms, such as *Serratia*, *Acinetobacter*, and amikacin-resistant gram-negative rods, decreased significantly.[29]

In another study the policies in a pediatric ICU required caregivers to put on clean gloves as previously described and wear a clean gown when in contact with patients.[23] The results suggested that these barriers provided protection (Table 6-1).

TABLE 6-1. Glove protection in pediatric intensive care unit

	Barrier use group	Control group
Average time to colonization	Day 12	Day 7
Proportion infected	2/32	12/38
Day of infection onset	Day 20	Day 8
Proportion of ICU days febrile	13%	23%

From Klein BS, Perloff WH, Maki DG: *N Engl J Med* 320:1714-1721, 1989.

Other researchers attempted to control an outbreak of *Clostridium difficile* diarrhea among patients.[22] The incidence of nosocomial *C. difficile* diarrhea was monitored for 6 months before and after an intensive program involving posters, education, and reminders for personnel on two wards who were instructed to wear vinyl gloves for contact with any moist body substances. The incidence of nosocomial *C. difficile* diarrhea decreased from 7.7 per 1000 to 1.5 per 1000 discharges. A pediatric study demonstrated decreased transmission of respiratory syncytial virus (RSV) when caregivers wore clean gloves and cover gowns to care for infants and toddlers. The investigators attributed the resulting decrease in RSV transmission to appropriate glove use rather than to the gowns.[26]

Some infection control experts have expressed concern that indiscriminate glove use will increase costs and the incidence of nosocomial infections instead of preventing them if they are not removed or changed when appropriate. This is a distinct possibility if caregivers believe that the only purpose for the gloves is to protect them from contact with moist body substances. However, the studies mentioned point out that nosocomial infections can be substantially reduced when gloves are used appropriately.

Guidelines for glove use follow:
1. Select gloves that are appropriate for the

procedure or task. Examination, surgical, or utility gloves may be used.

2. Wear appropriate gloves for anticipated contact with all moist body substances.
3. Use examination gloves that are clean at the time of use for contact with mucous membranes and nonintact skin sites that do not involve sterile tissue.
4. Wear sterile gloves for all procedures involving contact with normally sterile tissue.
5. Change gloves before moving to a new body site that requires use of sterile or clean gloves.
6. Wear gloves for phlebotomy and other situations that might result in puncture with a used sharp. One study has shown that a significant proportion of infectious particles will be removed by the glove when it is penetrated by a contaminated sharp.
7. Use double gloves for procedures involving sharp tools and bloody tissue. Two layers of glove reduce penetration of blood and contact with the wearer's skin.[14]
8. Remove gloves and discard after use. Kitchen or utility gloves are sturdy enough to be washed many times, and it is safe to do so as long as the gloves are not cracked or disintegrating.
9. Avoid reprocessing gloves if possible.

Masks

Surgical masks are designed to trap droplets from the wearer's exhaled breath and to prevent them from falling directly on the patient and to prevent splashes or droplets from reaching the wearer's facial mucous membranes or covered skin. Masks may be flat or molded in a cone shape. Flimsy tissue paper masks do not provide significant filtration or prevent droplets from soaking through.

Recently, both patients and caregivers have become more concerned about masks' ability to provide protection from airborne communicable microorganisms and aerosols such as tuberculosis. Aerosols are liquid or solid particles that remain suspended in air, unlike large-particle droplets that tend to fall rapidly, such as those generated by a sneeze.

Many people assume that surgical masks filter out bacteria and viruses, but this is not supported by research. Tuberculosis, measles, and chickenpox have all been transmitted to susceptible caregivers who wore surgical masks to care for patients with these diseases. Surgical masks do not filter tiny particles the size of viruses or tubercule bacilli from ambient air and they do not fit the face tightly enough to prevent the movement of air around the mask. The efficiency of air filtration, resistance to fluid saturation, and the tightness of the mask-face seal vary considerably, depending on the mask selected.[6]

When masks are worn to protect the caregiver from splatter of droplets, eyewear such as glasses or goggles are also necessary to protect the eyes. Plastic face shields that cover all the facial mucous membranes can be used as well. The U.S. Occupational Safety and Health Administration (OSHA) requires employers to supply and enforce use of facial protection whenever risk of splattering of body substances known to transmit HIV and HBV is likely. The employed caregivers must wear these barriers.[32]

Masks that protect against airborne transmission of microorganisms and laser plumes have been developed recently. Laser procedures produce plumes of smoke and debris from cell vaporization that contain fine particles of blood. The plume may be suspended in air and remain there for a long time and may contain infectious agents such as hepatitis B and C viruses, HIV, and human papillomavirus (HPV). Transmission of these organisms via this plume is theoretically possible.

The incidence of TB has increased worldwide and in the United States over the past decade[7] (see Clinical Study No. 7). Persons in families, hospitals, nursing homes, and jails have acquired TB because of inadequate infection control measures. The organisms' increased drug resistance prompts greater attention to engineering controls, personal protective equipment, and patient care practices that will reduce risk.

Respirators are recommended by the Centers for Disease Control and Prevention (CDC) for use when exposure to laser plumes or patients with infectious tuberculosis is anticipated.[4] These may be reusable or disposable. Respirators generally resemble surgical masks but are thicker and have a tighter face seal; breathing through one of these is more difficult than through a surgical mask. They are also more costly than surgical masks. It is not known whether the personal respirators actually reduce infection risk, but the size of particles that these masks can filter (1 to 5 μ) suggests that they may be effective. Routinely used surgical masks clearly are not effective.

The general rules for mask use follow:

1. Wear surgical masks to protect patients in surgical settings and anytime it is important to have a physical barrier between the droplets of caregivers and potentially susceptible patient sites (e.g., wounds, central line sites during insertion) and during performance of other invasive procedures, including dental work. These masks should be changed when wet or soiled to maintain their performance as filters because most mask materials decrease in effectiveness when wet. Discard after use.
2. Wear a surgical mask combined with eyewear or face shield to protect the facial mucous membranes and skin from splatter of moist body substances.
3. Wear respirator–type masks when caring for patients suspected or confirmed to have infectious TB. These are more expensive than surgical masks and do not deteriorate when worn for long periods.

The reusable masks may be used by the same person for at least 8 hours under normal conditions and unlike surgical masks can be taken off and put back on repeatedly.

Protective attire

Cover gowns of woven or nonwoven fabrics, plastic aprons, and laboratory coats are the protective attire most often used. Clothing is unlikely to play a major role in transmission of infectious microorganisms. Since a significant dose of organisms is almost impossible to transfer from clothing to a susceptible site on patients, except to children who are held or carried, attire is primarily intended to protect caregivers' clothing and skin from moist body substances. Protective attire does not play a role in preventing transmission of airborne communicable microorganisms that must be inhaled by the host. In two studies, use of cover gowns, caps, and masks in neonatal and pediatric intensive care units failed to decrease the rates of bacterial colonization or infections or to increase handwashing.[11,16] Except for these and the studies by Klein[23] and by LeClair,[26] protective attire has not been well studied. Soiled clothing should be covered or changed for aesthetic reasons and to prevent contamination of hands and devices used for invasive procedures.

Attire is important in surgical and other settings where large quantities of bloody fluids may soak through clothing and contact the skin of personnel. Several studies of disposable and reusable cover gowns have demonstrated that some fabrics are quite fluid resistant and others are not.[27] Intact plastic is very fluid resistant but tends to retain moisture and become uncomfortable when worn for long periods. However, it is excellent material for panels on gowns made of other fabrics. Certain nonwoven fabrics are also fluid resistant but are almost as hot and sticky as plastic. Some woven fabrics are reusable, fluid resistant, and comfortable. These fabrics withstand washing well, and when personnel laundering and disposal costs are considered, they may provide good protection at less cost than disposable gowns.

Selection of attire must be guided by the task to be performed. It is unacceptable for caregivers' skin or clothing to be in contact with moist body substances. When this occurs, it is a clear signal that caregivers underestimated their need for protective attire. On the other hand, it is unnecessarily expensive for caregivers to wear surgical-type fluid-resistant gowns to protect against minor spatter. Psychologic overdependence on special attire is costly and misleading.

Cover gowns' major role for years as part of isolation strategy reflects caregivers' fear of and lack of knowledge about transmission of organisms. One author reported that many nurses interviewed about their use of gowns when caring for AIDS patients said that they "felt safer" when gowned.[17] Infection prevention emphasis and resources should be directed toward prevention of contact with body substances and control of airflow when airborne pathogens are suspected.

Hair and shoe covers

Hair covers and shoe or leg covers are sometimes indicated in addition to gowns or aprons. Care providers should wear hair covers to protect the patient whenever hair is likely to fall onto patient wounds or open skin. Hair covers of plastic or fabric and leg or shoe covers of plastic and nonwoven fabric protect the wearer from contact with body substances. Surgical procedures that generate large quantities of blood or bloody irrigating fluid, trauma surgery, burn debridement, some urologic and orthopedic procedures, and some obstetric deliveries are examples of procedures that may require leg or shoe protection. The thin-fabric shoe covers traditionally worn during surgery do not reduce

risk of transmission of infectious agents to patients or personnel. Many operating rooms are discontinuing their use.

Protective eyewear

Glasses with side shields, goggles, and face shields keep spatter from the eyes. Many caregivers purchase their own eyewear to ensure fit, comfort, and optimal optical quality consistent with their personal needs. Eye protection must be provided by the employer to meet OSHA requirements.

General rules for attire

1. Wear a cover gown or apron suitable for the type and amount of body substances likely to be encountered during a particular task. Attire should cover the skin and clothing, prevent fluids from soaking through, and keep clothing and skin clean.
2. Wear a hair cover to prevent hair from getting on or in patients' wounds and to keep blood and fluids out of hair.
3. Wear shoe and leg covers to keep bloody fluids off the wearer's legs and feet.
4. Wear protective glasses, glasses with side shields, or a face shield to keep spatter from the eyes. Whenever a mask is indicated to protect facial mucous membranes, eyewear is also needed to protect eyes.

Selection of barriers

The barriers of the past, including muslin gowns, gauze masks, and rubber gloves, have been improved upon over time. Today, better technology is used in developing products, and more options are available to care providers.

Cover gowns made from woven and nonwoven fabrics offer varying degrees of fluid resistance. Some have a plastic lining in the sleeves and front panel to aid surgical staff and others who tend to get blood on their clothing in predictable places and need extra protection. Surgical masks filter more than 90% of droplets *from* the wearer, and recently masks have been developed to filter air *to* the wearer. These new masks may offer some degree of protection from organisms contained in droplet nuclei (e.g., *Mycobacterium tuberculosis*), which stay suspended in air and are tiny enough to pass through other masks. Gloves come in a variety of sizes and materials and as with the other barriers, need to be chosen for the particular anticipated task.

It is important to select barriers appropriate for the situation. Costs generally rise with the barrier's fluid resistance and the product's sturdiness. For example, vinyl gloves are less expensive than latex, but they are also less durable and therefore are unsuitable for prolonged, vigorous tasks. The most comfortable, sturdy gloves are sized surgical gloves, but they cost about 10 times as much as latex examination gloves. Utility gloves may be washed and disinfected. They are much more durable than examination gloves, but they are not appropriate for contact with mucous membranes or nonintact skin.

Another dimension to selecting barriers is determining when to use them. All health care facilities use two types of procedures to decrease risk for transferring organisms among patients and personnel:(1) routine patient care practices, such as individual respiratory therapy devices and sterile catheter insertion for all patients, and (2) special precautions for patients diagnosed or suspected of having particular infectious diseases.

In the past, barrier precautions and isolation strategies were used only in response to certain diagnoses. For a diagnosis-driven isolation system to be effective, the diagnosis must be made or suspected early, it must be highly likely the diagnosis is correct, and clinically recognizable cases must represent the major reservoir for the organism. This fortuitous combination of circumstances rarely occurs. Most infectious diseases have a very high proportion of unrecognized cases, and the major reservoir for the organisms includes moist body sites and substances of uninfected people. There is now a strong trend away from diagnosis-driven precautions and toward interaction-driven use of barriers for all patients. That is, blood and body substances of all patients are suspected of harboring microorganisms transmissable by direct contact; direct contact also plays a major role in transfer of microorganisms to particularly susceptible sites such as mucous membranes and nonintact skin on all humans. The specific interaction or encounter between caregiver and patient determines the protective attire used. This has several potential advantages:

1. Use of diagnosis-driven barrier precautions is inconsistent and frequently incorrect. Also, knowledge of a person's diagnosis is often difficult to obtain, and even when hospital personnel do know the diagnosis, they still may not use barriers correctly.

2. All humans are potentially susceptible to significant doses of new organisms placed on their mucous membranes or nonintact skin. Barrier precautions should always be used for these sites.

3. Caregivers who handle moist body substances with their bare hands may be unable to wash off the substances and the organisms effectively, even if they wash diligently. Gloves used before soiling the hands are more effective than handwashing afterward.

4. Caregivers who have contact with blood or bloody substances may become infected themselves, whether or not the patient is diagnosed with the disease. This concern led to the use of precautions to protect caregivers in all care situations, typically called *universal precautions*.

Finally, there are federal and state regulations concerning selection and use of barriers.[32] OSHA regulations specify that employers require their employed care providers and volunteers to wear protective attire when they are likely to have contact with blood and other moist body substances that may contain bloodborne pathogens such as HIV or HBV.[32] These requirements include wearing gloves. The OSHA regulations do not address transmission of other infectious agents or protection of patients or family members. They are only directed toward protecting health care employees. This narrow focus makes the OSHA rules and any control program established merely to meet these requirements insufficient to provide adequate patient and caregiver protection. OSHA requirements are enforced through unannounced inspections, citations, and large fines for facilities that fail to comply with the rules. Table 6-2 describes administrative requirements and indications for using barriers to meet OSHA regulations.

Precaution strategies

Infection precaution systems represent attempts to systematize decisions about caring for people with infectious diseases. The questions usually considered include the following:

1. When to wash hands
2. When to wear gloves and when to change them
3. Whether to put on a gown
4. Whether to put on facial protection and what type is indicated
5. Whether susceptible people may enter rooms of people with certain infectious diseases
6. How to select appropriate roommates

Several of these issues have been discussed previously in the context of barrier precautions for all caregivers and patients.

TABLE 6-2. Occupational Health and Safety Administration (OSHA) requirements for personal protective apparel to minimize exposure to bloodborne pathogens.*

Equipment	Indications for use	Must be:
Gloves	When contact with infectious material is likely During all vascular procedures Before contact with mucous membranes and non-intact skin	Suitable for task: general patient care, sterile surgical procedures Individualized: Various sizes, hypoallergenic, powderless
Clothing (Gowns, aprons, shoe covers, hats, hoods)	When splattering of clothing with body substances is likely	Suitable for task: Prevent blood, infectious materials from penetrating and reaching employee's skin or clothes
Facial protection (Masks, face shields, eyewear including glasses with side shields, goggles)	When splattering, splashing or spraying of eyes, nose or mouth with blood or other potentially infectious body substances is likely	Effective: in preventing infectious material from penetrating around barriers or under.

*All personal protective equipment must be conveniently located, accessible and provided free to employee. Employer is responsible for purchasing, repairing and laundering as appropriate. From Occupational Safety and Health Administration: *Federal Register* 56:64003-64182, 1991.

Isolating persons with infections

Historically, isolation techniques were derived from operating room and public health models of care that were standardized and ritualistic and that engendered poor compliance (see Suggested Readings). In fact, almost an inverse correlation existed between education and compliance: the more knowledgeable the persons, the less likely they were to comply with recommended isolation practices. Currently, there is more flexibility and choice of isolation or infection precaution systems. Also, considerable confusion surrounds what is really required to minimize risk for the patient and the care providers.

Formal, highly structured systems of infection precautions may be necessary in some hospitals and nursing homes when the complexity of care or staffing assignments make a highly flexible system difficult to administer. In less complex care settings the task-oriented precautions described earlier may be more practical. Nurses and other care givers must learn to assess quickly the planned task in terms of risk for transmission of microorganisms to themselves and their patients and must use the proper barriers. This approach of standard precautions is more effective than memorizing lists of infectious diseases and corresponding precautions.

Four precaution systems have been published: (1) category isolation, (2) disease-specific isolation, (3) universal precautions, and (4) body substance isolation.

Category isolation was last revised by the Centers for Disease Control (CDC) in 1983 and is scheduled for further updating in 1994. *Disease-specific isolation* was developed by the CDC at the same time as an alternative for facilities that did not want to use category isolation.[13] Both systems are intended to reduce transmission from diagnosed cases of infectious diseases, and both use posted signs to designate patients whose care requires special precautions. The Hospital Infection Control Practices Advisory Committee (HICPAC) of the CDC is currently updating the isolation guidelines. Publication is expected by early 1995.

The use of *universal precautions* is intended to reduce risk for transmission of bloodborne pathogens from infected patients to susceptible caregivers.[5] In the early 1980s, it became obvious that unrecognized cases of HBV and HIV infection were important sources of these diseases and that contact with infected blood resulted in the transmission of HBV to many health care workers. Previously, precautions were used only for diagnosed cases, which meant that precautions were not used with the most infectious patients. In one study, 30% of emergency department nurses had serologic evidence of previous HBV infection compared with only 5% of the general population.[9] This difference was clearly unacceptable. The CDC revised the previous category of "blood and body fluid isolation" from the category isolation system in 1987, and the precautions were applied to those body substances associated with transmission of bloodborne pathogens. This new designation did not apply to other body substances. Many elements of universal precautions have been incorporated into requirements of the OSHA Bloodborne Pathogens Standard.[32]

Body substance isolation (BSI) was first described in 1984 and revised in 1990.[29] It is intended to reduce risk for transmission of infectious agents to patients and caregivers. BSI is a comprehensive strategy that includes use of barrier precautions during contact with all moist body sites and substances. These precautions are task oriented, not diagnosis oriented, except for the management of airborne disease. Table 6-3 compares the four isolation systems.[20]

Air management

Air circulation systems in health care facilities must be appropriately managed if nosocomial transmission of tuberculosis and other airborne diseases is to be prevented. Many

TABLE 6-3. Comparison of four systems for infection precautions*

Situation	Category specific (CDC, 1983)	Disease specific (CDC, 1983)	Body substance isolation (Lynch, Jackson, et al, 1984-1990)	Universal precautions (CDC, revised 1988)
1. Patient known to have hepatitis B or C, human immunodeficiency virus (HIV) infection, acquired immunodeficiency syndrome (AIDS), or other bloodborne diseases	Category of blood and body fluid precautions was replaced by universal precautions in 1987 (revised 1988)	See universal precautions, revised 1988	Gloves: put on clean gloves immediately before contact with mucous membranes and nonintact skin; use gloves for contact with moist body substances Gown or plastic apron: use if soiling is likely Private room: assign if personal hygiene is poor Mask and eye protection: use if splashing is likely Trash and linen: bag securely to prevent leakage	Gloves: use for contact with blood and body fluids epidemiologically associated with transmission of bloodborne organisms or other bloody body fluids Use other protective barriers to reduce risk of exposure to blood or bloody body fluids Trash and linen: bag securely to prevent leakage
2. Patient *not* known to have hepatitis B or C, HIV infection, AIDS, or other bloodborne diseases	Use universal precautions	Use universal precautions	Same precautions as above; selection of barriers based on interaction with patient	Same as above
3. Patient with diagnosed enteric disease such as salmonellosis	Enteric precautions: gloves for contact with feces; gown if soiling is likely; private room if personal hygiene is poor; "Enteric Precautions" sign on door	See named disease in 1983 CDC guidelines (similar to enteric precautions); sign on door	Same precautions as above	Universal precautions do not apply to feces unless visibly bloody

Continued.

TABLE 6-3. Comparison of four systems for infection precautions*—cont'd

Situation	Category specific (CDC, 1983)	Disease specific (CDC, 1983)	Body substance isolation (Lynch, Jackson, et al, 1984-1990)	Universal precautions (CDC, revised 1988)
4. Patient *not* known to have salmonellosis	No special precautions because no diagnosis; routine patient care practices should be followed	No special precautions; routine patient care practices should be followed	Same precautions as above	Universal precautions do not apply except as above
5. Patient known to be colonized or infected with methicillin-resistant *Staphylococcus aureus*	Contact isolation: gloves for touching infective material; masks if close to patient; gowns if soiling likely; private room indicated; "Contact Isolation" sign on door	See named disease in 1983 CDC guideline (similar to contact isolation); sign on door	Same precautions as above	Universal precautions do not apply except as above
6. Patient *not* known to be colonized or infected with MRSA	No special precautions because no diagnosis; routine patient care practices should be followed	No special precautions; routine patient care practices should be followed	Same precautions as above	Universal precautions do not apply except as above
7. Patient diagnosed with varicella (chickenpox)	Strict isolation: for entering room whether or not contact occurs; gloves, gowns, gloves, gowns, masks, private room; immune persons do not need masks; "Strict Isolation" sign on door	See named disease in 1983 CDC guideline (similar to strict isolation); sign on door	Susceptible persons should not be assigned to care for patient; immune personnel should follow body substance isolation as above; sign on door to restrict entry	Universal precautions do not apply except as above

From Jackson MM, Lynch P. An attempt to make an issue less murky: a comparison of four systems for infection precautions. *Infect Control Hosp Epidemiol* 1991;12:448.

*Strategies characteristic of each system of infection precautions described are consistently applied in the same manner for other diagnosed or undiagnosed infections.

older facilities do not have adequate air exchanges or air movement systems and new facilities may recirculate warmed or cooled air in order to conserve energy.

Unfortunately, people with infectious airborne communicable diseases usually are not identified soon enough to prevent exposure of susceptible persons. Even when they are identified, airborne contamination may still result. The best approach is to include competent air systems in construction. Retrofitting filters or air handling systems in places where they are inadequate and where persons infected with potentially airborne microorganisms are likely to receive care should be considered. This includes AIDS diagnosis and treatment facilities where patients with HIV and *M. tuberculosis* may be seen, other in-patient units where patients with tuberculosis are cared for, emergency and radiology departments, some jails, some nursing home areas, and pediatric clinics where airborne viral diseases are frequent occurrences. Early suspicion and diagnosis of airborne communicable disease permits rapid initiation of precautions. Control of airflow is critical to prevent transmission. Surgical masks and personal respirators have been recommended to reduce transmission of *M. tuberculosis* but have not been tested and shown to be effective. When the organism is sensitive to the drugs used, chemotherapy typically reduces symptoms and infectivity within 1 to 3 weeks. When *M. tuberculosis* is resistant to the drugs used, infectivity may be prolonged despite chemotherapy (see Chapter 8, Chemotherapeutics). Whenever possible, caregivers who are immune to tuberculosis, varicella, measles and other airborne vaccine-preventable diseases should care for infectious patients. In some facilities, there may not be enough immune caregivers, and it will be necessary for susceptible caregivers with masks or respirators to provide care.

Spatial separation of patients has been reported to decrease infection risk for certain conditions. Although this arrangement reduces shared air space among patients and caregivers and may foster more frequent handwashing and glove changing between patients, spatial separation does not necessarily improve air circulation.

Selection of roommates for patients

Careful roommate selection for patients may help prevent transmission of some infectious diseases. Patient placement determines structural barriers provided by single versus multibed rooms. Patients with airborne communicable diseases should not room with susceptible persons. Patients who soil the environment with moist body substances should not have roommates who are likely to have contact with soiled articles. These guidelines include patients who are incontinent of feces, who have excessive wound or fluid drainage, and who have large or multiple draining lesions. Patients with these problems should be separated from other patients with open lesions or indwelling medical devices.

Soiled linen and supplies

In health care facilities, many people handle soiled supplies and linen after they are used. Consistent handling methods are advisable. Regulatory agencies may require special handling after items leave the facility. Soiled linen should be handled as little as necessary and be placed in bags that prevent leakage. Other linen management precautions should be based on the amount of contamination, not the diagnosis of the patient. Handlers should be instructed that all soiled linen contains potentially infectious material and may also contain sharp objects and other items. Double bagging (i.e., using two bags) for soiled linen from patients known to be infected has not reduced infection risk.[40] Water-soluble bags that contain the linen are placed directly in the washing machine, where the bags melt, avoiding handling of linen in the laundry. However, these bags are expensive and have not decreased infection risk, especially to laundry personnel who routinely wear gloves, gowns, aprons, and other barriers as necessary to prevent direct contact with body substances.

Dishes and utensils

At one time or another, most health facilities have used paper plates and disposable plastic utensils to serve food to patients in rooms with isolation precautions. The premise was that infected patients would contaminate regular utensils during meals, and microorganisms would be transferred to nurses or dietary staff during subsequent handling. To reduce this risk, food-service items were placed in the trash in the patient's room. There is no theoretic rationale for this practice and it does not reduce infection risk.[18]

Waste management

Bloody sharps, bloody fluid in containers, and pathologic waste from laboratories may transmit infectious organisms. These items should be handled carefully and rendered noninfectious by sterilization, incineration, or chemical disinfection. They may be packaged and transported to an appropriate disposal site.

Requirements for management of medical infectious wastes vary by state, county, and even municipality. Some jurisdictions require special handling and disposal of items not associated with risk for transmission, such as all trash from isolation rooms and bags used for intravenous fluids. The variation in definitions of potentially infectious waste reflects a combination of ignorance, fear, and financial incentive. Trash that requires special handling generates much more income for waste management companies than regular trash. OSHA has defined *regulated waste* in its Bloodborne Pathogens Standard. This document has set minimum standards for managing potentially

infectious regulated waste in the United States.[32]

Transmission of infectious organisms such as cytomegalovirus and bacterial and viral agents responsible for diarrhea among active toddlers is very common in day-care facilities. Diapering and diaper disposal have generated considerable discussion among many agencies, parents, and health care personnel. Disposable diapers are convenient and have been reported to reduce diaper rash in infants. In day-care facilities, toddlers diapered in disposable brands acquired fewer enteric diseases than children in cloth diapers.[39] Disposable diapers provided better containment than cloth, resulted in less fecal contamination of the environment, and required less handling by caregivers.[39]

Most studies of the relative effect of cloth and disposable diapers on infection risk have been biased in favor of one or the other and provide spurious conclusions. Soiled diapers are a source for potentially infectious organisms, but these organisms are ubiquitous in the environment and no evidence suggests that diapers in the landfill constitute an infection risk for waste handlers or will be a source of transmission from the landfill to other sites. Despite this lack of evidence, some agencies suggest that caregivers scrape feces off disposable diapers to reduce gram-negative and enteric pathogens that go into the landfill. However, this recommendation substitutes a weak, theoretic advantage of protecting the landfill for a real risk to caregivers handling feces.

Consumer Reports evaluated the life-cycle costs of cloth versus disposable diapers and found that reprocessing diapers used more water whereas landfill and paper costs increased with disposable diapers, which now constitute about 2% of municipal solid waste.[8] The overall costs at that time were about equal.

Fecal and urinary contamination of the environment frequently occurs in hospital ICUs, nurseries, and pediatric care centers. ICU patients are frequently incontinent of urine and feces and often have loose stools that soil the bed, linen, and other articles. This represents a major source of gram-negative organisms and may pose a significant infection risk. Disposable diapers may provide better containment and decreased environmental contamination with feces for incontinent patients who defecate in the bed linen or on absorbent pads. Even among adult patients who are alert and mobile, fecal contamination of the room, bathroom, and bed rails is common.[31]

Unresolved issues

Unanswered questions and unresolved issues still surround barrier precautions:

1. Are special practices indicated for immunocompromised patients? Protective or reverse isolation, consisting of gloves, gown, and mask worn by persons entering these patients' rooms, was intended to minimize patients' exposure to exogenous organisms. Since most infections in these patients result from endogenous microorganisms, these practices do not prolong their life span or reduce the number of infections. The CDC removed protective isolation from the category isolation system in 1983, but some facilities still use this category or elements of it.[13] Some hospitals require granulocytopenic patients to wear surgical masks in their rooms and whenever they go in the halls or outside the building, despite the lack of demonstrated efficacy. Others supply a private room when possible, exclude any staff with the slightest illness, defer invasive devices and procedures, and arrange staff assignments to avoid assigning staff on the same shift to patients with clinical infections and immunocompromised patients.

2. Do signs increase caregiver compliance with barrier precautions? Two reports suggest that compliance is not increased and that appropriate glove use may actually decrease when reminder signs are used.[15,28] Despite this, many facilities still use signs, and personnel say they "feel safer" when the known cases have labels differentiating them from unrecognized cases and other patients.

3. Are special precautions for patients with unusually drug-resistant organisms effective in reducing transmission? It is tempting to believe that placing patients from whom vancomycin-resistant enterococci or methicillin-resistant staphylococci have been recovered in isolation is valuable. Unfortunately, no controlled studies have demonstrated this to be true. Additionally, unrecognized cases are probably common (see Clinical Study 5).

4. Is it reasonable to use special precautions only for patients diagnosed with certain infectious agents and not for other patients with similar diseases caused by other organisms? In other words, are the well-studied diseases good markers or proxies for other organisms, or are they unique? For example, RSV is a viral agent that has been well studied. It is transmitted by droplets and is similar to other viral respiratory diseases of children. Some care facilities isolate patients after RSV is diagnosed even though many other patients, their families, and staff may have similar syndromes and remain unisolated.

Occupational Health

Policies to minimize the risk of transmission of infectious agents among personnel and patients should be coordinated by the occupational health service; the infection prevention and control program; the emergency department, which may have clinical responsibilities in the occupational health program; and other departments where patient contact or personnel exposure may occur. Some of the activities of the occupational health program include evaluating personnel for existing infections and susceptibility to infectious diseases, administering immunizations, keeping records, managing exposures, providing limited primary care, and providing health and safety education. A major focus is infection prevention.[35]

New hire and routine screening

New employees must be screened by laboratory tests or history for susceptibility to tuberculosis, hepatitis B, measles, rubella, and chickenpox. Immunization and retesting schedules should be established. For example, repeat screening of health care staff for tuberculosis is recommended at least annually.[4]

Immunizations

Immunizations are important for health care professionals. Those against measles (rubeola), influenza, rubella, and HBV should be provided (see Table 5-1.) Measles, rubella, and HBV can have severe health consequences for the health care provider (see Clinical Study 31). Morbidity and mortality associated with measles is high in adults. Rubella can be teratogenic to a fetus and induce abortion. HBV infection not only can produce initial acute infection, but also becomes chronic in up to 10% of those infected and produces prolonged illness or death. Some health care providers who are chronically infected with HBV have posed a continuing risk for transmission to patients. Recent standards from the U.S. Occupational Safety and Health Administration (OSHA) require that all employees in a health care facility with the potential for blood and body fluid exposure be offered HBV vaccine free of charge.[32]

Occupational exposures to blood among health care workers

For more than a decade, it has been recognized that health care workers who had contact with blood of patients were at increased risk for infections with bloodborne pathogens, including hepatitis B and C and HIV. Hospital-based studies identified activities associated with increased risk,[9,21,30] care facilities have responded to the information by developing programs to prevent blood contact and exposures and to reduce subsequent infections.

Caregivers themselves play a major role in reducing the frequency of blood exposures. Before beginning a task, caregivers must assess the nature of risk for the task and select prevention strategies that may include physical barriers such as gloves and other protective attire. These elements of risk were identified in one study:[19]

1. Potential route of exposure: higher risk is associated with punctures.
2. Experience of the health care worker and cooperation of the patient: risk increases when patients are unable to follow directions exactly and when health care workers are inexperienced at the task they are going to perform.
3. Prevalence of bloodborne pathogens in the population receiving care.
4. Difficulty of the situation. In emergencies and rushed or chaotic circumstances, the ability of the health care worker to manage blood and sharps are impaired.

Health care workers should assess each care situation for risk and consider the risk reduction methods that are available. For mucous membrane and skin contacts, barrier precautions are effective. For punctures, sometimes safer devices such as needleless IV connectors are available. When cooperation of the patient or inexperience are a problem, asking a more experienced person to assist is helpful.

The serious risk for bloodborne pathogen infection is often underestimated by health care workers. In 1989, the CDC estimated that approximately 200-300 health care workers die annually of the acute or chronic effects of occupationally acquired hepatitis B and that as many as 9000 cases of occupationally acquired hepatitis B may be prevented every year by the use of barrier precautions and hepatitis B vaccine required by OSHA.[32]

Punctures with contaminated sharps, particularly large-bore hollow needles, pose the greatest risk for transmission of HIV and HBV. The risk is less from small-bore needles, solid sharps, wires, scalpels, mucous membrane and small nonintact skin exposures, and least from blood in contact with intact skin.

Risk of exposure has been studied in two ways. Several investigators have studied incident and accident reports describing blood exposures.[21,30] In general, they found that exposures from needle manipulations—IV starts, phlebotomy, piggyback IVs, disassembly of injection cartridge sets, and two-handed recapping of needles were among the most common problems. These studies were hampered by poor reporting of blood exposures by personnel in operating room (OR) settings. Subsequently, OR-based studies using trained observers[34,38] or circulating nurses[14,35,41] to complete exposure reports have shown that blood contact may occur in as many as 30% of surgical cases, and punctures occurred during 7% of procedures. Table 6-4 shows the different rates from published studies in ORs. One study of nine collaborating hospitals demonstrated considerable variation among the participating facilities.[41] The lowest incidence was 4 contacts or exposures per 100 procedures in a small community hospital OR, and the highest was 32 per 100 procedures in a large university OR. Presumably, some of the variation is due to the success of prevention strategies among the ORs, though variation in the complexity of cases and the equipment used may have influenced their findings.

Two studies have raised a disturbing issue: they reported that 11%[41] and 29%[38] of personnel punctures in the OR result in exposure of the patient to blood from the health care worker. More research in this area is needed, but since patient exposures seem to be potentially serious and relatively common, facili-

ties that perform surgical services should establish post-exposure management policies for patients similar to those for employee exposures.

Post-exposure management

Potential exposures to infectious diseases should be promptly managed. Post-exposure management is usually circumstance-specific and organism-specific and each will require a somewhat different strategy. Written policies for post-exposure management should define exposure, provide algorithms for testing the source of the exposure (if appropriate), and provide guidelines for management of the exposed individual. These policies should address prophylaxis, therapy, follow-up, and counseling.

The algorithms for diagnosis and treatment of some infectious diseases including hepatitis B, HIV, and tuberculosis are quite complex. Personnel and managers should be familiar with the procedures for managing exposures, and have written procedures readily available. Delays in initiating therapy may reduce effectiveness. Personnel should be informed of the availability of prophylactic treatment with drugs, vaccines, or immune globulins; the risk of infection with and without therapy; and the side effects of therapy. In some cases such as exposure to *Neisseria meningitidis*, therapy must be initiated before

TABLE 6-4. Punctures with blood exposure during surgical procedures reported by five operating room studies

Investigator	Number of cases	Percent with punctures
Gerberding et al[14]	1307	1.7
Popejoy and Fry[36]	684	3.0
Panlilio et al[34]	206	4.9
Tokars et al[38]	1382	7.2
White and Lynch[41]	8502	1.6

the results of antimicrobial sensitivity testing are available.

Infections in health care workers

Since personnel in most health care settings are in contact with patients who have infectious diseases, occupationally associated infections may result. If personnel develop infections themselves, microorganisms may be transmitted to other personnel and patients. Occupationally acquired infections include chickenpox, conjunctivitis, cytomegalovirus, hepatitis A, B, and C, HIV, herpes simplex, influenza, measles, mumps, rubella, meningococcal disease, parvovirus, pertussis, respiratory syncytial virus, rotavirus, salmonella, shigella, scabies, staphylococci, streptococci, and tuberculosis.[35]

Usually when personnel have active infections, the signs and symptoms are apparent. This is often not the case for infections due to the bloodborne pathogens, HIV, and hepatitis B and C. Generally, personnel who have chronic infections need to use additional precautions to reduce risk for transmission to patients, or be reassigned unless epidemiologic evidence suggests transmission can occur. Post-exposure management of patients should be rigorous enough to identify personnel infected with any of these infectious agents.

The magnitude of potential exposures and the attendant human and financial cost provide powerful motivation for care facilities and personnel to reduce the risk as much as possible through employee health programs.

INFLUENCE OF SETTING ON BARRIER PRECAUTIONS

Strategies for using personal protection including barrier precautions and occupational health and safety procedures must be specific for the care setting.

A high incidence of infectious diseases has been reported among children in day-care centers[39] (see Clinical Studies 9 and 15). Ideally, all prodromal and ill youngsters should be excluded from attendance. Since this is unlikely, urine, feces, and airway secretions for all children should be managed as potentially infectious to minimize risk of transmitting disease to other children and staff. Containment requires gloves for diaper changes, disinfection of the changing table, proper disposal or handling of diapers and handwashing for the caregiver and child. Children in day care should not share eating or drinking utensils. Toys should be cleanable and should be washed frequently enough to provide a clean surface for the next child. Staff should use materials such as facial tissues and washcloths for a single child, then discard or launder. Infection control references for day-care settings are available.[10]

The same precautions should be used in hospitals, long-term care, home settings, clinics, group homes and infirmaries in prisons and schools. All caregivers should use appropriate barrier precautions when handling mucous membranes, moist body substances, and indwelling devices. Though many long-term care patients may require only assistance with meals, ambulation, dressing, and other daily activities, others require more intensive support including bathing, toileting, and invasive medical devices such as indwelling urinary catheters and intravenous catheters. In long-term care facilities, an effort is made to maintain a homelike setting, which encourages frequent social interaction between the patients, their families, and the staff. Patients who have difficulty managing their body substances present a particular challenge in these settings. The ambulatory care or home setting may not support management of the patient who has potentially airborne disease. Because negative pressure ventilation is not generally available, traffic may be high, and patients and families wait in close proximity to others who may have infectious disease(s) transmissible by the airborne, droplet, or contaminated fomite (toys) routes.

SUMMARY

Nurses and caregivers in all practice settings should assess the need for barrier precautions for each task they plan. They should also assess their perceived needs related to these special precautions and the appropriate protective measures for both patients and caregivers. The precautions will be most effective if they are based on this assessment and knowledge of the ecology of the host-environment interaction rather than on rigid isolation systems.

REFERENCES

1. Albert RK, Condie F. Handwashing patterns in medical intensive care units. *N Engl J Med.* 1981;304:1465-1466.
2. Birnbaum D. Personal communication, 1986.
3. Burke JF, et al. The contribution of a bacterially isolated environment in the prevention of infection in seriously burned patients. *Ann Surg.* 1977;186:377-385.
4. Centers for Disease Control and Prevention. Draft guideline for preventing the transmission of tuberculosis in health-care settings, 2nd ed. *Federal Register.* October 12, 1993;58:195. 52:810-854.
5. Centers for Disease Control. Recommendations for prevention of HIV transmission in health care settings. *MMWR.* 1987;36(suppl 2S). 15-185.
6. Chen CC, Welleke K. Aerosol penetration through surgical masks. *Am J Infect Control.* 1992;20:177-184.
7. De Cock KM, et al. Tuberculosis and HIV infection in sub-Saharan Africa. *JAMA.* 1992;268:1581-1587.
8. Diaper decisions. *Consumer Reports.* 1991;56:551-556.
9. Dienstag JL, Ryan DM. Occupational exposure to hepatitis B virus in hospital personnel: infection or immunization? *Am J Epidemiol.* 1982;115:26-39.
10. Donowitz LG, ed. *Infection Control in the Child Care Center and Preschool.* Baltimore: Williams and Wilkins; 1991.
11. Donowitz LG. Failure of the cover gown to prevent nosocomial infection in a pediatric intensive care unit. *Pediatrics.* 1986;77:35-38.
12. Garner JS, Favero MS. *Guideline for Handwashing and Hospital Environmental Control.* Atlanta: Centers for Disease Control; 1985.
13. Garner JS, Simmons BP. *Isolation Techniques for Use in Hospitals.* Atlanta: Centers for Disease Control; 1983.
14. Gerberding JL, et al. Risk of exposure of surgical personnel to patients' blood during surgery at San Francisco General Hospital. *N Engl J Med.* 1990;322:1788-1793.
15. Gerberding JL. Does knowledge of HIV infection decrease the frequency of occupational exposure to blood? *Am J Med.* 1991;91(suppl3B):308-311.
16. Haque KN, Chagla AH. Do gowns prevent infections in neonatal intensive care units? *J Hosp Infect.* 1989;14:159-162.
17. Jackson MM. Personal Communication.
18. Jackson MM. From ritual to reason with a rational approach for the future: an epidemiologic perspective. *Am J Infect Control.* 1984;12:213-220.
19. Jackson MM, Lynch P. Development of a health care worker risk assessment scale (HCWRAS) to evaluate potential for blood borne pathogen exposures. *AM J Infec Control* (In press).
20. Jackson MM, Lynch P. An attempt to make an issue less murky: a comparison of four systems for infection precautions. *Infect Control Hosp Epidemiol.* 1991;12:448-450.
21. Jagger J, et al. Rates of needlestick injury caused by various devices in a university hospital. *N Engl J Med.* 1988;319:284-288.
22. Johnson S, Gerding D, Olson MM, et al. Prospective, controlled study of vinyl glove use to interrupt *Clostridium difficile* nosocomial transmission. *Am J Med.* 1990;88:137-140.
23. Klein BS, Perloff WH, Maki DG. Reduction of nosocomial infection during pediatric intensive care by protective isolation. *N Engl J Med.* 1989;320: 1714-1721.
24. Larson EL. Persistent carriage of gram-negative bacteria on hands. *Am J Infect Control.* 1981;9:112-119.
25. Larson EL. Guideline for use of topical antimicrobial agents. *Am J Infect Control.* 1988;16:253-266.
26. LeClaire JM, et al. Prevention of nosocomial respiratory syncytial virus infections through compliance with glove and gown isolation precautions. *N Engl J Med.* 1987;317:329-334.
27. Lovitt SA, et al. Isolation gowns: a false sense of security? *Am J Infect Control.* 1992;20:185-191.
28. Lynch P, et al. Rethinking the role of isolation practices in the prevention of nosocomial infections. *Ann Intern Med.* 1987;107:243-246.
29. Lynch P, et al. Implementing and evaluating a system of generic infection precautions: body substance isolation. *Am J Infect Control.* 1990;18:1-12.
30. McCormick RD, et al. Epidemiology of hospital sharps injuries: a prospective study in the pre-AIDS and AIDS eras. *Am J Med.* 1991;91(suppl3B):301-307.
31. McFarland LV, et al. Nosocomial acquisition of *Clostridium difficile* infection. *Am J Med.* 1990;88: 137-140.
32. Occupational Safety and Health Administration. Occupational exposure to blood-borne pathogens: final rule, 29CFR Part 1910:1030. *Federal Register.* December 6, 1991;56:64003-64182.
33. Olsen RJ, et al. Examination gloves as barriers to hand contamination in clinical practice. *JAMA.* 1993;270:350-353.

34. Panlilio AL, et al. Blood contacts during surgical procedures. *JAMA*. 1991;265:1533-1537.

35. Polder JA, Tablan OC, Williams WW. Personal health services. In: Bennett JV, Brachman PS, eds: *Hospital Infections* 3 ed, Little Brown, Boston; 1993;31-62.

36. Popejoy SI, Fry DE. Blood contact and exposure in the operating room. *Surg Gynecol Obstet*. 1991;172:480-483.

37. Roth JA. Ritual and magic in the control of contagion. *American Sociological Review*. 1957;22(3):310-314.

38. Tokars JI, Bell DM, Culver DH, *et al*. Percutaneous injuries during surgical procedures. *JAMA*. 1992;267: 2899-2904.

39. Van R, et al. The effect of diaper type and overclothing on fecal contamination in day care centers. *JAMA*. 1991;265(14):1840-1844.

40. Weinstein SA, et al. Bacterial surface contamination of patients' linen: isolation precautions versus standard care. *Am J Infect Control*. 1989;17:264-267.

41. White MC, Lynch P. Blood contact and exposures among operating room personnel: a multicenter study. *Am J Infect Control*. 1993;21:243-248.

42. Weinstein RA. Epidemiology and control of nosocomial infections in adult intensive care units. *Am J Med*. 1991;91(suppl3B):1775-1845.

SUGGESTED READINGS

Austin DF, Werner SB. Epidemiology for the Health Sciences, 5th ed. Springfield, IL: Charles C. Thomas, Publisher; 1979.

Fedson D. Immunization for health-care workers and patients in hospitals. In: Wenzel RP, ed. *Prevention and Control of Hospital Infections* 2nd ed, Williams & Wilkins; 1993: 214-294.

Jackson MM, Lynch P. *At the interface: the nurse's role in risk reduction*, Marvik Educational Services, San Diego, 1993.

Jackson MM, Lynch P. Isolation practices: a historical perspective. *Am J Infect Control*. 1985;13:21-31.

Chapter 7

Antisepsis, Disinfection, and Sterilization

SUE CROW
NORANN Y. PLANCHOCK
EDDIE HEDRICK

More than 100 years have passed since the relationship between microorganisms and infectious diseases was recognized. Though Lister, Koch, Nightingale, Pasteur, and others introduced aseptic principles and practices to health care generations ago,[22] health care practitioners do not consistently use these principles. Thus infections continue to be caused by organisms transmitted from person to person and by contaminated medical instruments.[12,17,33]

Microorganisms are ubiquitous. Because they may pose an infectious hazard to patients and staff, it is important that nurses develop a second sense about the presence of microorganisms and a thorough understanding of the principles and methods of asepsis, cleaning, disinfection, and sterilization presented in this chapter.

Webster[47] defines *asepsis* as a condition free from pathogenic microorganisms. Hoeller[18] proposed that the term *asepsis* be used to describe the techniques of keeping the work area and personnel as free from microorganisms as possible with the intent of protecting the patient and the caregiver. Hoeller identified four steps as important for the practitioner:

- Know what is clean, disinfected, or sterile.
- Know what is *not* clean, disinfected, or sterile.
- Keep clean, disinfected, and sterile items separate from contaminated items.
- Take immediate action if contamination occurs.

This chapter focuses on Hoeller's first two components of asepsis, defining what is and what is not clean, disinfected, or sterile and describing the procedures that the nurse and other health care provider can use to clean, disinfect, and sterilize. Although patient care situations and settings vary, basic principles of asepsis dictate the proper course of action to reduce microbial contamination. It is important that the basic principles of asepsis be consistently incorporated into patient care.

The first section of this chapter demonstrates how asepsis, including cleaning, antisepsis, disinfection, and sterilization, relate to the interactions of the host, microorganism, physical environment, and social environment. The subsequent sections focus on selection and use of topical antiseptics; environmental cleaning, sanitation, and decontamination; products and processes of disinfection; and sterilization methods.

THE HOST-ENVIRONMENT INTERACTION

Asepsis, which includes the principles of cleaning, antisepsis, disinfection, and sterilization, influences and is influenced by host, microbiologic environment, physical environment, and social environment interactions.

The host

Antisepsis, disinfection, and sterilization practices determine the degree to which intrinsic host immunity will be challenged and thereby influence whether or not a person acquires an infection. The more compromised the host, the more important is the aseptic practice. For example, a patient who is elderly or has an immunosuppressive disease such as leukemia may be at significant risk if the principles of antisepsis, disinfection, and sterilization are violated.

The host's endogenous microorganisms are often the target of antiseptics. Paradoxically, the host tissues' tolerance to these agents can impose critical limitations on the use of these agents, which are specifically chosen for their ability to disrupt living cells.

The microbiologic environment

The mechanisms of antisepsis, disinfection, and sterilization are determined by characteristics of the target microorganisms. *Antiseptics* are chemicals applied to living tissues to remove, inhibit, or kill microbes. Handwashing, skin cleansing, and wound care using these agents reduces the number and type of microbes present and consequently the risk of infection. *Disinfectants* are chemicals applied to inanimate objects to destroy or reduce the growth of microorganisms to levels appropriate for the particular situation. *Sterilization* destroys all forms of microbial life and is used whenever possible for items intended to enter sterile tissues or body cavities. Appropriate cleaning, disinfection, and sterilization procedures should be selected for the specific clinical situation.

The physical environment

Cleaning, disinfection, and sterilization are important to reduce the risk of infection from instruments or medical devices.[16] The construction, materials, and clinical use of these devices affect microbial presence, the success of cleaning, disinfection, and sterilization, and the consequences of failed procedures. Infections have frequently been traced to the ineffective cleaning of patient care equipment.[38,39,43] For example, instruments used for invasive procedures such as flexible fiberoptic endoscopy, which may damage mucous membranes and provide a portal of entry into the vascular system, must be as free as possible of pathogenic microorganisms despite the fact that this equipment may be difficult to clean and unable to withstand the most reliable and economic sterilization procedures.[32]

The social environment

Aseptic practices are influenced by the social environment. Experience, study, and consensus have led to standard practices to support the delivery of safe, quality care. However, some situations tax the practitioner's ability to maintain these standards. Time constraints resulting from workloads and understaffing, cultural attitudes regarding asepsis, and rituals reflecting lack of integration of new information into clinical practice are examples of the social environment's effect on infection prevention. Maintenance of high-quality care requires that social and cultural value be placed on aseptic practices.

ANTISEPTICS

The host-microorganism relationship

It has been known for more than 140 years that disease-causing microorganisms can be carried on the skin.[22] For example, *Staphylococcus epidermidis*, a common inhabitant of normal skin, is the leading cause of nosocomial bacteremia and one of the primary causes of surgical wound infections.[42]

The Centers for Disease Control and Prevention (CDC) at one time related more than 50% of all nosocomial infections to inadequate handwashing practices.[16] Consequently, handwashing with an appropriate antiseptic is an essential part of patient care for all health care workers.

The skin, a multilayered surface covered by epithelial cells loosely attached to the deeper cell layers, provides an excellent place for some microorganisms to live. The numbers and types of microorganisms differ from one area of the body to another and may be resident or transient.[7] *Resident microorganisms*, also called *normal flora*, live and multiply on the skin. Most resident organisms are found in the superficial skin layers; approximately 10% to 20% live in the deep epidermal layers.[36] Resident organisms are not usually pathogenic, but they can cause infection if invasive procedures allow them to enter deeper tissues, if the patient's immune system is compromised, or if the patient has an implanted device.[16]

Transient microorganisms are those organisms acquired from another person or object. These organisms generally survive for a few minutes to hours or days on the skin but are not found in deeper tissues and do not remain indefinitely. Gram-positive organisms are predominant members of normal skin flora. However, several studies have shown that transient hand carriage of gram-negative bacteria by hospital personnel may be more prevalent than previously thought.[24,25] Factors that contribute to persistent hand carriage of transient microorganisms are not completely understood and need further study.[16,24]

The frequent use of broad-spectrum antimicrobials in health care facilities has been associated with the emergence of antibiotic-resistant strains of microorganisms. Therefore the microbiologic flora on the hands of health care professionals in these settings may be resistant to antibiotics.[48] If these microorganisms are transmitted to patients, they are difficult to treat with the usual antibiotic regimens.

Antisepsis uses chemicals (antiseptics) to reduce the number of microorganisms on the skin. When antiseptics are used appropriately to prepare the patient's skin and to clean the health care professional's hands, they can reduce skin colonization and subsequent clinical infection by inhibiting or destroying these microorganisms. Although it is not possible to remove all microorganisms from the skin, mucosa, or wounds, the number can be dramatically reduced when antiseptics are selected and applied correctly.

Selection of antiseptics

Health care providers should be aware of the types of solutions available and advantages or disadvantages of each if they are to choose the appropriate antiseptic for the situation. The labels of antiseptic handwashing agents and skin preparation solutions provide instructions for preparation and use, list the active ingredients, and note specific precautions to be taken during use.

Various antiseptic and nonantiseptic handwashing products are available. The valid indications for use of an antiseptic handwashing agent versus plain soap have not been objectively and comprehensively demonstrated. However, plain soap is generally used to remove transient microorganisms from the skin mechanically and is considered adequate for handwashing after most routine activities. No formulation of plain soap is preferred. It is available in several forms, including granules, leaflets, liquids, and bars. Selection of an appropriate soap depends on ease of use, personal preference, and ability to prevent contamination of the soap and its container. When bar soap is used, it should be placed on a rack that allows water to drain so it does not create a wet environment that would allow microorganisms to grow. When liquid soap is dispensed from reusable containers, the empty containers must be cleaned and refilled with fresh soap or discarded when empty. Reusable dispensers that have been refilled without cleaning or "topped off" can become reservoirs for microorganisms and have been identified as the source of microorganisms involved in many outbreaks. Contamination of liquid hand soaps is less likely when disposable containers are used. The box below lists some criteria to consider when selecting a plain soap for general use.

Antiseptic handwashing solutions are available as foams, liquids, sprays, and films. For locations that do not have sinks and running water (e.g., ambulances), waterless handwashing agents may be used as an interim measure until handwashing can be performed at a sink. Disposable hand-cleaning wipes that contain purported antiseptics are available but may or may not be appropriate, depending on the situation and the antiseptic activity of the agent found in the wipe. Antiseptic handwashing solutions do not replace physical removal of dirt and microorganisms; only soap, friction and running water can effectively remove such soil.

The U.S. Food and Drug Administration (FDA) defines seven categories of antiseptics.[13] These can guide selection of appropriate antiseptics (Table 7-1). Table 7-2 lists frequently used antiseptic ingredients and describes their activities.

SELECTION CRITERIA FOR PLAIN SOAP

Acceptable to user
Contains preservative to minimize contamination
Gentle to skin
Contains surfactant to help remove organic matter
Minimal price

Types of of antiseptic ingredients
Chlorhexidine gluconate

Chlorhexidine products are used often in health care settings. Some studies have shown a decrease in nosocomial infections associated with use of chlorhexidine gluconate for preoperative patient skin preparation.[6,28] Of the various formulations of chlorhexidine available, the 4% solution is used most frequently. Two characteristic advantages of chlorhexidine gluconate are that it remains active on the skin for up to 6 hours and does not hinder wound healing.[40] A disadvantage is that its activity is reduced by increased mineral content of water, some lotions, and soaps. In addition, ototoxicity has been reported if it is instilled directly into the ear, and keratitis may occur if it is used directly in the eye.[34]

Iodine and iodophors

Iodine has been a popular antiseptic for the past 50 years. Tincture of iodine is most effective as a 1% or 2% formula in 70% alcohol. The major advantages of iodine are its rapidity of action and low cost. Tincture of iodine is an excellent skin preparation agent to use before an invasive procedure. It continues to be the agent of choice for preparation of the skin before vein puncture to obtain blood for cultures. However, it is not as widely used as it once was because it can be irritating to the skin and has a tendency to cause stains. In most cases, tincture of iodine has been replaced by iodophors.

Iodophors were developed to take advantage of the antiseptic properties of iodine and to overcome the adverse effects of tincture of iodine. Iodophors consist of iodine complexed with a chemical carrier that slowly releases free iodine, which is the active antimicrobial agent. This process limits the irritation and staining but retains iodine's antiseptic properties. Interestingly, the release of free iodine increases as the solution is diluted. Consequently, dilution must be sufficient to release

TABLE 7-1. FDA's classification of antiseptics

Antiseptic	Description
Antimicrobial soap	Soap containing an ingredient with activity against skin flora
Health care personnel handwash	Broad-spectrum, antiseptic preparation that is fast-acting, nonirritating, and designed for frequent use
Patient preoperative skin preparation	Broad-spectrum, fast-acting antiseptic containing an antimicrobial that results in significant reductions in numbers of bacteria on intact skin
Skin antiseptic	Nonirritating preparation containing an antimicrobial ingredient to prevent clinical skin infection
Skin wound cleanser	Nonirritating liquid preparation used to remove foreign material from small, superficial wounds; may contain an antimicrobial ingredient and should not delay wound healing
Skin wound protectant	Nonirritating preparation containing an antimicrobial ingredient applied to clean, small wounds to form a protective physical and chemical barrier that neither delays healing nor favors microbial growth
Surgical hand scrub	Broad-spectrum, fast-acting, persistent, and nonirritating preparation containing an antimicrobial agent designed to reduce significantly the number of bacteria on intact skin

From Eiermann HJ. Antimicrobials: regulatory aspects. In Maibach H, Aly R, eds. *Skin Microbiology: Relevance to Clinical Infection.* New York: Springer-Verlag, 1981.

enough free iodine but not overdilute what is released. Iodophors have some disadvantages. They may:

1. Be absorbed into tissue and compromise wound healing if used on nonintact skin or tissue.[35]
2. Lose their effectiveness in the presence of organic material such as blood and body fluids.
3. Lose their antimicrobial properties rapidly after drying.

Iodophors are often used for routine and preoperative handwashing and skin site preparation before surgical incisions for invasive procedures.

Alcohols

Alcohols are among the safest, most effective antiseptics.[1] They act rapidly, have a broad spectrum of activity, and are inexpensive. The most frequently used alcohol solutions are 70% ethyl and 70% to 90% isopropyl. Alcohols vary slightly in their effectiveness, which is more a function of concentration than of type. The primary disadvantage of alcohols is their tendency to dry the skin. However, newer alcohol-based handwashing agents contain emollients that help to minimize the skin-drying effects. Also, alcohol's effectiveness may be decreased by organic material (e.g., blood, body fluids) and soil. Alcohol and alcohol-based products are flammable and must be used with care, particularly in the operating room. Alcohols are the active ingredient in many of the antiseptic rinseless handwashing agents and are frequently used as skin preparations before venous puncture or medication administration.

Chloroxylenol

Chloroxylenol (PCMX) has good antiseptic activity but is less effective than chlorhexidine and iodophors. It is relatively slow acting but only minimally affected by organic matter. PCMX is available in several handwashing products in concentrations of 1.5% to 3.5%.[26]

TABLE 7-2. Characteristics of six antiseptic ingredients

Agent	Gram-positive bacteria	Gram-negative bacteria	*Mycobacteria tuberculosis*
Alcohols	Excellent	Excellent	Good
Chlorhexidine	Excellent	Good	Poor
Hexachlorophene	Excellent	Poor	Poor
Iodine/iodophors	Excellent	Good	Good
PCMX (chloroxylenol)	Good	Fair	Fair
Triclosan (Irgasan, DP-300)	Good	Good (except for *Pseudomonas*)	Fair

Modified from Larson E. *Am J Infect Control.* APIC Guideline for use of topical antimicrobial agents. 1988;16(6):253-266.

Triclosan

Triclosan (Irgansan DP-300) is often used in deodorant soap to reduce body odor by inhibiting the growth of bacteria colonizing the skin. More data are needed before this antiseptic can be recommended for widespread use in health care. Triclosan is absorbed through intact skin but appears to be nonmutagenic. The recommended concentrations are 0.3% to 1%.[24]

Hexachlorophene

Hexachlorophene has good activity against gram-positive microorganisms but little activity against gram-negative microorganisms. It was often used to prevent staphylococcal infections in the newborn; however, rare instances of neurotoxicity associated with its use occurred, and that practice has been discontinued as a nursery routine.[26] Because chlorhexidine and other antiseptic solutions have a broader spectrum of antimicrobial activity and are safer, hexachlorophene is now rarely used in the health care setting.

Quaternary ammonium compounds

Quaternary ammonium compounds (e.g., benzalkonium chloride) are often found in "antiseptic" wipes. These compounds are easily inactivated by organic matter and can support growth of some potentially contaminating microorganisms such as *Pseudomonas* species.[31] They have relatively poor activity against gram-negative bacteria and have been implicated in nosocomial transmission of microorganisms.[31,35] Consequently, they are not recommended for use as antiseptics.[26]

Use of antiseptics
Routine and preoperative handwashing

The CDC recommends that plain soap be used for physical removal of transient microorganisms from hands.[16] However, an antiseptic is necessary when numbers of transient and normally resident bacteria must be reliably reduced in number.[24] The box below and Table 7-3 provide guidelines for use of antiseptics. Hands should be washed for 10 seconds or longer if soiled with dirt or organic matter.[16] A surgical scrub generally requires longer washing time for maximal effectiveness. The ideal surgical scrub time has not been objectively defined. Current recommendations for preoperative hand preparation require 2 to 5 minutes; however, this requirement is being reevaluated.[24] For surgical hand scrubbing, a timed or brush-stroke count method has traditionally been used to ensure standardized technique; specific recommendations for this procedure have been published.[2]

Effective handwashing includes lathering well, scrubbing all surfaces, rinsing, and drying. Despite its simplicity, handwashing is often performed incorrectly.[45] The surface areas most often missed are the back of the hands, between the fingers and thumb, under

Fungi	Viruses	Rapidity of action	Residual activity	Affected by organic matter?
Good	Good	Most rapid	None	Minimal
Fair	Good	Intermediate	Excellent	Minimal
Poor	Poor	Slow-intermediate	Excellent	Minimal
Good	Good	Intermediate	Minimal	Yes
Fair	Fair	Intermediate	Good	Minimal
Poor	Unknown	Intermediate	Excellent	Minimal

the fingernails, and the fingertips. Friction is vital to the mechanical removal of microorganisms. Hands should be rinsed under a stream of running water to remove soap and organisms. Care should be taken to avoid recontaminating the hands by touching the sink or faucet handles.

Health care personnel give many reasons for

GENERAL GUIDELINES FOR WHEN TO USE ANTISEPTIC SOAP

Before performing an invasive procedure

Before and after handling blood or body fluids or mucous membranes (wounds, orifices)

Before and after assisting with surgical procedures

Before direct contact with an immunocompromised patient

When moving from a contaminated site of patient's body to a clean area

When removing gloves

After touching inanimate surfaces that may have become contaminated with blood and body fluids

Between contact with patients in high-risk situations (e.g., patients with open wounds or invasive devices)

Modified from Garner JS, Favero MS. *Guidelines for the Prevention and Control of Nosocomial Infections: Guidelines for Handwashing and Hospital Environmental Control*. Atlanta: Centers for Disease Control; 1985.

not washing their hands. Some of the most common reasons are that their hands become irritated from excessive handwashing and harsh soap, that they have insufficient time for handwashing, and that facilities for handwashing are not readily available. Elliott[14] has listed additional influences on handwashing:

- Psychologic and physiologic stress of health care workers
- Emphasis on importance of handwashing by clinical managers
- Whether or not gloves are worn
- Degree of perceived personal gain or loss
- Degree of caregiver's education
- Caregiver's concern about skin integrity
- Childhood experiences
- Moral judgment of patient receiving care

Handwashing is the oldest, easiest, and traditionally considered one of the most effective strategies for the prevention of infection. It is important that all health care professionals adopt consistent, effective handwashing habits and participate in or encourage research aimed at influencing handwashing behavior (see Chapter 6).

Skin preparation for invasive procedures

The purpose of antiseptic preparation is to render the incision site for invasive or surgical procedures as free from microorganisms as possible, thereby reducing the likelihood that the skin will be a source of organisms that may produce infection. The skin must be cleaned to remove debris and organic material before the

TABLE 7-3. Indications for use of plain or antiseptic soap

Examples	Desired effect		
	Mechanical cleaning*	Rapid reduction of contaminating and colonizing flora†	Residual activity†
Routine patient bathing	x		
Routine handwashing in low-risk patient areas	x		
Routine handwashing in high-risk patient areas‡ (e.g., Newborn nursery, intensive care unit, areas with severely immunocompromised patients, transplant unit)	x	x	x
Preparation of hands before invasive procedures (e.g., venipuncture)	x	x	
Preoperative preparation of patient skin	x	x	
Surgical hand scrub	x	x	x

From Larson E. Guideline for Use of Topical Antimicrobial Agents. *Am J Infect Control.* 1988;16(6):253-266.
*If *only* this column is checked, plain soap is recommended.
†If this column is checked, antiseptics may be desired.

antiseptic is applied. The antiseptics most commonly used are similar to those used in antiseptic handwashing solutions and include iodophors, chlorhexidine, alcohols, and tincture of iodine (see Table 7-2). A variety of products containing these agents is available, and the manufacturer's recommendations should be followed when they are used.

CLEANING, DECONTAMINATION, AND SANITIZING

The primary purpose of cleaning is to decrease the amount of organic matter and soil and the associated microorganisms on environmental surfaces or instruments. The terms *cleaning, sanitization,* and *decontamination* are often used interchangeably. *Cleaning* is the removal of all visible dust, soil, and other foreign material. *Sanitization* and *decontamination* are often used to mean removal of sufficient numbers of disease-producing microorganisms to prevent infection in those who handle the object. Since the objective of each of these processes is to render items safe for use

or handling before disinfection or sterilization, the term *cleaning* is used in this chapter to refer to all these precautions.

Cleaning is a prerequisite to any type of disinfection or sterilization procedure.[15] Cleaning removes organic materials and soil that protect microorganisms and lowers the number of microorganisms present on the object. The cleaner the item, the greater is the chance of achieving disinfection or sterilization. A common misconception is that soaking a soiled instrument in disinfectant solution or sterilizer processing alone will accomplish disinfection or sterilization. On the contrary, if an item is not or cannot be cleaned first, it cannot be disinfected or sterilized reliably.

When to clean

In health care facilities, cleaning of patient equipment occurs in many locations, such as at the patient's bedside, in a clinic, or in a utility room. Although not always practical in all settings, cleaning, disinfection, and sterilization should be performed in a controlled environment. In most hospitals, this is the function of the central sterile processing department. Persons specifically trained to handle, clean, and disinfect or sterilize patient equipment generally staff this department. Staff nurses are seldom responsible for this process in most large facilities but many perform these functions in some settings where staff are limited. Regardless, nurses can assist by not allowing contaminants to dry on an instrument. When contaminated medical instruments are transported, they should be contained and labeled, consistent with U.S. Occupational Safety and Health Administration (OSHA) requirements, so as not to expose persons to the contaminants.[46]

How to clean

The first step in effective cleaning is to choose a solution designed for use on medical instruments. Effective cleaning products emulsify fats, contain an effective wetting agent, and break up proteinaceous material (blood, feces, saliva, etc.). Creation of suds is not necessary for effective cleaning. Enzymatic cleaners are often used to clean because they remove organic matter effectively. A common mistake is to use soaps designed for cleansing the skin to clean medical devices. In general, antiseptic hand soaps containing chlorhexidine and iodophors are not appropriate for use on medical instruments. The concentration of the ingredients in antiseptic soaps is not high enough to achieve disinfection, and these agents leave residual films on the instruments that tend to protect microorganisms. Abrasive cleaners should be avoided, since they can damage expensive medical instruments and decrease their life span.

Many systems are available for cleaning medical instruments, each with varying degrees of efficacy. These systems range from manual cleaning to sophisticated mechanical systems. Manual cleaning is often performed on instruments that are delicate and cannot withstand mechanical cleaning. In small facili-

ties, nursing homes, physicians' offices, and home health situations, this may be the only practical method available. Thorough cleaning must be followed by effective rinsing to remove any residual solution. The device should be visually inspected after cleaning to ensure that all soil is removed. When cleaning medical instruments by hand, health care professionals should avoid exposure to microbial contamination by wearing the appropriate personal protective equipment necessary for the type of exposure. Care must be exercised and forceps used as necessary to avoid punctures from sharp instruments or needles.

The preferred method of mechanical cleansing involves the use of an instrument-cleaning device. Many types of mechanical instrument cleaners are available, such as washer-decontaminators, instrument washers, ultrasonic washers, and washer-sterilizers. Each has its advantages and disadvantages. Mechanical cleaning devices that do not require instruments to be precleaned reduce the risk of exposing the worker to contamination, which may occur during manual precleaning. Individuals responsible for operating the equipment should be thoroughly familiar with the manufacturer's instructions for use.

Besides cleaning medical instruments before disinfection or sterilization, many areas of the health care environment must be cleaned. The most important aspects of cleaning are "elbow grease" and friction to remove organic matter and soil. Floors, furniture, walls, other flat surfaces, and visibly soiled areas must be cleaned as aesthetics and routine sanitation require. Disinfection is necessary only if there is contamination with blood or body substances. It is not necessary routinely to sterilize or high-level disinfect these surfaces, since the disinfectants are toxic and the inanimate environment plays a minimal role in transmitting microorganisms.[11,29]

Cleaning is a simple process, the importance of which is often underestimated. Disinfection and sterilization depend on correctly performed cleaning. An appropriate cleaning area, proper cleaning solutions and equipment, knowledge, diligence, and caution are necessary.

DISINFECTION

Disinfection eliminates pathogenic microorganisms on inanimate objects, with the exception of bacterial spores. This is generally achieved in health care settings by the use of liquid chemicals or wet pasteurization. Factors that influence disinfectant effectiveness include:[3,15]

- *Nature of the item.* The more crevices, joints, and hinges, the more difficult it is to disinfect. Disinfectants work only on areas they contact directly.
- *Number and type of microorganisms present on the object.* The higher the level of the item's contamination, the more difficult it is to disinfect. Some microbes are more difficult to kill than others. (The box on this page lists microorganisms in decreasing order of resistance to disinfectants.)
- *Amount of soil or organic matter present.* Soil protects microbes and may inactivate the disinfectant solution.
- *Contact time.* Disinfection requires direct contact with the agent for a specific time. For example, glutaraldehydes must be in contact with items for at least 20 minutes and up to 45 minutes for maximum effectiveness.
- *Concentration of solution.* The more concentrated the solution, the greater is its killing capacity. The solutions must be used at the concentration specified by the manufacturer to be most effective. Therefore, the manufacturer's dilution instructions must be followed.

Disinfectants vary in their ability to kill microorganisms. Three levels of disinfection commonly described are low, intermediate, and high (Table 7-4).

High-level disinfectants are effective against

RESISTANCE TO DISINFECTANTS IN DECREASING ORDER
(Most Resistant)
Prions (chronic infectious neuropathic agents, slow viruses)
↓
Bacterial spores: *Clostridium sporogenes*
↓
Mycobacteria: *Mycobacterium tuberculosis*
↓
Nonlipid or small viruses: adenoviruses, rhinovirus
↓
Fungi: *Candida* sp.
↓
Vegetative bacteria: *Pseudomonas, Staphylococcus*
↓
Lipid enveloped viruses: herpes, hepatitis B, human immunodeficiency virus
(Least Resistant)

Modified from Favero MS. Sterilization, disinfection, and antisepsis in the hospital. In Block SS, ed. *Disinfection, Sterilization, and Preservation,* 4th ed. Philadelphia: Lea & Febiger; 1991.

all vegetative bacteria, viruses, fungi, and TB, and most have a demonstrated level of activity against bacterial spores. High-level disinfectants are used primarily for such semicritical items as laryngoscopes, respiratory therapy and anesthesia equipment, and flexible fiberoptic endoscopes. The most commonly used high-level disinfectants are glutaraldehydes.

Intermediate-level disinfectants are more powerful and kill more resistant microorganisms than low-level disinfectants. In addition to vegetative bacteria, fungi, and lipid-enveloped viruses, they are effective against *Mycobacterium tuberculosis* and nonlipid viruses. They are not effective against resistant bacterial spores. Chlorine, iodophors, phenolics, and alcohols belong to this group.

Low-level disinfectants kill most vegetative bacteria, fungi, and lipid-enveloped viruses

TABLE 7-4. Levels of disinfection according to microorganism type*

	Bacteria			Fungi[1]	Viruses	
Levels	Vegetative	Tubercle-bacillus	Spores		Lipid or enveloped	Nonlipid
High	+[2]	+	+[3]	+	+	+
Intermediate	+	+	±[4]	+	+	±[5]
Low	+	−	−	±	+	−

[1]Includes asexual spores but not necessarily chlamydospores or sexual spores.
[2]Plus sign indicates that a killing effect can be expected when the normal use-concentrations of chemical disinfectants or pasteurization are properly employed; a negative sign indicates little or no killing effect.
[3]Only with extended exposure times are high-level disinfectant chemicals capable of actual sterilization.
[4]Some intermediate-level disinfectants can be expected to exhibit some sporicidal action.
[5]Some intermediate-level disinfectants may have limited virucidal activity.
Modified from Centers for Disease Control. Guidelines for the prevention and control of nosocomial infections. Guideline for handwashing and hospital environmental control. Atlanta, Georgia, 1985.

but do not kill spores or nonlipid viruses. They are less active against the *Mycobacterium tuberculosis* and some gram-negative rods, such as *Pseudomonas*. These disinfectants are typically used to wipe down items that will contact only intact skin or for environmental surface disinfection. Quaternary ammonium compounds, commonly called "quats," are low-level disinfectants.

Low-level and intermediate-level disinfectants for environmental sanitation

Low-level and intermediate-level disinfectants can be used to clean and disinfect the environment (floors, walls, beds, etc.) and some medical instruments. It is important to note that in general these solutions are designed for either environmental use or equipment processing and should not be used interchangeably. Environmental disinfectants can damage delicate instruments, and instrument disinfectants can be toxic if used in the environment. Since disinfectants are inherently toxic chemicals, appropriate protective attire should be worn to protect the user's skin and mucous membranes from exposure to these agents. Many disinfectant solutions are packaged in concentrated form, and one must

follow the manufacturer's recommendation for proper dilution.

The environmental disinfectants used on floors, walls, sinks, tabletops, instrument carts, and instrument knobs and handles should generally not be used on items for direct patient care.[10] Environmental surfaces play a much less significant role in disease transmission than medical instruments. Therefore, environmental cleaning agents usually are low-level to intermediate-level disinfectants.[15] The most popular environmental surface disinfectants are those that clean and disinfect in one step and require no rinsing. The most frequently used environmental disinfectants are reviewed below.

Common environmental disinfectants
Phenolic compounds

Lister was the first to use a phenolic solution as a germicide. This is one of the oldest agents for disinfecting environmental surfaces. Phenolic solutions are low-level to intermediate-level disinfectants when used in their recommended dilutions. They are effective in the presence of organic matter. However, they are not good cleaning agents and can be toxic if diluted improperly. Phenolics are absorbed by porous materials, and they leave an antimicrobial residual film on environmental surfaces.[3] Because they are difficult to rinse, their usefulness for disinfecting medical instruments is limited, and they are primarily used for environmental surface disinfection. These solutions can cause tissue irritation or depigmentation, and are possibly associated with hyperbilirubinemia in neonates.[45] Therefore, gloves should be worn during use and phenols are not recommended for use in nurseries. In some states, phenolics must now be managed as hazardous waste after use.

Quaternary ammonium compounds

Quaternary ammonium compounds are generally considered low-level disinfectants. However, they are good cleaning agents and are often preferred for environmental disinfection. However, the disinfection action is easily inactivated by organic matter and therefore they are of limited value for instrument disinfection. Some gram-negative bacteria, such as *Pseudomonas* species, will grow in these solutions once they are inactivated, creating a potential infection hazard. There have been many reports associating infections with contamination of these solutions. Consequently, the solutions must be discarded after each use.[27,31,35]

Activity against the relatively resistant mycobacteria has been proposed as a surrogate measure for activity against hepatitis B, HIV, and other bloodborne pathogens. Consequently, manufacturers have sought to demonstrate and claim their products are antituberculocidal. Unfortunately, attempts to substantiate these claims have often failed.[39]

Chlorine

The most common disinfectants used worldwide for environmental disinfection are *hypochlorites*. Sodium hypochlorite (bleach) in a concentration of 0.5% has broad germicidal activity. This agent is bactericidal, fungicidal, tuberculocidal, and virucidal. Hypochlorites

are inexpensive and fast acting. However, they are of limited use because of their corrosiveness, instability, and ineffectiveness in organic material.[3] Hypochlorites are often used for disinfection of surfaces after cleanup of blood or body fluid spills. In most United States health care facilities where other disinfectants are available, there is little need to use bleach, since its disadvantages outweigh its usefulness.

Iodophors

Most iodophors are manufactured as antiseptics; however, some iodophors are disinfectants.[9] An iodophor is a combination of iodine and a carrier that provides a sustained release of the active iodine. Iodophor disinfectants are intermediate-level disinfectants and are most active when appropriately diluted. Iodophors are corrosive to some metals, stain some products, and lose their effectiveness in organic material. These disadvantages make the iodophors a poor choice for environmental disinfection. They are occasionally used to clean environmental surfaces in food preparation areas because they are relatively nontoxic.

Alcohols

Alcohols are used both as topical antiseptics and disinfectants. They are considered to be intermediate-level disinfectants, although their effectiveness against viruses varies with the type of alcohol. Ethyl alcohol is broadly virucidal. Isopropyl alcohol only acts against lipid viruses. Alcohols evaporate quickly and have no residual activity. They are poor cleaners because they coagulate protein.[15] Although frequently used as environmental disinfectants, alcohols are not recommended for disinfecting large surfaces. Alcohol is very effective and convenient for small surfaces, such as stethoscope domes, intravenous (IV) site connections, and thermometers. These agents are flammable and must be stored in a cool, well-ventilated area.[3,39]

Disinfection of instruments

The complexity of the design and physical makeup of medical instruments often complicates the selection of an instrument disinfectant. Some instruments are delicate and can be damaged when an incompatible agent is used. Also, many disinfectants are toxic to the users. Occupational skin diseases and injuries have been associated with many of these agents. Those persons responsible for selecting and using disinfectants must understand the criteria for selecting an appropriate instrument disinfectant and the proper precautions to follow when using each agent.

Guidelines for the use of instrument disinfectants

- Use the disinfectant in a well-ventilated room.
- Make sure that items have been thoroughly cleaned before attempting disinfection.
- Disassemble all removable parts of the item.
- Thoroughly dry the item before placing it in the disinfectant.
- Mix the disinfectant as recommended on the label. Improper mixing can lead to injury of the patient, the instrument, and the person working with the solution. Read the directions for specific precautions.
- Completely immerse all parts of the item in the solution, ensuring that all lumens, creases, joints, and channels are in contact with the solution and that no trapped air bubbles are present.
- Do not leave the item in the disinfection solution for an undetermined time. The solution may damage the item and may also become a source of contamination.
- Close the container to prevent evaporation of the solution.
- Thoroughly rinse the item in at least two fresh rinse solutions to ensure adequate removal of the disinfectant. Sterile water rinses are best because tap water may contain large numbers of microorganisms.

Some fiberoptic scope manufacturers specify that the final rinse be alcohol.

- Thoroughly dry the disinfected item with a sterile towel, and place it in a dry, covered container until ready for use.

Many products and methods are used to disinfect instruments. A few are described below.

Alkaline glutaraldehyde 2%

Two-percent solutions are very effective high-level instrument disinfectants that can be sporicidal if the item is left in the solution for several hours.[39] Lengthy soaking, however, can damage items. Although these solutions have the ability to sterilize, the item should be considered disinfected instead of sterilized because no monitors adequately ensure sterilization. After the prescribed soaking time, remove the item and rinse thoroughly (at least two separate rinses). If there is a lumen in the instrument, an alcohol rinse or blowing of compressed air through the lumen may assist drying.[3] Glutaraldehydes have excellent antimicrobial properties, can work in the presence of some organic matter, and are noncorrosive when used properly.[15,41] They will not damage lensed instruments, rubber, or plastic items. These agents have had great popularity as high-level disinfectants. However, prolonged contact with them has been associated with skin and mucous membrane irritation. Gloves should be worn by those working with these solutions, and they should only be used in a well-ventilated area.

Formaldehyde

Formaldehyde is considered a high-level disinfectant.[15] However, it is seldom used in U.S. health care facilities today because of its irritating fumes, tissue toxicity, and potential carcinogenicity.

Pasteurization

Pasteurization is a method of thermal disinfection that involves immersion of precleaned items into water heated to approximately 75° to 100° C (167° to 212° F) for 30 minutes. This process is nontoxic and leaves no chemical residue. Even though it is a reliable, inexpensive method of disinfection, its use is limited to instruments that will withstand this type of wet heat. Pasteurization of respiratory therapy and anesthesia equipment is an effective alternative to chemical disinfection and is often used where ventilation is inadequate for chemical disinfection.

Problems with disinfectants

Selection of the appropriate disinfectant should include consideration of inherent problems:

- Lack of monitoring systems to ensure disinfection
- Lack of wrapping materials to keep the item clean or sterile before use
- Opportunity for human error (e.g., solutions not diluted or replaced appropriately can be ineffective, toxic, or a reservoir of microorganisms)
- Risk to staff (i.e., staff must use adequate personal protection and ventilation when mixing these solutions)

The selection of safe and effective agents is made difficult by the many agents available and the complexity and diversity of the health care environments and medical instruments. Nurses who are aware of the strengths and weaknesses of the various solutions are equipped to make appropriate selections to minimize infection risk and improve patient care. Table 7-5 is a guide to methods and agents for disinfection.

STERILIZATION

Sterilization is the only process that ensures that an item is free from all microbes and is the process of choice for items that will enter sterile body sites.[44]

Sterilization can be achieved with physical or chemical methods. Physical methods generally rely on moist or dry heat. The most common chemical used to achieve sterilization is ethylene oxide gas (ETO). Although soaking in high-level chemical disinfectants for long periods will achieve sterility, no practical test method is available for ensuring that sterility has been achieved.[44] Specific criteria must be established and met to ensure sterilization is effective.[3] As for all instrument and equipment processing, only appropriately trained personnel should be involved in this process.

Steam

Steam sterilization is the least expensive, most efficient, and least time-consuming method and is the method of first choice whenever possible. For the steam process to achieve sterility, the time, temperature, pressure, and moisture must be present in the correct proportions.[3] An imbalance in these components can result in the failure of the process.

Currently, two primary types of steam sterilizers are available: gravity sterilizers and high-speed (prevacuum) sterilizers. In the past, the *gravity sterilizer,* known as the *autoclave,* was the only type available. In the gravity sterilizer, the chamber fills with steam, displacing the air downward and forcing it out a drain until the thermal sensor probe detects that the preselected temperature and chamber pressure are reached. The minimum time for the entire cycle in the gravity sterilizer is 25 to 30 minutes at 121° to 132° C (250° to 270° F).[38]

It is possible to speed up the process in the gravity sterilizer by increasing the temperature, decreasing the time, and processing the item unwrapped. This method is called *flash sterilization.* Because the delicate balance among processing time, temperature, pressure, and moisture are changed, the probability that sterility will be achieved is reduced. For this reason, flash sterilization should be used only in an emergency (e.g., a surgical instrument has been dropped, no alternative

TABLE 7-5. Methods of sterilization and disinfection

	Sterilization		Disinfection		
	Critical items (will enter tissue or vascular system, or blood will flow through them)		*High level* Semi-critical items (will come in contact with mucous membranes or nonintact skin)	*Intermediate level* Some semicritical items[a] and noncritical items	*Low level* Noncritical items (will come into contact with intact skin)
Object	Procedure	Exposure time (hr)	Procedure (exposure time ≥20 min)[b,c]	Procedure (exposure time ≤10 min)	Procedure (exposure time ≤10 min)
Smooth, hard surface[d]	A[e]	MR	C	I	I
	B	MR	D	K	J
	C	MR	E	L	K
	D	6	F		L
	E	6	G[f]		M
	F	MR	H		
Rubber tubing and catheters[c]	A	MR	C		
	B	MR	D		
	C	MR	E		
	D	6	F		
	E	6	G[d]		
	F	MR			
Polyethylene tubing and catheters[c,g]	A	MR	C		
	B	MR	D		
	C	MR	E		
	D	6	F		
	E	6	G[f]		
	F	MR			
Lensed instruments	B	MR	C		
	C	MR	D		
	D	6	E		
	E	6	F		
	F	MR			
Thermometers (oral and rectal)[h]				I[h]	
Hinged instruments	A	MR	C		
	B	MR	D		
	C	MR	E		
	D	6	F		
	E	6			
	F	MR			

[a]Modified from Simmons BP. AM J Infect Control 1983;11:96–115.

[b]The longer the exposure to a disinfectant, the more likely it is that all microorganisms will be eliminated. Ten minutes; exposure is not adequate to disinfect many objects, especially those that are difficult to clean because they have narrow channels or other areas that can harbor organic material and bacteria. Twenty minutes' exposure is the minimal time needed to reliably kill *M. tuberculosis* and nontuberculous Mycobacteria with glutaraldehyde.

[c]Tubing must be completely filled for disinfection; care must be taken to avoid entrapment of air bubbles during immersion.

[d]See text for discussion of hydrotherapy.

Table footnote continued on next page.

exists, and the instrument is needed immediately). Devices to be implanted should not be flash sterilized because of the unreliability of the process, the lack of time to evaluate whether the sterilization process was effective before the item is used, and the serious consequences that result from infections involving these devices.

The *high-speed vacuum sterilizer* requires a shorter processing time than a gravity sterilizer because the air is pumped out of the sterilizer before the steam enters. These high-speed sterilizers develop fewer air pockets of uneven temperature and pressure because the air is mechanically withdrawn. These sterilizers are used when a brief processing time is important, since an entire cycle can be completed in as little as 15 minutes. However, some items cannot tolerate the vacuum and must be sterilized in the gravity sterilizer. Some steam sterilizers offer both gravity and high-speed sterilization in the same machine. Small tabletop sterilizers, often found in dental offices and clinics, are usually gravity sterilizers. These machines are essentially horizontal pressure cookers that achieve temperatures of about 121° C (250° F.). Since each sterilizer is unique, staff should always follow the manufacturer's instructions when operating them.

Ethylene oxide gas

Another frequently used sterilization method is known as *gas sterilization*. In this system, ETO is the sterilizing agent. ETO sterilization is complex and expensive. It is used to process heat-sensitive items that cannot withstand steam sterilization and has a much narrower margin of safety than steam.[44] Its effectiveness is a function of the ETO concentration, temperature, humidity, and duration of gas exposure.[15] Since excessive moisture can create a hazardous residue, items sterilized in ETO must be not only clean but also dry before sterilization. ETO can be toxic and carcinogenic; therefore, those working with this

---

Continued from previous page.

^{e}A, Heat sterilization, including steam or hot air (see manufacturer's recommendations).

B, Ethylene oxide gas (see manufacturer's recommendations).

C, Glutaraldehyde-based formulations (2%). (Caution should be exercised with all glutaraldehyde formulations when further in-use dilution is anticipated.)

D, Demand-release chlorine dioxide (will corrode aluminum, copper, brass, series 400 stainless steel and chrome with prolonged exposure).

E, Stabilized hydrogen peroxide 6% (will corrode copper, zinc, and brass).

F, Peracetic acid, concentration variable but ≤ 1% is sporicidal.

G, Wet pasteurization at 75°C for 30 minutes after detergent cleaning.

H, Sodium hypochlorite (1000 ppm available chlorine; will corrode metal instruments).

I, Ethyl or isopropyl alcohol (70%–90%).

J, Sodium hypochlorite (100 ppm available chlorine).

K, Phenolic germicidal detergent solution (follow product label for use-dilution).

L, Iodophor germicidal detergent solution (follow product label for use-dilution).

M, Quaternary ammonium germicidal detergent solution (follow product label for use-dilution).

MR, Manufacturer's recommendations.

^{f}Pasteurization (washer disinfector) of respiratory therapy and anesthesia equipment is a recognized alternative to high-level disinfection. Some data challenge the efficacy of some pasteurization units.

^{g}Thermostability should be investigated when appropriate.

^{h}Do not mix rectal and oral thermometers at any stage of handling or processing.

From Rutala WA: Disinfection, Sterilization, and Waste Disposal. In: Wenzel RP, ed: *Prevention and Control of Nosocomial Infections*. 2nd ed. Williams & Wilkins; 1993:461. Used with Permission.

agent must observe appropriate safety precautions.[8] These precautions include the following:

1. A minimum of 10 air changes per hour in the room where the sterilizer is located to remove any gas that escapes into room air
2. Door-locking devices on the machine
3. Cracking the door of the sterilizer open for 15 minutes after the cycle is complete to allow evacuation of residual gas
4. Use of a purge system to remove leftover gas from the machine
5. An alarm that alerts the user at the end of the cycle
6. A specifically designed ventilation cabinet for aeration of the processed supplies

ETO may be toxic to both patients and staff; therefore, ETO-sterilized items must be aerated over several hours to allow the gas to dissipate and be exhausted through a special ventilation system to prevent human exposure.

At least 12 hours are required to sterilize and aerate items when using ETO. If items sterilized by ETO are used frequently, this often necessitates a large inventory of supplies with the associated increased costs. Because of these issues and the potential for toxicity, alternatives to ETO technology are emerging.

Plasma sterilization

One of the newest available methods of sterilization is *plasma sterilization*.[19] Plasma can be produced when a chemical such as hydrogen peroxide is introduced into a strong electric or magnetic field and is "excited" into a state which is capable of disrupting the cell membranes and nucleic acids of microorganisms. The plasma thereby acts as a sterilizing agent. The sterilization cycle takes approximately one hour. Oxygen and water are the end products of the process. Thus there is no need for aeration as with ETO. This process has the potential to replace ETO for some

purposes. Its effectiveness and limitations are being evaluated.

Peracetic acid

Another method of chemical sterilization uses peracetic acid, normally corrosive in nature. This method combines acetic acid, hydrogen peroxide, and water in a noncorrosive form.[15] Its effectiveness depends on the proper concentration of peracetic acid, time, and temperature. Peracetic acid is less damaging to delicate instruments than other chemical agents and is compatible with a wide range of materials used in medical devices.[9] It also sterilizes at low temperatures and therefore can be used for heat-sensitive items such as fiberoptic endoscopes.

Peracetic acid is available in a sterilization system for instruments.[19] One advantage of this system is that it offers a quick processing time, approximately 30 minutes. However, as with all liquid chemical sterilants and high level disinfectants, items cannot be wrapped before sterilization and are slightly wet when removed from the sterilizer. Thus, care must be taken not to contaminate them after processing and before use. It is important to note that no biologic indicator test system has been approved by the FDA for marketing and use as recommended by the manufacturer of the sterilization system. To date, there are no independent, peer-reviewed studies to confirm the company data or claims for efficacy.[4,5,21,30] The peracetic acid sterilization system is used in some clinics, dental offices, and operating rooms.

Other sterilization and disinfection technologies being developed include 1) chlorine dioxide, 2) vapor-phase hydrogen peroxide, and 3) ozone.[19,32]

Dry heat

Dry heat, which sterilizes by cooking, is most often used in the dental setting in the United States. It is usually reserved for sterilizing powders and oils. In other countries, dry heat is often used for to sterilize sponges, bandages, and instruments. The major disadvantages of dry heat is that it penetrates materials slowly and unevenly. Consequently, a long exposure time is necessary and biologic indicators should be used.[38] Some sterilizers can be programmed to provide both steam and dry heat. (See Table 7-5 for methods of sterilization.)

Monitoring sterilization

Regardless of which sterilization method is used, the process should be monitored to determine that sterilization has occurred.[38] Mechanical, biologic, and chemical indicators help ensure that sterilizers are effective. The *mechanical monitor* is a recording chart or a computer that documents whether the specific conditions necessary to achieve sterilization have been met. The chart is read immediately after each sterilization cycle.

Biologic spores are the most accurate monitoring devices.[21] These indicators consist of spores of microorganisms that are most resistant to the process to be tested. Therefore, spore destruction indicates that all other organisms have been killed. For steam, the spore used is *Bacillus stearothermophilus*; for ETO, *Bacillus subtilis*. The frequency of biologic testing varies among practitioners and organizations and may be influenced by state or federal regulations or guidelines. Some monitor every sterilizer load; others monitor daily or weekly. Daily or weekly biologic monitoring of each steam sterilizer and each load that contains items to be implanted. (e.g., hip prosthesis) are commonly recommended routines. The biologic indicator should be placed in a test pack in the sterilizer where failure is most likely to occur and should be placed in each flash sterilizer load.

Chemical indicators consist of paper or tape containing chemical formulations that provide an immediate indication that a spe-

cific temperature has been achieved. These indicators do not document achievement of adequate pressures or exposure times and therefore do not assure that sterilization has taken place. Chemical indicators should be placed both inside and outside each pack. The item is not used if the test is positive. These indicators make it easy to determine that the item has been subjected to a sterilization process.

Each sterilized package should be labeled with a control number that designates the sterilizer used, date of sterilization, the sterilizer cycle of the day, and the expiration date. The label should be placed on the outside of the package before sterilization. When a monitoring device, whether mechanical, biologic or chemical, indicates inadequate sterilizer function, the test should be repeated. If a problem is still indicated, all items processed in the sterilizer since the last test indicating adequate sterilizer function should be identified by its control number, be recalled, and reprocessed. The sterilizer should be taken out of service until it is inspected, repaired, and retested. Health care providers of patients who may have been affected by the failure should be notified.

SELECTION OF DISINFECTION OR STERILIZATION METHODS

After an item has been cleaned, it is ready for either disinfection or sterilization. Choice of the appropriate process for an instrument is determined by its intended use and its construction. Recommendations from the manufacturer and, in hospital and long-term care settings, the central service staff, and infection control committee also guide this choice. These factors are discussed next.

Intended use

Spaulding devised a classification system to guide selection of disinfection and sterilization processes.[44] The system bases the choice on the degree of infection risk related to use of the items. He defined three broad categories of medical devices: critical, semicritical, and noncritical (Table 7-6).

Items are classified as *critical* when they enter a sterile body cavity. Spaulding specified that devices that enter sterile areas of the body or the vascular system should be sterilized. Some exceptions are made in the U.S. for expedience when there is insufficient equipment to allow the long turnaround times required for sterilization. This has resulted in endoscopes that enter sterile tissue, such as laparoscopes and arthroscopes, undergoing high-level disinfection rather than sterilization between patients.[39] High-level disinfection is recommended as a minimum for these devices when sterilization is not feasible.[16] No evidence suggests that this practice, when properly performed, has posed an infection risk to patients.

Semicritical items come into contact with mucous membranes or nonintact skin. These items must be free of all microorganisms, with the exception of numbers of bacterial spores typically present. Respiratory therapy and anesthesia equipment, flexible fiberoptic endoscopes, and diaphragm fitting rings are examples of objects classified as semicritical. *High-level* disinfectants may be used in these situations. These agents destroy all forms of microbial life but not necessarily all bacterial spores.

Spaulding's third category of items is *noncritical*. These come in contact with intact skin but not with mucous membranes, nonintact skin, tissue, or the vasculature. The risk of infection from these items is minimal. Examples of noncritical items include such patient care items as blood pressure cuffs, electrocardiogram electrodes, x-ray machines and environmental surfaces such as floors, walls, beds, and bedside tables. Intermediate-level or low-level disinfectants may be used for these noncritical items. *Intermediate-level* disinfection

TABLE 7-6. Classification of devices and processes

Device classification	Spaulding process classification
Critical (enters sterile tissue or vascular system): implants, scalpels, needles, other surgical instruments, etc.	Sterilization
Semicritical (touches mucous membranes): flexible endoscopes, laryngoscopes, endotracheal tubes, other similar instruments	High-level disinfection
Noncritical (touches intact skin): stethoscopes, table tops, floors, etc.	Intermediate-level disinfection (has tuberculocidal activity)
	Low-level disinfection (no tuberculocidal activity)

From Favero MS, Bond WW: Chemical disinfection of medical and surgical materials. In Block SS, ed. *Disinfection, sterilization, and preservation*, ed 4. Philadelphia, 1991, Lea & Febiger.

kills tubercle bacilli, vegetative bacteria, most viruses, and fungi. *Low-level* disinfection kills vegetative bacteria, some viruses, and fungi, but not tubercle bacilli.

Manufacturers' recommendations

Another factor that will influence the choice of instrument-processing method is the manufacturer's recommendations. Although these must be considered and are often followed, circumstances may require use of an alternative. For example, the manufacturer may recommend use of a product that does not achieve the desired level of disinfection or may damage the instrument. If this is the case, consult the manufacturer. The proper method of cleaning, disinfection, or sterilization should be determined before purchasing the instrument. This ensures that the appropriate system for processing the instrument is available.

Infection control committee consultation

In the United States the Joint Commission on the Accreditation of Healthcare Organizations (JCAHO) and some state laws assign the ultimate responsibility for infection control within a health care organization to an infection control committee.[20] This responsibility includes approval of disinfection and sterilization practices. When policies or procedures are developed for a specific instrument, or use of a specific cleaning, disinfection or sterilization process, this committee should be consulted. In the absence of an infection control committee, consultation with an in-house or external authority or a review of literature may be helpful. Some useful references are listed at the end of this chapter.

REUSE OF DISPOSABLE EQUIPMENT

In general, equipment intended for single use should not be reprocessed and used, since many disposable items cannot be adequately cleaned and sterilized or are made of materials that may be damaged by chemical or heat disinfection or sterilization. Many of these devices are made from plastics that may retain toxic levels of a chemical disinfectant. However, an institution may occasionally decide to reprocess an item following consultation with the manufacturer and review of the relevant literature and community standards and after performing in-house studies to ensure that a specific disposable product is not damaged or otherwise altered by cleaning, disinfecting, or sterilizing. Institutions choosing to reprocess disposable medical equipment assume the liability associated with use of the devices; therefore, all institutions should have a written policy regarding the reuse of disposable items.

ANTISEPSIS, DISINFECTION, AND STERILIZATION IN ALTERNATE CARE SETTINGS

The complexity of modern medical instrumentation requires proper training for those responsible for choosing and using disinfection and sterilization methods. When a central processing department is available, all equipment disinfection and sterilization should be performed in this area. However, in some practice settings nurses assume this responsibility (e.g., nursing homes, home health, and physicians' offices). Although the methods used in hospitals may be impractical for some situations, the principles of asepsis outlined earlier should not be compromised.

The methods chosen for disinfection or sterilization depend on available resources, circumstances, and review by a knowledgeable individual or committee designated to approve the selection. Clinics, physicians' offices, and nursing homes often have a steam sterilizer available on the premises. These devices should be used and monitored according to the manufacturer's recommendations. In these settings, the same antiseptics and disinfectants appropriate for use in hospitals can be used for handwashing, preparing the skin for invasive procedures, and instrument or environmental disinfection.

In home health care and other public health settings, flexibility and planning are necessary because sinks, handwashing facilities, and other equipment are not always readily available. Nurses working in these environments should carry a rinseless handwashing agent or antiseptic towelettes. Although sterilization cannot generally be performed in the home, disinfection can be achieved by boiling or using chemicals found in the home, such as a 1:10 dilution of household bleach. The limitations of these methods should be understood by practitioners who use them and will vary with the chemical, the item to be disinfected, and the ability to use them safely. Flexibility and ingenuity are important. For example, in the home setting, urinary catheters used for straight catheterization can be washed with soap and water and rinsed thoroughly or disinfected in the microwave oven. Alcohol can be flushed through the lumen to expedite drying and inhibit growth of bacteria. This same process can be used for other catheters, such as those for suctioning. These catheters can be wrapped in a freshly ironed towel to prevent contamination before reuse.

SUMMARY

Cleaning, antisepsis, disinfection, and sterilization are important components of infection prevention. Nurses should have a basic understanding of these principles to care effectively and safely for their patients. Nurses often perform these functions or use instruments processed by these methods and therefore must be familiar with the advantages and disadvantages of the agents and systems they use and must be able to detect and manage processing problems. Those directly responsible for instrument processing must understand the principles outlined in this chapter and should be familiar with the cited references.

REFERENCES

1. Altemeier WA. Surgical antiseptics. In Block SS, ed. *Disinfection, Sterilization and Preservation*, 3rd ed. Philadelphia: Lea & Febiger; 1983;493-506.
2. Association of Operating Room Nurses, Inc. *Standards and Recommended Practices for Perioperative Nursing.* Denver: AORN; 1990.
3. Bennett G, Shafer K. Section four: Sterilization, disinfection and sanitation. In Soule BM, ed. *The APIC Curriculum for Infection Control Practice.* 1983;1:517-551.
4. Bond WW. Biological indicators for a liquid chemical sterilizer: a solution to the instrument reprocessing problems? (editorial). *Infect Control Hosp Epidemiol.* 1993;14:309-312.
5. Bond WW. Biological indicators for a liquid chemical sterilizer. (Reply to a letter to the editor). *Infect Control Hosp Epidemiol.* 1993;14:565.
6. Brandberg A, Holm J, Hammersten J, Schersten T. Postoperative wound infections in vascular surgery: effect of preoperative whole body disinfection by shower-bath with chlorhexidene soap. In Maibach H, Aly R, eds. *Skin Microbiology: Relevance to Clinical Infection.* New York: Springer-Verlag, 1981.
7. Checko PJ. Section Two: Microbiology. In Soule BM, ed. *The APIC Curriculum for Infection Control Practice.* 1983; 1:212-219.
8. Code of Federal Regulations. Ethylene oxide. US Dept of Labor, Occupational Safety and Health Administration. July 1992. 29 CFR Part 1910.1047, 306-328.
9. Crow S: Product commentary: chemical disinfectants. *Infect Control and Hosp Epidemiology.* 1984;5(1): 53-54.
10. Crow S. Product commentary: housekeeping products, the choice is yours. *Infect Control Hosp Epidemiol.* 1988;9(1):40-41.
11. Delgado-Rodriguez M et al. Nonincreased risk of nosocomial infection during a 22-day housekeeping personnel strike in a tertiary hospital. *Infect Control Hosp Epidemiol.* 1993;14:706-712.
12. Dixon RE: Historical perspective: the landmark conference in 1980. *Am J Med.* 1991;91(suppl3B):65-75.
13. Eiermann HJ. Antimicrobials: regulatory aspects. In Maibach H, Aly R, eds. *Skin Microbiology: Relevance to Clinical Infection.* New York: Springer-Verlag, 1981.
14. Elliott PRA. Hand-washing: a process of judgement and effective decision-making. *Professional Nurse.* 1992;292-296.
15. Favero MS, Bond WW. Chemical disinfection of medical and surgical materials. In Block S, ed. *Disinfection, Sterilization and Preservation*, 4th ed. Philadelphia: Lea & Febiger, 1991.
16. Garner JS, Favero MS. CDC guidelines for the prevention and control of nosocomial infections; guidelines for hand-washing and hospital environmental control. Atlanta: Centers for Disease Control; 1985.
17. Goldmann DA. Contemporary challenges for hospital epidemiology. *Am J Med.* 1991;91(suppl3B):85-155.
18. Hoeller ML. *The Operating Room Technician.* St. Louis: CV Mosby; 1968;30-42.
19. Janssen DW, Schneider PM. Overview of ethylene oxide alternative methodologies in the clinical setting. *J of Healthc Mater Manage.* 1992;31-32, 34, 39.
20. Joint Commission for the Accreditation of Health Care Organizations. *1992 Accreditation Manual for Hospitals.* Chicago: JCAHO; 1992.
21. Kravolic RC. Use of biological indicators designed for steam or ethylene oxide to monitor a liquid chemical sterilization process. *Infect Control Hosp Epidemiol.* 1993;14:313-319.
22. LaForce MF. The control of infections in hospitals: 1750 to 1950. In Wentzel RP, ed. *Prevention and Control of*

Nosocomial Infections. Baltimore: Williams & Wilkins, 1987;1-12.

23. Larson E, Bobo L. Effective hand degerming in the presence of blood. *J Emerg Med.* 1992;20(1):11-15.

24. Larson E. APIC guideline for infection control practice, guideline for use of topical antimicrobial agents. *Am J Infect Control.* 1988;16(6):253-266.

25. Larson E. Persistent carriage of gram-negative bacteria on hands. *Am J Infect Control.* 1981;9:112.

26. Laufman H. Current use of skin and wound cleaners and antiseptics. *Am J Surg.* 1989;157:359-365.

27. Lee JC, Fialkow PJ. Benzalkonium chloride: source of hospital infection with gram-negative bacteria. *JAMA.* 1961;711:708-710.

28. Maki DG. Skin as a source of nosocomial infections. *Infect Control.* 1986;7:113-116.

29. Maki DG, et al. Relation of the inanimate hospital environment to endemic nosocomial infection. *N Engl J Med.* 1982;307:1562.

30. Malchesky PS. Biological indicators for a liquid chemical sterilizer (Letter to the editor). *Infect Control Hosp Epidemiol.* 1993;14:563-565.

31. Malizia WF, et al. Benzalkonium chloride as a source of infection. *N Engl J Med.* 1960;263:800-802.

32. Martin MA, Reichelderfer M. APIC guideline for infection prevention and control in flexible endoscopy. *Am J Infect Control.* 1994;22:19-38.

33. Martone WMJ, Jarvis WR, Culver DH, Haley RW. Incidence and nature of endemic and epidemic nosocomial infections. In Bennett JV, Brachman PS, eds. *Hospital Infections.* Boston: Little, Brown; 1992;579-581.

34. Morizono T, Johnston BM, Hadjar E. The ototoxicity of antiseptics. *J Otolaryngol Soc Aust.* 1973;3:550-559.

35. Plotkin SA, Austrian R. Bacteremia caused by pseudomonas sp. following the use of materials stored in solutions of a cationic surface-active agent. *Am J Med Sci.* 1958;235:621-627.

36. Price PB. New studies in surgical bacteriology and surgical technique. *JAMA.* 1938;111:1993-1996.

37. Rodeheaver G, et al. Bactericidal activity and toxicity of iodine-containing solutions in wounds. *Arch Surg.* 1982;117:181-186.

38. Rutala WA. Disinfection, sterilization and waste disposal. In Wenzl RP, ed. *Prevention and Control of Nosocomial Infections*, 2nd ed. Baltimore: Williams & Wilkins; 1993; 460-495.

39. Rutala WA. APIC guideline for selection and use of disinfectants. *Am J Infect Control.* 1990;18(2):99-117.

40. Sanchez I, et al. Effects of chlorhexidine-diacetate and povidone-iodine on wound healing in dogs. *Vet Surg.* 1988;17(6):291-295.

41. Scott EM, Gorman SP. Glutaraldehyde. In Block S, ed. *Disinfection, Sterilization and Preservation*, 4th ed. Philadelphia: Lea & Febiger, 1991.

42. Shaberg DR, Culver DH, Gaynes RP. Major trends in the microbial etiology of nosocomial infection. *Am J Med.* 1991;91(suppl3B):725-755.

43. Spach DH, Silverstein FE, Stamm WE. Transmission of infection by gastrointestinal endoscopy. *Ann Intern Med.* 1993;118:117-128.

44. Spaulding EH. Chemical disinfection and medical and surgical materials. In Block S, ed. *Disinfection, Sterilization and Preservation.* Philadelphia: Lea & Febiger; 1968;517-530.

45. Taylor LJ. An evaluation of hand-washing techniques. *Nursing Times.* 1978;74(2)54-55.

46. U.S. Dept. of Labor, Occupational Safety and Health Administration. Occupational exposure to bloodborne pathogens. Final Rule. *Federal Register.* Dec. 6, 1991;56:64004-64182.

47. Webster's Third New International Dictionary. Chicago: Meriam-Webster, Inc., 1981.

48. Weinstein RA. Multiple drug-resistant pathogens: epidemiology and control. In Bennett JV, Brachman PS, eds. *Hospital Infections.* Boston: Little, Brown; 1992;270-271.

49. Wysowski DK, et al. Epidemic neonatal hyperbilirubenemia and use of a phenolic disinfectant detergent. *Pediatrics* 1978;61:165-170.

SUGGESTED READINGS

Block S, ed. *Disinfection, Sterilization and Preservation*, 4th ed. Philidelphia: Lea & Febiger, 1991.

Chapter 8

Antimicrobial Chemotherapeutics

BRIAN W. COOPER

erhaps the most singular advance in medicine in the 20th century has been the development of antimicrobial compounds. Along with vaccines, these agents have played a major role in the decline of morbidity and mortality from bacterial infections during the past 50 years. Antimicrobial compounds have been used for more than 70 years and many new antimicrobial agents have emerged over the past 10 years. The extraordinary number of new drugs, such as aminoglycosides, ureidopenicillins, third-generation cephalosporins, macrolides, and quinolones, each with different spectrums of activity, pharmacokinetics, and adverse reactions, present challenges for nurses and medical practitioners in all practice settings. To integrate these very powerful tools properly into patient care practices, nurses must first familiarize themselves with the basic properties of various major classes of antimicrobial compounds.

The full effect of antimicrobial use cannot be considered in isolation. The ultimate effects of antimicrobial chemotherapy not only result from the pharmacologic and microbiologic properties of the drugs but also to a large degree from the interaction of these drugs with the physical environment and microbiologic populations that surround us, the patients for whom they are prescribed, and the constant social interactions that bring all elements together. These host-environment interactions, which determine disease causation, are considered here as they relate to chemotherapy.

THE HOST-ENVIRONMENT INTERACTION
Adverse effects of antimicrobial agents

It has been estimated that 5% of patients receiving an antibiotic will have an adverse reaction to the drug. Adverse effects may be mild and easily tolerated or may be life-threatening events. Although the frequency and types of adverse reactions vary from compound to compound, all drugs have been associated with some adverse outcomes. Often called therapeutic misadventure, patient injury resulting from therapy has also been termed medical friendly fire, a somewhat more evocative phrase.[4]

Hypersensitivity reactions

Allergy-mediated hypersensitivity reactions may be the most common antimicrobial side effects. Manifestations of hypersensitivity typically include one or more of the following: drug fever, skin rashes, pruritus, phototoxicity, and exfoliative dermatitis.

Immediate-type hypersensitivity reactions include anaphylactic reactions leading to hypotension, wheezing, or angioedema. Immediate-type hypersensitivity may occur in response to any antibiotic, although they are most often associated with β-lactam drugs. Evaluation of the patient with a history of hypersensitivity reactions is difficult, and patient histories regarding drug allergies are notoriously inaccurate. When a patient claims hypersensitivity to a β-lactam, drug sensitivity skin testing with penicillin G–derived antigens may be useful to confirm penicillin allergy.

Blood dyscrasias

Antimicrobial compounds may produce adverse hemopoietic effects by many mechanisms. Aplastic anemia is the most severe effect; anemia, leukopenia, and thrombocytopenia may also occur alone or in combination.

Adverse effects on specific organs

Virtually any organ may be affected by antimicrobial side effects. The most common reported adverse effects involve the gastrointestinal (GI) tract, kidneys, and liver.[5] In the GI tract, nausea and abdominal discomfort are reported most frequently, but antibiotic-associated diarrhea occurs often as well. The most severe form of diarrhea occurs after bowel organisms are suppressed, allowing overgrowth of *Clostridium difficile*. This toxin-producing organism can cause severe diarrhea that is often accompanied by pseudomembrane formation in the colon. Though first seen in association with clindamycin, *C. difficile* colitis has since been associated with all antibiotic classes (see Clinical Study 22). Reduction of normal bowel flora sensitive to antimicrobial therapy allows proliferation of resistant organisms to abnormal levels and establishes the gastrointestinal tract as a reservoir of potential pathogens.

Hepatitis and cholestatic jaundice may occur during treatment with numerous antibiotics but occurs particularly with erythromycin and sulfonamides. Isoniazid (INH) therapy for tuberculosis may cause an especially severe form of drug-induced hepatitis that may be fatal.

Renal toxicity caused by antibiotics may be manifested by glomerulonephritis, interstitial nephritis, or acute tubular necrosis. Interstitial nephritis has most frequently been reported with β-lactam drugs but has also been associated with tetracyclines and quinolones. Aminoglycosides cause nephrotoxicity by toxicity to tubular epithelial cells. Renal toxicity of aminoglycosides is most strongly associated with high serum trough levels of the drug; dosing of aminoglycosides must be adjusted according to renal function assessed by monitoring of serum creatinine.

Other organs may be adversely affected by antibiotics as well. Neurotoxicity may be manifested by central nervous system (CNS) disturbances secondary to quinolones and imipenem or as peripheral neuropathy, such as is seen during isoniazid therapy. Pulmonary toxicity can also occur, such as interstitial pneumonia secondary to nitrofurantoin.

Antimicrobial chemotherapy and the microbial environment
General resistance to antimicrobial drugs

Antimicrobial drugs are unique in the sense that once administered, they can affect not only the patient but other individuals and the environment as well. The ability of antibiotics to select for survival those microorganisms, which have resistance genes that can be shared and accumulated is the chief factor limiting the efficacy of antimicrobial chemotherapy.[12,15]

Organisms may become resistant to antibiotics through any of several mechanisms. To understand this process, it is useful to consider what an antibiotic must do to be effective. The antibiotic must first diffuse through tissues to the bacterial cell and achieve effective concentration. Then it must penetrate the bacterial cell wall and attack a target site within the organism. The target site varies with the antimicrobial. Bacteria are able to interdict this process in four main ways:

1. Bacteria may produce enzymes or other substances that destroy or degrade the antibiotic before it can penetrate. Examples include the destruction of

β-lactam molecules by the enzyme β-lactamase.

2. Bacterial cell wall structures may change so that penetration of the antibiotic is blocked. Protein structures such as porins in the cell walls of gram-negative bacteria allow selective passage of certain compounds, including some antibiotics. Changes in these porins' structure may effectively block penetration of some antibiotics.

3. The bacterial cell may develop efflux mechanisms. These are active pumps that shuttle the antibiotic out of the cell's cytoplasm as soon as it penetrates. Tetracycline resistance is mediated by this mechanism in some bacteria.

4. Genetic mutation may also alter the antimicrobial's target site or a metabolic pathway so that the antibiotic is rendered ineffective. Resistance to macrolide drugs (e.g., erythromycin) in gram-positive organisms is most often mediated by this mechanism.

Genetic resistance mechanisms

Genetically coded resistance determinants most effectively overcome antimicrobial therapy strategies when they are efficiently accumulated and transmitted to other bacteria of the same or other species. Bacteria display a remarkable genetic capacity to develop antimicrobial resistance by mutation or acquisition of deoxyribonucleic acid (DNA). The resistance genes may be passed on to other bacterial cells on nonchromosomal DNA structures known as plasmids or even smaller genetic units called transposons. *Plasmids* are small, closed, circular bits of extrachromosomal DNA that can carry and accumulate antimicrobial resistance genes. *Transposons* are genetic subunits that are able to excise themselves from the chromosomes and transfer to other chromosomes or plasmids. Resistance determinants coded on plasmids or transposons may be efficiently exchanged with other bacteria,

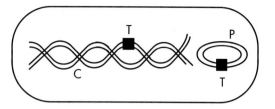

FIGURE 8-1. Bacterial genetics C-chromosome, P-plasmid, T-transposon.

including organisms of a different species or genus (Figure 8-1).

The social environment

Control of the spread of antimicrobial resistance is difficult. Three approaches have been used to minimize the effect of antibiotic-resistant organisms; each has been effective to limited degrees:

1. Control of antibiotic use
2. Use of antibiotic combinations
3. Enhancement of asepsis and infection control efforts

Control of antibiotic use

Studies have shown that a major influence on the prevalence of resistant organisms is the selective pressure imposed by the use of antimicrobial drugs.[13] Minimizing inappropriate use of antimicrobials can help reduce this selective pressure. Antibiotic prescribing patterns of practitioners vary widely, but several common errors in prescribing have been noted. The most frequent error is selection of an antibiotic inappropriate for the organism causing the infection. This may be selection of antibiotics to which the microorganism is resistant or with an unnecessarily broad spectrum of activity. Antimicrobials may also be selected inappropriately or administered ineffectively. For example, surgical antibiotic prophylaxis may be given after a surgical incision is made and surgery is under way instead of before incision, when it will be most effective in establishing a high tissue level of the drug when tissues are being manipulated. An antimicrobial may be continued for 1 or 2 days or more after the surgical procedure in an attempt to prevent surgical site infection when the greatest benefit is during and just after the procedure. Also, patients may discontinue antimicrobial therapy when symptoms subside and not complete the appropriate duration of therapy.

Other instances of antibiotic use do not involve the clinician directly but still significantly influence the global spread of resistant organisms. In some countries, antibiotics are sold "over the counter" to patients without a prescription by a care provider. The resulting huge volume of self-prescribed antibiotic use has facilitated emergence and global spread of numerous multiresistant organisms, such as *Shigella, Salmonella,* and penicillin-resistant pneumococci. Use of antibiotics in animal feeds has also been considered a factor in the spread of resistant bacteria, both in the United States and abroad.

Combination antimicrobial therapy

Antibiotic combinations have been used to overcome antimicrobial resistance. The strategy is to choose two or, rarely, more antibiotics with different mechanisms of activity or to increase the likelihood that an effective drug will be present should resistance to one or more develop. Although this strategy is often used, it has proved effective in only a few instances, including the treatment of tuberculosis and perhaps infections caused by *Pseudomonas aeruginosa* and certain other gram-negative organisms.

Asepsis

The careful application of infection control procedures does not directly limit the emergence of resistance but does prevent dissemination of resistant organisms from one colonized or infected patient to another. Appropriate handwashing, careful use of aseptic techniques, and judicious use of barriers such

as gloves, gowns, and masks can be critical. Barrier precautions are discussed in Chapter 6. Additional social factors that may lead to inappropriate antimicrobial use are listed in the box below.

GENERAL PRINCIPLES OF ANTIMICROBIAL CHEMOTHERAPY

Microbiologic issues

Physicians, nurse practitioners, and other clinicians must make a series of empiric decisions before selecting the antimicrobial

---

**SOCIAL FACTORS THAT MAY
LEAD TO INAPPROPRIATE USE OF
ANTIMICROBIAL AGENTS**

- Desire to prevent infection before it occurs
- Desire to provide optimal treatment using best drug available regardless of cost
- Fear of treating patient unsuccessfully
- Belief that large doses or extended use will be more effective than small doses of shorter duration
- Use of broad-spectrum agent or multiple drugs in lieu of single narrow-spectrum drug
- Pressure from the patient to receive an antimicrobial
- Pressure from pharmaceutical representatives to use a drug
- Pressure from health care facilities and third party payors not to use expensive diagnostic tools to evaluate need for antimicrobial
- Fear of malpractice litigation
- Inadequate knowledge of infectious diseases and related pharmacology

---

Adapted from Kunin CM. Problems in antibiotic usage. In Mandell GL, Douglas RG Jr., Bennett JE, eds. *Principles and Practice of Infectious Disease,* 3rd ed. New York: Churchill Livingston; 1990:431. Neu, HC. Antimicrobial agents: role in the prevention and control of nosocomial infections. In Wenzl RP, ed. *Prevention and Control of Nosocomial Infections,* 2nd ed. Baltimore: Williams and Wilkins; 1993:417.

compound most appropriate for the patient. First, they must conclude that the patient is likely to have an infection. Not every febrile patient requires antibiotic therapy, since fever has many causes besides infection.

When presence of an infection is established or suspected, the clinician must consider which organism(s) are most likely to be involved. Broad-spectrum "shotgun" antibiotic therapy, which may be effective against many possible organisms, may increase the likelihood that the therapy will be effective in a single situation. However, this strategy maximizes the selective pressure on the microbial flora, and should be avoided if at all possible. Reflexive use of broad-spectrum antibiotics increases the likelihood that resistant bacterial subpopulations will emerge.

Occasionally the prescriber has culture and sensitivity information already available, but in most cases the choice of antibiotic is based on an educated guess about the likely causative organisms. In making this guess, the practitioner applies knowledge of the characteristics of organisms known to cause the particular constellation of symptoms observed. For example, community-acquired biliary tract infection is usually associated with gram-negative rods or enterococci. The adult patient with bacterial meningitis is most often infected with *Streptococcus pneumoniae* (pneumococci) or *Neisseria meningitidis* (meningococcus). Host factors such as underlying illness, age, and previous hospitalization may be associated with particular pathogens or syndromes and therefore may influence the choice of antimicrobial agent.

Cultures of patient specimens are done to confirm the pathogenic agent's identity and allow testing of various antimicrobial agents against the microorganism. Thus, the likely effectiveness of therapy already begun can be determined and adjustments made. Proper collection and processing of culture materials is important. A simple Gram stain of purulent material may help determine whether infection is present and guide the choice of antibiotics. Other diagnostic methods that provide information more quickly than traditional culture techniques include direct fluorescent antigen testing, latex agglutination methods, and other immunologic and genetic probe assays, some of which can be performed directly on specimens.

A microbiologic culture report indicating growth of one or more organisms does not necessarily mean that the organism growing is the cause of the patient's infection. Specimens may easily become overgrown with contaminants. Consequently, the clinician must differentiate among contamination, colonization, and infection by a microorganism. *Colonization* is the relatively long-term presence and replication of a microorganism without the presence of clinically apparent infection. *Infection* is invasion of host tissues by microorganisms, usually accompanied by a host response to the invasion, which may be severe enough to define a clinically recognizable syndrome or disease.

When the identity of organisms that are likely pathogens in the patient is established, the clinician must also speculate on the organism's susceptibility to antimicrobials. This is guided by knowledge of microbial ecology as well as typical susceptibility of the local microorganisms to antimicrobial agents, which can vary greatly between geographic locales.

Frequently the microbiology laboratory tests the effectiveness of various antimicrobial agents against organisms grown in culture. Standards for in vitro susceptibility testing have been developed for many bacteria. Fungi, viruses, and bacteria with stringent growth requirements, such as strict anaerobes, are difficult to test for susceptibility in the typical laboratory, and results of susceptibility tests of these organisms are less reliable.

In clinical microbiology laboratories, two general methods of susceptibility testing are used most often: the disk diffusion and tube dilution methods[24] (see Chapter 2). These methods identify the antimicrobials to which the organism is sensitive and that offer the best therapy at the least cost.

Pharmacokinetics

Pharmacokinetics is the science that describes the distribution and metabolism of drugs in body tissues after administration. Pharmacokinetics defines the relationship between the drug's concentration in serum or tissues and its therapeutic or toxic effects. For antibiotics, the relationship between serum concentration and the drug's biologic effect is complex and poorly understood. Whereas pharmacokinetics describes concentration, distribution, and elimination of antimicrobial compounds in tissue, the science of pharmacodynamics relates these processes to antimicrobial effects.

A basic understanding of the terminology and the concepts of pharmacokinetics and pharmacodynamics allows the practitioner to dose antimicrobial drugs more effectively. This section presents a brief overview of several of these concepts. More detailed descriptions can be found in any of several references.[9,11]

CLASSES OF ANTIMICROBIALS
Penicillins

Sir Alexander Fleming's fortuitous discovery of penicillin in 1929 was the seminal moment in the emerging age of chemotherapy of infectious diseases. During his work with gram-positive cocci, Fleming noticed that growth of staphylococci was inhibited by *Penicillium* mold contaminants. He isolated from the molds small amounts of a substance that was responsible for this activity and designated it penicillin. Penicillin remained a laboratory curiosity for the next decade, until Florey, Chain, and colleagues defined the chemical and physical properties of the available form of penicillin, which turned out to be a mixture of substances. This work enabled clinical tests of penicillin treatment of infections in Great Britain and the United States in the 1940s. However, it was at the University of Illinois College of Agriculture in the late 1940s that a corn steep liquor fermentation process was developed that allowed large-batch production of purified penicillin.

Penicillin was the first antimicrobial having a core β-lactam key chemical structure (Figure 8-2). All β-lactam compounds inhibit bacterial growth by interfering with the synthesis of the bacterial cell wall. The box on p. 157 lists the most frequently used penicillins.

Benzylpenicillin

Benzylpenicillin, or *penicillin G*, is available as several different salts that vary in solubility. *Phenoxymethyl penicillin,* or *penicillin V,* is an acid-stable derivative of penicillin G that can be given orally. Penicillin G is susceptible to degradation by stomach acid and therefore is administered parenterally.

Penicillin G and V are highly active against most streptococci, staphylococci that do not produce penicillinase (an enzyme that inactivates β-lactam-based antimicrobials), many anaerobes, most *Clostridium* species (sp.), *Neis-*

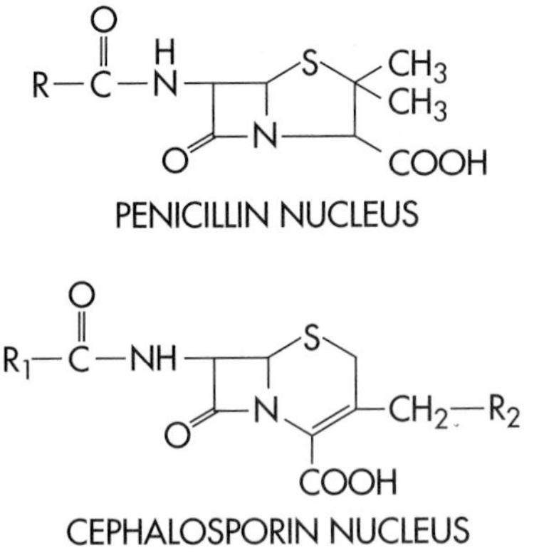

PENICILLIN NUCLEUS

CEPHALOSPORIN NUCLEUS

FIGURE 8-2. Basic chemical structures of penicillins and cephalosporins.

MAJOR PENICILLINS

PENICILLIN

Penicillin G
Penicillin G benzathine
Penicillin G procaine
Penicillin V

ANTISTAPHYLOCOCCAL PENICILLINS

Cloxacillin
Dicloxacillin
Methicillin
Nafcillin
Oxacillin

BROAD-SPECTRUM PENICILLINS

Amoxicillin
Ampicillin
Azlocillin
Carbenicillin
Mezlocillin
Piperacillin
Ticarcillin

---

seria sp., and spirochetes. *Bacteroides fragilis*–group anaerobes, gram-negative enteric aerobes, and *Haemophilus influenzae* are characteristically resistant. Enterococci are poorly susceptible to penicillin alone.

β-Lactamase and methicillin

Shortly after the introduction of penicillin, strains of resistant *Staphylococcus aureus* emerged. These organisms produced an enzyme, β-lactamase, that hydrolyzes and inactivates penicillin. Most *S. aureus* strains now produce this enzyme and are penicillin resistant.

To overcome this problem, chemists in the 1950s developed methicillin, a β-lactamase-stable penicillin. Because of toxicities, methicillin has been superseded by other β-lactamase-stable semisynthetic penicillins: oxacillin, nafcillin, cloxacillin, and dicloxacil-

lin.[18] Some staphylococci (both *S. aureus* and coagulase-negative staphylococci) have developed non–β-lactamase-mediated resistance to the semisynthetic penicillins. Methicillin-resistant strains of *S. aureus* are referred to as MRSA. Infections caused by methicillin-resistant staphylococci are most often treated with vancomycin.

Expanded-spectrum penicillins

The activity of penicillin G has been expanded by structural modification of the molecule to include some traditionally resistant organisms. The amino penicillins (ampicillin, amoxicillin) have expanded activity that includes *H. influenzae*, many *Escherichia coli* strains, *Salmonella*, *Shigella*, *Proteus mirabilis*, and enterococci. Unfortunately, these compounds are β-lactamase sensitive; consequently, β-lactamase-producing strains of *H. influenzae* are resistant. Other expanded-spectrum penicillins include carbenicillin, ticarcillin, mezlocillin, piperacillin, and azlocillin, which are active against *Pseudomonas aeruginosa* and several Enterobacteriaceae.

Adverse effects

The penicillins are generally very well tolerated by patients. The most common adverse effects are hypersensitivity reactions such as rash and drug-induced fever. Severe immediate hypersensitivity reactions such as anaphylaxis occasionally occur. Renal failure caused by vasculitis or interstitial nephritis occurs rarely.

Neutropenia, agranulocytosis, and other hematologic toxicities occur most often in patients receiving prolonged courses of penicillin but may occur after short-course chemotherapy as well. Overgrowth by and infection from resistant organisms may result from any antibacterial therapy, including that using β-lactams.

Most penicillins are eliminated by the kidney, and dosage must be reduced in patients who have diminished creatinine clearance. Nafcillin, which is an exception because it is also excreted in the bile, requires little dose adjustment in patients with renal failure.

Cephalosporins

The cephalosporins are β-lactam antibiotics derived from the *Cephalosporium* fungi.[19] These compounds are somewhat more β-lactamase stable than penicillins.

First-generation cephalosporins

The initially developed cephalosporins all have a similar spectrum of activity and are known as first-generation cephalosporins (see box at right). These drugs include cefazolin, cephalexin, cephalothin, cephradine, and others. All these agents have excellent activity against streptococci (except enterococci), *S. aureus*, and some coagulase-negative staphylococci. Methicillin-resistant staphylococci may appear susceptible in vitro but may be quite resistant in vivo. First-generation cephalosporins are also active against many *E. coli* strains, *P. mirabilis*, and *Klebsiella pneumoniae*. *Salmonella* and *Shigella* sp. often test susceptible to these agents in vitro, but clinical failures in the treatment of salmonellosis with first-generation cephalosporins have occurred regularly. *Listeria* sp. are not susceptible to cephalosporins.

Cephalexin and cephradine are first-generation cephalosporins that can be given orally. They are similar in spectrum and pharmacokinetics. Cefadroxil is another orally administered cephalosporin with a long half-life, which permits once-daily or twice-daily dosing. These orally administered cephalosporins are most often useful to treat minor skin and soft tissue infections caused by gram-positive cocci or urinary tract infection.

Second-generation cephalosporins

In the late 1970s, structural modification of the basic cephalosporin nucleus led to a group

---

MAJOR CEPHALOSPORINS*

FIRST GENERATION

Cephalothin
Cefazolin
Cephalexin†
Cephradine†
Cefadroxil†

SECOND GENERATION

Cefamandole
Cefuroxime‡
Cefoxitin
Cefotetan
Cefaclor†
Cefonicid
Ceforanide

THIRD GENERATION

Cefotaxime
Ceftizoxime
Ceftriaxone
Cefoperazone
Cefixime†
Ceftazidime
Cefpirome

*Parenteral administration except as noted.
†Oral administration.
‡Oral and parenteral administration.

---

of cephalosporins with activity broader than that of first-generation drugs (see box). Cefoxitin and cefotetan are active against *Bacteroides fragilis* and other anaerobes as well as certain enteric pathogens, such as indole-positive *Proteus* and *Serratia* sp. Cefamandole and cefuroxime are active against *H. influenzae*, including β-lactamase-producing strains. Cefuroxime is now available for oral administration. It retains all the in vitro activity of parenteral cefuroxime, but bioavailability is only 40% to 50%, and serum concentrations of the drug after oral administration tend to be low. Cefonicid is similar to cefuroxime except for its less impressive activity against *H. influenzae.* In general, the improvement of activity against anaerobes or *H. influenzae* has been at the expense of gram-positive coverage, although cefuroxime and cefamandole retain activity against *S. aureus.*

Cefaclor is an orally administered second-generation cephalosporin with improved activity against *H. influenzae* compared with first-generation cephalosporins. Its advantage is only modest, however, and cefaclor's moderate coverage of β-lactamase-producing *H. influenzae* (65% of these strains are susceptible) make it a poor choice for treatment of infections caused by this organism.

Cefixime is an oral cephalosporin with an in vitro spectrum similar to those of the third-generation cephalosporins. Although minimum inhibitory concentrations (MICs) to the common Enterobacteriaceae are excellent, the drug has no useful staphylococcal activity and poor activity against *Streptococcus pneumoniae* compared with the parenteral third-generation drugs.

Third-generation cephalosporins

The third-generation cephalosporins have a similar antimicrobial activity that outweighs their differences, and there is a confusing plethora of similar-sounding names.[2] Expanded activity against gram-negative bacteria is achieved at the expense of activity against some gram-positive organisms. The antimicrobials spectrum of each agent must be considered as each therapeutic choice is made. This situation worsens as additional cephalosporins are released.

Three drugs with similar antimicrobial activities but different pharmacokinetics comprise the most frequently used third-generation cephalosporins (see box). Cefotaxime and ceftizoxime are most similar. Ceftriaxone is characterized by its long half-life, which allows once-daily administration. The great advantage of these drugs is their superb activity against common Enterobacteriaceae such as *E. coli, Proteus, Providencia,* and *Klebsiella* sp., along with excellent tissue penetration and moderately good CNS penetration. These characteristics make the third-generation cephalosporins excellent drugs for the treatment of serious gram-negative infections when *Pseudomonas aeruginosa* has been ruled out.

Ceftazidime and cefoperazone are characterized by important activity against *P. aeruginosa.* Ceftazidime provides significantly better in vitro activity against *P. aeruginosa* than cefoperazone.

Other cephalosporins

Cefonicid has a spectrum most similar to second generation cephalosporins. It is characterized by a prolonged half life of >4 hours which permits once daily dosing. Its activity against gram-negative pathogens is usually weaker than that of other second generation agents.

Ceforanide is similar in activity to cefonicid with a half life of 3 hours and a dosing interval of every 12 hours recommended.

Cefpirome is a new third generation cephalosporin. In common with other third generation cephalosporins it has excellent activity against gram-negative microorganisms but it also has significant activity against *Pseudomonas aeruginosa* while retaining excellent coverage of *Staphylococcus aureus.* Clinical experience with this compound is limited at present.

Adverse effects

Adverse effects associated with the cephalosporins are similar to those seen with the penicillins. Hypersensitivity reactions are most common, but blood dyscrasias, hepatitis, and renal failure have been reported.

Because of the broad-spectrum nature of these compounds, suprainfections are often seen in patients after prolonged therapy. Suprainfection after cephalosporin use is most frequently caused by fungal organisms such as *Candida* sp. or enterococci.

Second- and third-generation cephalosporins have been associated with clinically significant bleeding, the risk of which is evidenced by prolonged prothrombin times in certain patients. Patients most at risk for this complication are elderly postoperative patients with poor nutritional status. Judicious prophylactic use of weekly vitamin K injections helps avoid this complication.

Other β-lactam antibiotics

Structural modification of the β-lactam nucleus has produced several unique compounds that differ significantly from penicillins and cephalosporins in both structure and pharmacologic properties. These drugs include the broad-spectrum agents imipenem and aztreonam, which are clinically useful only against gram-negative organisms.

Imipenem, the first of the thienamycin antibiotics, is a broad spectrum beta-lactam with excellent activity against a broad array of enteric rods including serratia and enterobacter. In addition, non fermenters such as *Pseudomonas aeruginosa* and *Acinetobacter* species are often susceptible. *Pseudomonas maltophila* is usually resistant.

The drug has clinically significant anaerobic activity and most species including *B. fragilis* group are susceptible. Gram-positive cocci such as staphylococci and streptococci are usually susceptible to imipenem. Failures in serious enterococcal infections have been reported and the drug should not be used in this situation.

After intravenous dosing, imipenem is quickly metabolized in the kidney and rapidly eliminated. Cilastatin, an inhibitor of the renal enzyme which degrades imipenem, is combined with the drug during formulation in order to improve the serum and tissue levels of imipenem. Cilastatin has no antimicrobial properties and serves solely to boost serum levels of imipenem.

Adverse reactions to imipenem are similar to those of other beta-lactams with the exception of neurotoxicity. Seizures occur infrequently but are most often seen in patients given large doses, patients with underlying central nervous system lesions, and patients with altered renal function.

Unlike other beta-lactam compounds, aztreonam has clinically useful activity only against gram-negative organisms. The drug has no gram-positive or anaerobic activity. Because of this rather narrow spectrum, when aztreonam is used for empiric coverage of seriously ill patients, it is combined with another cell wall active agent or clindamycin to provide activity against gram-positive cocci and anaerobes.

Clavulanic acid and sulbactam are so-called β-lactamase scavengers. These compounds have little useful intrinsic antimicrobial activity, but they bind and inactivate β-lactamase enzymes, thus preventing the destruction of β-lactam antibiotics. These drugs therefore are used in combination with other β-lactam antibiotics to provide synergistic activity. Drugs now available have combined these β-lactamase inhibitors with other active antimicrobials: amoxicillin/clavulanate, ticarcillin/clavulanate, and ampicillin/sulbactam. These compounds bind avidly to the common plasmid mediated beta-lactamases produced by *Staphylococcus aureus*, bacteroides, and many enteric rods. These combinations also have particularly good activity against oral gram-negative rods such as *Eikenella corrodens*, *Pasteurella multocida*, and DF-2 bacillus, which makes them excellent choices for treatment of infections caused by human or animal bites.

Aminoglycosides

The aminoglycosides inhibit bacterial protein synthesis at the ribosome.[18] Streptomycin, the first aminoglycoside, was developed in the mid-1940s and is still in used in the treatment of tuberculosis. Structurally, the aminoglycosides consist of two or more amino sugars linked to an aminocyclitol ring by glycosidic bonds.

Major aminoglycosides

The aminoglycosides most often used parenterally are gentamicin, tobramycin, amikacin, streptomycin, and netilmicin. Neomycin and paromomycin cannot be administered parenterally because they are severely toxic. Neomycin is used as an irrigating agent or as an oral nonabsorbable antibiotic for gut decontamination. Paromomycin is an oral nonabsorbable antibiotic used chiefly for its unique antiprotozoal activity. It is often recommended as an intraluminal agent for the treatment of intestinal protozoan infections such as amebiasis. Kanamycin was used for many years as the primary parenteral aminoglycoside, but the development of resistance by many clinically significant strains of bacteria has limited its utility in recent years. Kanamycin has been replaced by other aminoglycosides, except for occasional use as an irrigating solution in surgery. Spectinomycin is often grouped with the aminoglycoside class, although structurally it is composed solely of an aminocyclitol ring with no linked sugars.

Aminoglycosides have some activity against virtually all classes of bacteria, with the exception of anaerobes and streptococci. Most aminoglycosides are essentially equivalent against the Enterobacteriaceae. Activity against *P. aeruginosa* varies among the drugs. Aminoglycosides are active against staphylococci, but their relative toxicities compared with alternatives have limited their clinical utility in the treatment of staphylococcal infections.

Adverse effects

Aminoglycosides have been the mainstay of treatment for serious bacterial infections since they became available because of their excellent bactericidal activity against a broad array of gram-negative and gram-positive species. The clinical use of aminoglycosides is limited by their poor penetration of membrane barriers and limited availability in secretions (e.g., eye, CNS, bronchial secretions) and the relatively frequent toxic side effects. The major adverse effects of these compounds are renal toxicity and ototoxicity. Aminoglycosides are not absorbed orally and must be given parenterally. They are eliminated primarily through the kidneys; therefore, when renal insufficiency is present, doses must be carefully calculated and serum drug levels periodically monitored.

Because of the low therapeutic-to-toxic ratio of aminoglycosides and their lack of activity against streptococci and anaerobes, these drugs are often used in combination with other antibiotics (e.g., β-lactam and other drugs active against the bacterial cell wall) for the treatment of serious gram-negative infections and for empiric therapy of septic patients.

Sulfonamides

The sulfa drugs, first introduced in the 1930s, are azo dyes that were the first widely used class of antibacterial chemotherapeutic drugs. Hundreds of these compounds have been synthesized, but only a few remain in common clinical use.

Sulfa compounds are structural derivatives of paraaminobenzoic acid (PABA), which microorganisms need to synthesize folic acid. These drugs work by disrupting a precursor of folic acid.

Trimethoprim/Sulfamethoxazole

This agent, the most frequently used sulfonamide, consists of sulfamethoxazole combined with the folate antagonist trimethoprim. It is discussed here as the prototype compound of the class. Trimethoprim inhibits the reduction of dihydrofolic acid to tetrahydrofolate by interfering with the enzyme dihydrofolate reductase. Thus, sulfamethoxazole and trimethoprim act sequentially to interfere with folate synthesis. This sequential action helps prevent the emergence of resistant strains and promotes antibiotic synergy between the two compounds.[23]

The antimicrobial spectrum of Trimethoprim/Sulfamethoxazole (TMP/SMX) includes many gram-positive and gram-negative organisms. *S. aureus*, including methicillin-resistant strains; many streptococci, except enterococci; and most pneumococcal isolates are susceptible. Gram-negative organisms susceptible to TMP/SMX include respiratory pathogens such as *H. influenzae*, and *Moraxella (Branhamella) catarrhalis*, as well as many common Enterobacteriaceae such as *E. coli, Proteus*, and *Klebsiella* sp. *Salmonella* and *Shigella* are often susceptible, but resistant strains have emerged. TMP/SMX has no anti-anaerobic activity, and all *P. aeruginosa* species are resistant. In addition to common bacterial organisms, TMP/SMX has potent activity against more unusual organisms, such as *Pneumocystis carinii, Nocardia* sp., and *Mycobacterium marinum*.

TMP/SMX may be used for infections caused by these organisms at many different sites. The drug is most often used to treat urinary tract infections (UTIs) and upper and lower respiratory tract infections. TMP/SMX is highly effective against most community-acquired urinary tract pathogens. Three days of TMP/SMX is a gold standard for therapy of uncomplicated UTIs. The drug is well absorbed after oral administration, and an intravenous (IV) preparation is available as well. The half-life is long enough to allow twice-daily dosing, which may assist in patient compliance for completing prescribed regimens.

Adverse effects

The most common side effects of all sulfonamides is hypersensitivity manifested by diffuse rash and occasionally fever. The hypersensitivity may be severe enough to trigger Stevens-Johnson syndrome. Because of reactions with sunlight, photosensitive dermatitis occurs frequently with the sulfonamides. In high doses, some sulfa preparations can produce serious hematologic toxicity (e.g., bone marrow suppression) thought to result from antifolate activity. Early, relatively insoluble sulfa compounds typically produced crystalluria, which is rarely a problem with TMP/SMX. However, renal failure induced by other mechanisms may be associated with TMP/SMX.

Macrolides

The macrolide antibiotics are composed of a large lactone ring consisting of 12 to 16 carbon atoms with one or more sugar molecules attached by glycosidic linkage. Although many macrolides have been synthesized, until recently the only member of this class with widespread clinical use in the United States was erythromycin.[25]

Erythromycin

Erythromycin is active against many important pathogens, including most streptococci and community-acquired strains of *S. aureus*, pathogenic *Neisseria* sp., *Legionella*, and intracellular pathogens such as *Chlamydia* and *Mycoplasma*. Most enteric organisms are resistant.

Clinical use of erythromycin has been primarily for skin and soft tissue infections and for the treatment of lower respiratory tract infections. The drug is often employed to treat atypical pneumonia because of its activity against *Mycoplasma* and *Chlamydia*. It is the current drug of choice for treatment of *Legionella* infections. Additionally, erythromycin is an important alternative drug for treatment of staphylococcal and streptococcal soft tissue infection, pneumococcal pneumonia, streptococcal pharyngitis, and nongonococcal urethritis.

Other macrolides

Several other macrolide compounds similar in structure to erythromycin have been developed. Two of these compounds, clarithromycin and azithromycin, were released in 1992. These drugs are better absorbed than erythromycin and produce less gastric upset. Although their in vitro activity against *H. influenzae* is greater than that of erythromycin, little clinical data support their use for treatment of invasive *H. influenzae* infections. These new macrolides may play a role in the therapy of purulent urethritis because of their activity against *Chlamydia trachomatis*.

Adverse effects

GI reactions, including nausea, vomiting, and abdominal pain, are the most common adverse effects associated with macrolides. Up to 30% of individuals taking erythromycin will develop some form of GI reaction. Cholestatic hepatitis may occur with erythromycin administration, especially when the estolate salt is used in adults. This problem is rarely seen in children. Hearing loss may occur when erythromycin is administered in high parenteral doses. Macrolide-induced hearing loss is reversible, but hearing may take months to return to its baseline level.

Quinolones

The first quinolone antibiotic in clinical use was nalidixic acid. This drug was developed in the early 1960s for the treatment of UTIs caused by gram-negative aerobes. Its clinical use was restricted to the treatment of uncomplicated *E. coli* UTIs and complicated by the frequent occurrence of resistance. Although other quinolones were synthesized in the 1970s, no significant addition to the quinolone class occurred until the introduction of norfloxacin.

Major quinolones

Norfloxacin, the first fluorinated quinolone, has been followed by ciprofloxacin and ofloxacin. Fluorination significantly enhanced the spectrum of activity of the quinolones. These drugs are highly active against enteric gram-negative aerobes such as *E. coli, Citrobacter, Salmonella, Shigella*, and *Enterobacter*,[1] as well as *H. influenzae* and *B. catarrhalis*. These are also

the first oral agents with high-level activity against *P. aeruginosa*.

The activity of quinolones against gram-positive species is less consistent, but *S. aureus* is often inhibited. Clinical use of the quinolones in the treatment of staphylococcal infections has been limited by the rapid emergence of resistance. The quinolones are generally ineffective against streptococci, including β-hemolytic streptococci, α-hemolytic (viridans) streptococci, and enterococci. Although many strains of pneumococci are susceptible in vitro to the quinolones, clinical failures in the treatment of pneumococcal infections have occurred frequently.

Absorption of the quinolones from the GI tract may be blocked by medications such as antacids, which contain divalent cations such as aluminum, iron, and magnesium. The drugs penetrate tissues well, but ofloxacin is the only available quinolone that can significantly penetrate the CNS.

Quinolone antibiotics are highly effective against most organisms causing UTI. The quinolones work well in uncomplicated UTI, but other antibiotics are frequently as effective at much less cost. Most clinicians reserve the quinolones for the treatment of complicated UTIs. They are most useful as oral agents for the treatment of UTIs caused by difficult-to-treat organisms (e.g., multiresistant Enterobacteriaceae and *P. aeruginosa*).

The antimicrobial spectrum of the quinolones includes most organisms causing bacterial gastroenteritis. These drugs have superb activity against *Salmonella, Shigella, Campylobacter, Yersinia*, and enterotoxic *E. coli*. Their ease of administration, relative lack of side effects, and potent activity against GI pathogens have made quinolones frequent choices for the treatment of traveler's diarrhea, although clinical failures have occurred.

The quinolones may play a role in the treatment of certain sexually transmitted diseases. Although the drugs have no clinically proven activity against *Treponema pallidum*, most strains of gonococci remain susceptible to the quinolones. Although ciprofloxacin and ofloxacin are highly active in vitro against *C. trachomatis,* unfortunately none of the quinolones reaches sufficiently high urethral levels quickly enough to be effective single-dose therapy for *C. trachomatis* urethritis. In addition, their relative expense limits their usefulness against urethritis caused by gonococcus and *Chlamydia.*

Adverse effects

The quinolones are generally well tolerated. The most common side effects are mild GI disturbance, headache, and sleeplessness. CNS side effects appear to occur more often in the elderly. When administered in high doses to patients with impaired renal function, the quinolones may produce significant neurotoxicity, including seizures. Many quinolones interfere with the metabolism of methylxanthine compounds and lead to increased serum levels of theophylline.

Tetracyclines

The tetracyclines are broad-spectrum antibiotics effective against a wide range of microorganisms.[6] Clinical use of tetracycline antibiotics has decreased in recent years, however, because of the emergence of resistance in many common gram-positive and gram-negative bacterial isolates.

Major tetracyclines

Five tetracyclines are currently available for clinical use, including chlortetracycline, oxytetracycline, and tetracycline, as well as the newer synthetic agents doxycycline and minocycline.

Tetracyclines were initially highly effective against gram-positive bacteria, such as staphylococci, pneumococci, and other streptococci, and gram-negative organisms, including common community-acquired pathogens such as *E. coli* and *Klebsiella.* Nosocomial pathogens such as *Enterobacter* and *Pseudomonas* sp. have remained resistant to the tetracyclines.

Unfortunately, over the years many common gram-negative and gram-positive bacteria have become resistant to the tetracyclines. Tetracycline resistance may be mediated by a number of different mechanisms and is often transmissible on plasmid DNA.

These agents retain considerable clinical usefulness, however, for treatment of infections caused by rickettsiae, spirochetes, mycoplasma, and chlamydia, including *C. trachomatis* and *Chlamydia pneumoniae.* Most *Neisseria* sp., including meningococcus and some atypical mycobacterial specimens such as *Mycobacterium marinum,* are sensitive to tetracyclines.

Tetracyclines are not typically used for empiric therapy because of the prevalence of resistance. Tetracyclines are the preferred agents for treatment of rickettsial infections such as Rocky Mountain spotted fever, Q fever, and typhus. The antispirochetal activity of the tetracyclines allows their clinical use against *Borrelia* sp. responsible for relapsing fever and Lyme disease (see Clinical Study 1). Doxycycline is used in the prophylaxis of leptospirosis, but its usefulness in the treatment of this infection is debated. Because of their activity against *Chlamydia,* including strains causing lymphogranuloma venereum, and *Neisseria,* the tetracyclines have often been used to treat sexually transmitted diseases. In recent years, gonococcal resistance has limited the use of tetracyclines as single agents for the treatment of gonorrhea (see Clinical Study 11).

Adverse effects

Rash and photosensitive dermatitis are the most common side effects of tetracycline therapy. Suprainfection caused by overgrowth of *Candida* sp. as well as antibiotic-associated diarrhea have been associated with tetracyclines. These agents apparently increase amino acid catabolism and therefore must be dosed carefully in patients with chronic renal failure, or azotemia and acidosis will result. Dizziness and vertigo are possible side effects of minocycline therapy. Tetracycline can stain the teeth buds of the fetus so is not used to treat infections in pregnant women.

Major antimicrobial classes are summarized in Table 8-1.

OTHER ANTIMICROBIAL AGENTS

Clindamycin

Although unrelated structurally to erythromycin, clindamycin has a similar but somewhat expanded spectrum. The drug is active against staphylococci, streptococci, and many gram-negative anaerobes such as *Bacteroides fragilis*. It is highly effective when treating infections caused by *B. fragilis*–group organisms. Clindamycin has no activity against other gram-negative organisms. Most organisms that are resistant to erythromycin are also resistant to clindamycin.

Adverse reactions to clindamycin include hypersensitivity and blood dyscrasias. The most common adverse reaction to clindamycin is diarrhea. Antibiotic-associated diarrhea may be nonspecific or associated with *C. difficile* overgrowth.

Vancomycin

Vancomycin, a glycopeptide antibiotic with a complex structure, was introduced in 1956.

Initially, vancomycin was used to treat penicillin-resistant *S. aureus* infections. Clinical use was tempered by early recognition of ototoxicity and significant nephrotoxicity. In the early 1960s, vancomycin was replaced by methicillin and the other semisynthetic penicillins. Since then, methods have been developed to remove the chemical impurities that contaminated the original vancomycin preparations and were responsible for much of its toxicity. Vancomycin use has increased substantially in response to the emergence of methicillin-resistant staphylococci and enterococci.[16] Oral administration of vancomycin is used to treat *Clostridium difficile* colitis. Because the antibiotic is not absorbed, exceedingly high concentrations in the gut may be achieved. Although approximately 15% of patients with *C. difficile* colitis will fail the initial course of therapy, most can be cured with repeat courses.

Adverse effects

Nephrotoxicity and ototoxicity associated with high peak serum levels may occur during vancomycin therapy. Monitoring of serum drug levels may be necessary in patients with underlying renal insufficiency or patients at risk for nephrotoxicity, such as the elderly. Histamine-release reactions leading to flushing and hypotension (red man syndrome) are

TABLE 8-1. Major antimicrobial classes effective against bacteria other than mycobacteria

Drug class	Comments
β-Lactams	
Penicillins	Penicillin G and expanded spectrum penicillins
Cephalosporins	1st-, 2nd-, 3rd-generation agents generally increasing in gram-negative potency
Aminoglycosides	Superb bacterial killing, but ototoxicity and nephrotoxicity limit use
Sulfonamides	Chiefly used for UTI and pneumocystis carinii
Glycopeptides	Mainly active against gram-positive organisms
Macrolides	Chiefly used for respiratory tract, skin, and soft-tissue infections
Quinolones	Excellent gram-negative aerobic coverage; most don't cover gram-positive or anaerobic organisms
Tetracyclines	Useful against intracellular organisms such as chlamydia and Rickettsia

associated with too rapid an infusion of vancomycin. Parenteral antihistamines effectively treat this problem.

Metronidazole

Metronidazole was developed in 1960 for the treatment of parasitic infections, including those caused by *Trichomonas vaginalis, Entamoeba histolytica,* and *Giardia lamblia.* Subsequent evaluation in the 1970s revealed significant activity against most anaerobic species, including all *B. fragilis* sp. Gram-positive anaerobic cocci occasionally are resistant, as are certain other anaerobes such as *Propionibacterium acnes* and microaerophilic streptococci. Metronidazole is available in both oral and IV forms. The drug is almost 100% absorbed after oral administration and penetrates well into nearly all tissues and the CNS.

The most common adverse effects of metronidazole are nausea and an Antabuse (disulfiram)-like reaction with alcohol. Less common side effects include seizures and neurotoxicity, which usually occur when the drug is given at high doses.

Metronidazole is most often used in the treatment of parasitic and serious anaerobic intraabdominal, obstetric, and gynecologic infections. These infections are often caused by mixed organisms, so metronidazole is frequently combined with other antimicrobials in this situation. Metronidazole has revolutionized the treatment of pyogenic liver and brain abscesses by making cures possible in many patients without surgery.

Chloramphenicol

Chloramphenicol, a small-molecular-weight paranitrobenzene derivative, is now less often used than previously. Chloramphenicol was frequently used for the treatment of infections caused by *Haemophilus influenzae,* pneumococci, and meningococci because of its ability to penetrate tissue and the CNS. In recent years, this niche has been filled by the third-generation cephalosporins, since reactions to chloramphenicol include aplastic anemia in approximately 1:40,000 patients receiving the drug. Hematologic toxicity also includes reversible bone marrow suppression. In infants, a syndrome of respiratory depression lethargy, cyanosis, and circulatory collapse known as the gray baby syndrome can occur when oxidative phosphorylation is poisoned by high-dose chloramphenicol.

Chloramphenicol remains an excellent agent for parenteral therapy of rickettsial infections such as Rocky Mountain spotted fever; *Salmonella* infections, particularly typhoid fever; and as an alternative agent in the treatment of bacterial meningitis caused by *H. influenzae,* pneumococci, or meningococci. Chloramphenicol has also been successfully used in combination with penicillins for the treatment of brain abscesses.

Antimycobacterial drugs

Among the many compounds that show in vitro activity against *Mycobacterium tuberculosis,* 10 drugs have proven to be clinically useful in patients for treatment of tuberculosis (see box below). Five of these drugs are most often

---

DRUGS USED COMMONLY IN THE TREATMENT OF TUBERCULOSIS

PRIMARY DRUGS

Isoniazid (INH)
Rifampin
Ethambutol
Streptomycin
Pyrazinamide

SECOND-LINE DRUGS

Cycloserine
Capreomycin
Viomycin
Thiacetazone
Ethionamide

used and these are associated with few toxic side effects. Clinical usage of the other five drugs is limited by their lesser activity against *M. tuberculosis* or significantly greater potential for toxicity.[20,22]

Isoniazid

Isoniazid (INH) is the primary drug used in the treatment of *M. tuberculosis*. It is well absorbed orally and distributes well in all tissues, including the CNS.

The principal side effects of INH are hepatitis and peripheral neuritis. The incidence of hepatitis is age dependent; it is most frequent in elderly persons and quite rare in children. Mild elevation of serum transaminases occur in 20% of persons taking INH, and severe hepatitis occurs in 1% to 3% of persons, usually within the first 4 months of therapy. The hepatitis may be fatal. Peripheral neuropathy is most common in patients with altered renal function and may be avoided by concurrent prophylactic therapy with vitamin B_6. Hypersensitivity reactions may occur as well. Patients treated with INH should undergo periodic monitoring of serum transaminases.

INH is highly active against most strains of *M. tuberculosis* and should be a part of the therapeutic regimen of all patients undergoing therapy for TB. However, INH-resistant strains occur. Selection of resistant strains may be avoided when chemotherapy includes INH and one or more other antimycobacterial drugs.

Rifampin

Rifampin, an antibiotic obtained from a *Streptomyces* sp., is active against *M. tuberculosis*, *M. leprae*, and many gram-positive bacteria. Some gram-negative bacteria such as *Neisseria*, *Hemophilus*, and *Legionella* strains are susceptible to rifampin as well. The drug inhibits RNA polymerase in bacteria. It may be administered IV or orally.

The major side effect of rifampin is hepatitis, which occurs in 0.5% to 1% of patients. Hypersensitivity reactions, including drug fever, thrombocytopenia, and renal failure, may occur as well. The drug imparts an orange-red color to urine, sweat, and tears and may permanently stain contact lenses.

Rifampin is bacteriocidal. At present, it is primarily used in combination with INH for the treatment of TB. Rifampin is also used as an adjunctive drug in the therapy of *S. aureus* infections, *Legionella* infections, and to eradicate the meningococcal carrier state.

Ethambutol

Ethambutol is a bacteriostatic antituberculous drug with a long half-life. Like other antituberculous drugs, it may be administered once daily. It is primarily eliminated through the renal system. It is always used in combination with one or more other antituberculosis drugs. The most common toxicity is GI upset. Optic neuritis may occur when the drug is given at high doses. Patients with reduced renal function and those treated with high doses must have periodic ophthalmologic exams.

Streptomycin

Streptomycin, an aminoglycoside, has been used as an antituberculous agent since 1945. As with other aminoglycosides, it is poorly absorbed by mouth and must be given parenterally. The drug is administered as a single daily intramuscular injection. The standard adult dose is 1 g intramuscularly daily or twice weekly. The principal toxicities of streptomycin are those of the aminoglycosides. They include ototoxicity as well as nephrotoxicity.

Pyrazinamide

The oral drug pyrazinamide is another first-line agent used in the treatment of TB. It is well absorbed and has a long half-life, which allows single daily dosing. Pyrazinamide penetrates cells well and exerts its maximal effect at a slightly acidic pH such as that found in macrophages and within granulomatous tuberculosis lesions.

The primary toxicity of pyrazinamide is hepatotoxicity. Pyrazinamide-associated hepatitis may be severe and sudden. Consequently, liver function tests must be monitored. Additionally, serum uric acid levels often rise during pyrazinamide therapy and GI intolerance has been reported as well.

Second-line antituberculosis agents

The antituberculosis activity of this group of drugs is less well established than that of the first-line antituberculosis agents. In addition, many of these agents have highly significant side effects that limit their use.

Cycloserine inhibits most strains of *M. tuberculosis.* Orally administered, it distributes among most body tissues. Potent neurotoxicity, including both peripheral neuropathy and CNS side effects such as psychosis and seizures limit the broad use of this drug.

Capreomycin is a polypeptide antibiotic that is active only against mycobacteria. It is administered intramuscularly as a single daily injection. Though capreomycin is a modestly effective antituberculosis drug, many patients develop ototoxicity or nephrotoxicity.

Ethionamide is an orally administered drug with quite common GI side effects. Symptoms such as nausea, vomiting, anorexia, and abdominal pain may be severe enough to necessitate cessation of treatment. The drug has also been implicated as a cause of depression and acute psychosis. Because of its side effects, ethionamide is often considered a reserve drug in the treatment of TB.

Thiacetazone is well absorbed after oral administration and is popular in the developing world because of its low cost. Toxicities include GI side effects, hepatotoxicity, bone marrow depression, ototoxicity, and hypersensitivity reactions.

Viomycin, a polypeptide antibiotic, is rarely prescribed because of its side effects, limited antitubercular activity, and the need for intramuscular dosing. Side effects include nephrotoxicity, ototoxicity, and electrolyte imbalances. Viomycin should not be combined with any other potentially nephrotoxic drug such as streptomycin or capreomycin.

Antifungal compounds

The fungi are eukaryotic organisms. Their similarity to mammalian cells makes it difficult to develop antifungal drugs that will selectively kill or inhibit these organisms.[3]

Amphotericin B

Amphotericin B, developed in the 1950s, remains the most effective antifungal agent. It is poorly soluble, is not absorbable orally, and must be administered parenterally. It has serious side effects, and hypersensitivity reactions manifested as fever occur often. Because hypotension may develop, a test dose of 1 mg is often given to assess the patient's response to the drug. Nephrotoxicity predictably follows treatment with amphotericin B. Azotemia is dose related and generally reversible. Other manifestations of renal toxicity with amphotericin B include hypokalemia and hypomagnesemia. Bone marrow suppression is also possible with amphotericin B therapy. Anemia is most prominent, but neutropenia or thrombocytopenia may occur.

Amphotericin B is highly effective against many fungi. It acts by disrupting the fungal cell membrane. The drug is mainly used to treat deep infections caused by *Candida, Aspergillus, Mucor, Cryptococcus, Blastomyces,* and *Histoplasma.*

Azole compounds

The azole antifungal compounds are listed in the box on p. 169. Miconazole is a poorly absorbed azole that must be administered parenterally. Numerous serious side effects, including arrhythmias, hypotension, and anaphylaxis, are associated with the use of par-

---

AZOLE ANTIFUNGAL AGENTS

Clotrimazole
Fluconazole
Itraconazole
Ketoconazole
Miconazole
Terconazole

---

enteral miconazole. Because of the serious nature of these side effects, miconazole is rarely used.

Ketoconazole is available as an oral agent that is well absorbed. It has a broad spectrum of activity and may be used to treat both mucosal and cutaneous infections caused by *Candida* sp. as well as many dermatophytes such as *Trichosporon* and *Microsporum*. The drug is highly active against most *Candida* sp. and is standard therapy for the treatment of chronic mucocutaneous candidiasis. Other fungal infections that respond to ketoconazole include nonmeningeal forms of histoplasmosis and blastomycosis.

Ketoconazole is well absorbed after oral administration, but its absorption depends on gastric acidity. Patients with high gastric pH, such as those taking antacids or H_2 antagonists, will not absorb ketoconazole. It is distributed to most tissues and body fluids, with the exception of the urine and CNS, where achievable levels of ketoconazole are quite low.

GI toxicity manifested by nausea is the most common side effect of ketoconazole therapy. Serious hepatotoxicity occurs in approximately 1:12,000 patients, and ensuing hepatitis may be life-threatening. Ketoconazole interferes with the synthesis of steroid hormones, and endocrine suppression may lead to unwarranted side effects. Although adrenal insufficiency is rare in patients taking ketoconazole, suppression of testosterone synthesis is common, and side effects such as

gynecomastia, infertility, and loss of libido may occur.

Fluconazole is more water soluble than ketoconazole and achieves significantly better penetration into the CNS and urinary tract. It is effective in the treatment of vaginal candidiasis, esophageal candidiasis, and *Candida* UTIs. Because of its generally good activity against *Cryptococcus* in vitro, fluconazole has been used for the treatment of cryptococcal meningitis. It is a promising agent for maintenance therapy of cryptococcal meningitis after initial dosing with amphotericin B. The toxicity of fluconazole is low, and the most frequent adverse reactions are nausea and vomiting.

Itraconazole is an antifungal agent approved for the treatment of histoplasmosis and blastomycosis. Although its penetration into the CNS is relatively low, itraconazole may have a role in treatment of cryptococcal meningitis. Other fungi susceptible to this drug include most dermatophytes, *Candidia*, and agents of chromomycosis. Itraconazole has some activity against *Aspergillus* sp., but clinical trials for *Aspergillus* have not been completed.

5-Fluorocytosine

5-Fluorocytosine acts as a fungal antimetabolite. Its narrow spectrum of activity includes *Cryptococcus, Candida*, and the agents of chromomycosis.

Usually, 5-fluorocytosine is used in combination with amphotericin B because of the rapid emergence of resistance. When used in this combination, the drug may permit a lower dose of amphotericin B. When used to treat chromomycosis, 5-fluorocytosine is typically used alone.

Reactions to 5-fluorocytosine can involve the GI tract and bone marrow. Toxicity is exaggerated when serum levels rise during renal failure. Because the drug is usually administered with amphotericin B, serum

5-fluorocytosine levels may rise with the onset of amphotericin-associated azotemia.

Antiviral compounds

It is difficult to produce antiviral agents that are effective but have acceptable toxicity because viral functions are so well integrated into host cell functions. It is also difficult to diagnose many viral infections soon enough to institute effective therapy. Viruses can also develop resistance to antiviral agents. Administration strategies, such as sequential or combination administration of antiviral agents, are being studied.

Adenine arabinoside

Adenine arabinoside (vidarabine) was the first effective agent for the treatment of herpes simplex virus (HSV) infections and was initially used as a treatment for HSV encephalitis. It was also found useful for treatment of disseminated varicella-zoster virus infections in immunocompromised hosts.

Reactions to adenine arabinoside can affect the GI tract; CNS, as manifested by confusion and tremor; bone marrow, producing leukopenia; and kidney, producing azotemia. Adenine arabinoside has been replaced by the drug acyclovir.

Acyclovir

Acyclovir is a guanine nucleoside derivative that is effective in vitro against most herpesviruses.[8] A herpesvirus-specific enzyme phosphorylates the parent compound and renders it active intracellularly. Therefore, acyclovir has specific activity for virally infected cells. The drug is most effective against HSV and varicella-zoster virus. Although acyclovir does have some in vitro activity against other herpesviruses, such as Epstein-Barr virus (EBV) and cytomegalovirus (CMV), no clinically effective inhibition of EBV or CMV occurs in vivo.

Acyclovir can be administered orally, topi-cally, or parenterally. It is well absorbed after oral administration and is very well tolerated. The most common side effect after oral administration is mild GI disturbances. Renal toxicity may occur after parenteral administration, although this is relatively infrequent.

Gancyclovir

Gancyclovir, a nucleoside analog similar to acyclovir, is also active against most herpesviruses. Gancyclovir has mainly been used to treat CMV infections and has more than 10 times the activity of acyclovir against CMV.

Gancyclovir can be administered only parenterally and has potentially severe dose-limiting toxicities, including severe bone marrow suppression that results in neutropenia and thrombocytopenia. The effect of gancyclovir on the bone marrow is potentiated by concomitant use of other agents causing marrow toxicity, such as zidovudine.

Foscarnet

Foscarnet, a derivative of phosphonoformic acid, inhibits the DNA polymerase of all human herpesviruses. Its main clinical use has been in the treatment of CMV infections. Because of a lack of marrow toxicity, foscarnet is particularly useful as an alternative to gancyclovir therapy in the treatment of these infections. Unfortunately, renal toxicity and metabolic problems such as calcium and phosphorus disturbances limit foscarnet's clinical usefulness. An additional clinical use of foscarnet has been in the treatment of severe HSV infections that have become resistant to acyclovir.

Amantadine/rimantadine

Rimantadine, a structural analog of amantadine, is clinically as effective as amantadine in prevention and treatment of influenza A infections. It also may be better tolerated and may produce less frequent and fewer CNS side effects than amantidine.

Ribavirin

Ribavirin is a broad-spectrum antiviral agent with activity against both ribonucleic acid (RNA) and deoxyribonucleic acid (DNA) viruses. Aerosolized ribavirin has been used to treat severe respiratory syncytial virus infections in hospitalized children and adults. Several studies have noted clinical benefits, including decreased viral shedding and improved respiratory function in children. However, there is controversy over its cost, benefit, and safety, particularly potential teratogenic hazards to patients and care providers.

Ribavirin is generally well tolerated. No major side effects have been reported, but bronchospasm after aerosol administration has been noted. Ribavirin has been found to be teratogenic in several animal species, although no definite human teratogenicity has been reported. Because of this theoretic potential, ribavirin is contraindicated in pregnant women.

Zidovudine

Zidovudine, or AZT, is a thymidine analog that acts as an inhibitor of reverse transcriptase in mammalian retroviruses, including human immunodeficiency virus type 1 (HIV-1).[14] Viral reverse transcriptase is an RNA-dependent DNA polymerase that transcribes the viral RNA genome "message" to DNA that integrates into the host cell genome. AZT and other dideoxynucleoside anti-HIV agents inhibit reverse transcriptase.

The most common toxic reactions associated with AZT are anemia and granulocytopenia. These are dose dependent and most prominent at high doses. Other common side effects include headache, nausea, and hepatitis. Careful monitoring of blood components and liver function are required during therapy.

Randomized double-blind placebo-controlled trials have established the clinical utility of AZT in HIV-infected patients with T4 cell counts less than 500/ml. Clinical improvements include increases in T4 count, fewer opportunistic infections, weight gain, and decreases in viral titers as measured by level of serum viral P24 antigen. Studies indicate little difference in benefit between high-dose and low-dose therapy, and low-dose therapy is associated with significantly less toxicity (see Clinical Study 26).

Didanosine

Didanosine (ddI), the second nucleoside analog approved for therapy of HIV-infected patients, was released for clinical use in October 1991. It is approved for use by HIV-infected patients who are intolerant of or who no longer respond to AZT. Studies documenting ddI's effectiveness often have not included sufficient controls and have been less rigorous than those documenting efficacy of AZT; nonetheless, ddI appears to be beneficial. It is acid labile and must be administered with buffered tablets to limit drug degradation in the stomach.

Mild adverse effects to ddI are similar to those produced by AZT, including headache and nausea. The main advantage of ddI over AZT is the lack of significant hematologic toxicity. Peripheral neuropathy has developed in approximately 10% of patients taking ddI. Clinical pancreatitis and asymptomatic elevation of serum amylase occur frequently with ddI and should lead to discontinuation of therapy. Cases of fatal drug-induced pancreatitis have occurred.

Zalcitabine

As with ddI and AZT, zalcitabine (ddC) inhibits viral reverse transcriptase. It was released for clinical use in 1992 on the basis of several small uncontrolled trials that indicated beneficial effects when ddC was coadministered with AZT. It is indicated for the treatment of adult patients with advanced HIV infection who have demonstrated significant clinical or immunologic deterioration.

The major toxic effects of ddC are peripheral neuropathy and occasional pancreatitis. Moderate to severe neuropathy has been reported in up to 31% of patients taking the drug. Occasionally, mucositis and esophagitis have been attributed to ddC therapy. Hematologic toxicity associated with this drug appears to be minimal.

INFLUENCE OF PRACTICE SETTING ON ANTIMICROBIAL THERAPY
Long-term care

Therapy of infections in long-term care facilities is often empiric and, whenever possible, administered orally. Many long-term care facilities do not administer parenteral antibiotics. Several investigators have completed surveys of long-term care.[7,10] Some reports suggest that antibiotics may be overused in long-term care. In one study, 13% of catheterized patients were receiving antibiotics, and of these, 85% had at least one urinary bacterial isolate resistant to the antibiotic being administered. Antimicrobial resistance has been a major problem in long-term care, and these facilities may be significant reservoirs of resistant organisms. The combination of elderly, often debilitated clients with overuse of antibiotics may increase the likelihood that resistant organisms will emerge.

Important questions regarding the management of antimicrobials in long-term care remain unanswered. Antibiotic use must be correlated with the prevalence and emergence of resistant organisms and the development of infections. Antibiotic control programs similar to those proved effective in hospitals may facilitate appropriate use once standards for antibiotic use in long-term care, which may be quite different from those for acute care, are developed.

Home therapy

Driven by the trend toward shorter hospital stays, administration of IV antibiotics in the home has become commonplace. Home IV therapy was first attempted with patients who were being treated for bone and joint infections requiring many weeks of therapy. Subsequently, other infections, such as endocarditis, complicated UTIs, infected foreign devices, and intraabdominal infections, have been shown to be effectively managed at home.[21]

Along with the increasing use of IV antibiotics administered at home, a variety of other IV therapies have been developed for delivery outside the hospital. Hyperalimentation, blood products, and some forms of cancer chemotherapy now are administered to the patient at home.

To accommodate the increasing variety of IV medications given at home, vascular access devices have been developed. These devices lend themselves to easy home care or self-care and provide long-term IV access to the central circulation. Hickman, Groshong, and Broviac catheters as well as Portacath devices and other implantable products perform these functions well. Because of the increasing complexity of admixing medications and additives, manipulating IV access devices, and monitoring therapy for anticipated complications, a team approach to home IV care has become the most successful model for this therapy. Most often the home IV care team integrates pharmaceutical, medical, and nursing care to coordinate delivery of antibiotics and other medications.

Virtually any antibiotic may be administered in the outpatient setting; however, antibiotics with long half-lives are most popular. These drugs may be administered once or twice daily, a distinct convenience. Clinicians must often balance kinetics, microbiologic spectrum, and the potential for adverse events when selecting an antibiotic for outpatient therapy.

The monitoring of the quality of home IV therapy requires further development. When the patient leaves the hospital for the less structured situation in the home, it may be difficult to monitor adverse effects and intervene in a timely manner when a patient's condition is not improving or is deteriorating. Quality assurance procedures help to identify both deficiencies in home care policies and procedures that may lead to adverse outcomes and opportunities to improve care. At present, few standards for quality assessment of home IV care exist. With the large available market of patients, many commercial companies targeting home IV care have arisen and prospered in the United States. These commercial, for-profit concerns vary in commitment to quality control activities. Hopefully, methodical refinements and standardization of care incorporate procedures demonstrated to produce the best results will follow.

SUMMARY

Antimicrobial agents contribute significantly to our ability to prevent and manage infections. This is particularly true for bacterial infections.

Despite this contribution and our occasional inclination to think of antimicrobial agents as the major anti-infection therapy and prevention regimen, these agents have limitations which must be carefully considered. Cost, risk of side effects, disruption of the normal bacterial flora, and selection for survival of resistant microorganisms all increase with use of these agents. Consequently, antimicrobial chemotherapy may complement but cannot replace other patient care practices which contribute to infection prevention and management.

REFERENCES

1. Andriole VT. Clinical overview of the newer 4-quinolone antibacterial agents. In Andriole VT, ed. *The Quinolones.* London: Academic Press; 1988.
2. Barriere SL, Flaherty JF. Third generation cephalosporins: a critical evaluation. *Clin Pharm.* 1984;3: 351-372.
3. Benson JM, Nahata MC. Clinical use of systemic antifungal agents. *Clin Pharm.* 1988;7:424.
4. Brown P, Preece MA, Will RG. "Friendly fire" in medicine: hormones, homografts and Creutzfeldt Jakob Disease. *Lancet.* 1992;34:24-27.
5. Calderwood S, Moellering RC. Common adverse affects of antibacterial agents on major organ systems. *Surg Clin North Am.* 1980;60:65.
6. Chopra I et al. The tetracyclines: prospects at the beginning of the 1980s. *J Antimicrob Chemother.* 1981;8:5.
7. Daily PB, et al. A microbiologic survey of long-term care urinary catheters. *Nebr Med J.* 1991;76:161-165.
8. Dorsky DI, Crumpacker CS. Drugs 5 years later: acyclovir. *Ann Intern Med.* 1987;107:859.
9. Drusano GL. Role of pharmacokinetics in the outcome of infections. *Antimicrob Agents Chemother.* 1988;32:289.
10. Gaynes RP et al. Antibiotic resistant flora in nursing home patients admitted to the hospital. *Arch Intern Med.* 1985; 145:1804.
11. Gibaldi M, Levy G. Pharmacokinetics in clinical practice. Part I: *JAMA.* 1976;235:1864-1867. Part II: *JAMA.* 1976;235:1987-1992.
12. Holmberg SD, Solomon SL, Blake PA. Health and economic impacts of antimicrobial resistance. *Rev Infect Dis.* 1987;6:1065-1078.
13. Kunin CM. Problems in antibiotic usage. In Mandell GL, Douglas RG Jr., Bennett JE, eds. *Principles and Practice of Infectious Diseases.* New York: Churchill Livingstone Inc.; 1990.
14. Mathews SJ, Cersosimo RJ, Spivack ML. Zidovudine and other reverse transcriptase inhibitors in the management of human immunodeficiency virus related disease. *Pharmacotherapy.* 1991;11:419-449.
15. McGowan JE. Antimicrobial resistance in hospital organisms and its relation to antimicrobial use. *Rev Infect Dis.* 1983;5:1033-1048.
16. McHenry MC, Gavan TL. Vancomycin. *Pediatr Clin North Am.* 1983;30:31-47.
17. Moellering RC. Clinical microbiology and the in vitro activity of aminoglycosides. In Whelton A, Neu HC, eds. *The Aminoglycosides: Microbiology, Clinical Use, and Toxicology.* New York: Marcel Dekker; 1982.
18. Neu HC. Antistaphylococcal penicillins. *Med Clin North Am.* 1982;66:51.
19. Nightingale CH, Greene DS, Quintiliani R. Pharmacokinetics and clinical use of cephalosporin antibiotics. *J Pharm Sci.* 1975;64:1927-1988.
20. O'Brien RJ. Present chemotherapy of tuberculosis. *Semin in Respir Infect.* 1989;4:216.
21. Poretz DM. Home management of intravenous antibiotic therapy. *Bull N Y Acad Med.* 1988;64:570.
22. Reed MD, Blumer JL. Clinical pharmacology of antitubercular drugs. *Pediatr Clin North Am.* 1983; 30:177.
23. Salter AJ. Trimethoprim sulfamethoxazole: an assessment of more than 12 years of use. *Rev of Infect Dis.* 1982;4:196-236.

24. Thornsberry C. Antimicrobial susceptibility testing: general considerations. In Balows A, Hausler W Jr., Herrmann GJ, Isenberg HD, Shadomy S, eds. *Manual of Clinical Microbiology*, 5th ed. Washington D.C.: American Society for Microbiology; 1991.

25. Washington JA, Wilson WR. Erythromycin: a microbial and clinical prospective after 30 years of clinical use. Part I: *Mayo Clin Proc.* 1984;60:189-203. Part II: 1985;60:271-278.

SUGGESTED READINGS

1. Cohen ML. Epidemiology of drug resistance: implications for a post-antimicrobial era. *Science.* 1992;257:1050-1055.

2. Gilman AG, Goodman LS, Rall TW, Murad F. *The Pharmacological Basis of Therapeutics.* New York: Macmillan;1985.

3. Kunin CM. Resistance to antimicrobial drugs—a worldwide calamity. *Annals of Internal Medicine.* 1993;118:557-561.

4. Levy SB. Confronting multidrug resistance. *JAMA.* 1993;269:1840-1842.

5. Neu HC. The crisis in antibiotic resistance. *Science.* 1992;257:1064-1073.

6. Frontiers in Biotechnology: Resistance to Antibiotics. *Science.* 1994;264:360-397.

Chapter 9

Education and Behavior Change in Prevention and Control of Infection

BARBARA A. GOLDRICK and
JOAN G. TURNER

Nurses are in a position to influence positively others' behavior and to change their own behavior through health education. Effective educational interventions are based on needs mutually identified by the health care provider and patient. Health education activities have important applications and a common basis in clinical, school, home, and work settings.

Health education is a process which bridges the gap between health information and health practices. Health education motivates the person to take the information and do something with it—to keep himself healthy by avoiding actions that are harmful and by forming habits that are beneficial.[33]

As this definition implies, health education enables people to make changes in personal behavior that promote health or prevent disease. The educational needs assessment identifies factors that affect behavior as well as specific information needs important for promoting health among individuals and groups. Educational interventions based on such an assessment will be target specific and more effective.[33]

This chapter provides an overview of how methods of behavioral and educational diagnosis can be used as a framework to assess individuals or groups (hosts) within the context of host-environment interactions—biologic, physical, and social environments. This chapter uses assessment strategy to identify educational needs of health care providers and recipients. Examples of behavioral and educational diagnoses applied specifically to the area of prevention and control of infection are provided.

BEHAVIORAL AND EDUCATIONAL DIAGNOSES: AN OVERVIEW

If health education is defined as activities that encourage people to adapt their behavior to improve health,[33] the first step in planning an educational intervention is to diagnose or assess behavior and its health consequences. Behavioral and educational diagnoses involve all components of host-environment interactions, including microbiologic, biologic, physical, and social environments. This holistic approach to assessment is an integral part of the planning process for effective health education activities.

Behavioral diagnosis

A behavioral diagnosis can be accomplished by[33]

- Differentiating between behavioral and nonbehavioral causes of a problem

- Developing an inventory of behaviors
- Rating behaviors in order of importance
- Rating behaviors in order of changeability
- Choosing behavioral intervention targets

Nonbehavioral factors are personal and environmental conditions that are not controlled by the host but that may contribute to health or disease. These include genetic makeup, age, gender, underlying illness or disability, mental impairment, climate, workplace or school, and place of residence. Many of these factors are discussed in Chapters 1, 3, and 4.

Assessment of the nonbehavioral factors related to health problems enables the health care provider to (1) maintain a perspective on the multiple determinants of the problem being addressed and (2) identify factors, such as the environment, for which strategies other than education may be developed and used concurrently. Failure to identify nonbehavioral factors and recognize how they might affect outcomes may prevent the success of an otherwise sound program.[33] For example, age (a nonbehavioral factor) cannot be changed, but behaviors such as onset of sexual activity are changeable.

Once behavioral and nonbehavioral factors have been identified, specific behaviors contributing to the health problem can be identified and rated in order of importance and changeability.[33] This will help prioritize behaviors for intervention. Behaviors should be considered most important when (1) epidemiologic data clearly link the behavior to the health problem and (2) they occur frequently. Behaviors are considered less important when they are rare or are very indirectly related to a health problem. High changeability is probable when behaviors (1) are still in the developmental stages or have only recently been established and (2) are only superficially tied to established cultural patterns or lifestyles. Adolescent sexual activity that has not been initiated or has only recently been initiated is an example of behavior with high changeability.[33]

Behaviors have low changeability when they (1) have been established for a long time, (2) are deeply rooted in cultural patterns or lifestyles, or (3) have not been changed in previous attempts. Judgments about changeability must also include careful consideration of time management. How much time is necessary to intervene and show change? The more deeply rooted or widespread the behavior, the more time and effort are required to change the behavior.[33]

Health education is effective only if it influences behaviors found to be causally related to desired outcomes; for example, delay of sexual activity among adolescents and handwashing among health care providers. Therefore, the first task in the behavioral diagnosis is to establish a cause-and-effect relationship between behaviors and associated adverse outcomes[33] by reviewing the literature, collecting data, or talking with colleagues. For example, handwashing behavior of health care personnel has been shown to be one important determinant of nosocomial (institutionally associated) infections (the outcome).[48] Therefore a health education program designed to reduce nosocomial infections might be directed at maximizing handwashing behaviors of care providers.

Educational diagnosis

The second step is an educational diagnosis. The educational diagnosis takes into account the physiologic, psychologic, social, and physical environments that affect behavior. Green et al[33] classify these as predisposing factors, enabling factors, and reinforcing factors (Table 9-1). Any given behavior may be due to the collective influence of these three types of factors, which are an indispensable part of behavioral change.[33]

Predisposing factors

Predisposing factors are internal to the host and enhance or deter motivation for healthy decision making. Predisposing factors include

TABLE 9-1. Educational diagnosis: predisposing, enabling, and reinforcing factors

Type of factors	Examples
Predisposing factors	Knowledge, skills, maturation level, attitudes, beliefs
Enabling factors	Availability and accessibility of resources necessary for healthy behavior
Reinforcing factors	Rewards, incentives, peer/social support

Data from Green LW et al. *Health Education Planning: A Diagnostic Approach.* Mountain View, CA: Mayfield; 1980.

knowledge, skills, level of maturation, and physiologic functioning. People are more likely to change their behavior when or if they are aware of a need to change. For example, when people do not know that infections can be transmitted via sexual intercourse and that the correct use of condoms will decrease the likelihood of transmission, they may not use condoms. However, knowledge alone is insufficient to motivate healthful behavior.

Other predisposing factors, such as attitudes, opinions, and beliefs, provide a psychologic environment that also affects motivation and willingness to change behavior.[33] For instance, even though a person may know a condom will lower risk of infection transmission, decisions to use a condom will be strongly influenced by attitudes toward sexual activity and condoms as well as by attitudes toward health. If the person believes that condoms are a nuisance or that they diminish sexual pleasure, these factors will reduce the likelihood that condoms will be used, regardless of the level of knowledge. On the one hand, the adolescent may know that unprotected intercourse can lead to a sexually transmitted disease, but other contributions to behavior (e.g., emotional and/or physical need to have sex) combined with the adolescent's sense of invulnerability (i.e., "It can't happen to me"), may predispose him or her to

unprotected sexual behavior (see Clinical Studies 11 and 14).

Recent studies suggest that self-efficacy, one's assessment of personal capability, may be a strong predictor of risk behavior.[7,18,67,72] The concept of self-efficacy, which comes from social learning theory,[4] "is a perception of one's own capacity for success in organizing and implementing a pattern of behavior that is new, based largely on experience with similar actions or circumstances encountered or observed in the past (see Chapter 4)."[5] Self-efficacy refers to personal expectations about one's ability to carry out a specific behavior.[72] Self-efficacy influences behavior in that if individuals are highly confident about a behavior, they tend to perform it successfully. Seeman and Seeman[67] found that individuals with high self-efficacy were more apt to participate in preventive actions and initiate treatment for illness than individuals with low self-efficacy.

Enabling factors

Enabling factors, which are external to and not under the control of the host, can also affect motivation or aspiration toward healthful behavior.[33] The physical environment can enable the change to take place or can set up barriers that inhibit behavior change. Enabling factors include the resources necessary to perform health-promoting behavior, such as availability of condoms or money to buy them. Health behavior may be limited by the degree to which resources are available and accessible. For example, condoms are not available in some countries and not readily accessible in other settings. Although differing opinions exist regarding the desirability of providing availability of condoms to students in schools, surveys have shown that when students have access to condoms, they are more likely to practice safer sex.[70,84]

Reinforcing factors

Reinforcing factors are also external to the host. These factors occur following the behavior and provide a reward, incentive, or punishment for continuing a behavior, and they contribute to the behavior's persistence or extinction.[33,70] For example, a positive attitude about condoms in one's peer group and sexual partner will provide the necessary feedback to reinforce using condoms. Likewise, a negative attitude from a peer group will inhibit condom use.

In summary, studies have provided evidence that health education is often effective in changing health-related behaviors. For example, studies of the effects of school health education programs in 20 states indicated that such programs for children resulted in increased health knowledge, improved attitudes toward health, and more healthful behavior in such areas as nutrition and exercise.[11] However, for health education to be successful, it must take into account several factors. On one hand, the perceived benefits of changing behaviors exert a direct influence on one's predisposition to engage in health-promoting activities. On the other hand, potential or actual barriers to health-promoting activities affect health behavior. These barriers include inconvenience or difficulty of a particular health-promoting behavior[62] and low self-efficacy.[72]

AN APPLICATION OF BEHAVIORAL AND EDUCATIONAL DIAGNOSES IN PREVENTION AND CONTROL OF INFECTION IN THE COMMUNITY

Management of sexually transmitted diseases (STDs) illustrates the application of behavioral and educational diagnoses to create change among individuals, families, and communities. Considerable gains have been made in public knowledge about how the human immunodeficiency virus (HIV) is transmitted, but information alone is not sufficient to change behavior. Behavioral factors, including sexual activity at a very young age,[42] multiple sex partners,[69] and failure to use a condom,[84]

increase risk of acquisition of HIV and other STDs. Thus, altering these behaviors is the goal of health education intended to decrease the incidence of these diseases. In addition to these behavioral factors, nonbehavioral factors related to STDs include race,[68] socioeconomic status,[58,69] and place of residence (i.e., urban versus rural).[69] Obviously, the nonbehavioral factors are not amenable to change through health education, but knowing these factors is helpful in identifying high-risk persons to whom health education can be targeted.

Planners of educational programs about STDs, including HIV, should conduct a needs assessment, keeping in mind factors that are changeable among the identified target group.[33] If the problem of STDs is analyzed in terms of behavioral and nonbehavioral causes, educators should try to obtain the answers to certain questions: Are STDs related to age, sex, race, or other characteristics? Who is at risk? Once those at risk have been identified, questions about behavior can be addressed: What is the relative risk by age of initiation of sexual activity? What are the predisposing factors (e.g., knowledge, attitudes, beliefs) about the transmission of STDs among those at risk? These questions help educators select the behaviors that will be the subject of the intervention for the target population. To perform a behavior assessment that is requisite for planning health education interventions, it is necessary to consult current literature to identify behaviors associated with the health problem of interest. For example, the following information has been used to identify behavioral and nonbehavioral factors associated with STDs.

Epidemiologic data

Seidman et al[69] found that race, marital status, and early first intercourse were predictors for having multiple recent sex partners among 8,450 women 15 to 44 years of age in the United States. Nine percent of all unmarried women in the sample reported having sexual intercourse with two or more men in the previous 3 months compared with 0.4% of married women. Among the unmarried sexually active white women, most who reported having two or more recent partners were under 30 years of age; the unmarried, sexually active black women who most frequently reported having two or more sexual partners were 30 or older. Earlier age at first intercourse was found to be strongly associated with a higher rate of multiple recent partners for all never-married women. Among never-married white women, the percentage reporting multiple partners increased almost fivefold for those whose first intercourse was before age 15 (17.8%), compared with those whose first intercourse was after age 18 (3.8%). Likewise, a high percentage of never-married black women who reported first intercourse under age 15 (13.9%) reported having recent multiple sex partners compared with those with first intercourse at 18 or older (2.4%). Place of residence also was found to be a factor associated with multiple sex partners among never-married white women. A higher percentage of never-married inner-city white women reported multiple sex partners (11.3%) compared with never-married suburban white women (7.4%). However, no differences were found between never-married urban and suburban black women (6.2% for both groups). These findings illustrate the oversimplification introduced and erroneous conclusions that might be drawn by using race alone as a predictor of sexual behavior.[68]

Behavioral and nonbehavioral diagnosis

Given the previous epidemiologic data, health education interventions that promote safer sexual practices among certain groups (e.g., younger women, unmarried women whose first sexual intercourse was before age 15, never-married white women who live in a city) might be expected to reduce the morbidity associated with STDs. However, since the highest percentage of women who reported two or more sexual partners were those who were under age 15 at the time of first intercourse,[69] the primary target population for education about STD health problems would be adolescents aged 12 to 15 years. The secondary population would be adolescents aged 15 to 18; and tertiary populations would be parents of adolescents and school staff.

Behavioral factors for these groups include (1) sexual activity at a very young age (i.e., under 15 years), (2) sexual activity with more than one partner, and (3) failure to use protection during intercourse. Behavioral factors for parents and school staffs (the tertiary target groups) address the need for parents to communicate information about sex and sexual activity, lack of after-school supervision, lack of parental control over their children's dating practices, and failure of schools to provide sex education at an early enough age to be effective and to provide well-designed and well-taught sex education programs.[60] Using a priority-setting approach regarding changeability, a highly changeable behavior would be early sexual activity and an educational program behavioral objective would be "adolescents aged 12 to 15 years of age will delay the initiation of sexual activity by 2 to 5 years (depending on the adolescent's age) to age 17."

The nonbehavioral factors to consider in the primary and secondary target groups would include (1) family stability, (2) socioeconomic status, (3) peer pressure, (4) cultural norms, (5) place of residence, (6) age, and (7) race.

Educational diagnosis

The predisposing factors for STDs among this adolescent group include (1) lack of knowledge about reproduction and human sexuality,[40,60] (2) lack of knowledge about risks associated with sexual activity,[20,21,84] and (3) the perception that premarital sex is considered permissible and acceptable. [40,60]

Enabling factors for the primary (12- to 15-year-olds) and secondary (16- to 18-year-olds) target groups include developmental and cognitive skills regarding human sexuality and accessibility to information suited to the adolescents' stage of cognitive development.[60,84] Negative reinforcing factors to be addressed are peer pressure as a barrier to change and ambiguous behavioral and attitudinal signals from parents about sexual activity. Positive reinforcing factors include friends and family who support and provide reference regarding attitudes and beliefs about sex and delay of sexual activity.[60]

To determine whether self-efficacy among adolescents contributed to risk-reduction behaviors regarding STDs such as HIV, a survey was conducted among 1,720 randomly selected tenth-grade students.[43] Perceptions of self-efficacy were found to be significantly associated with condom use, and overall, self-efficacy explained the respondents' sexual intentions and behaviors. In another study that examined self-efficacy with respect to acquired immunodeficiency syndrome (AIDS) prevention behaviors among 181 ninth-grade students who resided near an AIDS epicenter, researchers found low self-efficacy to be common.[21] Students were unsure of their ability to do any of the following: (1) refuse sexual intercourse with a desirable partner under pressure or after drinking alcohol or using marijuana, (2) question sex partners about past risky behaviors, and (3) purchase or correctly and consistently use condoms. According to the researchers, students with lower self-efficacy for refusing sex were twice as likely to have had sexual intercourse, and those with lower self-efficacy for correct, consistent condom use were one-fifth as likely to have used condoms. These findings establish the link between the predisposing factor of self-efficacy and behavior. They also reinforce the need for educational programs that emphasize skill building along with providing the necessary information for behavior change.

APPLICATION OF BEHAVIORAL AND EDUCATIONAL DIAGNOSES TO PREVENT AND CONTROL INFECTIONS IN HEALTH CARE SETTINGS

Behavioral and educational diagnosis techniques described earlier may also target health care providers in the interest of preventing and controlling infectious diseases.

The problem of nosocomial infections has been well documented over the past 20 years* and most recently has been addressed by the U.S. Department of Health and Human Services (DHHS) in *Healthy People 2000*.[76] A goal of DHHS is to reduce the numbers of surgical wound infections and nosocomial infections in intensive care unit (ICU) patients by 10% by the year 2000.

There is no question that nosocomial infections are a leading cause of death in the United States[36] and are associated with significant morbidity.[35] In addition to the morbidity and mortality, the annual costs of nosocomial infections have been estimated at $1 billion.[36]

Nosocomial infections are a major source of morbidity and mortality in ICUs.[8,17,22] Risk factors associated with ICU patients include severe illness, immunocompromise, invasive devices, and multiple antibiotics that alter normal flora.[22]

Reduction of nosocomial infections has been made in the last 20 years.[53] Data from the Centers for Disease Control and Prevention (CDC) Study on the Efficacy of Nosocomial Infection Control (SENIC) indicated that effective infection control programs could reduce the incidence of nosocomial infection by 32%.[35] However, data from SENIC indicated that in 1976 only 6% of nosocomial infections were being prevented, leaving an additional 26% to be prevented.[35] A follow-up survey in 1983, using SENIC methodology, indicated that up to 9% of nosocomial infections were being prevented.[37] A recent U.S. Government Accounting Office (GAO) survey indicated that

---

*References 10, 24, 26-28, 35, 49, 52, 53.

99% of acute care hospitals have a multidisciplinary infection control committee and that 85% monitor patient care staff for compliance with specific patient care practices.[78]

Although SENIC examined the effectiveness of infection control programs, one of the study's weaknesses was the exclusion of long-term care facilities (LTCFs).[36] The CDC estimates that 1.5 million nosocomial infections per year occur in residents of LTCFs, which is equivalent to an average of one infection per resident per year.[71] Infections among residents in LTCFs are associated with a decline in activities of daily living, transfer to a hospital, and death.[61]

Behavioral diagnosis

The challenges of changing health care provider practices and compliance with infection prevention and control strategies have been well documented. Most studies have focused on improving handwashing, use of barrier equipment, and implementing universal precautions. Many have used some form of education to encourage health care providers to wash hands and use barrier techniques consistent with recommended guidelines.* However, educational programs designed to improve infection control–related behaviors have produced equivocal results.

Historically, compliance of health care providers with longstanding infection prevention and control procedures has been poor. In an early observational study, investigators reported that registered nurses failed to perform appropriate patient care handwashing 95% of the time.[26] Also using direct observation, Albert and Condie[1] reported that handwashing occurred after only 41% of patient contacts in an ICU. In 1983, Larson[47] reported that in less than half of contacts with patients known to be clinically infected did nurses, physicians, or other personnel wash their hands. In 1987 the CDC[12,13] recommended univer-

sal precautions as a means of preventing the transmission of HIV and other bloodborne pathogens.[12,13,14] Universal precautions were mandated in the 1991 U.S. Occupational Safety and Health Administration (OSHA) standard.[77] Although most hospitals have instituted universal precaution policies, many investigators have documented that health care provider compliance is substandard.† For example, a 1991 study found that universal precautions were practiced only 44% of the time in a large urban hospital emergency room.[44] Recapping of needles is specifically prohibited by universal precautions guidelines,[12,13] but health care providers continue to recap needles. In a longitudinal study on the relationship between reports of needle stick injuries and regular continuing education, one group of investigators concluded that educational programs over 3 years failed to produce a major reduction in needle stick injuries.[50] However, these educational sessions were not preceded by appropriate behavioral and nonbehavioral assessments. When instructional strategies are not preceded by assessments and guided by sound teaching-learning strategies, the message, or target information, may be lost. For example, in one study, more than half the nurse respondents said they were unaware that needles should not be recapped.[65]

Predisposing factors

It is assumed that nurses have basic knowledge regarding infection prevention and control. However, several studies have found that nursing students and nursing staff lack this knowledge.[2,30,31,66,75] One study conducted among third-year baccalaureate nursing students at two universities found a mean pretest score of 57% on an infection control knowledge test.[31] Another study conducted among third- and fourth-year baccalaureate nursing students at 10 colleges of nursing in Iowa found a mean correct response score of only 60% on

---

*References 3, 16, 23-28, 44, 50, 51, 73.

†References 44, 50, 55, 56, 65, 74, 83.

a test of knowledge of handwashing and isolation practices.[66] Nursing personnel at two Veterans Administration medical centers had a 70% mean pretest score on an infection control knowledge test.[30] A second study reported similar results among registered nurses, licensed practical nurses, and nursing assistants in two LTCFs. In a follow-up study among nursing assistants in LTCFs, the mean score on the infection control knowledge test was 65%.[2]

The health care providers' ability to render quality care to HIV-infected patients and their families may be compromised not only by knowledge deficits, but also by unresolved feelings, attitudes, and beliefs. Health care providers should be able to provide quality care to HIV-infected individuals, and supportive counseling and services to those at risk, if their knowledge levels about HIV transmission are increased. However, several investigators found that although health care providers were knowledgeable about HIV transmission, they needed to be sensitized to and educated about discussing human sexuality, obtaining a health history, and counseling. They also found that feelings and attitudes must be addressed in all AIDS-related education if changes in knowledge and behavior were to be realized.*

These findings reflect how feelings and attitudes, however irrational, can prevent behavior change despite increased information. It is not difficult to imagine that the care provider's behavior would be negatively influenced if patient or client were feared, disliked, or believed to be responsible for his or her own illness. However, when health care providers are given an opportunity to address and resolve these feelings, behavior change is possible.[81]

Enabling factors

In order to use handwashing and infection control skills, health care providers need the appropriate resources. The OSHA standards

---

*References 6, 9, 38, 45, 64, 80, 81.

require employers to take definitive steps to protect their employees from bloodborne hazards.[77] Almost half the respondents in a large emergency room indicated that there was not always sufficient time to put on protective garb; one-third believed that precautions interfered with performance of procedures; and nearly a quarter stated that the materials were uncomfortable.[44]

Reinforcing factors

Peers, colleagues, teachers, mentors, and supervisors provide the external feedback necessary to support behavior changes regarding infection control practices. When universal precautions were implemented in one facility after a hospital-wide training program, observers found that physicians and other employees were practicing consistently with the guidelines only 63% of the time. To improve practice, a system was developed that included feedback to employees regarding compliance and departmental enforcement.[56] When employees were observed not using universal precautions, they were taken aside and counseled. Additionally, infractions in universal precautions were made a part of employee performance evaluations. After departmental enforcement began, compliance increased significantly, from 63% to 82%.

The idea of using feedback as a reinforcement mechanism to change behavior or increase the quality of performance originated with Weiner.[82] The process of giving subjects feedback about past performance provides information that allows them an opportunity to change future behavior. Further, individuals generally are seeking a sense of competence about a task, and perception of competence (i.e., self-efficacy) is vital to behavior change.[19] Feedback has been successful in assisting nurses' professional development[41] and is recommended as an essential mechanism to achieve better performance among nurses.[15] Education reinforced through feedback has been found to be an effective method in sustaining infection control behavior change.[23,54]

In an attempt to identify determinants of handwashing behavior, effectiveness of an emollient soap was compared with feedback about the frequency of handwashing. Throughout a 16-week period, nurses and nursing assistants in medical and surgical ICUs were observed as they performed their usual clinical duties. Baseline observations without any intervention were conducted for the first 3 weeks of the study. In the next phase, one ICU served as a control while the other received a series of interventions. The first intervention involved using a new emollient soap in attractive dispensers. The second sequential intervention involved giving performance feedback to individuals that consisted of a daily memo in which handwashing mistakes or omissions made the day before were itemized. Use of the emollient soap produced no change in handwashing behaviors from baseline. However, an immediate and sustained increase occurred in handwashing frequency after the introduction of feedback. In fact, compliance with handwashing guidelines increased to 98% from a baseline of 63% after 3 weeks of performance feedback. Unfortunately, handwashing behaviors tended to approach the baseline or preintervention rate approximately 6 months after the termination of the feedback intervention.[54] These data emphasize the need for ongoing feedback to maintain compliance with infection control policies in the health care setting. However, ongoing formal educational programs are not practical or cost-effective. Other methods to increase compliance with infection control policies and procedures need to be considered.

Another approach was used to monitor the practice of universal precautions among employees in a large university emergency room through environmental safety rounds. Observers rotated among employees twice a month on a random schedule. If an infraction was observed, the employee was asked to stop the activity and was counseled immediately. The infractions were noted and the worker's supervisor notified. Investigators found that overall compliance with universal precautions improved from 44% to 72% after 1 year of environmental safety rounds.[44] In a similar study, after body substance isolation was adopted as hospital policy, some hospital departments made compliance with these guidelines a part of employee performance review. Although the process was not formally evaluated, compliance appeared to improve.[51]

Compliance with appropriate glove use among nurses following educational sessions on the implementation of body substance isolation exceeded 90% when head nurses were involved in the planning process, sought feedback on staff performance, and regularly reinforced performance with feedback.[51] The results observed in this study may have been the consequence of educational strategies that not only addressed predisposing factors (knowledge, attitudes, beliefs), but included performance feedback (reinforcing factor).

Feedback was also used to lower nosocomial infection rates associated with methicillin-resistant *Staphylococcus aureus* (MRSA). A team of investigators employed a combination of brief presentations on the importance of handwashing by the hospital epidemiologist and innovative performance feedback to physicians. When physicians were informed that they had a patient colonized or infected with MRSA, they were also reminded in the same communication that MRSA is most frequently spread by inadequate handwashing and that as managing physicians they were *the* role model for the rest of the team. Nosocomial infections with MRSA decreased by 50% over the 15 months of the study.[59]

In summary, failure to comply with accepted infection prevention and control standards and policies is a behavioral factor important to the assessment of education needs. The nonbehavioral factors to consider are (1) the physical environment, (2) equipment, and (3) peer pressure. The predisposing factors in the educational diagnosis include (1) lack of knowledge about infection transmission,* (2) lack of knowledge about the effectiveness of infection prevention and control practices,[44,47] and (3) attitudes and beliefs that certain behaviors such as handwashing[22,23,26,32,48] are not important, that isolation precautions are unnecessary, and that necessary equipment is inaccessible.[44,47] Educational and behavioral diagnoses provide the foundation for educational interventions for behavior change to prevent and control infections among clients and health care providers.

DESIGNING HEALTH EDUCATION PROGRAMS

Once a behavioral diagnosis based on the analysis of the predisposing, enabling, and reinforcing factors influencing the health behavior has been completed, the educator can plan the educational strategies most suitable for the target group.

Health education is intended to help people free themselves from factors that predispose them to unhealthful behaviors.[62] These predisposing factors may include knowledge or skill deficits, attitudes, and values. The purposes of health education, therefore, are to clarify values, improve one's understanding of personal motivation, and provide the information and skills necessary to make health-related decisions. As this chapter has illustrated, health education involves more than imparting knowledge and skills. Nonetheless, some knowledge is necessary before change and creation of attitudes conducive to healthy behavior can take place.[33] Although the influence of health education on health-related behavior and subsequently on the health status of individuals and groups has been challenged by some, an increasing number of studies provide evidence that health education

can in some cases result in sustained behavioral change.[11,29,57,62] Various learning experiences are used to motivate people to maintain or attain health-enhancing behaviors.[18,62]

The design and operation of an educational program for behavior change involves the following: (1) setting a climate for learning, (2) establishing a structure for mutual planning, (3) diagnosing needs for learning, (4) formulating directions (objectives) for learning, (5) designing learning experiences, (6) managing the execution of the learning experiences, and (7) evaluating results and rediagnosing learning needs.[46]

Setting a climate for learning

People bring to the learning situation unique personalities, established social interaction patterns, cultural norms and values, and environmental influences. Therefore, to facilitate behavior change and effectiveness of educational programs, persons' knowledge levels and attitudinal barriers should be identified as described in the first section of this chapter before designing educational programs.[33] Educators of adults also should be aware of the characteristics of the adult learner[46]:

- Previous experience, which provides a rich background to facilitate learning
- Preference for self-direction rather than dependency in the learning process
- Preference for problem-centered or interest-centered learning rather than subject-centered learning
- Priority for learning that leads to mastery of current developmental task[39]

A *developmental task* is one that arises at or about a certain period in one's life, the success of which leads to success with later tasks, or failure leading to difficulty with later tasks.[39] Each developmental task produces a readiness to learn, which at its peak presents a teachable moment. For instance, in early adulthood, one developmental task is to get a job. Having

---

*References 2, 30, 31, 38, 45, 64.

landed a job, the next task is to master it. At that point, one is ready to learn the special skills the job requires, the performance standards expected, and how to get along with fellow employees. This organizing principle, rather than the institution's needs, should be kept in mind when planning an orientation for new employees, which should deal with their real-life concerns: Where will I be working? With whom will I be working? What will be expected of me?

Both the psychologic and physical environments can enhance or inhibit the learning process.[46] Is there a climate of mutual trust and respect? Is the environment supportive and caring, warm and friendly? Is the physical environment comfortable and aesthetically pleasing? Does it facilitate interaction? For example, arranging seats to allow eye contact and enhance interaction among participants tends to promote an openness in which learning can be facilitated.

Establishing a structure for mutual planning

Most people tend to feel committed to a decision or activity to the extent that they have participated in planning or making it.[33,34,46] Educational programs designed without participation by the learners that impose planned activities on participants often result in apathy and resentment. Imposing the educator's will and desires on the learner is incongruent with the adult learner concept of self-direction.[46] When teaching family-planning participants about condom use, it would be inappropriate and counterproductive for an educator with strict religious opinions against condom use to provide only information based on his or her beliefs about the use of condoms.

Diagnosing needs for learning

Modifications in behavior can be accomplished through health education by (1) providing information about risk factors for specific diseases and how the level of risk can be

decreased and (2) motivating people to change their risky behavior. The more complex the causes of the behavioral problem, the greater is the need for different educational strategies. For example, a program to control STDs will require massive information-dispensing efforts and community-organizing strategies in schools, clinics, work sites, and other community locations. Furthermore, these activities should be coordinated with those of other health, educational, and economic development programs.[33]

Educational strategies addressing only predisposing factors, such as knowledge and skills, will generally have only short-term effects. Strategies that influence reinforcing factors will have intermediate effects; that is, the behavior will last as long as the reinforcing feedback is provided. However, programs designed to influence predisposing, reinforcing, and enabling factors will have the greatest effects on long-term behavioral change.[33]

Formulating objectives for learning

Once the behavioral and educational diagnoses are complete, educational goals can be identified. Goal identification enables the educator to identify the level of prevention to be addressed.[33]

Within the model of host-environment interactions, there are three levels of prevention: primary, secondary, and tertiary.[79] *Primary prevention* refers to interventions designed to eliminate accumulation of sufficient elements of cause in the host. For example, a goal of reducing the incidence of STDs among adolescents involves primary prevention. *Secondary prevention* directs actions toward early detection and treatment of disease. Therefore, the goal of increasing tuberculosis screening among health care personnel focuses on secondary prevention. *Tertiary prevention* focuses on limiting disability from disease or restoring function. Cardiac rehabilitation despite the presence of atherosclerotic disease and even after open heart surgery is an example of tertiary prevention.

Designing and managing learning experiences

Health education strategies can be planned according to (1) characteristics of the health problem (i.e., epidemiologic data); (2) characteristics of the health behavior (i.e., behavioral diagnosis); (3) factors that predispose, enable, and reinforce the behavior (i.e., educational diagnosis); and (4) administrative considerations (e.g., budget, personnel).[33]

Health educators have a broad range of educational methods at their disposal, including lectures, group discussions, role playing, games, case studies, audiovisual media, computer-assisted instruction, and mass media. In planning an educational program, the best possible combinations of educational approaches for the learners and the situations should be considered. Health educators should use a variety of learning experiences to facilitate change.[33] Three broad categories of educational strategies are discussed here: (1) strategies for individual learning, (2) strategies for group learning, and (3) strategies for community development or community education.[46]

Individual learning

Several strategies help individuals in self-directed inquiry. These include independent study, programmed instruction, and computer-assisted instruction (CAI). Independent study is a tailor-made program for an individual to pursue self-directed learning in a particular area of interest, which includes periodic consultations with a mentor to discuss progress and problems. This format is frequently accompanied by a learning contract.[46] Programmed instruction and CAI also are considered individual learning strategies. In both formats, material to be learned is presented in a series of carefully planned sequential steps. At each step, the learner is given feedback regarding mastery of the content and remedial content if necessary. The advantage of programmed instruction and CAI is they are self-paced, allowing for different levels of content mastery.

Group learning

Most organized learning takes place in groups, primarily because of the efficiency of this method and the richer resources and motivations for learning provided by a group.[46] Formats for group learning include courses, seminars, workshops, and conferences. Within these formats, several strategies, such as lectures, discussions, games, audiovisual media, and demonstrations, may be employed.

Community development or education

This method is largely related to social action of some sort and is a means to help communities learn how better to solve their problems.[46] It emphasizes the development of skills, abilities, and understanding in an entire community for the purpose of social improvement. Community development is based on the self-help approach to problems and works best with compatible social groups.[33]

Green et al[33] have reviewed the state of the art in the application of educational strategies to health education and have divided them into three broad categories: (1) communication methods, including lecture-discussion, individual instruction, and the four media techniques of mass media audiovisual aids, educational television, and programmed learning; (2) training methods, including skills development, simulations and games, inquiry learning, small-group discussion, modeling, and behavior modification; and (3) community development, including social action and organizational development. Health education strategies can be based on either a health problem or on the characteristics of a targeted group's health behavior. Information regarding a health problem is derived from epidemiologic data, and educational strategies are targeted toward primary, secondary, or tertiary intervention. Table 9-2 outlines recommended educational strategies according to characteristics of the health problem.

Information regarding the target group is based on behavioral and educational diagnoses, including the predisposing, enabling, and reinforcing factors causing the health behavior. The attitudes of family, employers, peers, and health providers (reinforcing factors) toward the target group also need educational attention and are specified as a secondary or indirect target group for the program.[33] Table 9-3 outlines educational strategies according to characteristics of the health behavior. There is much overlap among predisposing, reinforcing, and enabling factors. Although community development strategies are generally based on enabling factors, predisposing and reinforcing factors may also be relevant.[33]

The 13 strategies outlined in Tables 9-2 and 9-3 are based on research in psychology, education, and communication. They provide a general guide to educators who have attempted to choose their methods explicitly. Even if the guide does not result in the identification of methods that will have the greatest success, it ensures that the assumptions behind a selection are clear. "Given this, the failures and successes of health education can be examined more critically and programs improved more readily."[33]

When planning any health education program, it is important to keep in mind the following points:

1. Select a minimum of three educational strategies for any health education program, keeping in mind that people learn in different ways and that using a variety of educational strategies increases interest. The longer the program (both in terms of hours and number of sessions), the greater is the number of educational strategies that should be used.

2. Be sure that all factors—predisposing,

TABLE 9-2. Educational strategies selected according to cause of the health problem and stage of prevention

Educational strategies	Cause of problem		Stage of prevention		
	Primarily environmental/ economic	Primarily behavioral	Primary	Secondary	Tertiary
Audiovisual aids					
Lecture		x	x	x	x
Individual instruction		x	x		x
Mass media		x	x	x	
Programmed learning		x	x		x
Educational television		x	x		x
Skill development		x			
Simulations and games		x	x		
Inquiry learning		x			
Peer group discussion		x	x	x	x
Modeling		x	x		
Behavior modification		x		x	x
Community development	x				

Adapted from Green LW et al. *Health Education Planning: A Diagnostic Approach*. Mountain View, CA: Mayfield; 1980.

TABLE 9-3. Educational strategies selected according to desired outcome, complexity of health information and characteristics of the health behavior

Educational strategies	Educational outcome desired			Complexity of the health information		Complexity of the health behavior		Duration of the health behavior		Frequency of the health behavior		Prevalence of the health behavior	
	Cognitive: knowledge/comprehension	Affective: attitudes/beliefs	Psychomotor: skills	Simple	Complex	Simple	Complex	Short term	Long term	Infrequent	Frequent	Rare	Widespread
Audiovisual aids	X					X		X					
Lecture	X							X		X			
Individual instruction	X						X						
Mass media	X			X		X		X		X			
Programmed learning	X			X									
Educational television	X			X									
Skill development			X						X		X		X
Simulations and games	X	X											
Inquiry learning	X	X			X								
Peer group discussion	X	X			X				X		X		
Modeling			X								X		
Behavior modification			X				X		X		X		X
Community development									X				

Adapted from Green LW et al. *Health Education Planning: A Diagnostic Approach.* Mountain View, CA: Mayfield; 1980.

enabling, and reinforcing—receive attention.

3. The more complex the causes of the behavioral problem, the greater the range of educational strategies required.[33]

None of these approaches need be restricted to a particular setting. All can be adapted to various situations and settings.

Evaluating results and rediagnosing learning needs

The evaluation of a health education program generally assesses the degree to which the objectives of the program were initially met. Were the participants able to perform the stated behaviors at the expected level of performance? Long-term outcome evaluation in health education, on the other hand, requires larger groups, more time, and greater resources than short-term evaluations and is most useful when the incidence or prevalence of the clinical condition(s) of interest are measured and related to the program.[33]

SUMMARY

Health education has been identified as a process that bridges the gap between health information and personal health practices by attempting to influence behavior directly.[63] However, health education limited to sharing of information is often not enough to change behavior.

Epidemiologic data, along with educational and behavioral diagnoses, should be used to summarize predisposing, enabling, and reinforcing factors and to identify target groups for behavior change. The studies described in this chapter demonstrate the importance of thorough assessment of the target population when designing an educational intervention to change behavior intended to prevent transmission of infectious diseases in the community and health setting. To influence behavior, one must consider the factors that predispose (i.e.,

knowledge, skills, attitudes, beliefs, feelings), reinforce (i.e., feedback, support from family, peers, colleagues), and enable (i.e., availability, accessibility to resources) behavior change.

Two examples of applying the theory of behavioral and educational diagnosis to the prevention and control of infection are (1) prevention of STDs in the community and (2) use of infection control practices such as handwashing and universal precautions. Modification of behavior of health care providers, clients, families, and communities can be accomplished by providing information about relative risk factors for specific diseases and ways risk can be decreased and motivating people to change their behavior.

The principles outlined in this chapter can guide your identification of behaviors on which health education can have a direct, immediate influence. Through the use of behavioral and educational diagnoses, factors influencing behavior can be critically assessed as to their relative importance and changeability. Educational interventions in any setting should be based on mutual diagnosis and planning, which includes the health care provider as a change agent and the target patients, families, workers, or consumers who are contemplating or should contemplate change.

REFERENCES

1. Albert K, Condie F. Handwashing patterns in medical intensive care units. *N Engl J Med* 1981;304:1461.
2. Alvaran M. *Infection Control in Long-Term Care Facilities.* Baltimore, MD: Johns Hopkins University School of Nursing; 1991. Thesis.
3. Baird SC, Beardslee ND. Developing an inservice program on acquired immunodeficiency syndrome. *J Staff Develop* 1990;6:269.
4. Bandura A. *Social Learning Theory.* Englewood Cliffs, NJ: Prentice Hall; 1977.
5. Bandura A. *Social Foundations of Thought and Action.* Englewood Cliffs, NJ: Prentice-Hall; 1986.
6. Barrick B. The willingness of nursing personnel to care for patients with acquired immune deficiency syndrome: a survey study and recommendations. *J Prof Nurs.* 1988;4:366.

7. Basen-Engquist K, Parcel GS. Attitudes, norms, and self-efficacy: a model of adolescents' HIV-related sexual risk behavior. *Health Educ Q.* 1992;19:263.

8. Bauer TM, et al. An epidemiological study assessing the relative importance of airborne and direct contact transmission of microorganisms in a medical intensive care unit. *J Hosp Infect.* 1990;15:301.

9. Blumenfield M, et al. Survey of attitudes of nurses working with AIDS patients. *Gen Hosp Psychiatry.* 1987;9:58.

10. Brachman PS, Eikhoff TC, editors. *Proceedings of the International Conference on Nosocomial Infections.* Chicago: American Hospital Association; 1971.

11. Centers for Disease Control. The effectiveness of school health education. *MMWR* 1986;35:593.

12. Centers for Disease Control. Recommendations for prevention of HIV transmission in health care settings. *MMWR* 1987;36:285.

13. Centers for Disease Control. Update: universal precautions for prevention of transmission of human immunodeficiency virus, hepatitis B virus, and other bloodborne pathogens. *MMWR* 1988;37:377.

14. Centers for Disease Control. The HIV/AIDS epidemic: the first 10 years. *MMWR* 1991;40:357.

15. Chu LK, Chu GS. Feedback and efficiency: a staff development model. *Nurs Management* 1991; 22(2):28.

16. Conly JM, et al. Handwashing practices in an intensive care unit: the effects of an educational program and its relationship to infection rates. *Am J Infect Control* 1989;17:330.

17. Craven D, Regan AM. Nosocomial pneumonia in the ICU patient. *Crit Care Nurs Q* 1989;11(4):28.

18. Damrosch S. General strategies for motivating people to change their behavior. *Nurs Clin North Am* 1991; 6:833.

19. Deci EL. The effects of contingent and noncontingent rewards on intrinsic motivation. *Organizational Behavior Human Performance.* 1972;8:217.

20. DiClemente RJ, Zorn J, Temoshok L. Adolescents' knowledge of AIDS near AIDS epicenter. *Am J Public Health.* 1987;77:876.

21. DiClemente RJ, et al. Comparison of AIDS knowledge, attitudes, and behaviors among adolescents and a public school sample in San Francisco. *Am J Public Health.* 1991;81:628.

22. Doebbeling BN, et al. Comparative efficacy of alternative hand-washing agents in reducing nosocomial infections in intensive care units. *N Engl J Med.* 1992; 327(2):88.

23. Dubbert P, et al. Increasing ICU staff hand-washing: effects of education on group feedback. *Infect Control Hosp Epidemiol.* 1990;11:191.

24. Eickhoff TC. Nosocomial infections—a 1980 view: progress, priorities and prognosis. *Am J Med.* 1981; 70:381.

25. Fahey BJ, Kozoil DE, Banks SM. Frequency of non-parenteral occupational exposures to blood and body fluids before and after universal precautions training. *JAMA.* 1991; 90:145.

26. Fox MK, Langner SB, Wells RN. How good are hand-washing practices? *Am J Nurs.* 1974;74:1676.

27. Garner JS, Simmons BP. Guidelines for isolation precautions in hospitals. *Infect Control.* 1983; 4 (suppl):245.

28. Garner JS, Faveros MS. CDC guidelines for prevention and control of nosocomial infections; guidelines for handwashing and hospital infection control. *Am J Infect Control.* 1985;14:110.

29. Gioiella EC. Healthy aging through knowledge and self-care. *Aging Prev.* 1983;3:39.

30. Goldrick B. Programmed instruction revisisted: a solution to infection control inservice education. *J Contin Educ Nurs.* 1989;20:222.

31. Goldrick B, Appling Stevens S, Larson E. Infection control programmed instruction: an alternative to classroom instruction in baccalaureate nursing education. *J Nurs Educ.* 1990;29:20.

32. Graham M. Frequency and duration of handwashing in an intensive care unit. *Am J Infect Control.* 1990; 18:77.

33. Green LW, et al. *Health Education Planning: A Diagnostic Approach.* Mountain View, CA: Mayfield; 1980.

34. Greenberg JS. *Health Education: Learner-Centered Instructional Strategies.* Dubuque, IA: C. Brown; 1989.

35. Haley RW, et al. The efficacy of surveillance and control programs in preventing nosocomial infections in United States hospitals. *Am J Epidemiol.* 1985; 121:182.

36. Haley RW, et al. The nationwide nosocomial infection rate: a new need for vital statistics. *Am J Epidemiol.* 1985;121:159.

37. Haley RW, et al. Update on the SENIC project: hospital infection control: recent progress and opportunities under prospective payments. *Am J Infect Control,* 1985;13:97.

38. Haughey B, Scherer Y, Wu Y. Nurses' knowledge about AIDS in Erie County, NY. *J Cont Educ Nurs.* 1989; 20:166.

39. Havighurst RJ. *Developmental tasks and education.* New York: McKay; 1962.

40. Herceg-Baron R, et al. Supporting teenagers' use of contraceptives: a comparison of clinic services. *Fam Plann Perspect.* 1986; 18:61.

41. Huntsman AJ. A model for employee development. *Nurs Management.* 1987;18:50.

42. Jessor R, et al. Time at first intercourse: a prospective study. *J Perspect Soc Psychol.* 1983;44:608.

43. Kasen S, Vaughan RD, Walter HJ. Self-efficacy for AIDS prevention behaviors among tenth grade students. *Health Educ Q.* 1992;19:187.

44. Kelen GD, et al. Substantial improvement in compliance with universal precautions in an emergency department following institution of policy. *Arch Intern Med.* 1991;151:2051.

45. Kelly JA, et al. Nurses' attitudes toward AIDS and patients with AIDS. *J Contin Educ Nurs.* 1988;19:78.

46. Knowles MS. The modern practice of adult education, New York: Cambridge; 1980.

47. Larson E. Compliance with isolation technique. *Am J Infect Control.* 1983;11:221.

48. Larson E. A causal link between hand-washing and risk of infection? Examination of the evidence. *Infect Control.* 1988;9:28.

49. Larson E, Oram LF, Hendrick E. Nosocomial infection rates as an indicator of quality. *Med Care.* 1988;26:676.

50. Linnemann CC, et al. Effect of educational programs, rigid sharps containers, and universal precautions on reported needlestick injuries in health care workers. *Infect Control Hosp Epidemiol.* 1991;2:213.

51. Lynch P, et al. Implementing and evaluating a system of generic infection precautions: body substance isolation. *Am J Infect Control.* 1990;18:1.

52. Martone WJ. Year 2000 objectives for preventing nosocomial infections: how do we get there? *Am J Med.* 1991;91(suppl 3B):38.

53. Martone WJ, Garner JS, Duma RJ. Preventing nosocomial infections: progress in the 1980s; plans for the 1990s. *Am J Med.* 1991;91(suppl 3B):1.

54. Mayer JA, et al. Increasing handwashing in an intensive care unit. *Infect Control.* 1986;7:259.

55. Mazon D, McGeer A, Hierholzer W. *Assessing Compliance with Universal Precautions.* Presented at the Seventeenth Annual Education Conference of the Association for Practitioners in Infection Control; Washington, DC; 1990.

56. Mazon D, et al. *Does Department-Specific Monitoring of Universal Precautions Work?* Presented at the Nineteenth Educational Conference of the Association for Practitioners in Infection Control; San Francisco, CA; 1992.

57. Morisky DE, et al. The relative impact of health education for low- and high-risk patients with hypertension. *Prev Med.* 1980; 9:550.

58. Morton WE, Horton HB, Baker HW. Effects of socioeconomic status on incidence of three sexually transmitted diseases. *Sex Transm Dis.* 1979;6:206.

59. Nettleman MD, et al. Assigning responsibility: using feedback to achieve sustained control of methicillin-resistant *Staphylococcus aureus*. *Am J Med.* 1991; 19(suppl):228.

60. Panel on Adolescent Pregnancy and Childbearing. Risking the future: a symposium on the National Academy of Sciences Report on Teenage Pregnancy. *Fam Plann Perspect.* 1987;19:119.

61. Pearson D, Checko P, Hierholzer W. Infection control practices in Connecticut skilled nursing facilities. *Am J Infect Control.* 1990;18:269.

62. Pender NJ. Health promotion in nursing practice, 2nd ed. Norwalk, CT: Appleton Lange; 1987.

63. *Preventive Medicine USA. Health Promotion and Consumer Education.* New York: Prodist; 1976.

64. Prince NA, et al. Perinatal nurses' knowledge and attitudes about AIDS. *J Obstet Gynecol Neonatal Nurs* 1989;18:363.

65. Saghafi L, et al. Exposure to blood during various procedures: results of two surveys before and after implementation of universal precautions. *Am J Infect Control.* 1992;20:53.

66. Sangkardi K. *Assessment of Nursing Students' Knowledge of Infection Control: Implications for Nursing Education.* Presented at the Eighteenth Annual Education Conference of the Association for Practitioners in Infection Control; Nashville, TN; 1991.

67. Seeman D, Seeman T. Health behavior and personal autonomy: a longitudinal study of the sense of control in illness. *J Health Soc.* 1983;24:144.

68. Seidman SN, Aral SO. Race differentials in STD transmission. *Am J Public Health.* 1992;82:1297. Letter.

69. Seidman SN, Mosher WD, Sevgi OA. Women with multiple sexual partners: United States, 1988. *Am J Public Health.* 1992;82:1388.

70. Shafer M-A, Boyer CB. Psychosocial and behavioral factors associated with risk of sexually transmitted diseases, including human immunodeficiency virus infection, among urban high school students. *J Pediatr.* 1991;119:826.

71. Smith PW, Daly PB, Roccaforte JS. Current status of nosocomial infection control in extended care facilities. *Am J Med.* 1991;91(suppl 3B):281.

72. Strecher VJ, et al. The role of self-efficacy in achieving behavior change. *Health Educ Q.* 1986;13:73.

73. Talan D, Baraff L. Effect of education on the use of UP in a university hospital emergency room. *Ann Emerg Med.* 1990;18:1322.

74. Timm J, et al. *Measuring application of Standard Body Substance Precautions.* Presented at the Seventeenth Annual Education Conference of the Association for Practitioners in Infection Control; Washington, DC; 1990.

75. Turner J, Davis JH. Infection control competencies for nursing education. In Mirin S, ed. *Teaching Tomorrow's Nurse: A Nurse Educator Reader.* Wakefield, MA: Nursing Resources; 1980.

76. U.S. Department of Health and Human Services. *Healthy people 2000.* Washington, DC: U.S. Government Printing Office; 1990.

77. U.S. Department of Labor: OSHA standards: occupational exposure to bloodborne pathogens: final rules. *Federal Register.* December 6, 1991;255:64004.

78. U.S. General Accounting Office. *Infection Control:*

Military Programs Are Comparable to VA and Nonfederal Programs but Can Be Enhanced. Washington, D.C.: GAO; 1990.

79. Valanis B. *Epidemiology in Nursing and Health Care.* Norwalk, CT: Nursing Resources; Appleton-Century-Crofts; 1986.

80. Van Servellen GM, Lewis CE, Leake B. Nurses' responses to the AIDS crisis: implications for continuing education programs. *J Contin Educ Nurs.* 1988;19:4.

81. Wallack JJ. AIDS anxiety among health care professionals. *Hosp Community Psychiatry.* 1989;40:507.

82. Weiner N. *The Human Use of Human Beings: Cybernetics and Society.* Boston, MA: Mifflin; 1950.

83. Wong ES, et al. Are universal precautions effective in reducing the number of occupational exposures among health care workers? A prospective study of physicians on a medical service. *JAMA.* 1991; 265:1123.

84. Yoos L. Adolescent cognitive and contraceptive behaviors. *Pediatr Nurs.* 1987;13:247.

Chapter 10

Infection Prevention and the Policy Process

BARBARA M. SOULE

A society's health policies reflect its values and responses to "all the circumstances that lead to or detract from health, that foster or prevent disease."[54] Policy most often emerges from consensus and thus developing policy is rarely simple and straightforward. Influencing infection prevention and control policies requires an understanding of people's values, beliefs, biases, and personal agendas and the diverse interests of patients, health care providers, and policy makers who establish priorities and allocate resources. Science, economics, politics, and other forces that influence policy decisions are important and must be considered when designing a strategy to develop appropriate health policies.

This chapter presents three perspectives of policy making that offer nurses a variety of ways to influence, develop, or evaluate infection prevention policies. The first perspective describes how the components of the host-environment interaction (the host and the microbiologic, physical, and social environments) provide a basis to analyze policies affecting individuals, populations, or systems of care. The second perspective describes the sequential steps of policy development. These steps can be applied to health policy formulation on the national, state, or local level and in the public or private sector. The third perspec-

tive examines the conflicting and complementary roles of science and politics in policy development. Since epidemiology is integral to each of the perspectives presented, the chapter begins with a discussion of the role of epidemiology in health policy.

THE ROLE OF EPIDEMIOLOGY IN HEALTH POLICY

"Epidemiology is the study of the distribution and determinants of health-related states and events in specified populations and the application of this study to the control of health problems."[72] The term *epidemiology* comes from "epidemic," meaning "upon the people."[8] The control of communicable diseases, particularly epidemics, was the earliest application of this science in public health. More recently, epidemiologic methods have been used to evaluate other matters of health, such as malignant disease, psychiatric illness, occupational injuries, and the efficacy of health services. Epidemiologists use quantitative methods to count cases of illness, injury, or other health events. They seek relationships between those events and the distribution of exposure to possible causes that occur among members of the population in which the outcomes occur. This analysis provides a basis for evaluating the health of individuals and communities and planning health services. Epidemiology is fundamental to assessing the efficacy of infection prevention and control practices; thus, it plays an important role in health policy development.

Epidemiologic methods applied in surveillance and descriptive and analytic studies define the determinants, distribution, and effects of disease or health conditions. Surveillance is

The ongoing systematic collection, analysis, and interpretation of health data essential to the planning, implementation, and evaluation of public health practice, closely integrated with the timely dissemination of these data to those who need to know. The final link in the surveillance chain is the application of these data to prevention and control.[72]

Surveillance data have been extremely important in the design of infection prevention and control policies. For example, national surveillance data from the Centers for Disease Control, now called the Centers for Disease Control and Prevention (CDC), identified a problem with polio vaccine in 1955 and characterized the epidemiology of influenza in 1957.[33] Beginning in the late 1950s, surveillance data from hospitals began to define the epidemiology of nosocomial infections, particularly those caused by *Staphylococcus aureus*. This information led to an understanding of mechanisms of transmission of microorganisms in acute care facilities.

In each instance the surveillance information led to a specific policy response. Health policy decisions emerging from epidemiologic surveillance data in the past few decades include the implementation of mass immunization programs for school and day-care children and recommendations that persons limit their sexual contacts, and needle exchange programs be established for injection drug users. The latter programs help reduce the risk of acquiring the human immunodeficiency virus (HIV) and hepatitis B virus (HBV). Data from investigations of infection outbreaks led to

specific time intervals for changing intravenous infusion devices and respiratory therapy equipment to minimize nosocomial bloodstream and pulmonary infections in acutely ill hospitalized patients.

However, epidemiologic surveillance does not always result in new or changed health policy. Even though there is substantial documentation of tuberculosis (TB) outbreaks in long-term care settings, some nursing homes surveyed in 1990 did not require TB screening for employed health care providers or residents.[25] Additionally, although numerous epidemiologic studies have demonstrated that the elderly are at significant risk for influenza, and although the CDC has recommended influenza immunization for elderly residents of nursing homes and other chronic care facilities, only 1 of the 50 states in the same study required annual immunization for residents. Absence of a consistent policy in the face of convincing epidemiologic data may be the result of lack of knowledge about or belief in the data, resistance to new policies, personal value systems, economic factors, or a combination of all four.

Sometimes the role of epidemiology is to evaluate the effectiveness of a health policy decision. The epidemic of toxic shock syndrome (TSS) is an example. In 1980, 55 cases of a newly described disease, primarily in women, were reported to the CDC.[21] The disease appeared to be associated with *Staphylococcus aureus*. Onset occurred during menstruation in 95% of the women. An initial study suggested that one causative factor might be the synthetic material used in one brand of superabsorbent tampons.[65] That brand of tampon was removed from the market. Subsequently, an epidemiologic study confirmed decreased incidence of TSS.[33] These findings led to permanent changes in tampon composition that reduced absorbance and consequently the volume of habitat available to the staphylococcus.

The nature of a public health hazard appears to govern when and how epidemiologic information is used in policy making.[36] The more a health event or issue is perceived as harmful or urgent or results in events regarded by the public as horrifying or victimizing, the less understanding of the problem's epidemiology is needed before the issue is addressed in policy. During the TSS outbreaks, the deaths of young, otherwise healthy women alarmed the public. These women, with whom the public readily identified, were perceived as unwitting victims of a manufacturing error. Consequently, TSS prompted an immediate policy response based on preliminary and limited epidemiologic data. In contrast, if hazardous behavior is perceived as informed, voluntary risk taking, or if the exercise of personal choice and individual civil liberty has consequences only for the risk taker, the epidemiologic understanding of the problem must be more complete and convincing if it is to influence policy.[36]

The U.S. Occupational Safety and Health Administration (OSHA) mandate that health care workers who participate in vascular access procedures wear gloves became law only after employee unions pressured for a national standard to protect health care workers from exposure to HIV and HBV.[73] Interestingly, for many years strong epidemiologic evidence had indicated that the risk of becoming infected with HBV was significant for health care workers who were frequently exposed to blood.[28] Until the mandate, HBV was not perceived by workers as significant, immediate, or harmful enough to motivate them to change their work practices. The OSHA requirements expand the consequences of risky behavior to include fines for the employer. Chapter 9 explores the dynamics and strategies of behavior modification available to employers that might have influenced practitioners had they been implemented previously.

Epidemiologic data may also have limited influence when the evidence about the health effects is difficult to communicate or the solution to the problem is costly or unacceptable to well-organized interest groups. For example, requiring all HIV infections to be reported to public health authorities and restricting unimmunized children from attending school are public health interventions viewed by some as beneficial and desirable but by others as unacceptable compromises of civil liberties.[38] Consequently, the influence of surveillance information often depends not only on its quality or quantity but also on the specific nature of the health event and the balance between the forces for and against strict policy controls. In this regard, each health issue must be addressed individually to determine the usefulness of epidemiologic information.

PERSPECTIVES OF POLICY DEVELOPMENT
Host-environment interactions

The epidemiologic analysis of host-environment interactions that contribute to infection and determine patterns of infections in populations provides one perspective of policy development. Host-environment interactions that influence cause of disease are examined throughout this book.[57] They illustrate the interdependence and dynamic relationships among the host and the microbiologic, physical, and social environments as determinants of the infectious disease process. Knowledge of these interactions can serve as a basis for development or analysis of policies intended to prevent or manage infections and can be applied in two ways.

First, each of the four components (host, microbe, physical environment, and social environment) should be examined individually when policies are developed or reviewed. When a health issue first comes to the attention of a patient, group, caregiver, or policy maker, one of the four components of cause, such as the host or the social environment, may appear to merit primary consideration. However, factors that may not be initially evident can emerge as critical to considerations of policy.

Second, the four components should be explored as they interrelate and influence one another. For example, it is difficult or impossible to separate the social and microbiologic environments from one another when designing a policy to reduce transmission of sexually transmitted diseases.

An *Escherichia coli* 0157:H7 foodborne epidemic is an example of a health issue in which the microbiologic environment was the initial focus of investigation but the problem was eventually understood to be multi-faceted.[14] From November 1992 through February 1993, foodborne illness occurring in Washington, Nevada, Idaho, and California was traced to hamburgers prepared and served in a fast-food restaurant chain. The beef arrived at the restaurants heavily contaminated with *E. coli* 0157:H7 and was not consistently cooked to the required internal temperature (63° to 68° C, or 145° to 155° F). Hundreds of persons developed severe cramping and bloody diarrhea; some developed hemorrhagic uremic syndrome (HUS). Several young children died.

E. coli 0157:H7 has caused severe gastrointestinal infection in sporadic cases and small clusters of persons since 1982.[15] However, this was one of the few times in the United States that this species of *E. coli* was the agent in a dramatic, highly visible, widely distributed epidemic. *E. coli* 0157:H7 lives in the intestines of healthy cattle and can contaminate meat during slaughter. Grinding transfers the pathogens from the meat's surface to its interior. In this outbreak, routine inspections were inadequate to identify and eliminate contaminated meat. There was a rapid attempt to identify the source of contamination and initiate an interstate recall of the beef. The public was incensed that the

inspection process was insensitive. The government responded by ordering a review of meat inspection practices and making commitments to apply laboratory technology to quality control and to require warning labels on packaging to encourage appropriate cooking.

The focus on the microbiologic environment in this epidemic yielded the first significant information about the problem, and the causative organism was quickly identified and typed. However, other components of host-environment interaction had to be considered as new public health policy to prevent future outbreaks was developed.

Host factors were a significant influence in this epidemic. The ill persons ranged in age from infancy to 74 years, but all the deaths and much of the severe gastrointestinal illness and HUS occurred in children under age 7. Lack of age-related host defenses made the children more susceptible to severe renal failure.[15] The public reaction to ill and dying children was intense and visible.

The physical and social environments were also critical to policy consideration in this outbreak. This strain of *E. coli* may have colonized some cattle in the natural environment and subsequently contaminated the ground beef produced by the packinghouses. Investigators found that the physical environment in the processing plants was generally adequate but that factors related to the social environment were not. For financial reasons, the numbers of inspectors had been reduced. The meat inspection practices consisted of visual inspection only, which failed to identify and exclude contaminated carcasses. Inadequate cooking was ultimately implicated as the immediate cause of the outbreak. Employees at fast-food chains are under pressure to produce the food quickly after the order is placed in order to please the customer. Thus, the meat was sometimes cooked to temperatures below those required by the state health departments. Meanwhile, some establishment

Recognition and visibility

Once a health problem has been identified and defined, the nature and scope of the particular problem must be made visible.[5] Increasing visibility means clarifying, defining, characterizing, and communicating the issue so that it is understood and meaningful to decision makers and those affected by the decision. Visibility is achieved by collecting and disseminating epidemiologic information, publishing articles in academic and popular journals, books, and magazines and using various media to publicize the issue. Lobbying, demonstrating, and obtaining endorsements and opinions from high-profile businesses, agencies, and individuals, such as leading political figures and celebrities are often very effective strategies.

The challenge for nurses and other health care providers is to develop ways to increase the visibility of an infection problem and the accuracy of the information provided so that policy may be soundly based and involve the appropriate members of the society.

For every issue, some people or groups share the concern. Others are not interested in the problem, have competing priorities, are invested in the status quo, or find it politically expedient to have the issue remain invisible. The early years of the AIDS epidemic provide many examples of the effects of this diversity of opinion. The initial perception that AIDS threatened only marginalized members of society greatly affected the public health policy process during the first decade of the epidemic. Some journalists and activists who closely followed the epidemic and legislative events believed that powerful leaders in the federal administration found the gay-related disease a distasteful topic and ignored it.[67] The disease therefore remained "invisible"; it was not discussed in political circles except by a few knowledgeable members of Congress whose constituencies were affected.[66,67] The recognition of AIDS as an important policy issue

was delayed from 1981 until 1983, when some members of Congress realized that hemophiliacs and heterosexual women were becoming infected through the blood supply and "accepted" sexual practices. When it became apparent that AIDS was not restricted to the original risk groups, AIDS finally became a visible national health issue.

The experience of the AIDS epidemic can be contrasted with the advent of the epidemic of staphylococcal infections in newborns and surgical patients in hospitals in the late 1950s. Development of a health policy to address this infection problem met with little political resistance. Visibility was established through quantitative information from hospital medical records, death certificates, and reports from practitioners. Discussion of the morbidity and mortality in concrete, understandable terms helped increase the visibility and recognition of the seriousness of the problem. Physicians and nurses published their findings in scientific journals.[1,6,7,44,61,70] Both the CDC and the American Hospital Association (AHA)[3,30] viewed the resolution of this public health problem as consistent with their missions and sought an active role in education, scientific research, and policy development.[30]

Involvement of public figures, celebrities, and leaders in organizations adds visibility to a health issue. The Surgeon General's attention to HIV disease and AIDS did much to support visibility in public, academic, and political circles. Actor Rock Hudson's 1985 disclosure that he was dying of AIDS and Earvin "Magic" Johnson's announcement in 1991 that he was infected with HIV and would retire from basketball increased the visibility of HIV disease as a health issue.

Social construct

The social construct used to identify and define a health problem may affect the course of the policy process.[26] Early in the epidemic, AIDS was characterized by the CDC as a consequence of lifestyle of homosexual men and injection drug users. This social characterization promoted the belief that the disease could be attributed to certain groups of people whose inherent characteristics or behaviors made them responsible for their illness. Some social critics saw AIDS as "proof" of divine moral judgment of the lives of the afflicted.[9] Homosexuality, bisexuality, and illicit use of IV drugs were behaviors that were intolerable to many persons in the presiding administration, their constituents, and others in society. Consequently, many political leaders and members of the public ignored AIDS. It has been suggested that some leaders used their positions to prevent the epidemic from achieving recognition as a valid health policy issue.[39] Suppressing visibility and delaying definition of the problem postponed policy, education, testing, and employment security throughout the first decade of the epidemic.

In contrast, the staphylococcal epidemic was perceived as a serious medical illness not associated with issues of morality or marginalized persons. From the beginning, the disease affected patients without regard to their personal lifestyles or value systems. The patients who became ill were not perceived to be responsible for their illness and their illness not viewed as a consequence of their own "immoral" behavior, divine retribution, or guilt,[34] but as victims of the health care system. This difference in the social perception of the two epidemics affected the initial policy-making process. Social dynamics must be considered whenever health policies are developed.

Longevity

When a health issue persists for a long period, its definition may evolve over time, and each definition shift affects subsequent health policy decisions.[5,35] For example, early in the epidemic, AIDS was characterized by the CDC as a disease of homosexual men; the acronym GRID, gay-related immune disease,

was used. This label incorporated an association with a certain lifestyle into the disease's name. As the epidemic progressed, fear of contamination of the blood supply created a strong impetus for development of a test to detect HIV in serum. When heterosexual women and their newborn infants were shown to be infected as a consequence of sexual contact with bisexual or IV drug using men, characterization of the infection changed to fit a disease of both homosexual and heterosexual persons not necessarily related to sexual orientation or drug use. To some extent, this refocused educational efforts. In 1985, when the virus causing AIDS (HIV) was identified, another definition change, from lifestyle to microbiologic etiology, intensified the work to characterize further the causative agent. As more effective care prolonged the lives of persons with HIV or AIDS, the characterization of the natural history of the infection shifted from acute to chronic.[62] This change in perception was followed by increased efforts to develop care techniques for people living with an extended terminal illness rather than dying of an acute disease.

In comparison, the staphylococcal infections in the middle to late 1950s were clearly identified as an epidemic in the United States and a pandemic that included several other countries.[41] Once the initial outbreak was controlled, perception shifted so that these infections came to be considered endemic to hospitals and long-term care facilities. This change in emphasis led to creation of programs to prevent and control staphylococcal and other nosocomial infections. The policy support for reduction of nosocomial infections continues today through many state health care licensing laws and requirements of various accrediting agencies[46] and as part of the year 2000 health objectives for the United States.[56] In summary, the identification of a health condition as a focus for policy development depends on visibility and public and political perceptions of the significance of the issue.

Setting the agenda

Once a health policy issue has been identified and defined, the next step is to move it onto the policy agenda. The agenda consists of health issues, demands, or problems upon which decision makers feel compelled to act. These decision makers are the gatekeepers who decide which health issues will become part of the policy agenda[63] and which will be ignored or deferred. Gatekeepers exist at all levels of government and in health organizations and agencies. Identifying and influencing them presents considerable challenge to those who would influence policy regardless of setting.

Competition

Why do some public health problems, once identified, receive attention and action by policy makers, while others do not? One answer is that agenda building is competitive. There are more health problems than can be addressed at any given time. The list of problems that are candidates for intervention must be narrowed and priorities established. Raising the priority and increasing the possibility for a particular initiative to be given preferential consideration results from well-planned strategies that consider values, philosophies, and relationships of policy supporters and policy makers.[55]

As the policy process progresses to the agenda setting stage, a health issue must be brought to the attention of the public and policy makers, and be well articulated, publicized, and visible. If the policy identification process discussed previously has effectively moved the issue from ambiguity to clarity, created strong awareness that the issue is important for consideration, and appealed to the needs and concerns of the appropriate audience, then the issue may out-compete others for attention and action. For instance, administrators of hospitals and long-term care facilities are interested in preventing nosocomial infections in their patients as part of their quality of care programs. They also want to prevent occupationally acquired HIV and HBV and other infectious diseases in staff as a function of their concern for health and safety, insurance costs, implications for contract negotiations and assessment by regulatory agencies. As these issues are brought to the administrator's agenda each policy's importance to the health facility and the staff must be described to make it competitive with other pressing matters.

Political leaders and philosophy

Professionals and citizens who can expedite or prevent issues from becoming part of the agenda effectively influence health policy action. Political leaders such as the President, members of Congress, and public agency heads exert great personal influence over the agenda-setting process in the public arena.[5] In health organizations, administrators, program directors, professionals, and informal leaders exert that same influence. These persons may be motivated by public interest, altruism, personal advantage, economics, or philosophy to advocate for or obstruct an infection control policy.

In both the AIDS and the staphylococcal epidemics, the political philosophy of the national administration was a critical factor in how and when each was placed on the policy agenda. The conservative political ideology of the Reagan administration had a profound effect on policy related to HIV and AIDS during its 8 years in office. The epidemic surfaced when the political and economic climate did not favor financial commitment to the U.S. Public Health Service (USPHS) or federal solutions for health problems. The administration exercised power to keep AIDS off the national agenda. One analyst noted that

"President Reagan did not utter the word 'AIDS' until well into his second term in office."[39] It has been suggested that this policy of inaction caused a 2-year delay before the AIDS epidemic reached the policy agenda, postponing research, education, and funding that might have saved lives.[53]

The political philosophy was very different during the staphylococcal epidemic in the 1960s. Presidents Kennedy and Johnson believed that government could and should be socially active. Both presidents increased efforts to provide health care to the poor and elderly through Social Security and amendments such as the Kerr-Mills Act, Medicare, and Medicaid.[29] During their administrations the country was still enjoying the post–World War II economic boom, and the USPHS was viewed with favor following the successful resolution of the polio epidemic of the mid-1950s with a polio vaccine. The popularity of the PHS and the availability of fiscal resources provided a supportive environment for developing active public health care policies and a willingness to identify health problems as valid national policy issues. Thus, the staphylococcal epidemic reached the health policy agenda quickly, resources were allocated to study and resolve the problem, and the USPHS responded.

Dramatic events

Significant new scientific information, major crises (e.g., natural and social disasters), citizens' deaths, media pressure, grossly inequitable distribution of resources (particularly if "deserving" populations are affected), and civil disturbances are other triggering events that hasten the addition of an identified health issue to the agenda. The staphylococcal epidemics caused significant morbidity and mortality. Epidemiologic information was powerful enough to move the problem onto the U.S. national agenda in a fairly expeditious manner. Both the CDC and the AHA supported

relevant research through their agencies;[30] and there is little documentation of political interference in the roles taken by these agencies. In fact, had these agencies not addressed the issue, political pressure to do so might have ultimately been applied either by Congress, constituent members of the AHA, or others.

Special interest groups

Strong professional organizations, special interest lobbies, business groups, and the media can be powerful and successful influences on the policy agenda.[55,71] Occasionally, a respected individual with high visibility and stature can draw sufficient attention to an issue to establish it on the policy agenda. No single individual stands out as a champion for the staphylococcal epidemics, although several physicians, nurses, and researchers became spokespersons through publications and presentations at scientific meetings.[69,75,76] The AIDS epidemic produced an unexpected spokesperson during the mid-1980s when President Reagan instructed Surgeon General C. Everett Koop to prepare a report on AIDS. Koop called together leaders from all sectors of public and private communities, including those from the groups most affected by HIV and AIDS at the time. In 1986 he published an extensive report that supported funding for AIDS research and education.[49]

Proponents of health issues use many strategies to obtain a place on the agenda. Sometimes issues are defined ambiguously to broaden appeal and minimize offending special interests. Often a particularly controversial section of a policy may be removed to maximize potential for passage. Occasionally symbols are used to imbue the issue with legitimacy or common appeal.[63] For example, logos such as the heart and skull of the World Health Organization's AIDS Effort (Figure 10-1) can powerfully punctuate written or verbal messages.

Contemporary infection problems in acute

and long-term care include risk of occupational acquisition of bloodborne pathogens, TB prevention, management of patients and health care workers affected by HIV or AIDS, antibiotic use, and infectious waste management. The strategies previously outlined can be used to analyze and manage the social, political, and scientific components of health issues and facilitate their placement onto the appropriate agenda in any of these settings.

Step 2: Policy formulation

Once a health issue has reached the agenda, it must be fashioned into a specific proposal. This may require significant modification and compromise. Special expertise is required to design a health initiative so that it will be adopted by policy makers. The influence of key figures may be very important during this step.

An AIDS education policy was modified to its final form to make it acceptable to those in power. When the CDC recommended mass education about AIDS for the public in 1982, no funds were provided.[67] In 1983, the federal administration funneled a small amount of money into education indirectly through the U.S. Conference of Mayors but did not want to be associated with use of federal government funds to educate homosexuals. In 1985, Congress finally included educational funds with the $33.3 million appropriated for AIDS projects through the Department of Health and Human Services (HHS). However, the program content had to be designed so as not to appear to be "endorsing the gay lifestyle."[67] Each recipient of federal dollars had to appoint a program review panel to approve any educational materials and ensure compliance with the established guidelines. The formulation of the final policy changed the original scope and content of the educational offerings and illustrates that policy formulation and implementation occur in the context of the personal, political, and cultural values of decision makers.

Problem identification, agenda setting, and policy formulation constitute the initial stages of the policy process. These steps are important because they determine which issues will continue into final policy. The final three steps, policy adoption, implementation, and evaluation, involve more formal decisions that shape the eventual outcome of a particular policy.

Step 3: Policy adoption

Compromise is a reality of the policy process, regardless of whether the issue is implementing a new infection precaution system in a community hospital, designing attendance restrictions for infected children who attend a day-care center, or identifying whom to target

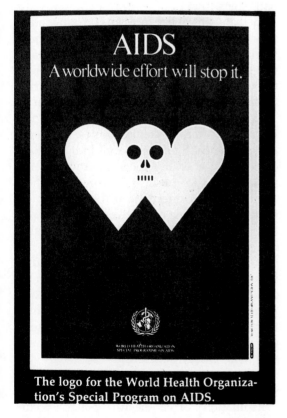

The logo for the World Health Organization's Special Program on AIDS.

FIGURE 10-1. World Health Organization (WHO) logo for AIDS.

for mass immunization in a public health outreach program.

Policy adoption involves decisions about alternatives. The basis for the decisions may be grounded in scientific evidence, the decision maker's value system, or a balance between the two. Regardless of the impetus, the process evolves by mandate, bargaining, compromise, persuasion, or a combination of these approaches. For instance, when Kimberly Bergalis and five other patients became infected with HIV after receiving dental care from a dentist with AIDS,[17-19] Bergalis made a passionate plea to legislators to require that all health care workers be tested for HIV. As the issue was debated in Congress, the legislators' personal views and feelings about HIV disease and AIDS, the scientific data regarding risk of transmission of HIV in the health care setting, concerns about public opinion, and the economic implications of testing were all considered. At first, emotions and public opinion played a dominant role. In the end, the scientific information, which established that appropriate infection control techniques would prevent infection, had a stronger influence on the decision process, and the proposed legislation failed. By contrast, voluntary implementation of infection control programs to reduce nosocomial infections occurred in the 1960s and 1970s in hospitals where nurses and physicians believed that risk for infections among patients could be reduced.[37,41] The variable support for these programs was associated with their promoter's ability and skill to persuade the administration that the programs were consistent with hospital priorities. Infection prevention and control programs are now mandated in health care facilities applying for various forms of accreditation,[46] by OSHA to comply with the Bloodborne Pathogens Standard,[73] and by most state regulations.

Step 4: Policy implementation

Implementation begins once a policy has been formally adopted as law, standard, recommendation, or guideline. Discretion, variability, and power exerted during the implementation phase continue to shape the policy as it is carried out.[5] If the legislature designs a policy to be vague or nebulous (a political tactic often used when proposals are controversial), the health agency responsible for implementation and oversight generally has more discretion, and thus more power, in the way the policy is implemented. For example, federal law grants state health departments the discretion to determine specific policies regarding practice parameters for HIV-positive health care workers during exposure-prone procedures.[16] OSHA grants states the right to develop stricter requirements than OSHA's for managing bloodborne pathogens.

In many instances, pressure groups, advisory bodies, and professional organizations work closely with the agency or administrator to influence implementation. Laws enforced through judicial action, such as those requiring the person's informed consent to perform an HIV blood test, accord the courts significant latitude to interpret statutes, rules, and regulations. In health facilities, a multidisciplinary committee generally has authority to determine criteria for nosocomial infections, how surveillance for infections will be performed, the action to be taken to prevent and control or eliminate infections and the resources allocated to this process.[46]

Nurses who wish to influence policy and its implementation must become proficient in the art of communication, negotiation and compromise. During these endeavors, it is essential to maintain clarity of the policy's purpose in one's own mind and in the minds of those who will make policy decisions.

Step 5: Evaluation

Evaluation of a health policy occurs throughout the development and implementation processes. Evaluation begins once the issue has moved on to the agenda, where it is scrutinized in the public sector by legislators, citizens, interest groups, the media, and others and in the health care arena by care providers, consumers, regulators, and payors. Evaluation continues throughout each policy phase either informally or formally once a policy has been implemented.[63] Generally, evaluation involves the assessment or approval of policy content and effect.[5]

Several quantitative and qualitative evaluation methods have been developed to aid health policy analysis. These include operational, systematic or summative, goal-free, and use-focused methods. Detailed review of these methods is beyond the scope of this discussion and can be found elsewhere.[5,55]

Many HIV/AIDS policies implemented during the AIDS epidemic have been evaluated. Once a serologic test for HIV became available in 1985, all donated blood was tested for antibody to the HIV. Subsequent evaluation indicates that this policy dramatically reduced the number of persons who acquire HIV from blood transfusion. Several states mandated that premarital HIV blood test be performed. However, the efficacy of this screening was not likely to have any significant effect on the course of the epidemic. Consequently, very few states have retained this policy. Recently, the CDC has suggested that in communities where the serologic prevalence rate of HIV is 1% or greater, hospitals consider offering HIV testing to all patients ages 15 to 54 years. This recommendation has not yet been evaluated.[13] The more radical proposal of placing HIV-infected persons in quarantine was considered briefly in the early years of the epidemic. The principle of separating diseased from healthy persons has been used as a basis for public health policy in the past, such as in efforts to prevent transmission of TB, which is spread by droplet nuclei transmitted through air. But HIV, unlike TB, is not transmitted through the air, by casual transmission, or from occupational duties such as food preparation. In fact, quarantine does

not successfully contain most diseases.[9,34] The quarantine of persons with AIDS would require lifelong incarceration of infected persons, and despite its proponents was evaluated and abandoned early in the policy process. It is the task of public health officials and epidemiologists to emphasize disease transmission patterns to the policy makers and the public so that sound health policy can be developed and evaluated.[9]

During the staphylococcal epidemic, stringent policies were adopted for asepsis and surgical technique in the operating room, and hand washing and cohorting were used in newborn nurseries. These policies were very successful in limiting transmission of staphylococci.[41,76] The post-intervention evaluation documented decreases in staphylococcal infections. Policies developed during the epidemic evolved into nosocomial prevention and control programs throughout the United States and in other countries. Eventually these programs were required by some accrediting organizations.[47] A massive nationwide evaluation study was undertaken in 1975 and 1976 to determine whether these programs actually prevented hospital-associated infections and to determine the characteristics of those programs that were most successful. The Study on the Efficacy of Nosocomial Infection Control (SENIC)[42] provided strong evidence that successful infection control programs using epidemiologic methods for surveillance and providing feedback and interventions could reduce the incidence of nosocomial infections by 32%. Unfortunately, only 6% of the hospitals had the components for a successful program at that time.

A sequential model of policy steps provides a set of road signs to follow as an infection prevention or control issue evolves from an idea or concern to policy. Generally, the policy process is more circular than linear and is complex rather than simple. The steps rarely occur in the straightforward sequence described here.[55] This complexity provides a special challenge. Table 10-2 presents a plan nurses can use to influence infection prevention and control policies.

Politics and science in health policy

A third perspective from which health policy can be studied views policy as the product of the interaction of politics and science. There is widespread consensus that both science and politics influence the policy process, but views about their interrelationship, relative value and the ethics of their interaction are debated. Lindblom[55] believes that policy does not evolve from an orderly and rational process, with a beginning, middle and end, where each stage is tied logically to each preceding one. He suggests, rather, that at every phase of the policy process the participants strive to balance information and analysis with considerations of personal values, economics, social justice, and political expediency. This is not an easy task, since science and politics overlap and intertwine. Nurses who understand and can work with the tools of both science and politics will be most effective in influencing or analyzing infection control policies.

Politics

Politics, broadly defined, is the total complex of activities related to the interactions and relations among persons living in a society. The political process brings together the competing interests, traditions, and aspirations of society's members. Perceptions, economics, questions of social justice, power, and ethics are all facets of the political process that shape health care policy.

The public does not consider all health risks to be equal.[60] Perception of risk is influenced by values and outcome. Risks are generally considered more serious if the outcome is immediate, direct, or personally frightening. The characteristics of the population at risk also influence public concern. The health problems of certain subgroups of a population may be given greater or lesser priority based on the value assigned to them by the influential. For example, drug users, homosexuals, women, and children received different levels of attention in the earliest years of the AIDS epidemic in the U.S.

Because health policies distribute valuable and limited resources and allocate advantages and disadvantages to different populations,

TABLE 10-2. Plan for influencing infection prevention and control policies

Steps	Action
Know the issue	Read, research, describe
Define your objectives	Recognize personal values, energy, commitment
Identify decision makers	Become familiar with policy makers, public, professionals, colleagues, others
Recognize influences	Learn about philosophies, values, biases, agendas, orientation, priorities, regulations
Know the policy process	Study policy steps: identification, agenda, adoption, formulation, identification, evaluation
	Increase visibility of issue
	Correlate science: epidemiology, other research, with politics: social, legal, economic issues
Take action	Join organizations; volunteer for committees; write letters; give speeches; attend hearings; testify
Persevere	Pace energy and time; acknowledge complexity of process

many analysts view the health policy process as adversarial and ultimately political. This is evident, for example, in the competition for research money. Cancer, Alzheimers' disease, heart disease, AIDS, vaccine-preventable illnesses and multidrug-resistant TB all have their advocates. From a business or governmental perspective, health policies that add costs, decrease revenues, or shift either from one responsible party to another may influence the decisions of policy makers regardless of the science available.

Legal considerations may also play an important role. For example, in the 1970s the CDC announced the possibility of an impending major influenza epidemic and lobbied strongly for funding for mass immunization. Congress sponsored legislation for mass immunization, and manufacturers began to develop influenza vaccines. Insurers, concerned about lawsuits resulting from adverse vaccine outcomes, began to withdraw coverage from manufacturers of influenza vaccines. Consequently, the manufacturers reduced production of vaccine. Committed to protecting the populace, the government agreed to accept liability for injuries associated with immunizations under a new law, the Swine Flu Immunization Act (Pub Law No. 94-380.90 1113 [1976]). After administration of the vaccine, Guillain-Barré syndrome appeared in a small number of vaccine recipients, which resulted in several lawsuits against the government.[52]

Science

Some policy analysts believe that scientific information should be the most influential determinant of health policy. Indeed, many health policy decisions rely heavily on sound, high quality research. However, for decision makers to rely wholly on scientific information would require that the data be infallible, totally believable, and capable of wholly resolving conflicts of values and interests.[5] Since scientific data cannot meet these requirements,

they are not a sufficient single component for health policy and infection control decisions.

Health policy designers have made use of social science data and empiric research for as long as these resources have been available. The oldest social databases are the census and vital (i.e., birth and death) statistics. Numerous governmental, professional, and trade organizations collect and disseminate health-related data to support policy analysis and decision making[43,58] (see box on p. 208). The use of data and research findings as a basis for policy decisions presents several challenges for the policy makers.

First, the sources of data, the data, and conclusions they support may be controversial. They may be influenced by the assumptions and biases of the researchers or advocates who suggest that the findings are valid and should form the basis for policy decisions. Therefore, research data offered to the policy arena by various organizations and interests must be viewed with their biases in mind.

Second, opinions differ as to when in the policy development process scientific information should be considered. Some believe that science is more useful during the preliminary and planning stages and when resources are being allocated, such as when federal dollars are being allocated for immunizations or sexually transmitted disease (STD) clinics.[11] Others contend that scientific data are more useful to defend or attack a health policy after it is formulated, for example, evaluating policies such as event-related shelf life for sterile surgical supplies.[59] Still others believe that the rationality science brings to a policy decision is unwelcome at any stage. This has been illustrated in the struggle among different parties who take positions on the confidentiality with which HIV test results should be managed. The differences in the influence of scientific information may relate to the nature of the particular policy issue, its urgency, importance, history, and the policy makers' intuition and personal experiences.

SELECTED GOVERNMENTAL AGENCIES, PROFESSIONAL ORGANIZATIONS, AND TRADE ASSOCIATIONS PROVIDING SCIENTIFIC DATA OR REGULATIONS, STANDARDS, GUIDELINES, OR OTHER POLICIES FOR INFECTION PREVENTION AND CONTROL

GOVERNMENTAL AGENCIES

Department of Health and Human Services
    Public Health Services
        Agency for Health Care Policy and Research (AHCPR)
        Agency for Toxic Substances and Disease Registry (ATSDR)
        Centers for Disease Control and Prevention (CDC)
            Hospital Infections Program (HIP)
            Advisory Committee on Immunization Practices (ACIP)
            National Institute for Occupational Safety and Health (NIOSH)
        Food and Drug Administration (FDA)
        Health Resources Service Administration (HRSA)
        National Institutes of Health (NIH)
    Health Care Financing Administration (HCFA)
Department of Labor (DOL)
Occupational Safety and Health Administration (OSHA)
Environmental Protection Agency (EPA)
Offices of Technology Assessment (OTA)
Government Accounting Office (GAO)
Congress

PROFESSIONAL NURSING ORGANIZATIONS

American Association of Critical Care Nurses (AACN)
American Association of Occupational Health Nurses (AAOHN)
American College of Nurse Midwives (ACONM)
American Nephrology Nurses Association (ANNA)
American Nurses' Association (ANA)
Association of Operating Room Nurses (AORN)
Association for Professionals in Infection Control and Epidemiology (APIC)
Intravenous Nurses Society (INS)
Nurses Association of the American College of Obstetricians and Gynecologists (NAACOG)

NONNURSING PROFESSIONAL ORGANIZATIONS

American Dental Association (ADA)
American Medical Association (AMA)
American Public Health Association (APHA)
American Society for Microbiology (ASM)
Society for Hospital Epidemiology of America (SHEA)
Surgical Infections Society (SIS)

TRADE ASSOCIATIONS

American Association for Advancement of Medical Instrumentation (AAMI)
American Hospital Association (AHA)
    American Society of Healthcare Central Service Personnel (ASHCSP)
    American Society for Healthcare Environmental Service (ASHES)
    American Society for Healthcare Risk Management (ASHRM)
    American Society for Hospital Engineering (ASHE)
American Institute of Architects (AIA)
National Committee for Clinical Laboratory Standards (NCCLS)

Adapted from McDonald LL, Pugliese G. Regulatory, accreditation and professional agencies influencing infection control programs. In: Wenzl RP, ed. *Prevention* and *Control of Nosocomial Infections*, 2nd ed. Baltimore: Williams & Wilkins; 1993.

The proposition that science contributes an impartial and rational foundation for policy making has been further challenged by those who propose that conclusions of scientific research are unduly influenced by (1) the values and assumptions of those who provide and interpret scientific data, (2) the elitism and conservative nature of the scientific community, and (3) the operational issues of condensing large quantities of information into easily digestible formats without compromising truth. These issues arise in the public and private arenas when legislators or administrators depend on experts or staff to collect and analyze data and base decisions on "executive summaries."[43]

Politics and science: The balance

The search for a rational strategy for decision making that integrates analytic and political forces has given rise to a new paradigm called *political epidemiology*. "Political epidemiology recognizes that political activities in resolving health problems . . . have a co-equal primacy with medical and epidemiological insights."[10] Political epidemiology suggests that in order to make appropriate social choices related to health hazards (which it is their job to make), policy makers must understand the limitations and significance of epidemiologic data and that epidemiologists and other scientists must become more skilled at presenting data. The following three examples illustrate this approach.

Epidemiologists and policy makers generally acknowledge that immunization of children is important. In 1990 the minimum cost to immunize a child fully in the United States was $82.90.[45] For many, the costs, bureaucracy and access problems posed major impediments to vaccination. The cost was a financial barrier for 6 to 8 million uninsured children, for those who were eligible for Medicaid but not yet enrolled, and for families with other pressing needs, such as food, shelter, clothing, and jobs. In addition, lack of coordination between separate programs caring for the same pediatric populations, such as the Women, Infants and Children (WIC) program and Aid to Families with Dependent Children (AFDC), led to assumptions by each that immunizations had been provided by the other.[45] Immunizations are recognized as important, but there are not yet effective measures to deliver them to all appropriate populations.

The search for strategies to control HBV infection in the general population provides another example of political epidemiology. Initially, U.S. policy makers believed that offering vaccination to persons known to be at high risk for HBV would reduce the incidence of HBV infection and disease. Unfortunately, it has been difficult to identify and vaccinate to those at high risk before exposure occurs. Up to 50% of HBV cases reported to CDC have reported no identifiable risk of infection.[2,23] However, many individuals at high risk did not seek the vaccine even when it was available at little or no cost. Consequently, no significant decline in the total number of acute HBV cases reported annually to CDC occurred in the first decade during which the vaccine was available. Since a policy based on availability and voluntary participation did not reduce the incidence of HBV infection, policy makers, with input and encouragement from epidemiologists and research scientists, recommended immunization of infants and suggested immunization of teenagers against HBV.[20] This was based on the premise that immunizations given early, before the person has an opportunity to be exposed, are most likely to prevent HBV infections.[68]

Epidemiologic data have provided the basis for the strategy of universal HBV immunization. Studies in which immunized infants were followed for a decade have shown that the vaccine is highly effective in preventing perinatal infection. It reduces the incidence of chronicity in infected neonates and is likely to be effective up to and through young adulthood, when probability of exposure is highest. In addition, follow-up studies of high risk adult vaccinees who seroconverted indicate that most adults are protected for at least 10 years after immunization[68] and that anamnestic response may provide protection from chronic carriage of hepatitis B even when antibody drops below detectable levels. Using this scientific information, the Advisory Committee of Immunization Practices[20] and the American Academy of Pediatrics have proposed a national policy to immunize all infants as one part of a comprehensive program to eliminate HBV.[20]

Political and social forces such as compliance and cost will influence the success of this policy proposal. First, the recommended schedules for HBV do not coincide precisely with the schedules for other childhood immunizations. This could increase the need for visits to physicians' offices or public health clinics and thereby add cost and inconvenience. To resolve this problem, research to adjust the administration protocol to match the schedule for other childhood immunizations is under way. If the administration time of HBV could be adjusted to coincide with that of other immunizations, such as measles, mumps, and rubella (MMR) or diphtheria and tetanus (DT), it may be possible to mix the vaccine formulations.

Some hospitals give the first dose of HBV vaccine in the hospital before the newborn is discharged. This raises questions about (1) vaccine reimbursement for health facilities, (2) reduction of income of pediatricians and family practice physicians who might otherwise see the infant at the office or clinic, and (3) documentation of administration of the vaccine series, which will ensure completion on schedule without costly repeat administration resulting from lost or inaccessible records of previous doses. The comprehensive vaccine program for HBV illustrates how science and politics are linked in the design of public health infection control policies.

Public concern regarding the management of potentially infectious medical waste provides another example of political epidemiology. Infectious waste is medical waste that has the potential to transmit an infectious disease. Before the 1980s, medical waste generated as a result of patient diagnosis or treatment (e.g., soiled dressings from wounds, IV tubing, microbiologic cultures, sharp instruments, blood, and body fluids) was of little interest to the general public.

However, interest in waste disposal practices increased during the past decade when children were found playing with discarded tubes of blood or poking each other with needles from trash receptacles or dumpsters of health clinics, when medical waste washed ashore on popular eastern U.S. beaches, and as anxiety about the transmission of AIDS intensified among the public.

This health policy issue drew different reactions from health professionals, waste managers, politicians, and the public. Health professionals generally supported the existing requirements for waste disposal and opposed additional regulation of wastes. This opposition was based on the lack of evidence that hospital waste is more infective than residential waste. In fact, in one study[48] the microbiologic content of residential waste was demonstrated to be 10 to 100,000 times higher than hospital waste. Second, no epidemiologic evidence links hospital waste disposal practices to disease in any community.[64] Third, with the exception of sharps, there are only rare instances of in-hospital transmission of infection associated with waste.[40] Fourth, agencies such as the U.S. Environmental Protection Agency (EPA) and the CDC had addressed appropriate disposal of medical waste years before[24,31] and most hospitals followed these protocols as routine practice. A survey conducted by the AHA and an independent researcher in 1988 found that at least 80% of U.S. hospitals were in compliance with infectious waste guidelines from the CDC or the EPA.[64] Finally, hospital representatives in particular noted that compliance with proposed regulations could cost U.S. hospitals an additional $385 million annually in the absence of added safety.

Nonetheless, many legislators and the public favored strict legislation. Politicians responded to concerns and pressure from their constituents, whose fear of infectious wastes centered on the perceived risk of transmission of HIV and HBV. Firms in the waste disposal business involved with transportation, incineration, or landfill disposal of infectious wastes also applied pressure in favor of more stringent disposal regulations. Policy makers were lobbied strongly by environmental groups, such as those in air pollution control agencies who were concerned about the risk of aerosolized pathogens and breakdown products from plastic. Lastly, those who generate income from tourism joined with the politicians to encourage legislation to protect the recreation industry (i.e., beaches).

The main challenges to balancing science and politics for this policy were delineating the real and the perceived risks posed by infectious waste and the differences between fact and illogical fear. The epidemiologic information indicated that the risk of disease transmission from medical wastes handled in a prudent manner was low despite the fact that concerns were high.

Congress passed interim legislation to evaluate the management of medical waste from certain health care facilities.[32] They heard extensive public and professional debate and testimony about concerns and proposals for public and environmental safety. In addition, many states implemented regulations to control the management of medical waste.

Scientists, policy makers, and the public reached a compromise. New regulations regarding waste handling in health care facilities were incorporated into the OSHA Bloodborne Pathogens Standard.[73] These regulations were based on some factual information and potential for risk. They were more stringent and

expensive than in the past and carried the threat of large fines. They appeased much public fear, demonstrated governmental response to the public, and provided guidelines for waste generators.

These examples clearly show that infection prevention and control policies do not evolve from a single perspective. While these policies may be based on methodic observation and research, they are usually implemented and evaluated within the political arena. Since science and politics bring together many different perspectives, policy making is often fraught with conflict and misunderstanding. However, it is critical that both perspectives be brought to bear on health policy issues. Science is a tool used to test alternative theories, but it alone cannot address value judgments and issues of social justice.[51] Politics is the process through which these issues are addressed in the policy development process.

THE POLICY PROCESS IN SPECIFIC HEALTH CARE SETTINGS

Each of the three policy perspectives presented in this chapter can be applied to the design and analysis of infection control policies in many health care settings. The dynamics of the host-environment interactions, the steps in policy making, and relevant elements of science and politics will vary in importance depending on the circumstances.

In acute, long-term, and other care settings that provide day care or basic services to high-risk patients, administrators and professional health care personnel are responsible for the care rendered and the financial well-being of the organization. Pressure to provide high-quality, cost-effective care is forcing changes in health services delivery that may drive infection control or prevention policies onto the policy agenda. For example, providing needles and syringes with protective devices that will protect health care workers from occupational injury or additional immunizations that may reduce their risk of infection will require evidence that the policy meets performance criteria. This may include the potential to promote wellness, prevent illness, improve quality of care, minimize risk, satisfy patients, and reduce or minimally increase costs. For some policies one criterion will be significantly more important than the others. Other policies will have to satisfy several requirements.

Economics is an important, influential feature of all health policy because resources are generally limited. This was the case in the building of the Volga dam in Ghana, is evident in other countries where only $1 or $2 is available each year for the health care needs of each person in the society, and is increasingly true in the United States. At times, social dilemmas may be the catalyst for policy decisions. Issues of civil rights and discrimination have influenced policies related to the HIV/AIDS epidemic, such as HIV testing, patient or caregiver confidentiality, and reporting of HIV status to health authorities.

In the public health setting, the need to provide primary care for the greatest number of people will have a strong influence on policy formulation. In the private sector, decisions about the types and range of services offered may be strongly influenced by consumer demands, caregiver preferences or financial implications. For example, resources may be managed by using only generic drugs or emphasizing low cost or high-revenue-producing services. In litigious environments, policies may be developed to protect those who are vulnerable to malpractice suits.

SUMMARY

Regardless of setting, health policy development may be studied by applying general models. Three perspectives have been discussed in this chapter: the ecologic model of host-environment interactions, the sequential pattern of action model, and the science versus politics thematic model. Understanding and applying these perspectives will prepare nurses to have an important influence on the design, implementation, and analysis of infection prevention and control policies.

REFERENCES

1. Adams R. Prevention of infections in hospitals. *Am J Nurs.* 1958;58(3):344-348.
2. Alter MJ, Hadler SC, Margolis HS, et al. The changing epidemiology of hepatitis B in the United States. *JAMA.* 263;1218-1222, 1990.
3. American Hospital Association. Infection Control in the hospital. Chicago: American Hospital Association; 1968.
4. American Organization of Nurse Executives. Nursing, health care prevention and political influence: a winning combination. *Nursing Management.* 24(3):28-32, 1993.
5. Anderson JE. Public policy making: an introduction. Boston: Houghton Mifflin; 1990.
6. Anonymous. A national conference on staphylococcal diseases. *Am J Nurs.* 58:1537, 1958.
7. Blair JR, Carr M. Staphylococci in hospital-acquired infections. *JAMA.* 166:1192-1196, 1958.
8. Brachman PS. Epidemiology of nosocomial infections. In Bennett JV, Brachman PS, eds. Hospital infections, 3rd ed. Boston: Little, Brown; 1992.
9. Brandt AM. AIDS in historical perspective: four lessons from the history of sexually transmitted diseases. *Am J Public Health.* 78:367-371, 1988.
10. Brownlea A. From public health to political epidemiology. *Soc Sci Med.* 15D:57-67, 1891.
11. Campbell AG. The application of science to health policy-making. *Health Management Forum.* Autumn 1983;4:50-59.
12. Centers for Disease Control and Prevention. Draft guidelines for preventing the transmission of tuberculosis in health care facilities. U.S. Dept. of Health and Human Services. *Federal Register.* Oct 12, 1993; 58;195.
13. Centers for Disease Control. Recommendations for HIV testing services for inpatients and outpatients in acute-care hospital settings. *MMWR.* 42(rr-2):1-6, 1993.
14. Centers for Disease Control. Preliminary report: foodborne outbreak of *Escherichia coli O 157:H7* infections from hamburgers—Western United States, 1993. *MMWR.* 42(4):85-86, 1993.
15. Centers for Disease Control. Update: multistate outbreak of *Escherichia coli O 157:H7* infections from hamburgers—Western United States, 1992-1993. *MMWR.* 42(14):258-63, 1993.

16. Centers for Disease Control. Recommendations for preventing transmission of human immunodeficiency virus and hepatitis B virus to patients during exposure-prone invasive procedures. *MMWR.* 40:1-8, 1991.

17. Centers for Disease Control. Update: transmission of HIV infection during invasive dental procedures—Florida. *MMWR.* 40:21-27,33; 1991.

18. Centers for Disease Control: Update: transmission of HIV infection during invasive dental procedures—Florida. *MMWR.* 40:377-381, 1991.

19. Centers for Disease Control. Possible transmission of HIV infection during invasive dental procedure—Florida. *MMWR.* 1991;40:489-493.

20. Centers for Disease Control: Protection against viral hepatitis: recommendations of the Immunization Practices Advisory Committee. *MMWR.* 39(rr-2), 1-26, 1990.

21. Centers for Disease Control. Reduced incidence of menstrual toxic-shock syndrome—United States, 1980-1990. *MMWR.* 39(25),421-23, 1990.

22. Centers for Disease Control. Guidelines for preventing the transmission of tuberculosis in health-care settings, with special focus on HIV-related issues. *MMWR.* 39(rr-17):1-29, 1990.

23. Centers for Disease Control. Changing patterns or groups at high risk for hepatitis B in the United States. *MMWR.* 37;429,437; 1988.

24. Centers for Disease Control. *Disposal of Solid Wastes from Hospitals.* Bacterial Disease Division, Bureau of Epidemiology. Atlanta: U.S. Department of Health and Human Services; 1980.

25. Crossley K, Nelson L, Irvine P. State regulations governing infection control issues in long-term care. *J Am Geriatr Soc.* 40:251-54, 1992.

26. Crystal S, Jackson M. Health care and the social construction of AIDS: the impact of disease definitions. In Huber J, Schneider BE, eds. The social context of AIDS. (American Sociological Association Presidential Series.) Newbury Park, CA: Sage Publications; 1992.

27. Desowitz RS. New Guinea Tapeworms and Jewish Grandmothers: Tales of Parasites and People. New York: W W Norton & Co; 1981.

28. Dienstag JL, Ryan DM. Occupational exposure to hepatitis B virus in hospital personnel: Infection or immunization? *Am J Epidemiol.* 1982;115:26-39.

29. Dobson A, Bialek R. Shaping public policy from the perspective of a data builder. *Health Care Financial Review.* 6:117-34, 1985.

30. Eickhoff TC. Standards for hospital infection control. *Ann Intern Med.* 89(pt2):829-31, 1978.

31. Environmental Protection Agency Guide for Infectious Waste Management. Washington D.C.: Office of Solid Waste, U.S. Environmental Protection Agency. May 1986;EPA/530-SW-86-014.

32. Environmental Protection Agency. Standards for the tracking and management of medical waste. *Federal Register.* March 24, 1989; 54:12326-95.

33. Foege WH. Uses of epidemiology in the development of health policy. *Public Health Rep.* 1984;99:233-236.

34. Fox DM. Chronic disease and disadvantage: the new politics of HIV infection. *J Health Polit Policy Law.* 15:341-55, 1990.

35. Fox DM. The history of responses to epidemic disease in the United States since the 18th century. *Mt Sinai J Med.* 58:223-29, 1989.

36. Frank JW. Public health policy and the quality of epidemiological evidence: how good is good enough? *J Public Health Policy.* 1985;6(3):313-321.

37. Garner JS, Emori TG. Nosocomial infection surveillance and control programs. In Lennette EH, et al, eds. *Manual of Clinical Microbiology,* 4th ed. Washington, DC: American Society for Microbiology; 1985;105-109.

38. Gostin L, Curran WJ. The limits of compulsion in controlling AIDS. *Hastings Cent Rep.* December 1986;24-29.

39. Gostin L. A decade of a maturing epidemic: an assessment and direction for future public policy. *Am J Law Med.* 1990;16:1-32.

40. Grieble HB, et al. Chute hydropulping waste disposal system: a reservoir of enteric bacilli and pseudomonas in a modern hospital. *J Infect Dis.* 130:602-607, 1974.

41. Haley RW. The development of infection surveillance and control programs. In Bennet JE, Brachman PS, eds. *Hospital Infections,* 3rd ed. Boston: Little, Brown; 1992;63-77.

42. Haley RW, Schachtman RH. The emergence of infection surveillance and control programs in United States hospitals: an assessment, 1976. *Am J Epidemiol.* 111:574-91, 1980.

43. Hanft RS. Use of social science data for policy analysis and policy-making. *Milbank Mem Fund Q.* 59:596-613, 1981.

44. Harder HI, Panuska M. Staphylococcal infections. *Am J Nurs.* 58(3):349-351, 1958.

45. Hinman AR. Immunizations in the United States. Pediatrics 86(suppl):1064-1066, 1990.

46. Joint Commission on Accreditation of Hospitals. *Accreditation Manual for Hospitals.* Chicago: Joint Commission on Accreditation of Hospitals; 1993.

47. Joint Commission on Accreditation of Hospitals. *Accreditation Manual for Hospitals.* Chicago: Joint Commission on Accreditation of Hospitals; 1976.

48. Kalnowski G, Wiegand H, Ruben H. The microbial contamination of hospital waste. *Zbl Bakt Hyg.* I. Abt Orig B. 178:364-79, 1983.

49. Koop CE. Surgeon general's report on acquired immune deficiency syndrome. Washington, DC: Department of Social and Health Services, U.S. Public Health Service, 1986.

50. Kunes E. The trashing of America. Omni, VOL 10, 1988:40-42.

51. Lanes SF, Poole C. 'Truth in packaging': The unwrapping of epidemiologic research. *J Occ Med.* 1984;26: 571-574.

52. Landwirth J. Medical-legal aspects of immunization: policy and practices. *Pediatr Clin North Am.* 37(3):771-783, 1990.

53. Lee PR, Arno PS. The federal response to the AIDS epidemic. *Health Policy.* 6:259-67, 1986.

54. Lee PR, Silver GA, Benjamin AE. Health policy and the politics of health. In Last JM, Wallace RB, eds. *Public Health and Preventive Medicine.* Norwalk, VA: Appleton & Lange; 1992:1165-1172.

55. Lindblom CE. *The Policy-Making Process,* 2nd ed. Englewood Cliffs, NJ: Prentice-Hall; 1980.

56. Martone WJ. Year 2000 objectives for preventing nosocomial infections: how do we get there? *Am J Med.* 1991;91(suppl3B):3b-39S,

57. Mausner JS, Kramer S. *Epidemiology: An Introductory Text.* Philadelphia: W B Saunders; 1985:22-42.

58. McDonald LL, Pugliese G. Regulatory, accreditation, and professional agencies influencing infection control programs. In Wenzel RP, ed. *Prevention and Control of Nosocomial Infections,* 2nd ed. Baltimore: Williams & Wilkins; 1993:58-69.

59. Mitsunaga BK. The use of knowledge and health policy planning: forms and functions of the relationships. *Community Nursing Research.* 14:1-8, 1981.

60. Morrison AB. Public policy on health and scientific evidence—is there a link? *Journal of Chronic Diseases.* 37(8):647-52, 1984.

61. Nahamias AJ, Eickhoff TC. Staphylococcal infection in hospitals: recent developments in epidemiologic and laboratory investigation. *N Engl J Med.* 1961;265:74-81, 120-128, 177-182.

62. Osborn JE. AIDS: challenges to our health care systems. *Cleve Clin J Med.* 57:709-714, 1990.

63. Palumbo DF. Public policy in America: government in action. San Diego, CA: Harcourt Brace Jovanovich, 1988:33-56, 176-204.

64. Rutala WA, Odette RL, Samsa GP. Management of infectious waste by United States hospitals. *JAMA.* 262:1635-40, 1989.

65. Schlech WF, Shands KN Ringold AL, et al: Risk factors for development of toxic shock syndrome: association with a tampon brand. *JAMA.* 1982;248:835-839.

66. Shilts R. And the band played on: politics, people, and the AIDS epidemic. New York, NY: St. Martins Press; 1987.

67. Sorian R. The bitter pill: tough choices in America's health policy. New York, NY: McGraw-Hill; 1988: 203-237.

68. Stevens CE, et al. Prospects for control of hepatitis B virus infections: implications of childhood vaccination and long-term protection. *Pediatrics.* 1992;90(1): 170-173.

69. Streeter S, Dunn H, Lepper M. Hospital infection—a necessary risk? *Am J Nurs.* 67:526-33, 1967.

70. Thompson LR. *Staphylococcus aureus. Am J Nurs.* 58(8):1098-1100, 1958.

71. Tierney JT. Organized interests in health politics and policy-making. *Med Care Rev.* 44:89-118, Spring 1987.

72. Tyler CW, Last JM. Epidemiology. In Last JM, Wallace RB, eds. *Public Health and Preventive Medicine.* Norwalk, CT: Appleton & Lange; 1992:11-40.

73. U.S. Dept. of Labor, Occupational Safety and Health Administration: Occupational exposure to bloodborne pathogens, final rule. *Federal Register.* December 6, 1991;56:64004-182.

74. U.S. Dept. of Labor, Occupational Safety and Health Administration: Memorandum: Enforcement Policy and Procedure for Occupational Exposure to Tuberculosis, Washington DC, October, 1993.

75. Williams REO. Changing perspectives in hospital infection. In Brachman PS, Eickhoff TC, eds. *Proceedings of the International Conference on Nosocomial Infections.* Chicago: American Hospital Association; 1971:1-10.

76. Williams REO. Summary of Conference. In Brachman PS, Eickhoff TC, eds. *Proceedings of the International Conference on Nosocomial Infections.* Chicago: American Hospital Association; 1971:318-321.

SUGGESTED READINGS

Ashford NA. New scientific evidence and public health imperatives. *Am J Public Health* 1987;316:1084-1085.

Crooks GM. Shaping public policy. U.S. Public Health Service, Department of Health and Human Services, Washington, DC. Public Health Rep 1987;Jul-Aug Suppl:85-90.

Dever GEA. *Epidemiology in Health Services Management.* Rockville: Aspen, 1984.

Gerberding JL, Henderson DK. Design of rational infection control policies for human immunodeficiency virus infection. *J Infect Dis.* 1987 Dec;156(6):861-4.

Ibrahim M. *Epidemiology and Health Policy.* Rockville: Aspen, 1985.

Institute of Medicine, National Academy of Sciences. Confronting AIDS: Directions for public health, health care and research. Washington: *National Academy Press,* 1986.

Institute of Medicine, National Academy of Sciences. Confronting AIDS: update 1988. Washington: *National Academy Press,* 1988.

Institute of Medicine. The future of public health. Washington: *National Academy Press,* 1988.

Kuller LH. Epidemiology and health policy. *Am J Epidemiol.* 1988 Jan;127(1):2-16.

Lave LB, Seskin EP. Epidemiology, causality, and public policy. *Am Sci.* 1979;67:178-186.

Litman TJ, Robbins LS, eds. *Health Politics and Policy.* 2nd ed. Albany: Delmar, 1991:3-37.

Miller GH, Turner CF, Moses LE, eds. AIDS: the second decade. National Research Council. Washington: *National Academy Press,* 1990.

Modan B. Epidemiology and health policy: prevention initiatives, resource, allocation, regulation, and control. *Public Health Rep.* 1984 May-Jun;99(3):229-33.

Report of the Presidential Commission on the Human Immunodeficiency Virus Epidemic. Submitted to the President of the United States, June 24, 1988.

Stivers C. The politics of public health: The Dilemma of a public profession. In: Litman TJ, Robins LS, eds. *Health Politics and Policy.* 2nd ed. Albany: Delmar, 1992: 356-367.

Terris M. Epidemiology as a guide to health policy. *Annu Rev Public Health.* 1980;1:323-44.

Tesh SN. *Hidden Arguments: Political Ideology and Disease Prevention Policy.* New Brunswick: Rutgers University Press, 1988.

Clinical Studies

This section consists of 35 clinical studies illustrating host-environment interactions and applying the tools of infection prevention and management introduced in Sections One and Two. These presentations of typical infectious diseases demonstrate how an understanding of these interactions and use of the tools form a basis for nursing care.

Each study includes a clinical presentation and an analysis of host, microbiologic, physical environment, and social factors that influence the process and outcome of the infection. The summary table at the end of each clinical presentation itemizes some of the significant factors influencing the epidemiology, clinical considerations, and patient care strategies. The reader may identify additional factors or interactions that expand this summary and serve as a basis for discussion.

The clinical studies vary in emphasis and complexity. They cover a broad range of human conditions, infections, and care settings. This diversity provides opportunities to illustrate the consistency with which host-environment interactions are at work in these settings and demonstrate prevention and management techniques that may apply to care decisions.

Clinical studies

No	Title	Setting	Population	Micro-organism	Origin of infection
1	Lyme Disease at a Boy Scout Camp	Community	Infant/Child	Bacterium	Community
2	Nursing Home Resident with Post-Antibiotic Oral Candidiasis	Long Term Care	Elderly	Fungus	Nosocomial
3	Staphylococcal Food Poisoning in a University Cafeteria	Community	Adolescent	Bacterium	Community
4	*Pseudomonas* Bloodstream Infection in an Arterial Line	Acute Care	Adult	Bacterium	Nosocomial
5	Methicillin-Resistant *Staphylococcus aureus* (MRSA) in a Sternal Wound	Acute Care	Adult	Bacterium	Nosocomial
6	Varicella (Chickenpox) in a Pediatric House Officer	Acute Care	Adult	Virus	Community/Nosocomial
7	Pulmonary Tuberculosis in a Homeless Person	Community	Adult	Bacterium	Community
8	Intensive Care Patient with Ventilator-Associated Pneumonia	Acute Care	Elderly	Bacterium	Nosocomial
9	Two Children with *Haemophilus influenzae* Disease from a Day-Care Home	Day Care	Infant/Child	Bacterium	Community
10	Nosocomial Aspergillosis during Hospital Remodel	Acute Care	Adult	Fungus	Nosocomial
11	Penicillin-Resistant Gonorrhea in a Teenage Male	Community	Adolescent	Bacterium	Community
12	Burn Patient with *Pseudomonas* Infection	Acute Care	Adult	Bacterium	Nosocomial
13	Herpetic Whitlow in a Critical Care Nurse	Acute Care	Adult	Virus	Nosocomial
14	Adolescent Female with *Chlamydia* Infection	Community	Adolescent	Bacterium	Nosocomial
15	Rotavirus in a Day-Care Center	Day Care	Infant/Child	Virus	Community/Nosocomial
16	Measles (Rubeola) in an Immunized Child	Community	Infant/Child	Virus	Community
17	Kidney Transplant Patient with Staphylococcal Sepsis	Acute Care	Adult	Bacterium	Nosocomial
18	Influenza in an Elderly Resident of a Nursing Home	Long Term Care	Elderly	Virus	Nosocomial

Clinical studies—cont'd

No	Title	Setting	Population	Micro-organism	Origin of infection
19	*Chlamydia Trachomatis* Conjunctivitis and Pneumonia in Two Infants	Acute Care	Infant/Child	Bacterium	Nosocomial (Maternal)
20	Community-Acquired Aspergillosis in a Cancer Patient	Community	Adult	Fungus	Community
21	*Giardia* in a Traveler	Community	Adult	Protozoan	Community
22	*Clostridium difficile* in a Nursing Home Resident	Long Term Care	Elderly	Bacterium	Nosocomial
23	Infection in a Child with Hydrocephalus and a Ventricular Shunt	Acute Care	Infant/Child	Bacterium	Nosocomial
24	*Proteus mirabilis* Urinary Tract Infection in an Elderly Person at Home	Community	Elderly	Bacterium	Nosocomial
25	Cholera in a 3-Year-Old Child in Bangladesh	Community	Infant/Child	Bacterium	Community
26	Human Immunodeficiency Virus in a Female Who Injects Drugs	Community	Adult	Virus	Community
27	Bone Marrow Transplant Patient with Cytomegalovirus Infection	Community	Adult	Virus	Community/ Nosocomial
28	Presumptive Pneumococcal Pneumonia in an Elderly Woman	Community	Elderly	Bacterium	Community
29	Respiratory Syncytial Virus in a Special Care Nursery	Acute Care	Infant/Child	Virus	Community/ Nosocomial
30	Pertussis in an Infant	Community	Infant/Child	Bacterium	Community
31	Occupationally Acquired Hepatitis B in a Health Care Worker	Acute Care	Adult	Virus	Nosocomial
32	Tuberculosis Transmission in a Pediatric Hospital	Acute Care	Infant/Child	Bacterium	Community/ Nosocomial
33	Legionnaires' Disease: Possible Acquisition on a Cruise Ship	Community	Adult	Bacterium	Community
34	Group B Streptococcal Disease in an Infant	Acute Care	Infant/Child	Bacterium	Community
35	Schoolteacher with Malaria Glossary	Community	Adult	Protozoan	Community

Lyme Disease at a Boy Scout Camp

PATRICIA J. CHECKO

CLINICAL PRESENTATION

Steve Franklin, a 12-year-old boy, spent a week at a Boy Scout camp in southeast Connecticut in mid-June. One day before leaving camp he found an engorged tick on his thigh.

He wasn't certain how long the tick had been there or where he had picked it up, but he had been hiking most days. Steve went to the camp nurse who carefully extracted the tick with tweezers and cleaned the area. About 2 weeks after returning home from camp he complained of headache, achy joints and muscles, a stiff neck, and fever. He showed his mother a large red lesion at the site of the tick bite. Over the next few days there was an expanding area of erythema that was tender, warm, and pruritic. Steve was examined by a pediatrician, who diagnosed his condition as probable Lyme disease on the basis of the unique skin lesion, erythema migrans (EM), the classical presentation of early Lyme disease. Approximately two-thirds of persons infected with *Borrelia burgdorferi*, the etiologic agent of Lyme disease, develop EM.

When he was seen, Steve had several secondary annular skin lesions on both legs. The original EM lesion measured 15 cm. The pediatrician prescribed oral doxycycline for 21 days. Steve's uneventful recovery was accompanied by total resolution of symptoms. After completion of therapy, approximately 5 weeks after infection, serum submitted for ELISA testing was positive for IgM antibody. A year later Steve had no evidence of late complica-

tions, which might have included neurologic, cardiac, and arthritic manifestations.

HOST-ENVIRONMENT INTERACTION
The host

No specific host factors are known to predispose a person to Lyme disease. Persons of all ages are susceptible (known age range is 2 to 88 years). Reinfection has occurred in those treated with an antibiotic for early disease.

Like other spirochetes, *B. burgdorferi* can cause multisystem disease. Spirochetes transmitted from the tick to human skin migrate outward, causing the unique expanding skin lesions. Subsequent hematogenous dissemination to secondary sites may cause major organ system involvement.

Approximately 15% of untreated persons will develop neurologic abnormalities within 2 to 8 weeks of onset of symptoms. These include aseptic meningitis, encephalitis, peripheral neuropathy, peripheral radiculoneuritis, and Bell's palsy, a paralysis of the seventh cranial nerve. Fortunately, Steve did not suffer any of these complications.

Lyme carditis, which occurs in 5% to 10% of untreated patients within 2 to 6 weeks of infection, may be the first manifestation of Lyme disease. The most common feature of cardiac involvement is first-degree heart block, which may be so severe as to require a temporary pacemaker. Myocarditis and cardiomegaly are much less common.

Arthritis is the most common sequela of untreated Lyme disease. Months to years after erythema migrans, 60% of untreated persons will develop joint manifestations ranging from migratory arthralgias to chronic destructive arthritis. The most common syndrome is intermittent inflammatory arthritis of one or more large joints lasting from several days to a year. The knee is most often involved. About 10% of patients with arthritis will develop chronic arthritis, which may involve permanent joint destruction.

The microbiologic environment

Lyme disease is a tick-borne infection caused by the spirochete *Borrelia burgdorferi*. Infection is transmitted from wild animals to humans by the bite of ticks of the genus Ixodes. The *I. dammini* tick is found primarily along coastal areas from Delaware to Massachusetts and in Wisconsin and Minnesota. In the Southeast, *I. scapularis* is the vector. On the Pacific Coast, *I. pacificus* is the vector. Recent information suggests that *I. dammini* may be the same species as *I. scapularis*.[5] *I. dammini* is a small, reddish brown to dark brown tick. There are three active stages of the tick: immature larvae, nymphs, and sexually mature adults. Larvae (0.5 mm) are not considered to play a major role as vectors of the disease to humans. Nymphs, about the size of a pinhead or freckle (1.2 mm), are responsible for most Lyme disease cases. Most active from May to early July, they account for the marked seasonality of the disease. Adults are somewhat larger (2 to 3 mm) and are active in the fall and in early spring.

The first cluster of Lyme disease was seen in Lyme, Connecticut. It is now the most common arthropod-borne disease in the United States.[3] In 1991, over 9000 cases were reported to the Centers for Disease Control and Prevention (CDC). Incidence and patterns of transmission reflect differences in the vectors and vector ecology in different geographic regions. The prevalence of infection in Ixodes ticks in the northeast and north central United States is 30% to 50% versus infection rates of only 1% to 2% on the Pacific coast.[1]

Reservoir hosts for the spirochetes include rodents, other mammals, and even birds. White-footed mice (*Peromyscus leucopus)* are particularly important reservoirs, and white-tailed deer appear to be crucial for maintaining tick populations. Transmission of *B. burgdorferi* is directly related to the duration of attachment by an infected tick. It is rarely transmitted when ticks are attached for less than 48 hours.[6] Lyme borreliosis has been diagnosed in dogs, cats, cattle, and horses. Pets may also expose humans to infected ticks.

Diagnosis is based on clinical findings and serologic tests. However, the serologic tests are poorly standardized and insensitive during the first several weeks of infection. These include IFA and ELISA procedures for total immunoglobulins (Ig) or IgM and IgG antibody. Test sensitivity increases markedly as patients progress to later stages. Antibodies may cross-react in patients with syphilis or relapsing fever, giving false positive results. As in Steve's case, the diagnosis of early disease is normally based on clinical characteristics, specifically EM, and disease-specific serologic testing is more useful during later stages of the illness.

The physical environment

Humans encounter ticks in woodlands, grassy and shrubby areas along beaches and in parks, in yards around homes, and even inside houses after domestic animals or humans have carried ticks inside. The best way to prevent Lyme disease is to avoid tick-infested areas when *I. dammini* nymphs are active in May, June, and July. The tick is most abundant in woodlands, especially in areas of transitional vegetation where mammalian and avian hosts for the tick flourish. In endemic areas, undeveloped woodlands and parks have been demonstrated to be heavily infested with ticks.

The emergence of Lyme disease is directly related to changes in land use. During this century land previously cleared for farming has undergone reforestation, especially along the east coast. Deer populations increased at the same time, and people began to visit or live in forested rural areas. The range of the tick and associated Lyme disease is growing as more houses are built in woodlands and as birds and other animals distribute ticks inland.[2]

The social environment

As residential development in woodlands and outdoor recreation increases, people must learn to coexist with the tick, learn more about recognizing it, and take proper precautions while outdoors. The proximity of deer, mice, ticks, and people supports opportunity for human infection.[2]

Humans are usually exposed to ticks as part of leisure or social activities such as camping, hiking, and hunting. Housing developments and vacations take many people to wooded areas. Ticks are likely to be found in wooded areas and in coastal areas with transitional tall grasses and shrubs, where mammalian and avian hosts flourish. On the east coast many persons become infected at the beach. Personal prevention measures can substantially reduce the risk of acquiring tick bites in these areas.

PREVENTION AND CONTROL

Since the risk of infection is directly related to the duration of attachment of a tick, use of personal protection is the most practical strategy to prevent infection. Host management, habitat modification, and chemical control of tick populations are generally impractical on a large scale.

Personal preventive measures can substantially reduce the risk of tick bites in tick infested areas. Wearing light-colored clothing allows ticks to be seen. Long-sleeved shirts and pants help, although they may be inconvenient and uncomfortable in the summer. The camp nurse and counselors had advised the boys about these precautions, but Steve wore shorts at camp because it was hot. This increased his risk of exposure during camp outings. Ticks are unlikely to crawl under clothing if pants are tucked into socks and closed shoes are worn. Most ticks are picked up on lower legs or feet and crawl upward. People walking in wooded areas or high grass should avoid overhanging grass and brush by walking in the center of trails. They should carefully inspect themselves and their pets for ticks and should brush off clothing and pets before entering the house. If a tick attaches, prompt removal with tweezers will reduce the chance of infection. Ixodes ticks are very small, and even when fully engorged may be no larger than 1/4 inch.

Insect repellents can reduce the risk of tick bites. Diethyltoluamide repellents (Deet, Autan) can be applied to clothing and skin. The camp managers had provided counselors with a supply of repellent to make available to the boys prior to hikes in the woods. Products containing 30% or less Deet are recommended, since that compound can be toxic at higher concentrations. Permethrin repellents should be applied to clothing only, not to skin.

Early recognition of Lyme disease and appropriate antibiotic treatment shorten the duration of EM and generally prevent the later manifestations of Lyme disease. No data support the common practice of prescribing prophylactic antibiotics after Ixodes tick bites, even where Lyme disease is known to be endemic.

Researchers using decision analysis methods have suggested that empiric therapy with doxycycline is indicated if the probability of infection after a tick bite is 3.6% or greater but is not recommended if probabilities of infection are 1% or less.[4] A double-blind placebo-controlled trial to assess the risk of infection with *B. burgdorferi* and the efficacy of prophylactic antimicrobial treatment after a deer-tick bite revealed that even in an endemic area the risk of infection after a recognized deer-tick bite is very low (less than 5%) and does not warrant routine antimicrobial prophylaxis.[4,7]

SUMMARY

Lyme disease is a multisystem infection transmitted by Ixodes ticks and caused by the spirochete *B. burgdorferi*. It occurs mainly in the northeast, upper midwest, and California, but cases have been reported from 48 states, Canada, Asia, and Europe, and it affects all age groups. Factors associated with the risk of Lyme disease after a deer-tick bite include the probability that the tick is infected, the developmental stage of the tick, and the length of time the tick was attached.

Transmission does not occur until the tick has fed for several hours, so identification and removal of ticks within 48 hours may be important in interrupting the chain of transmission.

SUMMARY TABLE 1. Lyme disease at a Boy Scout camp

Host-environment model	Case presentation	Factors that influence infectious process	Prevention and control
Host factors	12-year-old healthy male	All ages susceptible	No vaccine
Microbiologic factors	*Borrelia burgdorferi*	Tickborne transmission occurs after tick has been attached for several hours (usually >48 hrs) No transmission person to person Nymphs most active May-July	Treat with doxycycline or amoxicillin
Physical environment	Boy Scout camp	Woodland, grassy and shrub-like areas where *Ixodes* tick is found Summer seasonality	Avoid tick-infested areas Wear covering clothes Use insect repellents Check skin for ticks after possible exposure Identify and remove ticks with tweezers
Social environment	Children in a recreational setting in wooded areas	Recreational activities associated with warm weather Visiting or living in wooded area	Educate children and adults about disease and how to avoid ticks

The estimated risk of contracting Lyme disease after a tick bite in an endemic area ranges from 1.2% to 5%.[4] The marked seasonality, with initial cases primarily during the summer, reflects the life cycle of the tick.

Carditis occurs in roughly 8% of untreated persons within 2 to 6 weeks of infection. Neurologic abnormalities occur in about 15% of patients within 2 to 8 weeks of disease onset. Some 60% of infected persons develop manifestations of joint disease ranging from migratory arthralgias to chronic destructive arthritis months to years after EM.

Prevention and control strategies consist primarily of education and personal prevention to reduce the risk of acquiring tick bites. Avoiding heavily tick-infested areas, using insect repellents, wearing proper attire for outdoor activities in wooded areas, and doing tick checks are also important prevention tactics.

Strategies to control the vector or eradicate hosts on a large scale are impractical. A vaccine may eventually be the best control measure. Currently, early recognition and treatment of Lyme disease to prevent late manifestations of disease are critical. Serologic testing may confirm the diagnosis, but antibodies may not be detectable until 4 to 6 weeks after infection.

REFERENCES

1. Dennis DT: Epidemiology. In Coyle PK, editor: Lyme disease. St. Louis, 1993, Mosby–Year Book.
2. Institute of Medicine: factors in emergence. In Lederberg J, Shope RE, Oaks SC, Jr. (editors): *Emerging infections: microbial threats to health in the United States.* Washington, 1992, National Academy Press.
3. Lyme disease—United States, 1991-1992. *MMWR* 42:345-348, 1993.
4. Magid D, et al: Prevention of Lyme disease after tick bites: a cost-effectiveness analysis, *N Engl J Med* 327:534-541, 1992.
5. Oliver JH, et al: Conspecificity of the ticks *Ixodes scapularis* and *I. dammini* (Acari: Ixodidae), *J Med Entomol* 30:54-63, 1993.
6. Piesman J, et al: Duration of adult female *Ixodes dammini* attachment and transmission of *Borrelia burgdorferi* with description of needle aspiration isolation method, *J Infect Dis* 163:895-897, 1991.
7. Shapiro ED, et al: A controlled trial of antimicrobial prophylaxis for Lyme disease after deer-tick bites. *N Engl J Med* 327:1769-1773, 1992.

SUGGESTED READINGS

Barbour AG, Durland F: The biological and social phenomenon of Lyme disease. *Science* 260:1610-1616, 1993.
Rahn DW, Malawista SE: Lyme disease: recommendations for diagnosis and treatment, *Ann Intern Med* 114:472-481, 1991.
Treatment for Lyme disease. *Med Lettr Drugs Ther,* 34:95-97, 1992.

Nursing Home Resident with Post-Antibiotic Oral Candidiasis

T. GRACE EMORI

CLINICAL PRESENTATION

Maud Sanders is an 81-year-old African-American woman and a resident of the Sunny Hills Nursing Home. After the death of her husband about 2 years ago, her children sold her home and moved her into the nursing home. She has her own room, which is decorated with many of her personal belongings, and she enjoys hosting other residents who frequently stop by to visit. Mrs. Sanders has non-insulin-dependent diabetes that is reasonably well controlled. She has been under treatment for a recurrent urinary tract infection and was begun on a 10-day course of oral cephalexin, to be taken 4 times a day. On the eighth day of antibiotic treatment she complained that her mouth was sore and irritated. When the charge nurse examined Mrs. Sanders's mouth, she found her tongue coated with adherent white patches. Although Mrs. Sanders had no other complaints, the nurse examined her throat and skin, paying particular attention to the moist areas between skin folds.

The staff physician at the nursing home was notified. She ordered a direct microscopy examination using a potassium hydroxide (KOH) preparation of a scraping of the material on the patient's tongue and discontinued the antibiotic. She also prescribed nystatin oral suspension 4 times a day, requested that Mrs. Sanders remove her full-mouth dentures for 3 days, and ordered a soft diet. The next day the laboratory reported budding yeasts on the smear, which with the clinical manifestations, confirmed the diagnosis of oropharyngeal candidiasis.

HOST-ENVIRONMENT INTERACTION
The host

In Mrs. Sanders's case, candidiasis was likely a superinfection resulting from the broad-spectrum antibiotic therapy, which suppressed the competing bacteria and permitted the *Candida* species (sp.) to overgrow.[15] Mrs. Sanders's superficial candidiasis will probably resolve without further treatment because most of these infections are self-limiting.

Thrush is an alternate term for candidiasis of the mucous membranes, regardless of its location on the body. Invasive candidiasis may involve the bloodstream (*candidemia*) or almost any deep organ in the body. Patients receiving immunosuppressive therapy to prevent rejection of transplanted organs or as cancer chemotherapy are particularly susceptible to invasive candidiasis. In these patients, a *Candida* infection can be life-threatening. The treatment of choice for invasive candidiasis is amphotericin B, which is expensive and potentially toxic. Patients with diabetes, the elderly, and newborns are also known to be predisposed to *Candida* infection as a consequence of compromised or immature cellular immune function.[1,2,16,18] Recently, considerable attention has been given to oropharyngeal *Candida* infection in persons with the human immunodeficiency virus (HIV).[12] Approximately 90% of patients with acquired immunodeficiency syndrome (AIDS) develop oral candidiasis.

The microbiologic environment

The major agent of candidiasis is *Candida albicans.* It constituted approximately 76% of all *Candida* sp. isolated from nosocomial infections reported to the National Nosocomial Infections Surveillance (NNIS) system between 1980 and 1990.[3] Although more than 80 *Candida* sp. are known, only 8 are believed to be clinically important.[7]

Candida sp. are yeasts typically found in the normal microbial flora of humans, predominantly in the oropharynx, gastrointestinal tract, and female genital tract. *Candida* sp. are also normally found in the environment, such as soil, food, and animals. As commensal organisms, most *Candida* sp. are not pathogenic unless the host is immunosuppressed or microbial competition eradicated.

Fungal elements can be detected microscopically in the laboratory after tissue and cellular debris have been removed by heating the specimen mixed with KOH. This process can be completed in 5 to 10 minutes. Because most *Candida* sp. grow aerobically at room temperature, laboratory specimens should not be permitted to remain at that temperature for an extended period before they are analyzed.[11,17] The diagnosis of invasive candidiasis may be more difficult, particularly since a positive blood culture may not be evidence of disseminated infection.[14] Further, *Candida* growth in blood culture may result from contamination from *Candida* sp. present on the skin. The diagnosis of some invasive candidiasis may require a biopsy of the tissue. In a nursing home, oral candidiasis in an immunocompetent patient is likely to be diagnosed clinically and treated without laboratory confirmation.

The physical environment

Mrs. Sanders's oral candidiasis was almost certainly caused by her own endogenous *Can-*

dida sp. Carriage of *Candida* sp. in the mouth is common in normal healthy people. Little is known about factors that cause variation of strains of *Candida* sp. colonizing an individual. The infant may acquire *Candida* sp. from the mother during passage through the birth canal or from the mother's skin during nursing. Other factors that have been suggested include intimate contact with a carrier, hospitalization, and consumption of certain foods such as fruit juices, uncooked vegetables, and meats contaminated with *Candida* sp.

Colonization of indwelling medical devices, such as an intravascular line or a urinary catheter, may occur, usually by the patient's own endogenous flora. In one study of *Candida* bloodstream infection in hospitalized nonleukemic patients, the two most important infection risks were central lines and bladder catheters.[4] The indwelling urinary catheter may act as a conduit to transfer the *Candida* sp. on the patient's perineal area to the bladder. A well-documented exogenous source of *Candida* bloodstream infection is hyperalimentation fluid, which supports the growth of *Candida* sp. once it has been contaminated.[19] Although oral candidiasis in patients with dentures may occur on the hard palate under the upper dentures, it is not clear whether dentures are a predisposing factor.

A single case of oropharyngeal candidiasis, as with Mrs. Sanders, does not warrant further investigation. However, nosocomial outbreaks of invasive candidiasis, although rare, have been reported.[5,8,10] The study of the epidemiology of *Candida* sp. is hindered by the lack of a convenient or reliable biotyping system, which would allow clearer identification of relationships between epidemiologically linked isolates.[7,9]

The social environment

In the nursing home, where people at high risk for infection intermingle constantly, transmission of many microorganisms, including *Candida* sp., is possible. One of the most important aspects of nursing home life is socialization among residents. Consequently, residents may be exposed to pathogens in the common living areas and from other residents. Factors that may promote the transmission of *Candida* sp. in such settings include fecal incontinence, contamination of the hands after toileting or touching the mouth, and contamination of fixtures and furnishings in the nursing home by ambulatory patients with poor hygienic practices. However, the importance of these exogenous sources in causing *Candida* colonization or infection has not been established.

PREVENTION AND CONTROL

Extraordinary measures to prevent exposure of nursing home residents to *Candida* sp. are not warranted, since most residents are probably already colonized. The guidelines from the Centers for Disease Control and Prevention do not recommend specific precautions (i.e., private rooms, masks, gowns, or

SUMMARY TABLE 2. Nursing home resident with post-antibiotic oral candidiasis

Host-environment model	Case presentation	Factors that influence infectious process	Prevention and control
Host factors	81-year-old woman Noninsulin dependent diabetes	Incompetent or waning immunity resulting from old age and diabetes	Use good hygiene
Microbiologic factors	*Candida* sp.	Probable endogenous infection	Administer oral antifungal therapy Discontinue antibiotic, or if UTI* has not cleared, change antibiotic.
Physical environment	Nursing home	Likely not relevant, except patient's dentures may have promoted candidiasis	Provide appropriate supplies to clean and store dentures, and assist patient as necessary Practice handwashing between patients and certain activities.
Social environment	Elderly patient in a setting with frequent social interaction; person-to-person and environmental transmission possible	Probably not relevant in this case	None

*Urinary tract infection.

gloves) when caring for patients with any form of candidiasis.[6] Promoting good hygienic practices with particular emphasis on good hand-washing by the care staff between patients is among the techniques for preventing the transmission of many pathogens, including *Candida* sp. Although it is not clear how effective hygienic measures such as meticulous mouth care or special attention to moist skin areas are in preventing or at least mollifying superficial candidiasis, they should be part of long-term nursing care. Patients with dentures should be provided with supplies to clean and store their dentures. Such patients must be assisted with denture care when necessary.

Preventing or reducing the effect of candidiasis should be a goal. If immunosuppression is a part of the patient's underlying condition or if the therapy given for another condition will lead to immunosuppression or cause fungal overgrowth, as in Mrs. Sanders's case, care providers must be vigilant for the symptoms of candidiasis. The patient can be spared considerable discomfort by early detection and treatment with an effective antifungal agent. The use of antifungal prophylaxis for certain high-risk patients may be effective but remains controversial.[13,20]

SUMMARY

Candida sp. are commensals, and most healthy individuals are normally colonized with at least one species. *C. albicans* is by far the most common *Candida* sp. causing infection.

Candidiasis results primarily from immunosuppression as the result of a disease, such as AIDS; immature or waning host resistance, as in newborns or the elderly; or therapy, as during immunosuppressive therapy in organ transplantation. Deep, disseminated *Candida* infections are life-threatening and require treatment with toxic and expensive agents. Candidiasis may also be a superinfection when antibiotic therapy eliminates competing bacterial flora and permits resistant *Candida* sp. to flourish.

Most superficial candidiasis in healthy individuals is self-limiting, as it is in others when the cause of immunosuppression or superinfection is removed. Such infections can also be effectively treated with topical solutions.

The prevention and control of candidiasis focuses on (1) preventing *Candida* sp. already present in the host from becoming invasive and (2) limiting the extent and duration of the infection. Nursing care should emphasize good hygiene by patients and staff and observation and examination of high-risk patients for evidence of candidiasis.

REFERENCES

1. Aly FZ. Factors influencing oral carriage of yeast among individuals with diabetes mellitus. *Epidemiol Infect.* 1992;109:507-518.
2. Bartholomew GA, Rodu B, Bell DS. Oral candidiasis in patients with diabetes mellitus: a thorough analysis. *Diabetes Care.* 1987;10:607-612.
3. Beck-Sague CM, Jarvis WR: Secular trends in the epidemiology of nosocomial fungal infections in the United States, 1980 to 1990. *J Infect Dis.* 1993; 167:1247-51.
4. Bross J, et al. Risk factors for nosocomial candidemia: a case-control study in adults without leukemia. *Am J Med.* 1989;87:614-620.
5. Burnie JP, et al. Outbreak of systemic *Candida albicans* in intensive care unit caused by cross infection. *Br Med J.* 1985;190:746-748.
6. Centers for Disease Control. *CDC Guidelines for Isolation Precautions in Hospitals.* HHS Pub (CDC) 83-8314, Atlanta: Centers for Disease Control; 1983.
7. Crislip MA, Edwards JE Jr. *Candida albicans* and related species. In Gorbach SL, Bartlett JG, Blacklow NR, eds. *Infectious Diseases.* New York: W. B. Saunders Co.; 1992.
8. Doebbeling BN, et al. Restriction fragment analysis of a *Candida tropicalis* outbreak of sternal wound infection. *J Clin Microbiol.* 1991;29:1268-1270.
9. Hunter PR. A critical review of typing methods for *Candida albicans* and their applications. *Crit Rev Microbiol.* 1991;17:417-434.
10. Hunter PR, Harrison GA, Fraser CA. Cross-infection and diversity of *Candida albicans* strain carriage in patients with nursing staff on an intensive care unit. *J Med Vet Mycol.* 1990;28:317-325.
11. Kwon-Chung KJ, Bennett JE. *Medical mycology.* Philadelphia, PA: Lea & Febiger; 1992.

12. McCarthy GM. Host factors associated with HIV-related oral candidiasis: a review. *Oral Surg Oral Med Oral Pathol*. 1992;73:181-186.

13. Meunier F. Prophylaxis of fungal infections. In Bennett JE, Hay RJ, Peterson PK, eds. *New Strategies in Fungal Disease*. Edinburgh: Churchill Livingstone; 1992.

14. Meunier-Carpentier F, Kiehn TE, Armstrong D. Fungemia in the immunocompromised host. *Am J Med*. 1981;71:363-370.

15. Roberts SOB, Hay RJ, MacKenzie DWR. *A Clinician's Guide to Fungal Disease*. New York, NY: Marcel Dekker, Inc.; 1984.

16. Sharp AM, Odd FC, Evans EG. *Candida* strains from neonates in a special care baby unit. *Arch Dis Child*. 1992;26(1 spec no):48-52.

17. Warren NG, Shadomy HJ. Yeast of medical importance. In Balows A et al, eds. *Manual of Clinical Microbiology*, 5th ed. Washington, DC: American Society for Microbiology; 1991.

18. Wilkieson C, et al. Oral candidiasis in the elderly in long term hospital care. *J Oral Pathol Med*. 1991; 1:13-16.

19. Williams WW. Infection control during parenteral nutrition therapy. *J Parenter Enter Nutr*. 1985;9:735-746.

20. Winston DJ, et al. Fluconazole prophylaxis of fungal infections in patients with acute leukemia. *Ann Intern Med*. 1993;118:495-503.

Staphylococcal Food Poisoning in a University Cafeteria

KAYE BENDER

CLINICAL PRESENTATION

Stephanie Edwards is a 19-year-old sophomore at a local university. She lives on campus in one of the dormitories. After dinner one evening, she became ill with nausea, vomiting, diarrhea, and abdominal cramps. Five other women who live in Ms. Edwards' building developed similar symptoms that same evening. When others in the dorm found out about the symptoms, most of them thought a gastrointestinal virus was making the women ill. None of these six women was ill enough to seek medical attention.

That same evening Mary Lang, a 20-year-old woman who lives in another dormitory, also came down with nausea, vomiting, and severe abdominal cramps. Ms. Lang was not able to control the vomiting, so her roommate took her to the local hospital emergency room. Ms. Lang was hospitalized and given replacement intravenous fluids and medications for nausea and diarrhea. The hospital, which serves the university town, is relatively small, and the admission of nine individuals, all students from the university, for similar symptoms within approximately 6 hours that evening was recognized as unusual by the hospital staff. The emergency department physician contacted the campus clinic physician at home to report that she had treated eight students that same evening for nausea, diarrhea, and abdominal cramps. The next morning she notified the local county health department that she suspected a foodborne illness outbreak but could not offer any suggestions about the common food that the students might have consumed, since there had not been a major school activity that evening.

The school clinic and county health department personnel interviewed the ill students to obtain a 24-hour dietary history. An analysis of the common foods from the histories indicated that the students had all eaten at the university cafeteria a few hours before developing the symptoms and that every ill student, including Ms. Lang and Ms. Edwards, had eaten either hamburgers or omelets. No students who ate any other foods at the cafeteria became ill, and not all students who ate hamburgers and omelets became ill. Of the 4,000 students, 22 developed gastroenteritis within a few hours of eating in the school cafeteria; only Ms. Lang was hospitalized.

A second-level food history recall revealed that students who were ill and who had eaten either hamburgers or omelets had also eaten mushrooms served on the condiment bar with their hamburgers or omelets. Both Ms. Lang and Ms. Edwards had eaten omelets with mushrooms.[10] Students who did not become ill did not eat the mushrooms. Samples of the implicated mushrooms were taken to the public health laboratory for analysis. Staphylococcal enterotoxin was identified in the sample taken from the condiment bar as well as from previously unopened cans from the same lot. A complete review of the food handling, preparation, and storage procedures maintained by the university cafeteria staff did not reveal any deficiencies such as poor hygiene practices, lack of stock rotation, or inappropriate temperatures during holding periods.

The outbreak was assumed to have occurred as a result of staphylococcus enterotoxin contamination of the canned mushrooms served at the condiment bar of the university cafeteria.

HOST-ENVIRONMENT INTERACTION
The host

Humans are the primary host for staphylococcal food poisoning. This common foodborne illness is rarely fatal. There are no known host-specific factors associated with risk of staphylococcal enterotoxin–induced foodborne illness, though it is speculated that persons who are otherwise ill may be more susceptible. Persons who ingest foods requiring handling after cooking may be at greatest risk.

Typical symptoms include severe nausea, abdominal cramps, vomiting, lethargy, and diarrhea. Both Ms. Lang and Ms. Edwards had most of these symptoms, as did many of the others who visited the local emergency room that evening. Symptoms usually occur 2 to 4 hours after the toxin-containing food has been ingested. Some persons also develop a low-grade fever and slightly lowered blood pressure. Because the symptoms are similar to those of other conditions and may be mild, reported cases may underestimate the actual incidence of foodborne illness. In this outbreak, six women who lived in the dorm exhibited the same symptoms but did not visit the emergency room because they thought they had a gastrointestinal virus. The duration of the symptoms is typically 1 to 2 days and usually only the most severely ill patients are hospitalized. Diagnosis usually is made when several cases are seen in a short time and the common food item can be identified. When symptoms are severe, the differential diagnosis includes other types of microbiologic and chemical contamination of food. Both can be evaluated by public health laboratory analysis of the implicated food and emesis and/or fecal specimens from ill individuals.[10] Laboratory findings must be correlated with the clinical symptoms of those who are ill.

The microbiologic environment

Illness may follow consumption of food or water contaminated with preformed bacterial enterotoxins or toxin-producing bacteria such as *Staphylococcus aureus*. Staphylococcal enterotoxin is heat stable and is formed in cooked foods contaminated by certain strains of staphylococci. Staphylococcal food poisoning, one of the more common food-related illnesses, is not an infection. It is a toxic reaction to poison in food, not the result of staphylococcal infection of the host. Diagnosis is made by culture of a significant number of staphylococci from a sample of the suspected foods, feces, or emesis. Significant contamination is defined as greater than 10^5 enterotoxin-producing *S. aureus* per gram of food. If the food has been heated, and organisms rendered unculturable, a Gram stain of the food samples may expedite identification.[2,1,6]

Foods most commonly contaminated are those in frequent contact with the preparer's hands. Many of these foods are not cooked after handling. The organisms are transferred to the food from the preparer's hands, typically from an infected finger, eye, nasal secretion, abscess, facial pimple, or other colonized or infected break in the skin. Once the bacteria have been introduced into the food, they multiply and produce toxin, especially if the food remains at room temperature or is held in a warmer before consumption.

In this outbreak, the implicated mushrooms were purchased in 68-oz. cans containing pieces and stems. Epidemiologic study determined that the problem was widespread enough for the product to be recalled by the Food and Drug Administration; however, the origin of the staphylococcal contamination was never identified.[3]

The physical environment

Two primary environmental factors are associated with foodborne illness outbreaks. The most significant is the temperature at which the food is held. Once the organism is introduced into the food, it will multiply if held at or above room temperature. Cafeterias, restaurants, and other places where food is prepared for large groups of people and left to stand for an indefinite period are most commonly implicated in outbreaks of staphylococcal foodborne illness. In this outbreak, the condiment bar was prepared before meals and left until the last student had been served. However, the preformed toxin may have been present in the commercial product and not a consequence of growth of staphylococci at the salad bar.[8,9]

The second important environmental factor is the transmission of the organisms from the handler to the food. This transmission may be from an infected open wound (e.g., pimple, cut, abscess) during the food preparation process. Though the source of staphylococcal contamination was not identified in this investigation, it may have occurred during the precanning preparation. Once bacterial contamination has occurred, toxin is more likely to be produced in foods such as sandwiches, salad dressings, cold cuts, and pastries, which require no cooking after the handling and contamination. Many foods hospitable to staphylococcal growth are high in salt or sugar. Occasionally, foods may be contaminated as they are placed in their commercial containers.[9]

The social environment

People often eat commercially prepared foods in convenience or fast food settings. Economic circumstances and workplace pressure may prompt people to work when they have wounds or other illnesses. Preparation of large volumes of food plus pressure to work in spite of illness presents opportunity for contamination of food products leading to possible toxin production, and intoxication of large numbers of consumers.

The hurried pace of today's lifestyle, the routine use of disposable utensils, and the availability of antibiotics may contribute to a widespread though inaccurate perception that individual attention to hand washing and personal hygiene are unimportant to the transmission of microorganisms. To counter this perception, many of the educational sessions presented to food handlers as part of restaurant licensure and worker certification requirements include emphasis on hygiene and food handling techniques.[6,7,11]

PREVENTION AND CONTROL

Prevention of *S. aureus* foodborne illness includes thorough education of food handlers. The community health nurse has a vital role in working with public health sanitarians to prepare educational materials for establishments that handle and prepare food. Temporarily excluding from food preparation those who have open wounds, abscesses, or other sources of purulent drainage will minimize contamination of food. Food handlers in many states are required to use plastic gloves at all times during food preparation to minimize food contamination. Hand washing before handling of each food item during preparation also reduces the possibility of food contamination. It is essential to provide frequent education and reminders to food handlers about the dangers of working with food if they have skin or eye infections. In this outbreak, however, a review of the procedures and physical inspection of food handlers in the cafeteria and cannery failed to reveal any source of contamination or lapses in procedures.[5,7-9,11]

Food establishment managers should periodically evaluate procedures. For example, the time required to process and serve foods should be measured regularly and holding times reduced as necessary to prevent the growth of any microorganisms. Potentially hazardous foods should not be held between 45° and 140° F (10° to 60° C) for more than 4 hours between the beginning of food preparation and consumption. If the food is not consumed within that period, it should be discarded. Perishable foods should be held below 10° C (40° F) or above 60° C (140° F). Containers for storage should be shallow, to allow for quicker cooling, and not covered. Foods commonly held for intermittent consumption are salads in

SUMMARY TABLE 3.   Staphylococcal food poisoning in a university cafeteria

Epidemiologic model	Case presentation	Factors that influence infectious process	Prevention and control
Host factors	Healthy young adults	All humans susceptible	Vaccine not available
Microbiologic factors	*Staphylococcus aureus,* enterotoxin	Contamination of food during preparation or holding period	Minimize food preparation and holding times Cook and hold food at appropriate temperatures
Physical environment	University cafeteria	Large groups to be fed Large amounts of food prepared	Avoid handling food when open wounds present Wash hands Wear gloves Store and handle food properly
Social environment	Mobile society Large-volume food preparation Inadequate food handler preparation	Increased numbers of individuals eating away from home More foods available in group settings More workers handling food	Educate handlers about food preparation, storage, and temperatures Institute effective outbreak control measures Regulate and assess food services

ice beds and hot foods in tubs over hot water.[1,8]

Control of foodborne illness outbreaks requires rapid identification of the source and interruption of transmission. A careful history of the onset of the symptoms and a complete dietary recall are invaluable.[4] Comparison of the histories and recall lists of several ill individuals will often reveal common items once contaminated food is identified. Food-handling techniques, methods of storage, and health status of food handlers should be assessed. All suspected outbreaks and individual cases of foodborne illness are reportable to local health authorities in all 50 states and territories of the U.S.[9,11]

SUMMARY

Staphylococcal foodborne illness is the most common food poisoning in the United States. The onset occurs approximately 2 to 4 hours after the contaminated food has been ingested. Typical symptoms include nausea, vomiting, abdominal cramps, and diarrhea. The symptoms last for 1 to 2 days. Simultaneous presentation of a number of ill individuals who share a food history suggests foodborne illness.

S. aureus may be introduced into food from a cut in the finger or other wound of the food handler. If the contaminated food is allowed to remain at or above room temperature, the organism will multiply and produce toxin. Enterotoxin may be identified in the emesis or stool of the affected individual and from the contaminated food.

Control of an outbreak requires careful case finding and history taking to identify the food source and perhaps the associated food handler or processing problem. In this university outbreak, histories revealed that the students who became ill, including Ms. Lang and Ms. Edwards, had eaten hamburgers or omelets from the cafeteria, but only those who added mushrooms to their food became ill. A review of the food-handling techniques did not indicate that food preparation procedures were the problem. The history taking and case finding afford the community health nurse an excellent opportunity to provide health teaching related to the transmission of foodborne illnesses. The education of food handlers must include a review of the importance of proper food handling and storage techniques as well as the importance of excluding infected food handlers from food preparation.

REFERENCES

1. Angelotti R, Foter MJ, Lewis KH: Time-temperature effects on salmonellae and staphylococci in foods, *Am J Public Health* 51:76-83, 1961.
2. Beneson AS: Control of communicable diseases in man. Washington, 1990, American Public Health Association.
3. Centers for Disease Control: Multiple outbreaks of staphylococcal food poisoning caused by canned mushrooms, *MMWR* 38(24), 1989.
4. Centers for Disease Control: Self-Study Training Course No. 3016-G. Atlanta, Georgia.
5. Clemen-Stone S, Eigsti DG, McGuire S: *Comprehensive family and community health,* ed 3, Chapter 10. St. Louis, 1991, Mosby.
6. Fuerst R: *Microbiology in health and disease,* Chapter 28. Philadelphia, 1983, Saunders.
7. Holmberg SD, Blake PA: Staphylococcus food poisoning in the United States: New facts and old misconceptions, *JAMA* 251(4):487-89, 1984.
8. Longree K, Armbuster G: *Quantity food sanitation,* Chapter 4. New York, 1987, Wiley.
9. Mausner J, Kramer S: *Epidemiology: An introductory text,* Chapter 11. Philadelphia, 1985, Saunders.
10. Mississippi State Department of Health: Internal Case Reports, Jackson, Mississippi, 1988.
11. Werner SB: Food Poisoning. In Last W, Wallace RB, eds: *Public health and preventive medicine,* Connecticut, 1992, Appleton and Lange.

Pseudomonas Bloodstream Infection from an Arterial Line

CANDACE FRIEDMAN

CLINICAL PRESENTATION

Thomas Applegate, age 72, was admitted to the intensive care unit after he was seen in the emergency room with chronic obstructive pulmonary disease (COPD), acute pneumonia, and hypotension. Mr. Applegate had a 40-year history of smoking and had been hospitalized several times within the past 3 years, most recently for a severe respiratory infection. The night before this admission he complained of mild dyspnea, fever, cough, severe pleuritic pain, and a shaking chill. The emergency room staff inserted a central venous catheter (CVC) and Mr. Applegate was started on cefuroxime for suspected pneumococcal pneumonia.

On Mr. Applegate's admission to the intensive care unit a 20-gauge arterial catheter was inserted percutaneously into his right radial artery to allow for continuous hemodynamic monitoring. The arterial site was prepared by the intravenous therapy nurse specialist, who applied an iodophor solution that was allowed to dry before the catheter was inserted. The nurse washed her hands, wore gloves and a mask, and used a sterile drape during the procedure. After insertion, the catheter was firmly anchored to the skin and the insertion site covered with a sterile dressing.

Mr. Applegate's physician ordered frequent blood gas analyses during the first 48 hours of his ICU care. During each sampling procedure the stopcock on the arterial system was opened for withdrawal of the blood specimen. Mr. Applegate had low-grade fevers and a WBC of 11,900/mm^3 during the first 2 days in the ICU. On day 3 his temperature rose to 39.5° C (103.1° F), and he became flushed and complained of chills. His white blood cell count was elevated to 18,500/mm^3 with a white blood cell differential showing an increase in the proportion of young forms of polymorphonuclear leukocytes ("left shift"). Mr. Applegate's physician was called. Suspecting a bloodstream infection, she ordered that blood cultures be obtained via peripheral venipuncture.

There was no apparent source for the bloodstream infection, such as a wound, urinary tract infection, or empyema. However, bacteremia is often related to the use of vascular devices. Mr. Applegate had both a CVC and arterial catheter. As part of the routine assessment of the catheter site, his nurse found that the exit site of the CVC looked clean without redness or drainage, but the exit site of the arterial catheter was reddened and inflamed. Because of the risk of serious infection, the arterial catheter was removed, and its tip cultured, and blood cultures were obtained. Mr. Applegate's fever subsided; his blood culture grew *Pseudomonas aeruginosa*.

The host

The first report of septic endocarditis originating from an arterial catheter was published in 1970. Since then there have been many reports of infections resulting from the use of such catheters. Arterial catheter–associated sepsis is reported to occur in 1% of patients in whom these devices are used.[6]

Patients with serious underlying disease develop nosocomial bloodstream infection more frequently than other patients.[9] The incidence of nosocomial bacteremia is two to three times as high in elderly patients as in younger persons.[5] Thus, Mr. Applegate's age, COPD, and other health problems placed him at significant risk for nosocomial infection. Many patients who are critically ill require invasive devices such as urethral catheters, endotracheal tubes, vascular access devices, and other devices that bypass normal body defense mechanisms. These may serve as points of entry for microorganisms.

The microbiologic environment

Pseudomonas aeruginosa is a gram-negative, aerobic, motile, straight or slightly curved rod-shaped bacterium. Some strains produce fluorescent pigments. The bluish-green pigment pyocyanin, found in more than half of clinical isolates, is the origin of the name *aeruginosa.* This pigment produces a characteristic sweet grapelike odor in culture or in body secretions containing the organism.

Pseudomonas is a ubiquitous inhabitant of water, vegetation, and moist soil. It has been isolated from the feces of approximately 5% to 10% of healthy persons, sporadically in moist areas of skin (axilla, groin), and the nose and throat. Most strains require minimal nutrients with only one organic compound as an energy source. Because *Pseudomonas* can thrive in most moist environments, it has been found in medications, whirlpool baths, incubators, antiseptic soaps, eye drops, and intravenous fluids.

Although most healthy persons are not colonized with *Pseudomonas,* broad-spectrum antibiotics may alter normal bacterial flora and allow this relatively resistant organism to flourish. Many patients in intensive care units become colonized by this mechanism.

P. aeruginosa produces toxic substances that enhance its pathogenicity, including endotoxins, proteases, extracellular slime, and leukocidin, which interferes with host defense mechanisms by killing white blood cells. *Pseudomonas* is identified in the laboratory by culture, antibiotic susceptibility, and pyocin, serologic, or DNA typing.

The physical environment

Arterial catheters are used to obtain valuable clinical information, such as blood for O_2 and CO_2 analysis, without the need for repeated punctures. However, these catheter systems may admit microorganisms to the bloodstream and they constitute a foreign body to which organisms can adhere. The components of an arterial line system are the catheter, flush solution, pressure tubing, flush devices, stopcock, and transducer. Bloodstream infection may result from contamination of any of the components. Factors that influence the risk of bacterial contamination to the arterial line include insertion technique and site of placement, preparation of the intravenous system, duration of use of administration tubing and flush solutions, duration of catheterization, maintenance and care techniques, and line access techniques.

Antibiotic therapy also influences risk of infection. Many patients with arterial catheters receive systemic broad-spectrum antimicrobial therapy while the catheter is in place. This was true for Mr. Applegate, who received antibiotics for treatment of pneumonia. Antibiotics often suppress the patient's microbial flora and permit acquisition of hospital microorganisms or organisms from other anatomic sites such as gram-negative bacilli from the gastrointestinal tract. Severe illness and immobility also predispose the patient to a shift in microbial flora to a predominance of gram-negative bacilli.

The heavy use of antimicrobials in hospitals may contribute to nosocomial infections by encouraging emergence of resistant strains. Resistance may make treatment of infections difficult. The genetic determinants of resistance may be transmitted between organisms, and the resistant strains themselves may be transmitted to other patients.

The social environment

Arterial catheters must be placed and maintained using meticulous aseptic practice. It is vital that the nurses who tend Mr. Applegate follow hospital policy regarding maintenance of his catheters and other invasive devices and practice barrier precautions during care.

PREVENTION AND CONTROL

The manipulation that occurs with insertion, delivery, and use of arterial line monitoring systems provides opportunity for contamination and subsequent development of bloodstream infection. Prevention and control efforts focus on avoiding contamination of the system.

Insertion technique and site of placement

The risk of sepsis is more likely with cutdown procedures because of the extent of tissue damage. Percutaneous catheter placement presents a lower risk of infection and is the technique of choice. Mr. Applegate's catheter was inserted in his radial artery percutaneously using aseptic technique.

Most vascular catheter–related infections are caused by microorganisms that invade the intracutaneous tract during or after catheter insertion. It is important to cleanse the skin properly prior to puncture to prevent the catheter from being colonized. Vascular catheter–associated bloodstream infection may begin as a local infection of the catheter site caused by microorganisms that invade the intracutaneous tract during insertion of the catheter or any time thereafter. To remove any microorganisms present and decrease the potential for contamination, the site should be prepared with a skin antiseptic such as povidone iodine or chlorhexidine solution[7] and aseptic technique. The solution should be allowed to dry before the catheter is inserted.

Maintenance of the intravenous system

Mr. Applegate's arterial catheter system was inserted using aseptic technique to prevent contamination. His nurses maintained catheter patency by infusing heparinized 0.9% saline solution through a continuous-flow device distal to the transducer.

Studies suggest that tubing should be changed every 72 to 96 hours and flush solution replaced every 24 to 48 hours.[2,8,11] Mr. Applegate's nurse changed the flush solution daily and changed the administration set at 72 hours the morning of the onset of his bacteremia.

A standard time of 4 days has been recommended for changing peripheral catheters, but at least one study has demonstrated that arterial catheters may be left in place for up to 7 days with no increase in risk of infection.[11] Ducharme et al[4] have proposed that routine replacement of arterial catheters in children is unnecessary. Changing catheters over a guidewire does not appear to influence infection or colonization rates.[10] Mr. Applegate's arterial catheter had been in place 3 days when he developed bloodstream infection.

The site should be kept clean and dry, inspected daily, and dressings changed every 48 to 72 hours. Mr. Applegate's gauze and tape dressing had not been changed before the onset of infection. A closed system accessed through an inline port is preferred to a stopcock system because stopcocks may become contaminated through manipulation. Mr. Applegate's arterial system contained stopcocks for blood sampling. After taking blood gas measurements, the staff thoroughly flushed any accumulated blood from the stopcock and tubing to eliminate a favorable medium for bacterial growth.

Arterial infusions have been associated with an increased risk of nosocomial bacteremia caused by contaminated infusion fluid, presumably because of fluid stagnation due to slow infusion and the numerous manipulations of the system.[8] If contaminated, a dextrose solution provides a readily available source of carbon for bacterial growth. Saline is the safest solution for arterial infusions, because it is relatively inhospitable to bacterial growth.

Outbreaks of infection have been related to inadequate reprocessing of reusable transducer domes, contamination of the transducer head, and contamination of the impermeable membrane in the reusable transducer dome.[1,8] If transducers and domes are reused, they must be sterilized or receive high-level disinfection between each use with strict protocols for drying and storage. The introduction of the sterile disposable transducer dome was a major breakthrough in the prevention of infections.

Another potential source of contamination is the fluid within the transducer assembly. Recommendations for the care of transducers specify that sterile saline or water be used as the interface between the dome membrane and the transducer head.

The arterial system is frequently opened for blood sample withdrawal and manipulated for calibrations. In addition, heparinized fluid is used to maintain patency. Typically excess fluid is withdrawn and discarded before a blood sample can be obtained. The frequency and complexity of these manipulations require concentration and skill. Stopcocks used as blood sampling ports in arterial pressure monitoring systems can be contaminated with bacteria and allow entry of microorganisms into the system.[3] Risk of contamination is increased by frequent manipulations. Stagnant blood within the stopcock may enhance bac-

SUMMARY TABLE 4. *Pseudomonas* **bloodstream infection from an arterial line**

Epidemiologic model	Case presentation	Factors that influence infectious process	Prevention and control
Host factors	72-year-old man with COPD and pneumonia	No immunity Age Underlying illness Break in integument	No vaccine
Microbiologic factors	*Pseudomonas aeruginosa*	Colonization Entry into vascular system	Treat with antimicrobials
Physical environment	Intensive care unit	Arterial catheter system	Select appropriate site Wash hands Wear gloves Carefully prepare insertion site Maintain catheter system aseptically Discontinue catheter as soon as possible
Social environment	Contact with hands of caregiver	Compliance with aseptic technique	Comply with policies, procedures

terial growth if not properly flushed after use.

Stopcocks should be flushed after use until no blood remains, and ports should be covered when not in use. Stopcocks should be placed far enough from the hub of the catheter to allow for easy manipulation during blood withdrawal and to reduce risk of contamination. The number of stopcocks in the system should be minimized. Closed-needle and needleless sampling systems that permit entry through a rubber diaphragm eliminate the use of stopcocks. These administration and sampling systems remain closed once in place and should be discontinued as soon as clinical circumstances permit.[3]

The cooling of syringes for blood gas studies in ice water before specimen withdrawal may lead to contamination of the system. This problem has been eliminated by methods that do not require iced syringes.

Bacteremia has also resulted from transmission of organisms from hands of caregivers.[1] Hand washing before touching any part of the pressure monitoring system is an important element of prevention of contamination.

SUMMARY

The long-term indwelling arterial catheter is commonly used for accurate hemodynamic monitoring and to provide vascular access to critically ill patients. Though these catheters minimize blood vessel damage when many arterial specimens are required, thrombosis and infection can occur. Devices such as completely disposable transducers have greatly reduced the infection risk associated with arterial lines. Many institutions' policies require change of the entire disposable administration system, including tubing, transducer, and stopcocks, every 72 to 96 hours.[8] As new studies are performed and better information

is available, recommendations will continue to change.

REFERENCES

1. Beck-Sague CM, Jarvis WR: Epidemic bloodstream infections associated with pressure transducers: a persistent problem. *Infect Control Hosp Epidemiol* 10:54, 1989.
2. Covey M, et al: Infection related to intravascular pressure monitoring: effects of flush and tubing changes. *Am J Infect Control* 16:206-213, 1988.
3. Crow S, et al: Microbial contamination of arterial infusions used for hemodynamic monitoring. *Infect Control Hosp Epidemiol* 10:557-561, 1989.
4. Ducharme FM, et al: Incidence of infection related to arterial catheterization in children: a prospective study, *Crit Care Med* 16:272-276, 1988.
5. Gross PA, Levine JF: Infections in the elderly. In Wenzel RP, editor: *Prevention and control of nosocomial infections,* ed 2. Baltimore, 1993, Williams & Wilkins.
6. Maki DG. Infections Due to Infusion Therapy. In Bennett JV and Brachman PS: *Hospital Infections,* ed 3, Boston, 1992, Little, Brown.
7. Maki DG, Ringer M, Alvarado CJ: Prospective randomised trial of povidone-iodine, alcohol, and chlorhexidine for prevention of infection associated with central venous and arterial catheters, *Lancet* 338:339-342, 1991.
8. Mermel LA, Maki DG: Epidemic bloodstream infections from hemodynamic pressure monitoring: signs of the times (editorial). *Infect Control Hosp Epidemiol* 10:47-53, 1989.
9. Pittet D: Nosocomial bloodstream infections. In Wenzel RP, editor: *Prevention and Control of Nosocomial Infections,* 2nd ed. Baltimore: Williams & Wilkins, 1993:512-555.
10. Snyder RH, et al: Catheter infection: a comparison of two catheter maintenance techniques. *Ann Surg* 208:651-653, 1988.
11. Widmer AF: IV-related infections. In Wenzel RP, editor: *Prevention and control of nosocomial infections,* ed 2. Baltimore, 1993, Williams & Wilkins.

SUGGESTED READINGS

Banerjee SN, et al: Secular trends in nosocomial primary bloodstream infections in the United States, 1980-1989. *Am J Med* 91:3B-86S, 1991.

Norwood SH, et al: Prospective study of catheter-related infection during prolonged arterial catheterization, *Crit Care Med* 16:836-839, 1988.

Methicillin-Resistant *Staphylococcus aureus* (MRSA) in a Sternal Wound

JEAN M. POTTINGER

CLINICAL PRESENTATION

Edward Michaels is a 70-year-old man admitted to the hospital for a coronary artery bypass graft. He has chronic obstructive pulmonary disease (COPD) and he frequently requires antibiotic therapy for respiratory infections. He controls his adult-onset diabetes with diet and oral medication. The nurses observed a stasis ulcer on his left ankle but no evidence of infection.

Mr. Michaels was transferred to the intensive care unit after surgery. He had postoperative respiratory distress, and weaning him from the ventilator was difficult. Antibiotics were prescribed on the second postoperative day, when he developed a fever of 101.6 F (38.7 C). He was transferred out of the intensive care unit on the fifth postoperative day. The next day his sternal incision was reddened and one day later purulent drainage from the incision was noted. Methicillin-resistant *Staphylococcus aureus* (MRSA) was cultured from the sternal incision and sputum. Mr. Michaels was treated with vancomycin and his infection resolved. Eighteen days after developing the infection he was discharged from the hospital. During Mr. Michael's stay in the ICU, MRSA was cultured from the sputum and wound drainage of two other patients in the same unit.

HOST-ENVIRONMENT INTERACTION
The host

Humans are the primary reservoir of *S. aureus*, but the organism can also be found in the environment. *S. aureus* is part of normal human flora and can be cultured from the nose, throat, and skin of about 20% to 50% of healthy adults. It is not known why *S. aureus* colonizes only certain people or why some individuals are only intermittently colonized. *S. aureus* can persist in the nose, throat, perineum, conjunctiva, tracheostomy, gastrostomy, and wounds. The host defense response is primarily nonspecific. Although circulating antibodies to *S. aureus* are produced during infection, they do not seem to play a major role in overcoming the infection.

Patients at highest risk for MRSA colonization and infection are those with a history of injection drug abuse, serious underlying illness, prior antimicrobial therapy, previous hospitalization, admission to an intensive care unit, or prolonged stay in a health care institution.[3] Medical devices such as intravenous catheters, urinary catheters, and mechanical ventilators place patients at increased risk of colonization and infection with MRSA.

Mr. Michaels had several factors that predisposed him to infection. He was elderly, had two chronic diseases—COPD and diabetes—and often required antibiotics to treat respiratory infections. Because the antibiotics caused nausea, Mr. Michaels often stopped taking them without completing the entire course of therapy. This may have contributed to the development of drug resistance in *S. aureus* already present as part of his endogenous flora. Alternatively, since Mr. Michaels had an extended stay in the intensive care unit, he may have acquired MRSA while there. During Mr. Michael's ICU stay, two other patients were also shown to be colonized and infected. The organism may have been transmitted on the hands of health care workers, as has been demonstrated in investigations of outbreaks of MRSA.[6,10,16]

The microbiologic environment

A member of the family *Micrococcaceae, S. aureus* is a gram-positive coccus that resembles a cluster of grapes when viewed under a microscope (see Clinical Study 17). The species name *aureus* refers to the organism's golden colored colonies on blood agar. The organism is resistant to drying and heat. *S. aureus* produces the enzyme coagulase, which clots plasma and produces thrombi. It is not entirely clear whether antimicrobial-resistant strains of *S. aureus* have specific virulence factors since their virulence appears to be similar to that of sensitive strains.[7,8,13]

S. aureus is a common cause of nosocomial and community-acquired colonization and infection. In 1880 a surgeon identified *S. aureus* as the cause of most abscesses among his surgical patients. The mortality from staphylococcal bacteremia was as high as 80% prior to the discovery of antibiotics.[17] All forms of *S. aureus,* including MRSA, can quickly invade and infect minor breaks in the skin or mucous membranes. The most common sites of staphylococcal infection are surgical wounds, skin, and the respiratory tract. Bloodstream infection develops in about 20% of infected patients.[18]

The progressive development and dissemination of antimicrobial resistance of *Staphylococcus aureus* illustrates the ecologic interactions of the host, physical, social, and microbiologic environments. In 1943 penicillin was found to be an effective treatment for *S. aureus* infections. However, soon after the introduction of penicillin, some strains of *S. aureus* were noted to produce the enzyme

penicillinase, which inactivates B-lactam antimicrobials such as ampicillin, cephalosporins, and penicillin (see Chapter 8). Methicillin, introduced in 1959, was the first penicillinase-resistant semisynthetic penicillin used to treat infections caused by *S. aureus.* In the early 1960s resistance to methicillin was reported in Europe. In the U.S. methicillin-resistant strains of *S. aureus* were first identified in large teaching facilities. The earliest nosocomial outbreak of MRSA infections in the United States was reported at Boston City Hospital in 1968.[1] Since then, MRSA has become prevalent and outbreaks have been reported in many acute and long-term care facilities. Once a strain is introduced into a health care institution, it may be extremely difficult to eradicate. Infections caused by MRSA are of concern because methicillin resistance, often accompanied by resistance to other antimicrobials, leaves few alternative drugs available, making treatment difficult and expensive. Unfortunately, MRSA's prevalence is increasing in the United States, in both acute and long-term care settings.[4]

Resistance to the B-lactamase resistant penicillins confers resistance to oxacillin and nafcillin as well as methicillin. Although strains of *S. aureus* may be resistant to all the semisynthetic penicillins, it is common practice to refer to them collectively as MRSA rather than use the name of specific antimicrobials.

Resistance to methicillin is conferred by a gene carried on the bacterial chromosome (MEC A) that codes for an abnormal penicillin binding protein (PBP). This abnormal PBP has a lower affinity for all penicillins so very little methicillin binds to it. Hence, all B-lactam antibiotics, which must bind to a PBP to disrupt cell wall synthesis and kill the bacteria, are ineffective.[9,11,14]

Some strains of MRSA acquire plasmids or mutations that confer resistance to aminoglycosides and antimicrobials other than methicillin. Resistant strains can become prevalent in the presence of these antimicrobials. Of recent concern is the potential for MRSA to acquire the gene conferring vancomycin resistance from vancomycin-resistant enterococci (VRE). Since vancomycin may be the only drug available to treat some MRSA infections, resistance to this antimicrobial would present serious problems if widespread.

Identification of strains can be important in determining whether a cluster of MRSA infections, such as the one in the ICU where Mr. Michaels received care, is caused by the same or different strains and to link strains to their sources. *S. aureus* strains can be distinguished by bacteriophage typing, restriction endonuclease digestion of plasmids or whole chromosomal DNA followed by electrophoresis, or polymerase chain reaction.[15]

The physical environment

The physical environment can play an important role in the transmission of MRSA. Transmission of *S. aureus* including MRSA occurs primarily by direct contact. Colonized patients and health care providers can harbor MRSA. Transient carriage of the organism on the hands of hospital personnel can lead to transmission from one patient to another. Staphylococci can also be transmitted short distances by aerosols, but the frequency of such transmission is much lower than for direct contact.[3]

MRSA can become established in acute and long-term care facilities. Transmission can occur through contact with contaminated fomites, but this route is much less efficient than direct contact. Physical proximity of colonized patients, especially in long-term care settings, may increase the endemic levels of colonization.

The social environment

MRSA colonization and infection occurs in the community, and community sources have been associated with nosocomial outbreaks. Factors contributing to risk of acquiring MRSA in the community include serious underlying disease and antimicrobial therapy. Injection drug use and sporadic noncompliance with antibiotic treatment also influence risk. Community-acquired colonization is often unrecognized because identification of MRSA requires a culture that is not usually prompted unless signs and symptoms of infection are present.

PREVENTION AND CONTROL

The epidemiology and control of MRSA in acute and long-term care settings have been studied and many measures are reported to control transmission. However, experts disagree about the intensity of interventions required to control the spread of MRSA, and recommendations for management of outbreak and nonoutbreak situations vary widely.[2,5,12,18]

Hands of health care professionals are important in transmitting MRSA between patients.[18] Therefore, hand washing and use of gloves during contact with moist body substances is recommended to prevent its spread. Precautions to prevent the transmission of MRSA include private rooms or cohorting. During outbreaks, surveillance cultures of staff and of patients upon admission and periodically thereafter have been used to identify MRSA carriers. Patients' records have been flagged as part of a strategy to identify colonized persons. Efforts to prevent the spread of MRSA have included policies that prohibit admission of colonized individuals to health care facilities, but this practice is impractical and inappropriate.

Antimicrobial therapy has been used to treat patients and health care professionals colonized with MRSA, especially during periods of high incidence of clinically significant infection. Culture surveys of health personnel are not indicated unless part of an epidemiologic investigation. When surveillance cultures are necessary, it is important to obtain surveillance culture specimens from at least the nares. Other sites (e.g., hands) may be appropriate in some circumstances.

The pattern of antibiotic use can affect the emergence of antibiotic resistance. Policies that limit use of antimicrobials to significant infections, restrict the use of certain antibiotics when narrower spectrum alternatives are available, and encourage specific combinations and dosages of antimicrobials known to be effective but least likely to facilitate emergence of resistance are critical.

Staff education is commonly cited as important for terminating MRSA outbreaks, but it seems to provide only short-term benefits. An education program that provides feedback to staff about incidence of MRSA and monitors compliance with control measures may reduce the incidence of infection.[16]

Because factors contributing to outbreaks vary by institution, there are no standard control measures beyond meticulous attention to hand washing and gloving. Control measures must be evaluated and revised as necessary during the outbreak. In this case study, the infection control practitioner and nurse coordinator of the intensive care unit began an investigation when the cluster of patients with MRSA was recognized. First they reviewed laboratory data for similarities of antibiotic susceptibilities among strains isolated and observed care practices to identify any obvious deficiencies. Although hand washing prior

SUMMARY TABLE 5.   Methicillin-resistant *Staphylococcus aureus* (MRSA) in a sternal wound

Host-environment model	Case presentation	Factors that influence infectious process	Prevention and control
Host factors	70-year-old man History of COPD and diabetes	Age Chronic disease Surgery Past frequent use of antibiotics Universal susceptibility	No vaccine
Microbiologic factors	MRSA	Transmission by direct contact	Prevent inappropriate antibiotic use Treat with vancomycin or rifampin
Physical environment	ICU stay Prolonged hospital stay	Other patients on unit colonized with MRSA	Wash hands and use gloves Cohort patients
Social environment	Noncompliance with antimicrobial therapy in past Inadequate barrier technique used by ICU staff	Noncompliance with antibiotic therapy at home Noncompliance of ICU staff with barrier precautions	Encourage compliance with antibiotic regimen Reinforce appropriate patient care practices and barrier precautions

to each invasive procedure and after each patient contact was unit policy, staff also wore gloves for patient contact during the outbreak. Education sessions were held for all personnel, and unit nursing staff were assigned to monitor compliance with precautions and care practices and to report breaks in technique to the observed individual health care professional. No other patients with MRSA were identified over the next few months. Since the outbreak was contained, cultures of personnel to identify carriers and the environment were not done.

SUMMARY

S. aureus is a cause of significant morbidity and mortality in the community and in health care settings. The most common manifestations of infection include skin infections (abscesses, boils, burns, decubiti) and surgical wound infections. Less common are respiratory infections and sepsis. The prevalence of multiple-resistant, β-lactamase–producing strains like MRSA has increased steadily over the past three decades. MRSA is now endemic in many acute and long-term care facilities. Since transmission is usually by direct contact, successful management of this organism requires consistent application of basic infection control measures such as hand washing and gloving by the entire health care team. In some instances, antimicrobial therapy may be used to eliminate carriage.

REFERENCES

1. Barnett FF, McGehee RF, Finland M: Methicillin-resistant *S. aureus* at Boston City Hospital, *N Engl J Med* 279:441-447, 1968.
2. Bennett ME, et al: Recommendations from a Minnesota task force for the management of persons with methicillin-resistant *S. aureus*, *Am J Infect Control* 20:42-48, 1992.
3. Boyce JM: Methicillin-resistant Staphylococcus

aureus: detection, epidemiology, and control measures. *Infect Dis Clin North Am* 3:901-913, 1989.
4. Boyce JM: Increasing prevalence of methicillin-resistant *S. aureus* in the United States, *Infect Control Hosp Epidemiol* 11:639-642, 1990.
5. Boyce JM: Should we vigorously try to contain and control methicillin-resistant *S. aureus*? *Infect Control Hosp Epidemiol* 12:46-54, 1991.
6. Boyce JM: Methicillin-resistant *S. aureus* in hospitals and long-term care facilities: Microbiology, epidemiology, and preventive measures, *Infect Control Hosp Epidemiol* 13:725-737, 1992.
7. Duckworth GJ, Jordens JZ: Adherence and survival properties of an epidemic methicillin-resistant strain of *S. aureus* compared with those of methicillin-sensitive strains, *J Med Microbiol* 32:195-200, 1990.
8. French GL, et al: Hong Kong strains of methicillin-resistant and methicillin-sensitive *S. aureus* have similar virulence, *J Hosp Infect* 15:117-125, 1990.
9. Gerberding JL, et al: Comparison of conventional susceptibility tests with direct detection of penicillin-binding protein 2a in borderline oxacillin-resistant strains of *S. aureus, Antimicrob Agents Chemother* 35:2574-2579, 1991.
10. Goetz AM, Muder RR: The problem of methicillin-resistant *S. aureus:* a critical appraisal of the efficacy of infection control procedures with a suggested approach for infection control programs, *Am J Infect Control* 20:80-84, 1992.
11. Hackbarth CJ, Chambers HF: Methicillin-resistant staphylococci: genetics and mechanisms of resistance, *Antimicrob Agents Chemother* 33:991-994, 1989.
12. Haley RW: Methicillin-resistant *S. aureus:* do we just have to live with it? *Ann Intern Med* 114:162-164, 1991.
13. Jordens JZ, Duckworth GJ, Williams RJ: Production of virulence factors by epidemic methicillin-resistant *S. aureus* in vitro, *J Med Microbiol* 30:245-252, 1989.
14. Jorgensen JH: Mechanisms of methicillin resistance in *S. aureus* and methods of laboratory detection. *Infect Control Hosp Epidemiol* 12:14-19, 1991.
15. Maslow JN, Mulligan ME, Arbeit RD. Molecular epidemiology: Application of contemporary techniques to the typing of microorganisms, *Clin Inf Dis* 17:153-164, 1993.
16. Nettleman MD, et al: Assigning responsibility: using feedback to achieve sustained control of methicillin-resistant *S. aureus, Am J Med* 91 (suppl 3B):228S-232S, 1991.
17. Sheagren JN: *Staphylococcus aureus*: The persistent pathogen. *N Eng J Med* 310:1368-1373, 1984.
18. Wenzel RP, et al: Methicillin-resistant *S. aureus:* implications for the 1990s and effective control measures, *Am J Med* 91(suppl 3B):221S-227S, 1991.

SUGGESTED READINGS

Brumfitt W, Hamilton-Miller J: Medical progress: methicillin-resistant *S. aureus. N Engl J Med* 320:1188-1196, 1989.

Kauffman CA, Bradley SF, Terpenning MS: Methicillin-resistant *S. aureus* in long-term care facilities. *Infect Control Hosp Epidemiol* 11:600-603, 1990.

Morita MM: Methicillin-resistant *S. aureus:* past, present, and future. *Nurs Clin North Am* 28:625-637, 1993.

Mulligan ME, et al: Methicillin-resistant *S. aureus:* a consensus review of the microbiology, pathogenesis, and epidemiology with implications for prevention and management, *Am J Med* 94:313-328, 1993.

Opal SM, et al: Frequent acquisition of multiple strains of methicillin-resistant *S. aureus* by health care workers in an endemic hospital environment. *Infect Control Hosp Epidemiol* 11:479-485, 1990.

Pritchard VG, Sanders N: Universal precautions: how effective are they against methicillin-resistant *S. aureus? J Gerontol Nurs* 17:6-11, 1991.

Varicella (Chickenpox) in a Pediatric House Officer

EMILY RHINEHART

CLINICAL PRESENTATION

On May 3 the infection control department in a children's hospital was called by a senior house officer who had identified primary varicella in Charlie Hawkins, an intern. The intern had no history of previous varicella infection. He had worked the month before in the hospital's emergency department (ED) and since May 1 had been working in the medical intensive care unit (MICU) caring for critically ill children, some with immunosuppressive illnesses. He had not felt well for the past 24 hours and complained of malaise, loss of appetite, and mild fever. The senior resident who examined Dr. Hawkins noted vesicular lesions on his face, neck, and upper trunk that looked like typical varicella lesions. Dr. Hawkins was an only child who had spent most of his childhood in Puerto Rico. He was married without children. Based on history and physical examination, the senior house officer diagnosed probable chickenpox.

Dr. Hawkins was sent home and advised to rest and take acetaminophen for his fever, tepid baths for the itchy rash, and to use benadryl, calamine lotion, or a similar product to reduce itching. Although his varicella appeared to be typically mild and self-limited, varicella can occasionally be life threatening in an adult, especially if varicella pneumonia develops. Dr. Hawkins was advised to inform his own primary care physician of his illness in the event he should require hospitalization and treatment with acyclovir. Dr. Hawkins was advised to remain at home until his lesions were crusted. He was told by the occupational health nurse he could not work or come to the hospital for any purpose while he had uncrusted lesions. Dr. Hawkins remained at home for 7 days and returned to the hospital when his lesions were crusted and dried. Upon his return, the occupational health nurse examined his lesions and cleared him to return to duty.

Since Dr. Hawkins had been working with several immunosuppressed children in the MICU, the physicians evaluated each child and gave varicella-zoster immune globulin (VZIG) to 3 of 16 children. Two of the immunized children had leukemia and one had HIV. Nurses were instructed to watch the exposed children for early signs of varicella such as fever and vesicular rash. Those children who remained hospitalized longer than 8 days following exposure were placed in airborne precautions. Two secondary cases developed in children in the unit who reported no prior infection. Fortunately, these were not the immunosuppressed patients. The hospital's occupational health nurse performed follow-up surveillance on staff to determine who was exposed and susceptible. All of the staff had already had chickenpox and no secondary cases occurred in employees.

HOST-ENVIRONMENT INTERACTION
The host

Chickenpox is the primary infection caused by the varicella-zoster virus (VZV), one of the human herpesviruses.[2] A very common infection, it usually occurs during early childhood, frequently in children aged 4 to 7 years who have entered day care or elementary school. Varicella affects males and females equally and persons of all races.[9] In temperate climates the vast majority (95% to 98%) of persons have had a primary infection by adulthood. However, for unexplained reasons, persons raised in tropical climates are less likely (approximately 50%) to have had chickenpox during childhood.[2,3]

A susceptible person who is exposed to varicella has a high probability of becoming infected.[1] This is true especially when the exposure is to a member of the household, such as a sibling. Once the primary infection has occurred, an individual almost always develops lifelong immunity to chickenpox. Immunity can be demonstrated by the detection of serum IgG antibody to the virus. A carefully obtained clinical history of chickenpox is considered by some to be a fairly reliable determinant of immunity.[3]

Chickenpox in children is usually mild and rarely causes serious systemic complications. Infection in adults can be more serious and results in mortality of approximately 4.3 of 100,000 cases.[2] In immunosuppressed patients, such as those with lymphoma and leukemia, the infection may be quite aggressive and lead to disseminated or fulminant disease and death in more than 5% of cases.[9] Perinatal varicella can occur in children born to mothers with infection during the first trimester of pregnancy. Infants born to mothers who are infected 5 days to 48 hours before delivery have a 20% risk of infection. Approximately 30% of these infants die.[7]

The hallmark of chickenpox is a characteristic vesicular rash that may be accompanied or preceded by a mild fever. The generalized rash frequently begins on the trunk and occurs in crops over the course of 2 to 5 days. Lesions can develop on any mucosal surface, including the oropharynx and vagina. Initially, superficial macular lesions appear. These evolve into fluid-filled vesicles commonly described as "teardrop on a rose petal", which are easily recognized by an experienced clinician. The vesicles usually rupture and eventually evolve into crusted lesions. Vesicles that do not rupture become purulent, dry, and crusted. The crusts are not infectious and may remain intact for 1 to 3 weeks. An infected child or adult may have lesions at various stages of the illness.[3,9]

Various varicella vaccines have been developed and undergone clinical trials in the United States and other countries. A live attenuated vaccine has been tested in normal and immunocompromised children and adults in the United States with encouraging results.[5] However, so far no vaccines have been licensed in the United States.

The microbiologic environment

VZV is a double-strand DNA virus with a lipid envelope. It is one of the human herpesviruses which also includes herpes simplex, cytomegalovirus, and Epstein-Barr virus. These viruses are ubiquitous throughout the world.

Although the diagnosis of chickenpox is most commonly based upon history and clinical findings, fluid from a vesicle can be obtained for microscopic examination. A Tzanck smear, which reveals multinucleated giant cells, confirms the presence of herpesvirus.[10] Specific serologic tests for VZV such as direct fluorescent antibody to membrane antigen (FAMA) or enzyme-linked immunosorbent assay (ELISA) can be performed by some laboratories in a few hours.[2] VZV can be isolated in tissue culture. However, viral culture is not used for diagnosis. Serum antibody testing may identify susceptibles but is not usually used for diagnosis.

Once VZV infects a susceptible host, it replicates in the respiratory epithelium.[2] The virus is shed in the respiratory secretions for 1 or 2 days prior to the onset of the vesicular rash, when shedding reaches its peak. Transmission occurs most commonly via respiratory droplets, airborne droplet nuclei, and direct contact with fluid from vesicular skin lesions.[2] Communicability declines as the illness progresses, and contagiousness from a host with normal immune function is limited to 5 to 7 days after the onset of rash.[2]

A susceptible individual like Dr. Hawkins should be considered exposed if he has had face-to-face contact with a contagious person. Children who play in the same closed space or room are also considered exposed. Secondary infections may occur in as many as 70% to 90% of susceptible household contacts.[1,9]

The incubation period for chickenpox ranges from 10 to 21 days, with the majority of cases occurring between 11 and 14 days of exposure. Dr. Hawkins may have unknowingly had significant exposure via face-to-face contact with an emergency department patient who was incubating varicella, or he could have unknowingly been exposed by sharing the same air with an infected patient or family member for whom he did not provide direct care. The patient or the patient's parents may not have been aware of an exposure or Dr. Hawkins may have failed to obtain an exposure history. Dr. Hawkins, in turn, exposed some of his coworkers and patients in the MICU during the 48 hours before he became symptomatic and chickenpox was diagnosed.

VZV remains latent in a host after primary infection, residing in ganglion nerve cells. Reactivation of the virus commonly results in a local rash, shingles, in the dermatome or skin innervated by the chronically infected ganglion. Disseminated infection may also occur in immunosuppressed patients.[9]

The physical environment

Chickenpox is seen throughout the year, especially in nontemperate climates. In temperate climates chickenpox occurs most fre-

quently during the late winter and early spring.[3]

Airborne and respiratory droplet spread, the most common modes of transmission, are enhanced by crowded living conditions such as may occur in homes or in day care facilities, where outbreaks frequently occur. Airborne spread has been described in hospitals where air handling systems have allowed circulation of air from an infected patient to susceptible hosts.[6]

The social environment

Primary varicella infection most frequently occurs during childhood. The widespread prevalence of this disease results in a periodic high incidence of absenteeism from school, parental leave from work to care for sick children, and medical costs.[9] Although some parents may feel it prudent to attempt to avoid chickenpox, infection at an early age is usually mild and usually provides lifelong immunity, which eliminates the possibility of acute varicella infection later in life.

PREVENTION AND CONTROL

Prevention of primary varicella infection in the community is difficult in the absence of vaccine. However, prevention of nosocomial chickenpox is a critical element of infection control programs, especially in pediatric hospitals. A Varicella outbreak in the community may result in introduction of the virus to the hospital. Consequently, all children should be assessed upon admission for immunization status and history of infectious disease, including chickenpox. Susceptible children and their parents should also be questioned about recent exposure to chickenpox in case the child is incubating the disease and may become contagious during hospitalization.

Preventing exposure and transmission within the health care setting requires placement of the infected patient in a single room with negative pressure relative to adjacent spaces with the door kept closed. This strategy should be used in the ambulatory as well as inpatient setting. Many clinics, emergency departments, and hospitals do not have appropriate room and air handling systems to prevent transmission of airborne organisms. This is changing as the importance of controlled airflow has been reemphasized during the resurgence of tuberculosis. These accommodations to prevent transmission of tuberculosis will provide facilities appropriate for managing other airborne organisms, including varicella.

Since chickenpox can be transmitted via the air, management of airflow has a significant role in its control. Like tuberculosis, chickenpox can be transmitted if susceptible individuals breathe recirculated air that has been contaminated by airborne droplet nuclei from an infected person. Consequently, rooms with negative-pressure unrecirculated airflow are necessary for control and prevention of transmission. These rooms must provide a negative airflow in relationship to the corridor and must exhaust air from the room directly outdoors, without recirculation away from any air intake vents (see Chapter 3).[6,8]

Patients with active chickenpox or disseminated VZV infection and susceptible persons exposed 8 to 21 days earlier should be managed with the airborne-disease precautions described above. Health care providers who are known to be immune to chickenpox may care for the patient, using routine precautions when working with body substances, including skin lesion drainage. Those known to be susceptible should be excluded. Gowns and gloves are used for direct contact with lesions. Antibody testing of exposed health care workers who are unsure of their immunity can confirm immunity and limit exclusion from work to those who are susceptible.

A verbal history of chickenpox should be obtained from health care workers at the time of employment. In some health care facilities, antibody testing to determine immunity is part of the routine assessment of all new staff. Other facilities test only when the information will be immediately useful, since past results may not reflect current immune status. Judicious testing may benefit both the health care worker and patients by guiding infection control management, which protects each from exposure and subsequent infection.

Charlie Hawkins probably exposed many of the MICU patients who were in the unit on May 1 or 2. Although those with whom he had direct contact were at greatest risk, other patients, staff, and visitors would be considered exposed if they had been in the area and sharing the same air supply. Patients who were exposed and susceptible should be managed with airborne precautions from the eighth day following the first exposure (e.g., May 9) through the 21st day following the last exposure (e.g., May 23). The precautions include a single room with appropriate negative ventilation and a closed door. Staff who are susceptible should not enter the room.[1]

All exposed immunosuppressed patients should receive varicella-zoster immune globulin (VZIG) as soon as possible, within 72 hours of exposure.[1] Varicella hyperimmune globulin contains high titers of antibody against varicella and can prevent or ameliorate infection. It is especially important for immunosuppressed patients, who may be at risk for mortality due to a primary varicella infection. If susceptible patients receive VZIG, the incubation period may be prolonged; so airborne disease precautions for these patients should be extended to 28 days following the last exposure.[1]

SUMMARY

Varicella is very common worldwide. The primary infection, chickenpox, occurs in most people before adulthood and most commonly

SUMMARY TABLE 6. Varicella (Chickenpox) in a pediatric house officer

Host-environment model	Case presentation	Factors that influence infectious process	Prevention and control
Host factors	Susceptible house officer in pediatric hospital Susceptible children in MICU	All persons susceptible to Infection confers immunity Some children in MICU immunosuppressed Passive immunization may lengthen incubation period	No vaccine Infection produces immunity Give to VZIG for immunosuppressed and susceptible children
Microbiologic factors	Varicella-zoster virus, (VZV) chickenpox	Inhalation of respiratory droplets or droplet nuclei Direct contact with infected fluid from lesions	Check VZV history and recent exposures Know or determine immune status of health care workers Assign immune workers to care for infected patients Triage admissions in health facility
Physical environment	Seasonal in temperate climates; Airborne communicable disease	Crowded living, work, play conditions Close contact in MICUs Air-handling systems	Place infected patients in single rooms with door closed, or cohort Ensure negative airflow with exhaust away from intake
Social environment	Work in pediatric setting	Close contact of susceptibles with those infected during patient care activities	Comply with airborne disease precautions

during early childhood. In children it is usually a mild illness. However, it is a significant concern in health care settings because it can cause serious disease in immunosuppressed children and adults and is extremely contagious. An accurate history and recognition of exposed and susceptible patients and staff are important to prevent and control infections. These measures help identify those who may be incubating chickenpox and those who are susceptible. A varicella vaccine is expected to be available soon in the United States.

REFERENCES

1. American Academy of Pediatrics: Report of the Committee on Infectious Diseases (*The Red Book*). 22nd edition. Elk Grove Village, IL, 1991, American Academy of Pediatrics.

2. Brunell P: Varicella-zoster infections. In Feigan R and Cherry J, editors: *Textbook of Pediatric Infectious Diseases*, ed 3. Philadelphia, 1992, Saunders.

3. Fehrs LJ, Preblud SR: Chickenpox. In Last JM, Wallace RB, editors: *Public Health and Preventive Medicine*, ed 13. Norwalk, 1992, Appleton-Lange.

4. Garner J, Simmons BP: Guidelines for isolation precautions in hospitals. *Infect Control* 4:245-325, 1983.

5. Gershon AA: Viral vaccines of the future. *Pediatr Clin North Am* 37(3):689-707, 1990.

6. Leclair J, et al: Airborne transmission of chickenpox in a hospital. *N Engl J Med* 302:450-453, 1980.

7. Prober CG, et al: Consensus: varicella-zoster infection in pregnancy and the perinatal period. *Pediatr Infect Dis J* 9:865-869, 1990.

8. Rhinehart E, Leclair J: The physical environment. In Berg R, editor: The Association for Practitioners in Infection Control Curriculum, vol 111. Dubuque, 1988, Kendall Hunt.

9. Whitley RJ: Varicella-zoster virus. In Mandell G, Douglas RG, Bennett J, editors: *Principles and practice of infectious diseases*. New York, 1990, Wiley.

Pulmonary Tuberculosis in a Homeless Person

MARGUERITE McMILLAN JACKSON

CLINICAL PRESENTATION

John Seward is a 36-year-old man with a history of mental depression who lost his job 3 years ago and has been homeless since that time. For the past 4 months he has been spending the nights and receiving breakfast and dinner at a shelter for the homeless in a large city. The shelter houses 48 persons. The staff noted that Mr. Seward was coughing and asked him about other symptoms. Mr. Seward stated that he had had a productive cough and night sweats for about 3 weeks. The staff called the public health department tuberculosis clinic and had him escorted to his appointment. The staff at the clinic noted that Mr. Seward had a record in the clinic file of a documented positive tuberculin skin test at age 14, but the record showed he had not completed preventive isoniazid therapy. A chest x-ray showed a left upper lobe cavity. Because active tuberculosis was suspected and Mr. Seward was quite ill, he was admitted to the hospital, placed in airborne-disease precautions, and started on four antitubercular drugs. Two days later his sputum smear was reported positive for acid-fast bacilli. Six weeks after that, a culture of his sputum grew *Mycobacterium tuberculosis* that was sensitive to isoniazid.

After 2 weeks in the hospital, Mr. Seward's cough subsided, his chest radiograph cleared, and his sputum smears were negative on 3 consecutive days. Because sputum cultures may remain positive even when smears are negative, he was discharged to a designated shelter that had adequate facilities, ventilation, and staff to provide proper care for homeless persons with tuberculosis. After completion of the first 8 weeks of therapy and when his culture results were known, his medication regimen was changed to two drugs three times a week for 16 weeks. His medications were given to him by shelter staff at mealtimes which allowed them to observe him taking the medication.[3,4] This strategy is often referred to as "directly observed therapy" (D.O.T.). Mr. Seward will continue to have periodic sputum smears and cultures and medical care at the tuberculosis clinic until his tuberculosis is classified as cured.

HOST-ENVIRONMENT INTERACTION
The host

Host defenses against *M. tuberculosis* are modulated primarily by cell-mediated immunity. Once the pulmonary alveoli become infected with the tubercle bacillus, macrophages, which are attracted to the site of infection by lymphocytes, ingest and kill the bacilli. If the bacilli are not all killed, additional macrophages accumulate, encase the microorganisms, and create a granuloma in the lung. The granuloma may become necrotic (caseate). The organisms may be contained in the granuloma for years and the infection classified as latent tuberculosis (infection with no disease). Alternatively, the organisms can excavate and form cavities, which is classified as active pulmonary disease (box). This immune response also induces development of a delayed hypersensitivity reaction in most persons, which can be measured by tuberculin skin testing within 2 to 10 weeks.[2,6,7]

In the first few weeks of infection, prior to the development of hypersensitivity, the *Mycobacterium* bacilli ingested by the macrophages may not be killed. The infected macrophages may spread to regional lymph nodes and disperse via the lymph system to infected distant body sites. An extrapulmonary lesion may develop promptly or after a period of latency. Extrapulmonary, non laryngeal tuberculosis is usually not transmissible, since aerosolization of droplet nuclei does not occur under usual circumstances.[6,7]

Certain segments of the population in the United States have a high prevalence of tuberculosis infection, including some racial and ethnic groups, homeless persons, current or past prison inmates, alcoholics, injecting drug users, the elderly, persons from nations with a high prevalence of tuberculosis, and close contacts of persons with active tuberculosis.[6]

Approximately 10% of persons with latent tuberculosis eventually develop active pulmonary tuberculosis.[2] For Mr. Seward, the period between infection and development of active disease was 22 years. The risk of developing active disease is greatest the first 2 years after infection. In contrast, persons who are also infected with the human immunodeficiency virus (HIV) have an 8% to 10% annual risk of developing active pulmonary tuberculosis.[14]

Others who face a relatively high risk of progression from latent infection to active disease include persons with silicosis, prior gastrectomy or jejunoileal bypass surgery, malnourishment ($\geq$10% below ideal body weight), chronic renal failure, diabetes mellitus, some malignancies, and those who have received immunosuppressive therapy. Also, persons who have had *M. tuberculosis* infection within the past 2 years, pulmonary fibrotic lesions, and children 5 years old or less may progress more readily to active disease.[7]

Although the true incidence of new infections is not known, screening studies of the homeless have found the prevalence of active tuberculosis to range from 1.6% to 6.8% and the prevalence of latent tuberculosis infection to range from 18% to 51%.[5]

AMERICAN THORACIC SOCIETY CLASSIFICATION OF PERSONS EXPOSED TO OR INFECTED WITH *M. TUBERCULOSIS*

Class 0. No tuberculosis exposure; not infected
No history of exposure and a negative reaction to the tuberculin skin test

Class 1. Tuberculosis exposure, no evidence of infection
History of exposure; negative reaction to tuberculin skin test

Class 2. Tuberculosis infection, no disease
Positive reaction to the tuberculin skin test, negative bacteriologic studies, no clinical or radiographic evidence of tuberculosis.

Class 3. Tuberculosis, clinically active
Clinically active tuberculosis with clinical and/or radiographic evidence of current tuberculosis; bacteriologic isolation of *M. tuberculosis* or positive reaction to the tuberculin skin test

Class 4. Tuberculosis, not clinically active
History of previous tuberculosis or abnormal radiographic findings in a person with a positive reaction to tuberculin skin test, negative bacteriologic studies (if done), and no clinical or radiographic evidence of current disease.

Class 5. Tuberculosis suspect (diagnosis pending)
Diagnosis of tuberculosis is being considered, whether or not treatment has begun.

(Adapted from Jackson MM: Tuberculosis in infants, children and adolescents: new dilemmas with an old disease. *Pediatr Nurs* 19:438, 1993.)

Microbiologic environment

M. tuberculosis is the primary cause of Mycobacterial pulmonary infection in the United States. Pulmonary infection of variable pathogenicity and clinical importance is rarely caused by other members of the *Mycobacterium* genus (e.g., *M. bovis, M. africanum, M. kansaii*). *M. avium* can also cause pneumonia but this organism is not transmitted person-to-person via the airborne route.[7]

M. tuberculosis is an aerobic, non–spore forming, nonmotile bacillus with a lipid-containing cell wall. It is an obligate parasite that infects humans, some primates, and mammalian species in close contact with humans. Humans are the primary reservoir of the organism.

Detection of characteristically shaped acid-fast bacilli (AFB) in laboratory smears of specimens usually indicates *Mycobacterium*. Identification of the species depends on growth on culture medium. *M. tuberculosis* grows slowly, and visible appearance of colonies on solid culture medium usually takes 4 to 6 weeks. Radiometric, liquid media culture techniques and nucleic acid probes have reduced the time required for organism growth and identification, diagnosis, and implementation of appropriate therapies but these techniques are not yet widely available.

Resistance to antitubercular drugs was observed in mycobacteria soon after the introduction of chemotherapy for the disease. *M. tuberculosis* becomes drug resistant through random, spontaneous genetic mutation. These mutations occur frequently enough that treatment with multiple drugs is standard therapy. The resistant organisms may become predominant if the patient does not comply with medication regimens, or the treatment regimen is inadequate. Successful treatment of active infection requires simultaneous administration of multiple drugs consistently for the full course of therapy.

The number of new cases of tuberculosis has increased in the United States since the mid-1980s.[1,6] Much of the increase is attributable to tuberculosis among persons with HIV infection and immigrants from countries with a high prevalence of tuberculosis. In these groups, there has also been an increase in drug-resistant tuberculosis. Outbreaks of organisms resistant to two to seven antitubercular medications[2,3] have occurred in hospitals and correctional institutions in several states, where appropriate precautions were not used.

Transmission of *M. tuberculosis* almost always results from inhalation of droplet nuclei, which are particles of respiratory secretions aerosolized from an infectious person who is coughing, sneezing, or talking. These airborne droplet nuclei are formed from droplets that dry while airborne. They can remain suspended for long intervals, and are small enough to reach the terminal alveoli in the lungs. The likelihood of transmission is associated with prolonged exposure to contaminated air. The number of organisms in the air is a function of the site of infection (pulmonary, laryngeal), forcefulness of cough, number of organisms in the sputum, effectiveness of containment and/or removal of droplet nuclei, and the length of time the infected person has been on chemotherapy.[2,5,7]

At age 14 Mr. Seward acquired his infection from his grandfather, who developed active tuberculosis while living with Mr. Seward and his parents. Mr. Seward was coughing and producing droplet nuclei while he was staying in the shelter for prolonged periods. Transmission from Mr. Seward to other persons could also have occurred there.

The physical environment

Management of the physical environment is important to prevent transmission of *M. tuberculosis*. Controlled airflow can exhaust contaminated air to the outdoors and prevent recirculation. Ultraviolet light, including sunlight, can kill the organism.[7,13]

In the health care setting, biomedical devices have been implicated in transmission: two incidents during autopsies on a caseous lesion,[9,11] an electronic irrigation device used for irrigation of an open tubercular abscess,[8] bronchoscopes and their accessories used for the diagnosis of pulmonary disorders,[12] and hypodermic needles.[10] Fomites such as bed linens have not been implicated in transmission of tuberculosis. Several environmental factors may be associated with the transmission of tuberculosis in homeless shelters. The organisms can survive in droplet nuclei for long periods and are dispersed via air currents.[7] Ventilation systems in shelters do not usually adequately dilute and remove contaminated air. Shared dining, recreational, and sleeping spaces allow for high numbers of persons to be exposed to a coughing person in the same area. The size of the rooms and the number of persons sharing the space affect the probability of transmission. In winter months in cold climates shelters are likely to be crowded, and ventilation from the outside may be diminished,[5] which supports transmission of *M. tuberculosis*.

The social environment

Persons who live in crowded environments, which are conducive to the spread of tuberculosis, may be economically disadvantaged and medically underserved.[5] Consequently, tuberculosis infection or disease in such settings may not be readily recognized in a timely manner or properly treated.

Control of tuberculosis in persons in homeless shelters may be complicated by substance abuse, fear or distrust of medical institutions, mental illness, substandard housing, poor nutrition, communal living spaces, intermittent incarceration or use of shelters and frequent moves from shelter to shelter.

Compliance with drug therapy over long periods may be difficult for the homeless, when concern for physical needs such as shelter, food, and safety take precedence over antitubercular therapy. Further, carrying medications can be dangerous for a homeless person because the medications may be assumed to be illicit drugs.

PREVENTION AND CONTROL

Prevention and control of tuberculosis for the homeless require identification, evaluation, and reporting to the local public health department to ensure appropriate therapy for the patient and to provide assistance in the evaluation of possibly exposed clients, staff, and volunteers. If Mr. Seward had had preventive isoniazid therapy when infected at age 14, his risk of developing active disease would have been considerably reduced—by 69% after 6 months of therapy and by 93% after a year of it.[1]

Environmental measures that may be implemented in shelters for the homeless include evaluation and improvement of ventilation, supplemental air cleaning measures (e.g., high-efficiency particulate air filtration or ultraviolet germicidal irradiation), and smaller community rooms. Shelters that maintain confidential records in accordance with local and state regulations, record the client's name and dates of stay. These records assist in tracking patients for follow-up medical care.

Education of clients, staff, and volunteers should describe the epidemiology of tuberculosis and the local resources for tuberculosis care. Shelter staff and volunteers should receive at least annual skin testing.[5]

Special facilities, innovative programs, and incentives to complete therapy may be needed to ensure compliance and completion of therapy for homeless populations.

Many recommendations for prevention and control of tuberculosis had been adopted by the shelters in Mr. Seward's community because the prevalence of tuberculosis was high. The shelter staff had been educated by the public health department about tuberculosis control, procedures had been developed to ensure that persons with symptoms received proper medical evaluation, and the public health department and community groups had been consulted to assure proper care for homeless persons with tuberculosis. The ventilation systems had been checked and it was determined that additional air-cleaning devices were not needed.[2] All exposed staff, volunteers, and clients in the shelter during the 2 weeks that Mr. Seward was coughing received baseline tuberculin skin tests if recent results were not available and were retested 12 weeks after the date of their last exposure if the baseline test was negative. Those with positive skin tests at 12 weeks (converters) were evaluated for symptoms and had a chest radiograph to rule out active pulmonary infection. Persons with positive chest radiographs had sputum specimens collected and were treated for active disease if the diagnosis of pulmonary tuberculosis was confirmed by culture. Persons who converted were provided preventive isoniazid therapy.[2,5,6]

SUMMARY

Tuberculosis disproportionately affects certain segments of society, such as the homeless,

SUMMARY TABLE 7. Pulmonary tuberculosis in a homeless person

Host-environment model	Case presentation	Factors that influence infectious process	Prevention and control
Host factors	36-year-old man History of UTB infection	Human is major host All humans are susceptible to infection, but some are more likely to develop disease	Recognize infection and disease early, especially in groups known to be at high risk of disease
Microbiologic factors	*Mycobacterium tuberculosis*	Airborne transmission of droplet nuclei Cell wall resists host immune response	Use early therapy for new, inactive infection Encourage compliance with multi-drug therapy for active disease
Physical environment	Homeless shelter	Inadequate ventilation systems Crowded living spaces, creating prolonged contact with susceptible persons	Evaluate ventilation systems Reduce crowding Isolate persons with disease Consider supplemental air-cleaning devices
Social environment	Exposed persons difficult to follow-up for contact investigation and therapy	Congregate living Limited access to care and treatment supervision	Identify persons with disease Facilitate appropriate treatment Educate shelter clients, staff, and volunteers

and can cause extremely serious disease among persons with severely impaired cellular immunity, especially those with HIV infection. Inhalation of droplet nuclei, which are the airborne residual of droplets expelled from an infected host, is the primary means of transmission. Factors associated with transmission in shelters for the homeless include crowding, inadequate ventilation, and poor compliance with drug therapy.

One of the greatest challenges to treatment of this infection among the homeless is the provision of adequate follow-up of patients who have begun therapy. Many individuals do not complete their treatment regimen. This creates an environment in which the transmission of tuberculosis, including multi–drug-resistant strains, can occur.

Prevention strategies should focus on rapid identification and treatment of persons with active disease and latent tuberculosis infections. Ventilation with good exchange of fresh air or the addition of air cleaning devices may aid in reducing risks of transmission of disease.

REFERENCES

1. American Thoracic Society, Centers for Disease Control and Prevention: Control of tuberculosis in the United States, *Am Rev Resp Dis* 146:1624-1635, 1992.
2. Centers for Disease Control and Prevention: Draft guidelines for preventing the transmission of tuberculosis in health care facilities, ed 2. Federal Register 58:195; Oct. 12, 1993.
3. Centers for Disease Control and Prevention: Initial therapy for tuberculosis in the era of multidrug resistance: recommendations of the Advisory Council for the Elimination of Tuberculosis, *MMWR* 42(RR-7), 1993.
4. Centers for Disease Control and Prevention: Management of persons exposed to multidrug-resistant tuberculosis, *MMWR* 41(RR-11):61-171, 1992.
5. Centers for Disease Control and Prevention: Prevention and control of tuberculosis among homeless persons: recommendations of the Advisory Council for the Elimination of Tuberculosis, *MMWR* 41(RR-5):13-23, 1992.
6. Centers for Disease Control and Prevention. Guidelines for prevention of TB transmission in hospitals, *MMWR* 39(RR-17):1990.
7. DesPrez RM, Heim CR: *M. tuberculosis*. In Mandell GL, Douglas RG Jr, Bennett JF, editors: *Principles and practice of infectious diseases,* ed 3. New York, 1990, Churchill Livingstone.
8. Hutton MD and others: Nosocomial transmission of tuberculosis associated with a draining tuberculosis abscess, *J Infect Dis* 161:286-295, 1990.
9. Kantor HS, Poblete R, Pusateri SL: Nosocomial transmission of tuberculosis from unsuspected disease. *Am J Med* 84:833-838, 1988.
10. Kramer F, et al: Primary cutaneous tuberculosis after a needlestick injury from a patient with AIDS and undiagnosed tuberculosis, *Ann Intern Med* 119:594-595, 1993.
11. Lundgren R, Norrman E, Asberg I: Tuberculosis infection transmitted at autopsy, *Tubercle* 68:147-150, 1987.
12. Nelson KE, et al: Transmission of tuberculosis by flexible fiberbronchoscopes, *Am Rev Respir Dis* 127:97-100, 1983.
13. Riley RL, Permutt S: Room air disinfection by ultraviolet irradiation of upper air, *Arch Environ Health* 22:208-219, 1971.
14. Selwyn PA, et al: A prospective study of the risk of tuberculosis among intravenous drug users with human immunodeficiency virus infection, *N Engl J Med* 320:545-550, 1989.

SUGGESTED READINGS

American Thoracic Society, Centers for Disease Control and Prevention: Diagnostic standards and classification of tuberculosis, *Am Rev Resp Dis* 142:7215-7735, 1990.

Rieder HL, et al: Epidemiology of tuberculosis in the United States, *Epidemiologic Reviews* 16:79-98, 1989.

Intensive Care Patient with Ventilator-Associated Pneumonia

MARJORIE J. STENBERG

CLINICAL PRESENTATION

George Moore is a 70-year-old ambulatory resident of a state soldiers' home. He was admitted to the hospital after developing severe right lower quadrant pain and altered mental status. He has had six hospital admissions in the past 5 years. His medical history includes hypertension, chronic obstructive pulmonary disease (COPD), a pack-a-day smoking habit, and sleep apnea. He was admitted to the surgical intensive care unit (SICU), where a pulmonary artery catheter was placed for hemodynamic monitoring.

Mr. Moore was suspected to have a bowel obstruction, and the day after admission he underwent an exploratory laparotomy. The surgeon found carcinoma of the cecum with associated bowel necrosis and performed a right hemicolectomy. After surgery Mr. Moore returned to the SICU supported by a mechanical ventilator, a pulmonary artery catheter, a nasogastric tube, and an indwelling urinary catheter.

Mr. Moore's postoperative course was complicated by the fact that his endotracheal tube extended into his right mainstem bronchus. Subsequently he developed a right middle lobe atelectasis. The endotracheal tube was repositioned, but he required repeated bronchoscopies for the removal of mucous plugs. He extubated himself on postoperative day 3 and tolerated extubation for 48 hours. Two days later he was noted to be increasingly lethargic. Blood gases demonstrated respiratory acidosis, and he was reintubated for ventilatory support.

Eight days after surgery Mr. Moore was febrile. Gram stain of sputum showed 50 polymorphonuclear leukocytes (polys) per low-power microscopic field, 2+ gram-positive cocci in clusters, 4+ gram-negative rods, and 1+ gram-negative coccobacilli. The cultures grew 2+ *S. aureus* and 4+ *Klebsiella pneumoniae* resistant to ampicillin and gentamicin but sensitive to other aminoglycoside antibiotics. Mr. Moore's white blood cell count was 26,000/mm^3 with 70% polys, 10% bands, and 20% lymphocytes. Additional cultures obtained the next day grew the same organisms plus *Acinetobacter lwoffii*. With appropriate antibiotics, Mr. Moore's temperature returned to normal and his respiratory status improved. He was weaned from the respirator 2 weeks after surgery. Despite a urinary tract infection with *Candida albicans*, Mr. Moore was transferred from the SICU to the surgical aftercare floor 18 days after surgery. He continued to progress well, and on postoperative day 23 was discharged to the soldiers' home.

HOST-ENVIRONMENT INTERACTION
The host

Nosocomial pneumonia is a leading cause of morbidity and mortality in ICU patients and those on mechanical ventilation. Mr. Moore had the following signs and symptoms: (1) purulent sputum (more than 25 polys, low-power field), (2) significant respiratory or nosocomial pathogen in a culture of a tracheal aspirate, (3) a white blood cell count above 10,000/mm[3], and (4) a fever above 38.3° C (101° F). These signs and symptoms are consistent with the Centers for Disease Control and Prevention (CDC) definition of nosocomial pneumonia.[3]

Mr. Moore had many of the host factors that predispose a mechanically ventilated patient to pneumonia. Advanced age (over 60), possibly cancer associated with some immune deficiencies, and abdominal or thoracic surgery are risk factors for pneumonia.[2,6] Postoperative pain and resultant guarding reduce lung excursion and gas exchange and promote atelectasis and pooling of secretions in the lungs. Some intubated patients are prone to gastric stress ulcers. These are treated with histamine-2 blockers and antacids in order to reduce the risk of gastric ulcers. Change of the stomach from acid to alkaline supports the growth of bacteria normally killed by acid stomach secretions. A nasogastric tube permits gastric reflux of this bacteria-rich fluid to the oropharynx, colonization of the oropharynx, and possible aspiration into the lungs.[2]

Most patients undergoing surgery incur some degree of nutritional deprivation because of surgery-related fasting. This restriction in food intake may render the patient unable to meet the high caloric demands of breathing and wound healing. Though not present in Mr. Moore's case, nosocomial pneumonia is also associated with prior antimicrobial therapy, failure to elevate the head of the intubated patient, and extended duration of mechanical ventilation.

The microbiologic environment

Pneumonia acquired in the health care setting, unlike that originating in the community, is frequently polymicrobial (i.e., involves more than one organism).[2] These bacteria may originate from the patient's endogenous flora or from the hospital environment. Bacteria from the hospital environment may originate from an adjacent patient and be transmitted to other patients on the hands of health care workers or contaminated invasive equipment. In many health care settings these exogenous bacteria are resistant to the usual antibiotics as a consequence of the selective pressure of previous exposure to antibiotics. Bacteria found on the walls, furniture, and air usually are not associated with nosocomial pneumonia.

More than 60% of hospital-acquired pneumonias are caused by gram-negative bacteria.[7] These organisms are introduced from the skin or mucous membranes into the upper airway, the trachea, and ultimately the lungs, where they colonize the patient in small or moderate numbers. Relatively innocuous colonization can progress to life-threatening infection if the number of specific organisms becomes large, predominate, or is delivered to a susceptible site.

The three bacteria cultured from Mr. Moore's sputum all can cause pneumonia and other infections. Many laboratory reports use a quantification system ranging from 1+ to 4+ to indicate the numbers of bacteria seen on Gram stain or colonies grown on culture plates.

K. pneumoniae, a gram-negative bacillus or rod (GNR), was the bacterium isolated in the largest amounts from Mr. Moore's sputum. This GNR is found in animals, humans, and food and will survive in water or any moist environment. It is found on human skin and is part of the normal gastrointestinal flora. Bowel colonization is an important factor predisposing to Klebsiella infections at other sites. Klebsiella commonly colonizes the upper respiratory tract, particularly that of the immobile patient, which probably accounts for its frequent association with nosocomial pneumonias.[5]

S. aureus was present in Mr. Moore's sputum in somewhat smaller numbers than the Klebsiella. Staphylococci colonize skin, the nose, gastrointestinal tract, and the perineum. These bacteria secrete a variety of extracellular substances which may be toxic and produce abcesses, wound infections, food poisoning, and toxic shock syndrome[5] (see Clinical Study 3). The primary source of *S. aureus* in hospitals is the skin of patients and caregivers; 20% to 50% of health care providers in hospitals are colonized with this organism, but very few are shedders who efficiently transmit the organism to their patients. Colonization in most healthy persons can be of short duration and end without treatment. In some individuals, newly acquired bacteria persist and become part of the permanent flora.[1]

The third organism identified in Mr. Moore's sputum was *A. lwoffii*, a gram-negative coccobacillus widely distributed in nature, water, food, animal sources and sewage. It can be part of the normal flora of the colon, skin, and mouth; it can cause conjunctivitis, ear infections, and pneumonia. Clusters of infections caused by Acinetobacter may indicate a common source outbreak such as contaminated water in humidifiers[5] or serial transmission from patient to patient.

All the previous Acinetobacter isolates from the SICU in this hospital were *A. anitratus*. Three days after the first *A. lwoffii* isolate was identified in Mr. Moore's sputum, the sputum of the patient in the bed next to him also was reported by the laboratory to have *A. lwoffii*. The infection control practitioner, alerted by this second isolate of Acinetobacter in the SICU, began a cluster investigation. As the charts of all patients in the unit were being reviewed, the microbiology laboratory called to report a third isolate of *A. lwoffii* in the SICU. All three patients were on ventilators.

The infection control practitioner's investigation included observation of respiratory care techniques and culture of the hands of Mr. Moore's caregivers using a plastic bag filled with broth media. The cultures revealed *A. lwoffii* on the hands of one respiratory therapist who did not routinely wear gloves when providing respiratory care. His large hands made it difficult for him to find comfortable sterile or examination gloves. Subspecies typing, which compared genetic fragments of the four Acinetobacter strains strongly suggested the therapist and three patients shared a common organism. It could not be determined whether the respiratory therapist was colonized from a patient or if the *Acinetobacter* were part of his own flora. He was advised to wash and shower with an antimicrobial soap and use the proper size gloves, which were ordered for him. During the investigation, personnel in the unit became more aware of their own technique, washed their hands more frequently, and analyzed procedures to identify where breaks in technique might be occurring. Following the investigation and interventions, no additional isolates of this organism were identified in the SICU.

The physical environment

The two most important environmental risk factors that led to Mr. Moore's nosocomial pneumonia were his admission to the SICU and mechanical ventilatory support.

Severely ill patients may be closely clustered in most intensive care units, where multiple invasive life support and monitoring devices breach two important body defenses against infection—skin and the airway. While critical care beds comprise only 8% of hospital beds, one study of 7,367 nosocomial infections identified during a 14-year period found that 26% of nosocomial infections and 41% of the nosocomial pneumonias occurred in ICUs.[7]

Monitoring and fluid administration devices such as central and peripheral intravenous lines have multiple access ports and are manipulated by many individuals. Each manipulation creates some risk for the entry of bacteria into the system. Some compromised patients are unable to clear transient bacteria from the bloodstream. These episodes may lead to sepsis. Organisms can spread via the blood (hematogenously), resulting in or contributing to pneumonia.

The incidence of pneumonia in mechanically ventilated patients is 7 to 21 times that in patients not requiring mechanical respiratory support.[2] Pneumonia is associated with one-third of deaths related to nosocomial infection.[4] The ventilator system can contribute to the introduction of bacteria deep in the lungs. The endotracheal tube (ET) bypasses the upper airway defenses associated with nasal breathing such as filtration and natural humidification of air provided by the nasal passages, reduces ciliary activity, and allows secretions to pool around the ET cuff. The mucosa of the trachea is traumatized by the ET and cuff pressure may cause erosion. The nasogastric (NG) tube, used for feeding and administration of medications, allows oropharyngeal colonization by gastric bacteria and possible reflux of feedings into the lungs. The NG tube may also contribute to the risk of acute sinusitis in mechanically ventilated patients.

Condensate in the expiratory circuit of the ventilator may contain up to 200,000 colony-forming units/ml of bacteria that most often originate from the patient. Manipulation of the circuitry can disturb the flow of the condensate and deposit a large innoculum of organisms into the patient's airway or into the environment. Another potential source of contamination is the respiratory (Ambu) bag placed at the bedside to aerate the patient's lungs during suctioning or transport without the ventilator. The connector from the bag to the patient may be heavily colonized. The practice of leaving these bags attached to flowing oxygen can create a spray of microdroplets containing bacteria into the environment. Spirometers and oxygen analyzers may transmit organisms if inadvertently used on more than one patient without adequate decontamination.

Mr. Moore required frequent bronchoscopies to clear secretions and mucous plugs while in the unit. This procedure requires passage of the bronchoscope through the heavily colonized oropharynx into the lower respiratory tract, and increases the risk of delivery of microorganisms to the lower respiratory tract and pneumonia.[6]

The social environment

The social environment also influenced the course of events in Mr. Moore's hospitalization. In the ICU, he was at risk for acquiring bacteria from caregivers who failed to wash their hands or wear gloves between patient contacts and from breaks in aseptic technique that accompany the emergencies common to intensive care settings. The failure of the respiratory therapist to wear gloves when giving treatments to patients may have transmitted organisms to Mr. Moore, which were ultimately responsible for his nosocomial pneumonia.

Some of the risk for nosocomial pneumonia is not attributable to the hospital. Mr. Moore lives in the assisted-living section of a long-term care facility, where he receives meals and supervision of his medications. He and his friends are free to come and go as they please. They socialize at a local club where they play cards. Mr. Moore smokes on these outings, which compromises his already impaired respiratory status.

When he becomes ill, he is transferred to the nursing section, where he usually occupies a double room. There he may be exposed to the bacteria and viruses of other residents who have been recently hospitalized. Exacerbations of his COPD, which require his admission to the hospital, expose him to still more organisms.

During his most recent hospitalization his children were very concerned about him; they visited frequently but felt they would be unable to care for him in their home. They hoped he could return to the soldiers' home, where the staff and his friends were a source of support.

PREVENTION AND CONTROL

The prevention and control of ventilator-associated pneumonia depend on decreasing the risks imposed by mechanical ventilation, prospectively managing host or social factors amenable to interventions, recognizing and treating infections as they occur, and using surveillance data to identify and interrupt the transmission of organisms to patients by personnel or equipment.

All health care facilities that provide mechanical ventilation should develop standards of care. These should be followed by all personnel. Care should be documented, and all deviations from the standard protocol documented on appropriate flow sheets. It is helpful to maintain the patient in a 30-degree upright position as much as can be tolerated to help reduce gastric reflux and subsequent aspiration. Using sucralfate instead of H_2 blockers for gastric ulcer control can substantially reduce the proliferation of bacteria in gastric contents and minimize the consequences of aspiration. Assigning equipment and instruments to a single patient will reduce opportunities for organism transmission from these sources. The expiratory side of the ventilator tubing must be managed carefully to prevent environmental contamination and accidental backflow of secretions into the patient's lungs. Respirator bags should be changed daily if used frequently or are visibly contaminated or when the breathing circuits are changed.[6] Sterile fluids must be used in humidifiers and nebulizers to prevent these devices from becoming reservoirs of bacteria. Strict ventilator maintenance standards are important and should include a clear delineation of the responsibilities of respiratory therapists and nursing staff. Bronchoscopy of ventilated patients should be used only when necessary, as this procedure has been correlated with the subsequent development of pneumonia.[6]

Infection precaution strategies must be observed in the ICU as elsewhere for all patient contacts. Hand washing and wearing gloves should be emphasized. More sophisticated methods of microbiologic control can be negated by failure to implement adequate cleansing between patient contacts or to wear gloves when administering respiratory treatments or handling the equipment. Aseptic or sterile techniques must be maintained for all manipulations of indwelling lines or invasive equipment. In addition to using these basic infection precautions to protect the patient and staff, caregivers should wear a mask when they suction patients or perform any other procedures that might produce droplets which might reach their face.

Some research has indicated that selective gut decontamination may be accomplished with an oral paste composed of selected antibiotics; however, antibiotic-resistant microorganisms may emerge as a consequence of the selective pressure imposed by such methods. Judicious use of antimicrobial therapy can limit emergence of resistant organisms and disruption of patients' normal flora.

Assessment and change of the patient's social environment may provide opportunities for prevention of infection. Mr. Moore might benefit from the use of nicotine patches that would help ease him through the smoking cessation necessitated by his emergency surgery. Management of pain and anxiety promotes comfort and respiratory competence. Elective surgery provides an opportunity to assess and support the patient's nutritional status. When a patient has major thoracic or abdominal surgery that requires him or her to be mechanically ventilated or have a long period of recovery, some surgeons insert a gastric feeding tube at the time of surgery. The feeding tube eliminates the NG tube and its contribution to the risk of pneumonia.

SUMMARY

The natural history of ventilator-associated pneumonia in surgical patients illustrates the

SUMMARY TABLE 8.   Intensive care patient with ventilator-associated pneumonia

Host-environment model	Case presentation	Factors that influence infectious process	Prevention and control
Host factors	70-year-old man COPD Emergency abdominal surgery Cancer of bowel Pain, and anxiety	Immune dysfunction of advanced age and cancer COPD Pain-impaired clearing of secretions	Assess patient frequently Assist in secretion clearance Manage pain
Microbiologic factors	S. aureus K. pneumoniae A. Iwoffi Probably a mix of patient and hospital bacteria	Antimicrobial resistance Bacteria may colonize skin or mucous membranes, then invade	Minimize risk of colonization with careful aseptic technique
Physical environment	ICU is location of highest risk in hospitals Mechanical ventilation Emergency care increases risk	NG and endotracheal tubes are aspiration risk for bacteria-rich fluids in alkalinized stomach Lines to blood or bladder can be portals to lungs	Adhere to standards of care for ventilated patients Discontinue ventilator as soon as practical Do not share care items
Social environment	Regular smoker and occasional drinker who lives in a long-term care facility Frequent hospital admissions in recent past	COPD-impaired lung function Exposure to antimicrobials and nosocomial microorganisms	Have patient discontinue smoking preoperatively

critical interplay of the host and the microbiologic, physical, and social environments. These ill patients challenge the knowledge, assessment and technical skills, and creativity of nurses, respiratory therapists, and physicians. Not all ventilator-associated nosocomial pneumonias are preventable, but it is important to minimize the risk of this serious complication of hospitalization.

REFERENCES

1. Boyce JM, et al: Spread of methicillin-resistant *S. aureus* in a hospital after exposure to a health care worker with chronic sinusitis, *Clin Infect Dis* 17:496-504, 1993.

2. Craven DE, Stegar KA, Barber TW: Preventing nosocomial pneumonia: state of the art and perspectives for the 1990s, *Am J Med* 91(suppl 3B):44S-53S, 1991.

3. Goldmann DA: Contemporary challenges for hospital epidemiology, *Am J Med* 91(suppl 3B):85-155, 1991.

4. Horan TC, et al: Nosocomial infections in surgical patients in the United States, January 1986–June 1992, *Infect Control Hosp Epidemiol* 14:73-80, 1993.

5. Jorgenson JH, Rinaldi MG: *A Clinician's Dictionary of Bacteria and Fungi.* Indianapolis IN: Eli Lilly and Company, 1986.

6. Joshi N, Localio AR, Hamory BH: A predictive risk index for nosocomial pneumonia in the intensive care unit, *Am J Med* 93:135-142, 1992.

7. Wenzel KP, et al: Hospital acquired infections in

intensive care unit patients: an overview with emphasis on epidemics, *Infect Control* 4(5):371-375, 1983.

SUGGESTED READINGS

Craven DE: Nosocomial pneumonia: new concepts on an old disease. *Infect Control Hosp Epidemiol* 9(2):57-58, 1988.

Daschner MD, et al: Stress ulcer prophylaxis and ventilation pneumonia: prevention by antibacterial cytoprotective agents? *Infect Control Hosp Epidemiol* 9(2):59-65, 1988.

Fagon JY, et al: Nosocomial pneumonia in ventilated patients: a cohort study evaluating attributable mortality and hospital stay, *Am J Med* 94:281-288, 1993.

George DL: Epidemiology of nosocomial ventilator associated pneumonia, *Infect Control Hosp Epidemiol* 14:163-169, 1993.

Hanson LC, Weber DJ, Rutala WA: Risk factors for nosocomial pneumonia in the elderly, *Am J Med* 92:161-169, 1992.

Thompson AC, Wilder BJ, Powner DJ: Bedside resuscitation bags: a source of bacterial contamination, *Infect Control* 6(6):231-232, 1985.

Two Children with *Haemophilus Influenzae* Disease from a Day-Care Home

BETH HEWITT STOVER

CLINICAL PRESENTATION

Danny Elden is a healthy 5-month-old boy who receives day care in a private home. Four other children under the age of 3 years are cared for in the same home. The care provider has a 12-year-old daughter and 9-year-old son. After school they assist their mother with the care of the infants and toddlers. Danny received one dose of *Haemophilus influenzae* type B (Hib) conjugate vaccine at age 2 ½ months.

On November 10 Danny's parents took him to the pediatrician because of irritability. He had not been taking formula well for the past 12 hours. His temperature was 41.2° C (103.6° F). He was irritable and had bulging fontanel and nuchal rigidity. He had circumoral cyanosis, pale skin, and rapid and shallow breath sounds. His chest was clear. His heart rate was 166, blood pressure 100/50, and respirations were 44. Danny's WBC was elevated to 34,800 with a left shift showing 76% segmented neutrophils, 14% lymphocytes, 8% monocytes and 2% eosinophils. The pediatrician admitted him to the children's hospital. Danny's cerebral spinal fluid (CSF) findings were: glucose 12, protein 137, WBC 5200, RBC 100, polymorphonuclear cells 96%, and monocytes 4%. Urine and CSF latex antigen tests were positive for Hib. Gram stain of CSF showed gram-negative pleomorphic rods. Danny was given dexamethasone followed immediately by cefotaxime and ampicillin. His fever gradually subsided, his fontanel became flat, his neck be-

came supple, and he showed steady improvement. By the third day of hospitalization, his CSF and blood culture had grown Hib, β-lactamase negative and ampicillin sensitive. Cefotaxime was discontinued that afternoon and the physician prescribed 10 days of parenteral ampicillin, 4 days of rifampin, and completion of the Hib vaccine regimen. The local health department was informed of the case within 48 hours of diagnosis and told that he had received one dose of Hib vaccine.

Ellen Andrews, a 3-month-old previously healthy girl who received care in the same home as Danny, was brought to the emergency department on November 16. Ellen was the second child of 32-year-old parents who also had a 3-year-old daughter. Both girls received day care in the same home. On November 16 Ellen vomited after her morning feeding, then vomited her next feeding as well. The day care provider called Ellen's mother, informed her of the vomiting episodes, and told her that she thought Ellen had a fever. The mother took Ellen to the emergency department of the local children's hospital. Ellen's temperature was 40.5° C (103.2° F); her heart rate was elevated to 166 with respirations of 42 and a blood pressure of 100/54.

The physicians ordered laboratory work. Analysis of CSF showed a glucose of 10 and protein of 254. The CSF white blood cell count was 7800, with 89% polymorphonuclear leukocytes (PMNs) and 11% lymphocytes, which suggested a bacterial disease. Her white blood cell count was 15,400 with some immature cells present. Urine and CSF latex antigen tests were positive for Hib. Like Danny, Ellen received dexamethasone, cefotaxime, and ampicillin. Her CSF grew β-lactamase negative, ampicillin sensitive Hib. Cefotaxime was discontinued on the third day of hospitalization and she completed a 10-day course of parenteral ampicillin. Her fever gradually subsided. Ellen and her family members received rifampin prophylaxis. The county public health department was informed about Ellen and determined that she represented the second case of Hib at the day care home within a week. The health department recommended that all day care children, their immediate families, the caretaker and her family receive rifampin prophylaxis.

HOST-ENVIRONMENT INTERACTION
The host

Humans are the only known host of *H. influenzae*. The nasopharynx is the primary site of colonization; however, conjunctival and genitourinary tract colonization can occur. Up to 80% of people may have been colonized with *H. influenzae*,[13,14] most with unencapsulated strains (i.e., not type B). Hib, an encapsulated strain, may colonize up to 5% of the population. Factors associated with risk of invasive disease from nonencapsulated strains and Hib are poorly understood, but young children and individuals with certain immune deficiencies are most susceptible.[13]

Meningitis is the most common manifestation of Hib, which has been the major cause of bacterial meningitis in infants in the United States.[1,13-15] Nonencapsulated *H. influenzae* is a recognized cause of early-onset sepsis, pneumonia, and meningitis in neonates.[14] Nonencapsulated strains have been associated with otitis media in infants and young children; risk of infection probably is related to lack of immune experience with *Haemophilus* in this age group and the immature anatomy of eustachian tubes. Two-thirds of Hib meningitis cases in the United States occur in infants under one year of age. Some studies have shown a slightly higher incidence of infection in males, blacks, Navajo Indians, and Native Alaskans.

Some patients with Hib meningitis have a recent history of otitis media or upper respiratory infection. Bacteremia is thought to precede meningitis. Positive blood cultures commonly accompany positive CSF findings. Clinical symptoms include fever and altered central nervous system function, as evidenced by irritability and vomiting. Seizures, nuchal rigidity, tense and bulging anterior fontanel, obtundation, or coma may be present. Coagulopathy, purpura fulminans, and shock occur in some patients.[13,14,17]

In children over the age of 2 years, epiglottitis is the most common manifestation of Hib. Epiglottitis usually presents with a fulminating onset including fever, sore throat, dyspnea, and drooling. Maintaining a patent airway is critical. Orotracheal intubation is preferred to tracheostomy.

Presenting cellulitis is usually preseptal. A warm, raised, reddish-blue area of discoloration is generally present. Arthritis, cellulitis, and pneumonia are most common in children under 2 years of age. Pneumonia with empyema is another major manifestation of Hib. In nearly 50% of cases, pneumonia accompanies other manifestations of Hib (i.e., meningitis, epiglottitis, and otitis). Infections at other sites occur less commonly.[13,14]

Microbiologic environment

H. influenzae is a nonmotile gram-negative pleomorphic coccobacillus and a facultative anaerobe. *H. influenzae* has many phenotypic properties that are used to divide the species into eight biotypes. *H. influenzae* is categorized by biotype and capsule type. The capsule may be associated with virulence. Hib is generally biotype I and, by definition, type b capsulation.[13,14]

Diagnostic methods include Gram stain of the infected body fluid culture, latex agglutination, and capsular antigen detection.[13,17] The two latter techniques can rapidly identify the organism in blood, urine, CSF, or other infected body fluids. Urine of recent recipients of Hib vaccine can also contain Hib antigen.

Antibiotic-resistant Hib has been reported in recent years.[13,14] During the early 1970s ampicillin-resistant strains of Hib emerged in the United States. A plasmid-produced enzyme, β-lactamase, confers ampicillin resistance and occurs in 13% to 50% of Hib. Resistance to chloramphenicol and trimethoprim-sulfamethoxazole, which have also been used in Hib therapy, has been reported. Third-generation cephalosporins such as cefotaxime and ceftriaxone are usually effective against Hib, although resistance has been documented.[13]

Colonization occurs following intranasal inoculation with *H. influenzae*. The individual can become a carrier and occasionally, subsequent infection develops. *H. influenzae* produces compounds that inhibit ciliary activity of epithelial cells. The type b capsule confers resistance to phagocytosis. Children aged 3 months to 3 years lack antibody against the organism. The submucosa of the nasopharynx is penetrated and Hib invades the bloodstream. Studies in animals have shown that bacteria appear in the bloodstream 12 to 24 hours after nasal inoculation. Meningitis usually is a result of hematogenous spread through the choroid plexus, which separates the brain from the sinuses.

Physical environment

Human-to-human transmission of Hib occurs when the mucosa is inoculated with nasal secretions or respiratory secretion droplets from a colonized or infected individual.[17] Hib has been found on environmental surfaces;[8] however, fomites have not been identified in the chain of transmission. Outbreaks of Hib infections, including meningitis, have occurred in day care centers, hospitals and other settings.[2,9-12] Transmission to members of households and among children in close contact with cases are well documented. Healthy adults, including household members and health care contacts of children with invasive Hib disease, have developed Hib epiglottitis and bacteremia after unprotected exposure. However, this is an infrequent event. Invasive Hib infection occurs with bimodal seasonality, which peaks during the spring and fall.

Social environment

Infants and young children who develop invasive Hib are usually from families with older siblings. Infants such as Danny and Ellen, who attend day care, are at increased risk of Hib disease because of close contact with other children who are asymptomatically colonized.[11] Unimmunized infants such as Ellen and incompletely immunized infants such as Danny may develop invasive disease when exposed to Hib.[11]

PREVENTION AND CONTROL

Hib vaccines have been available since 1985.[17] Initially, these were recommended for children 24 months of age or older; however, most cases of invasive Hib disease occur in infants younger than 2 years. Conjugate vaccines, developed since then, are useful in preventing Hib infection in younger infants.[3] Vaccination can now begin when the infant is 2 months of age. A three-dose series is given at 2-month intervals. A fourth dose at 15 months is recommended. The FDA has also approved use of a combined diphtheria-tetanus-pertussis and *H. influenzae* b conjugate vaccine for use in infants and young children.[4] The Centers for Disease Control and Prevention recently published recommendations for use of the Hib conjugate vaccines and the combined DTP and Hib vaccine.[5] The American Academy of Pediatrics[17] and the Centers for Disease Control and Prevention Advisory Committee on Immunization Practices have made specific recommendations for infants and children with chronic illnesses and immunosuppressive diseases.[6]

Medical management includes antimicrobial therapy. Cefotaxime, ceftriaxone, ampicillin, and chloramphenicol are antimicrobials used for treatment of invasive Hib infection.[13,14,16,17] β-lactamase–producing strains are resistant to ampicillin, so therapy usually is begun with an alternative antibiotic either alone or in combination with ampicillin. If the organism is susceptible to ampicillin, ampicillin may be preferred because it may be less costly. The third-generation cefalosporin ceftriaxone has been approved for parenteral administration in one daily dose. When total costs for administering antimicrobials are considered, once-a-day therapy with ceftriaxone may cost less than four daily doses of alternatives. A course of 7 to 10 days is recommended.[10,12,17] When complications associated with meningitis occur, therapy may be extended beyond 10 days. Dexamethasone therapy may be considered for patients 2 months of age and older because it reduces complications of cerebral edema associated with bacterial meningitis. It is begun with the first dose of antibiotic.

Rifampin prophylaxis is recommended for individuals who have Hib infection or who have been exposed to the respiratory droplets of infants and children with Hib disease.[13,14,17] These include infants who have been immunized as well as household contacts where there are other children under 48 months of age who are not fully vaccinated against Hib. Rifampin is given to prevent Hib colonization of the upper respiratory tract. Recommendations for prophylaxis in day care settings are controversial. However, if two or more cases occur among attendees within 60 days, it is generally agreed that attendees and staff should receive prophylaxis.[17]

Patients hospitalized with invasive Hib disease require a private room, and caregivers who have close contact should wear masks.[7] These precautions should be continued for 24 hours after initiation of appropriate antibiotics. The staff should instruct parents and visitors about meticulous hand washing. Some hospitals require family members to wear a mask to standardize management of visitors and on the chance that a family member may have escaped colonization.

SUMMARY

Hib is a common bacterial agent causing life-threatening infection in infants and young children under the age of 5 years. Until recently, Hib has been the most common cause of bacterial meningitis in this age group. Secondary cases of Hib disease have been reported in hospitals, affecting both patients and staff, in day care settings and in siblings and adult household contacts. Immune-deficient individuals are at increased risk for invasive Hib disease. Hib conjugate vaccines have proven effective. A profound reduction in Hib disease in the United States and other countries is attributed to the widespread use of Hib conjugate vaccines. Combination vaccines containing Hib vaccine plus diphtheria, pertussis, and tetanus vaccines are routine for infant immunization. More effective initiatives are needed to increase immunization levels. Agreement regarding indications for prophylaxis of contacts is not universal. Once disease is suspected, patients should be placed in a private room, and staff having close patient contact should mask. Antimicrobial management should include coverage for β-lactamase–producing strains until resistance

SUMMARY TABLE 9.   Two children with *Haemophilus influenzae* disease from a day care home

Host-environment model	Case presentation	Factors that influence infectious process	Prevention and control
Host factors	5-month-old healthy boy 3-month-old healthy girl	Humans are only known host Young age, incomplete immunization series, or vaccine failure	Immunize on recommended schedule
Microbiologic factors	*Haemophilus influenzae* type b	Droplet and direct mucosal contact with colonized secretions	Administer antimicrobial therapy Consider rifampin prophylaxis for contacts
Physical environment	Day care in home setting	Close contact with other potentially colonized and susceptible hosts	Exclude children with known infection
Social environment	Older sibling in home	Older sibling a potential asymptomatic carrier	Report infection to local health department Require vaccine before acceptance to home care

is demonstrated to be absent. All cases of invasive Hib disease should be promptly reported to the public health authorities.

REFERENCES

1. Adams WG, et al: Decline of childhood *H. influenzae* type B disease in the Hib vaccine era, *JAMA* 269:221-226, 1993.
2. Barton LL, Granoff DM, Barenkamp SJ: Nosocomial spread of *H. influenzae* type B infection documented by outer membrane protein subtype analysis, *J Pediatr* 102:820-824, 1983.
3. Centers for Disease Control: Haemophilus b conjugate vaccines for prevention of *H. influenzae* type B disease among infants and children 2 months of age and older: recommendations of the Immunization Practices Advisory Committee. United States Department of Health and Human Services. *MMWR* 40(RR-1):1-7, 1991.
4. Centers for Disease Control: FDA approval of use of a new Haemophilus b conjugate vaccine and a combined diphtheria-tetanus-pertussis and haemophilus B conjugate vaccine for infants and children, *MMWR* 42:296-297, 1993.
5. Centers for Disease Control and Prevention: Recommendations for use of Haemophilus B conjugate vaccines and a combined diphtheria, tetanus, pertussis and Haemophilus B vaccine, *MMWR* 42(No. RR-13):1-15, 1993.
6. Centers for Disease Control and Prevention: Recommendations of the Advisory Committee on Immunization Practices: use of vaccines and immunoglobulins in persons with altered immunocompetence. *MMWR* 42(No. RR-4):1-18, 1993.
7. Garner JS, Simmons BP: Guidelines for isolation precautions in hospitals, *Infect Control* 4(suppl):316-349, 1983.
8. Gilsdorf JR, Herring G: Recovery of *H. influenzae* B from hospital and environmental surfaces, *Am J Infect Control* 15:33-35, 1987.
9. Glode MP, et al: An outbreak of *H. influenzae* type B meningitis in an enclosed hospital population, *J Pediatr* 88:36-40, 1976.

10. Howard AJ: Nosocomial spread of *H. influenzae, J Hosp Infect* 19:1-2, 1991.

11. Makintubee S, Istre GR, Ward JI: Transmission of invasive *H. influenzae* type B disease in day care settings, *J Pediatr* 111:180-186, 1987.

12. McGechie DB: Nosocomial bacteremia in hospital staff caused by *H. influenzae* type B. *J Hosp Infect* 20:159-160, 1992.

13. Mendelman PM, Smith AL: *H. influenzae.* In Feigin RD, Cherry JD, editors: *Textbook of pediatric infectious diseases,* ed 3. Philadelphia, 1992, Saunders.

14. Moxon ER: *H. influenzae.* In Mandell GL, Douglas RG Jr., Bennett JE, editors: *Principles and practice of infectious diseases,* ed 3. New York, 1990, Churchill Livingston.

15. Murphy TV, et al: Declining incidence of *H. influenzae* type B disease since introduction of vaccination, *JAMA* 269:246-248, 1993.

16. Peltola H, et al: Randomized comparison of chloramphenicol, ampicillin, cefotaxime and ceftriaxome for childhood bacterial meningitis, *Lancet* 1:1281-1287, 1989.

17. Peter G, Lepow ML, McCracken GH, Phillips CF, editors: Report of the Committee on Infectious Diseases, ed 22. Elk Grove Village, IL, 1991, American Academy of Pediatrics.

SUGGESTED READINGS

Deitch SR, editor: Health in day care: a manual for health professionals. Elk Grove, IL, 1987, American Academy of Pediatrics.

Donowitz LG, editor: *Infection control in the child care center and preschool.* Baltimore, 1991, Williams & Wilkins.

Marlow DR, Redding BA, editors: *Textbook of pediatric nursing,* ed 6. Philadelphia, 1988, Saunders.

Plouffe JF, Powell DA: Serious infections in adults exposed to children with *H. influenzae* type B meningitis, *Ann Intern Med* 94:785-786, 1981.

Nosocomial Aspergillosis during Hospital Remodel

ROSEMARY BERG

CLINICAL PRESENTATION

Elizabeth Berglune, a 42-year-old woman with acute myelogenous leukemia, was hospitalized for an allogenic bone marrow transplant. She was admitted to a private room on the oncology unit three days prior to the transplant procedure. Ten days after the procedure she suddenly became ill with a fever, chills, and a cough. Her initial chest radiographs were clear, but 4 days later, on post-transplant day 14, her chest radiograph showed bilateral pulmonary infiltrates. The physician began cephalosporin and aminoglycoside antibiotic therapy. The initial cultures of blood and sputum were negative. However, on post-transplant day 16, blood cultures were positive for *Aspergillus fumigatus*. The patient's compromised immune status, the clinical symptoms and culture results led the physician to suspect invasive bronchopulmonary aspergillosis. He began amphotericin B therapy. Ms. Berglune died 22 days after the transplant in spite of aggressive medical care. Within several days of her positive blood culture, *A. fumigatus* was isolated from the blood of two other patients on the same oncology unit. An investigation established that remodeling of the radiology department adjacent to the oncology unit was the probable source of contamination.

HOST-ENVIRONMENT INTERACTION

The host

Two major factors determine the risk of invasive *Aspergillus* infection: the degree of immunosuppression of the patient and the level of aspergillus contamination of inspired air. Nosocomial aspergillosis is seen most often in immunosuppressed patients with granulocytopenia. Patients with acute myelocytic leukemia and those who have undergone allogenic bone marrow transplantation are at greatest risk of nosocomial aspergillosis as a consequence of cytotoxic chemotherapy, antimicrobial therapy, and prolonged granulocytopenia. In recent years the spectrum of underlying diseases predisposing to aspergillosis has expanded. Long-term administration of high-dose adrenal corticosterioids also predisposes to this infection because these drugs interfere with macrophage function. Immunosuppression associated with renal or cardiac transplantation, lymphoma, or burns also places patients at risk for aspergillosis.

The probable incubation period for invasive aspergillosis is a few days to weeks. Since *Aspergillus* spp. most readily reach the host via the respiratory tract, the most common forms of infection are pneumonia and sinusitis. Pulmonary aspergillosis may extend to contiguous organs or lead to disseminated infections. Other forms of aspergillosis include primary cutaneous infection at intravascular device insertion sites[1] and allergic bronchopulmonary aspergillosis (see Clinical Study 20.)

Diagnosis of pulmonary infection is usually difficult because the organism may not be cultured from the sputum despite respiratory infection and, conversely, may be cultured from sputum but represents contamination and not infection. The "classic" clinical presentation of pulmonary aspergillosis is sudden onset of pleuritic chest pain, fever, hemoptysis, and a pleural friction rub, suggestive of pulmonary embolus and infarction. Unfortunately, this syndrome occurs in fewer than 30% of patients.[2] Often the only evidence of infection is prolonged fever with noncharacteristic pulmonary infiltrates that fail to respond to antibacterial therapy.

The microbiologic environment

A. flavus and *A. fumigatus* are important causes of invasive, often fatal fungal disease in immunocompromised patients. After *Aspergillus* organisms have penetrated mucocutaneous barriers, they may cross other natural barriers, including cartilage and bone. They have a propensity to invade blood vessels, causing thrombosis and infarction. Outbreaks of nosocomial aspergillosis may include patients infected by more than one species.

No definitive test for serologic diagnosis of aspergillosis is available at present. Enzyme-linked immunosorbent assay (ELISA) and other serologic tests are being investigated.[6] Histologic examination of infected tissues may confirm the diagnosis, but often post mortem.

The physical environment

The inanimate environment is the source of the organism. *Aspergillus* species are ubiquitous in soil, decaying vegetation, and air. Outside air has 1 to 10 *Aspergillus* colony-forming units per cubic millimeter.[5] Increases in the numbers of *Aspergillus* spores in ambient air in hospitals are related to environmental disturbances, such as construction, renovation,

window air conditioners, and fireproofing. Disturbance of dust above false ceilings also is a significant risk to susceptible patients. Immunocompromised patients usually acquire invasive aspergillosis in the hospital by inhalation of spores. Several clusters of aspergillosis reported among bone marrow transplant recipients have been attributed to faulty ventilation systems.

Routine cultures of environmental samples, such as air, are not indicated because recovery of ubiquitous organisms such as aspergillus is inevitable. In an outbreak, however, cultures of air or other samples may help to identify the probable source of the organism.

The social environment

Social factors affect the risk of nosocomial transmission of disease as they relate to design, construction, maintenance and management of the environment. Those who develop or implement construction policies must collaborate and communicate. In this case, the chief engineer failed to inform the nurse manager of the planned remodel and the construction supervisor failed to install adequate barriers to exclude spore-laden air from the oncology unit. When the nurse realized the patients were at risk, the engineer stopped the construction until barriers were in place. Unfortunately, Ms. Berglune and the two other patients were already infected.

PREVENTION AND CONTROL

Infection control surveillance systems should monitor for aspergillosis, particularly if severely immunocompromised patients are cared for in the hospital.[3] Clusters or small outbreaks may be difficult to recognize because of the small number of patients who become infected. Should an outbreak be identified, a common source may not always be detected; however, construction, defective or contaminated heating, ventilation or air conditioning (HVAC) systems, and other possible environmental disruptions should be investigated.

Prevention of nosocomial aspergillosis requires the participation of many persons—architects, hospital designers, housekeepers, maintenance staff and engineers. Prevention also requires reduction in the spore content of the patient's ambient air. This is achieved by a combination of filtration of supply air, reduction of infiltrating and introduced spores and maintenance of adequate or increased numbers of air exchanges.

The ambient spore content in a patient's room can be reduced by filtration, air exchanges, and general air control. Several studies have demonstrated that high-efficiency air filters (HEPA) can reduce the risk of nosocomial aspergillosis.[2] Maintaining air exchange rates of at least 10 per hour, preventing infiltration of air from surrounding adjacent inside or outside areas, and upgrading corridor air filtration minimize the presence of spores. Aspergillosis may occur even with these controls and a low spore content of air.[4] Further reductions in spore counts can be accomplished with laminar airflow rooms, which maintain 100 exchanges per hour of HEPA filtered air. For some facilities it is desirable to minimize the ambient air content of aspergillus throughout the facility. However, this is a costly endeavor.

The best strategy for reducing the risk of

SUMMARY TABLE 10. Nosocomial aspergillosis during hospital remodel

Host-environment model	Case presentation	Factors that influence infectious process	Prevention and control
Host factors	42-year-old woman immunocompromised	Degree of immunosuppression	No vaccine
Microbiologic factors	*Aspergillus* spores	Airborne transmission	Therapeutic use of antibiotics (amphotericin B)
Physical environment	Construction in radiology department adjacent to oncology unit	Construction barriers not installed; exposure to spores in ambient air	Filter supply air Increase air change rate Seal off construction areas Move immunocompromised patients away from construction areas Clean areas thoroughly after construction
Social environment	Failure to notify oncology staff of construction	Lack of communication resulted in unnecessary exposures	Collaborate when planning construction activities Establish surveillance systems to detect possible clusters of infections

aspergillosis in neutropenic patients remains to be defined. In general, exposure of seriously immunocompromised patients to construction activity should be minimized. Patient care areas should be sealed off from construction activity with impermeable barriers. Hospital ventilation systems should be installed and maintained to provide the proper air exchange rates and pressure relationships in critical areas near construction activity. Air should not be circulated from construction areas into other hospital areas. Hospital engineers should adapt filter maintenance and ventilation system cleaning procedures to maintain safety during construction. After construction, the ventilation systems should be balanced to design specifications and filters should be examined for integrity. Hospital construction areas should be thoroughly cleaned before patients are admitted. The most important prophylactic measure is careful attention to the ventilation system within the hospital.

Treatment of nosocomial aspergillosis in highly immunosuppressed patients is often unsuccessful, and amphotericin B is the only agent with significant activity. Very few leukemic patients have recovered from invasive aspergillosis despite amphotericin B therapy unless their neutrophil count has returned to normal.

SUMMARY

The risk of aspergillosis in hospitalized patients has increased in recent years. This has coincided with longer survival of highly immunocompromised patients, such as those with acute leukemia and other hematologic malignancies and immunosuppressed organ transplant recipients. Careful attention to the management of the air supply to susceptible patients is important to prevent outbreaks, especially when construction is taking place. It is difficult to establish a diagnosis of invasive aspergillosis, but a high index of suspicion often results in empiric use of antifungal therapy. A reliable serologic test may be available soon.

REFERENCES

1. Allo MD, et al. Primary cutaneous aspergillosis associated with hickman intravenous catheters. *N Engl J Med*. 1987;317(18):1105-1108.
2. Bodey GP, Vartivarian S. Aspergillosis. *Eur J Clin Microbiol Infect Dis*. 1989;8(5):413-437.
3. Carlisle PS, Gucalp R, Wiernik PH. Nosocomial infections in neutropenic cancer patients. *Infect Control Hosp Epidemiol*. 1993;14(6):320-324.
4. Iwen PC, et al. Nosocomial invasive aspergillosis in lymphoma patients treated with bone marrow or peripheral stem cell transplants. *Infect Control Hosp Epidemiol*. 1993;14(3):131-139.
5. Klimowski LL, Rotstein C, Cummings KM. Incidence of nosocomial aspergillosis in patients with leukemia over a 20-year period. *Infect Control Hosp Epidemiol*. 1989;10(7):299-305.
6. Spreadbury C, et al. Detection of *Aspergillus fugigatus* by polymerase chain reaction. *J Clin Microbiol*. 1993; 31(3):615-621.

SUGGESTED READINGS

Anaissie E, Bodey GP. Nosocomial fungal infections: old problems and new challenges. *Infect Dis Clin North Am*. 1989;3(4):867-882.

Arnow PM, et al. Endemic and epidemic aspergillosis associated with in-hospital replication of aspergillus organisms. *J Infect Dis*. 1991;164(11):998-1002.

Beyer J, et al. Strategies in prevention of invasive pulmonary aspergillosis in immunosuppressed of neutropenic patients. *J Antimicro B Chemother*. 1994;38(5):911-917.

Meunier F. Prevention of mycoses in immunocompromised patients. *Rev Infect Dis*. 1987;9(2):408-416.

Rhame FS. Nosocomial aspergillosis: how much protection for which patients? *Infect Control Hosp Epidemiol*. 1989;10(7):296-298.

Sherertz RJ, et al. Impact of air filtration on nosocomial aspergillus infections. *Am J Med*. 1987;83:709-718.

Wadowsky RM, Benner SM. Brief report: distribution of the genus aspergillus in hospital room air conditioners. *Infect Control Hosp Epidemiol*. 1987;8(12):516-518.

Weems JJ, et al. Construction activity: an independent risk factor for invasive aspergillosis and zygomycosis in patients with hematologic malignancy. *Infect Control Hosp Epidemiol*. 1987;8(2):71-75.

Penicillin-Resistant Gonorrhea in a Teenage Male

HALA FAWAL

CLINICAL PRESENTATION

In May 1993 James Allen, a 19-year-old man, went to an inner city health center complaining of dysuria and urethral discharge. He first noted some scant, somewhat cloudy urethral discharge 2 days prior to his clinic visit. Within 24 hours the discharge became profuse and very cloudy and was accompanied by burning on urination. This progression of symptoms prompted him to seek care. Mr. Allen had unprotected sexual intercourse with a new female partner about 4 days before his symptoms started.

Mr. Allen was examined by the health center physician, and the urethral discharge was Gram-stained and cultured. The Gram stain showed gram-negative intracellular diplococci. A provisional diagnosis of gonorrhea (GC) was made. Mr. Allen was given ceftriaxone IM and tablets of doxycycline to be taken twice daily for 7 days. Mr. Allen was instructed to refer to the health center for evaluation and treatment all partners with whom he had had sexual contact within 30 days of his onset of symptoms. He was counseled to refrain from sexual activity until he and his partner(s) had completed therapy and were free of symptoms and to return to the clinic if symptoms persisted. Two days later the culture results were reported as *Neisseria gonorrhoeae*, or gonococcus, the agent of gonorrhea. The gonococci produced penicillinase, an enzyme that inactivates penicillin.

HOST-ENVIRONMENT INTERACTION

The host

The major host and demographic factors associated with gonorrhea are adolescence, low socioeconomic level, poor education, inner city residence, young age at initiation of sexual activity, single marital status, large number of sexual partners, inconsistent contraceptive use, mobility, history of gonorrhea, illicit drug use, and recidivism.[6,7,10,11] Gonococcus readily infects humans,[5] and susceptibility is universal. However, not all exposures result in infection because virulence, amount of inoculum, and the presence or absence of nonspecific resistance, or specific immunity, all vary.[11] Reinfection commonly occurs among both men and women, and persons may remain infected for months in the absence of appropriate treatment.[5,10] No vaccine is available.

Gonorrhea, a bacterial infection, is one of the oldest known human diseases.[6,14] It is endemic throughout the world, and in the United States is the most frequently reported infectious disease.[4,5,8] Although it can infect persons of all ages, those under age 30, especially teenagers with multiple sexual partners, are at highest risk.[8,12]

The gonococcus initially infects mucous membranes of the urogenital tract, rectum, oropharynx, or conjunctivae. Usually the infection is localized to the site of original inoculation, but serious morbidity may result if the organism ascends the genital tract to

TABLE 11-1. Clinical manifestations of gonococcal infections

Site of infection	Uncomplicated	Complicated
Urethra	Symptomatic: ranges from scant clear discharge to copious purulent discharge	Epididymitis*
	Asymptomatic	Penile edema, abscess of Cowper's, Tyson's glands, seminal vesiculitis
Various		DGI† manifestations: bacteremia, fever
		Skin lesions: macular, erythematous, pustular, necrotic, hemorrhagic
		Tenosynovitis joints: septic arthritis
		Endocarditis meningitis
Cervix	Symptomatic: red, friable cervical os; purulent discharge from os; bilateral or unilateral lower abdominal tenderness	PID‡ manifestation: endometritis, salpingitis, tuboovarian abscess, pelvic peritonitis, ectopic pregnancy, infertility
	Asymptomatic	DGI
Rectum	Symptomatic: Copious purulent discharge; burning, stinging pain; tenesmus; blood in stools	DGI
	Asymptomatic	
Pharynx	Symptomatic: mild pharyngitis; mild sore throat; erythema	DGI
	Asymptomatic	
Conjunctiva	Symptomatic: copious purulent discharge	Keratitis and corneal ulceration: perforation, extrusion of lens
		Scarring: opacification of lens; blindness

From *Atlas of Sexually Transmitted Disease* by Morse SA, Moreland AA, and Thompson SE, Gower Medical Publishing, London, UK.
*Syndromes listed in parentheses occur infrequently.
†Disseminated gonococcal syndrome.
‡Pelvic inflammatory disease.

cause salpingitis or epididymitis. Infection may extend to the bloodstream to produce bacteremia.[7] Acute salpingitis from gonorrhea is one of the most common causes of female infertility in the world.[6]

There is usually a rapid, local neutrophilic response to mucosal infection, which clinically manifests as a purulent discharge or exudate.[8] The most frequently infected sites are the urethra in men and the endocervical canal in women.[6,7] Symptomatic infection at these sites is characterized by a purulent discharge, usually accompanied by dysuria.[6-8] The infecting strain influences the severity of symptoms (Table 11-1).[7]

Microbiologic environment

Neisseria is one of four genera in the family Neisseriaceae. The genus includes two species, *N. meningitidis* and *N. gonorrhoeae*, that are well recognized human pathogens.

N. gonorrhoeae are aerobic gram negative kidney-shaped cocci that characteristically grow in pairs (diplococci). Gonococci are traditionally differentiated from other *Neisseria* by their capacity to grow on media containing certain antimicrobial agents, to reduce nitrites, and to use glucose but not maltose, sucrose, or lactose. They cannot grow well on simple nutrient agar. The optimal temperature for growth of most strains is 35° to 37° C (95° to 98.6° F).[6]

Humans are the only natural host for *N. gonorrhoeae*,[11,14] which is almost exclusively transmitted by sexual contact or from mother to infant during delivery. Transmission through nonsexual contact or by fomites is extremely rare. The efficiency of gonorrhea transmission depends on the sites infected and exposed and the number of exposures.[7]

The incubation period for acute gonococcal urethritis in men ranges from 1 to 14 days, occasionally longer. Most men develop symptoms within 2 to 5 days. Left untreated, the infection generally resolves within several weeks.[6,7] However, individuals may still be infectious even after symptoms have resolved.

In women, the incubation period for urogenital gonococcal infection is more variable than in men, but most women who develop symptoms do so within 10 days of exposure.[6,7] The clinical assessment of women is often hindered by the lack of specificity of the signs and symptoms and the high prevalence of concomitant cervical or vaginal infections with

Chlamydia trachomatis (see Clinical Study 14), *Trichomonas vaginalis*, *Candida albicans*, herpes simplex virus, and other organisms.[7] Efforts to eradicate gonorrhea are complicated by its short incubation period, the large number of carriers of asymptomatic infection, and the emergence of multiple antibiotic resistance.[4]

Culture of *N. gonorrhoeae* is the standard tool to confirm the diagnosis.[6] DNA probes and other rapid identification tests applied to cultured organisms or directly to specimens are available[7,8,9] and may prove to be important diagnostic tools. Provisionally, a diagnosis may be made by a Gram stain from urethral, cervical, or rectal specimens if gram negative diplococci are seen intracellularly in neutrophils. A presumptive laboratory diagnosis can be made in cervical and rectal specimens if the organism grows on the appropriate selective media and is oxidase positive.[8]

Several methods for typing gonococci have helped define the pathogenesis and epidemiology of these organisms. Two techniques used to differentiate strains are auxotyping and serotyping. Auxotyping distinguishes strains by nutritional requirements. Serotyping distinguishes strains according to the antigenic diversity of protein I, the protein present in the greatest amount in the gonococcal outer membrane. Using these methods, scientists have been able to map the geographic and temporal occurrence of gonorrhea in communities, analyze the patterns of antibiotic resistance, and study disease transmission.[6,7,9]

N. gonorrhoeae resistance to penicillins was identified in the early 1950s.[7] Penicillinase-producing *N. gonorrhoeae* (PPNG), first described in 1976, inactivate penicillins and other β-lactam antibiotics.[6,7,8,11] At least five β-lactamase–producing plasmids of various sizes have been identified and used to track the geographic spread of PPNG. PPNG became endemic in the United States in 1981, has increased dramatically since 1984, and can now be found in almost all major metropolitan areas.[8] As the number and variety of strains resistant to antibiotics increases, there is a decrease in cases caused by penicillin-sensitive organisms.[12] PPNG strains accounted for over 11% of gonococcal infections in the United States in 1991.[3]

The physical environment

N. gonorrhoeae, a very fastidious organism, does not survive long outside the body. It is rapidly killed by drying, heat, disinfectants, and antiseptics.[4]

In the United States gonorrhea is seasonal. The highest incidence occurs in late summer and the lowest in late winter and early spring.[6,7] There are also seasonal fluctuations in antimicrobial susceptibility. The proportion of gonococcal isolates resistant to penicillins and tetracycline is highest in late winter, possibly as a result of seasonal variation in antibiotic usage, access to health care, and in sexual activity.[7]

The social environment

The epidemiology of gonococcal infections is influenced by a number of social factors. The behavioral response to symptoms influences the transmission of gonorrhea. Since symptomatic individuals are more likely to cease sexual activity and seek treatment, infected asymptomatic individuals contribute disproportionately to the transmission of gonorrhea.[7] Most commonly, gonorrhea is contracted from a sexual partner who has minimal or no symptoms, who ignores the symptoms, or who does not realize their significance.[6,8]

The behavioral response is linked to education, demographics, and sociocultural factors.[6] Incidence of infection is highest in males, nonwhites, and inner city populations,[6,7,8] where risk may be associated with poverty, lack of education, and limited access to health care. The reported cases in the United States are tenfold higher in nonwhites than whites. This is partially explained by nonwhites'

greater use of public health centers, from which reporting is more complete than from private practice.[6,7]

The number of cases of gonorrhea reported annually in the United States has declined since 1975, with nearly all of the decrease since 1981 occurring in the white population. Concurrently, the incidence among African-American teenagers increased between 1981 and 1991.[3,12] Illicit drug use and prostitution heightened the risk of gonorrhea and other STDs during the 1980s.[6,7] In the United States, for reasons that are unclear, infection with PPNG has been uncommon in homosexual men with gonorrhea.[6] Furthermore, risk of gonorrhea to homosexually active men has decreased because of a change in sexual behaviors intended to prevent transmission of human immunodeficiency virus (HIV). The use of hormonal rather than barrier contraceptives by women may increase the risk of contracting gonorrhea. A spermicide and/or a diaphragm protect against infection.[7]

The prevalence of gonorrhea in the community may be sustained not only by transmission from asymptomatically infected individuals but also by core group transmitters, who are more likely than other members of the community to contract gonorrhea and transmit the organism to their sexual contacts. Members of the core group are often geographically clustered, usually within inner cities, and of low socioeconomic status. They include individuals who have had repeated episodes of gonorrhea, who fail to abstain from sexual activity despite symptoms or awareness of recent exposure, and who engage in high-risk behavior such as prostitution, prostitute patronage, illicit drug use, or unprotected sex.[7] Many individuals who transmit gonorrhea and other STDs fail to cease sexual activity spontaneously and seek medical care. This underscores the importance of partner notification to bring the sexual partners of infected individuals to treatment.[6,7]

SUMMARY TABLE 11.   Penicillin-resistant gonorrhea in a teenage male

Host-environment model	Case presentation	Factors that influence infectious process	Prevention and control
Host factors	19-year-old man	Age under 30 years Host universally susceptible	Vaccine not available
Microbiologic factors	*Neisseria gonorrhoeae* resistant to penicillin (PPNG)	Repeated exposure from frequent sexual activity Readily invades mucous membranes of urogenital tract Contact transmission	Treat with ceftriaxone
Physical environment	Contact with organism during sex	Seasonal variation	Not applicable
Social environment	Member of a sexually active age group	Inner-city resident Low socioeconomic status Limited access to health care and information Sexually transmitted	Provide education Encourage behavior change Notify and treat partners Promote safer sex practices, including abstinence, condoms, spermicide, and barrier contraceptives

PREVENTION AND CONTROL

Strategies for prevention and control of gonorrhea, including PPNG, are the same as those for other STDs. These include (1) education of persons at risk about risk reduction; (2) screening to detect infection in both asymptomatic persons and in those who are symptomatic but are not likely to seek further evaluation; (3) effective diagnosis and treatment of persons who are infected; and (4) evaluation, treatment, and counseling of sex partners of persons with an STD.[1,2] Also, in the United States, a primary measure used to prevent gonorrhea is to screen high-risk women, since gonococcal infections in women are often asymptomatic. The method and intensity of partner notification, or contact tracing, for gonorrhea varies by locale according to the priorities and resources of the public health sector, but in general is less actively pursued than in the past. One reason for this change is that funds previously used to support gonorrhea control efforts are now being used to combat the HIV epidemic.

Prompted by increasing prevalence of antimicrobial resistance and the findings of the Centers for Disease Control and Prevention's (CDC) Gonococcal Isolate Surveillance Project, treatment recommendations were changed in 1989 from penicillin as the drug of choice to a third-generation cephalosporin.[12,13] The CDC's 1993 guidelines recommend ceftriaxone IM in a single dose or one of several other oral antibiotics in a single dose. These are cefixime, ciprofloxacin, or orofloxacin.[2] Further, because of a high incidence of coexisting chlamydial infection, treatment for gonorrhea includes simultaneous coverage for *Chlamydia*, such as doxycycline.[1,2,13]

Education about risk and behavioral choices should be considered primary prevention measures. Patients should be counseled about strategies to lower their risk of acquiring STDs, including sexual abstinence, monogamy, careful selection of sexual partners, proper use of condoms, vaginal spermicides and barrier contraceptives, and periodic examinations.[1,2]

Early identification and treatment of asymptomatic infection in women is important to prevent complications of asymptomatic gonococcal infection such as disseminated gonococcal infection and pelvic inflammatory disease.[8] When persons seek care for other reasons but are also at high risk for STDs, nurses should evaluate these individuals for risk factors and screen for asymptomatic infections.[1,2]

Diagnosis of gonorrhea or any other STD suggests that the person is engaging in unprotected sex. Therefore, patients such as Mr. Allen should be closely evaluated for other sexually transmitted infections including syphilis, HIV, and *Chlamydia*.[1,2] In Mr. Allen's community, gonorrhea and chlamydial coinfection is common, so he was given doxycycline as antichlamydial therapy.

SUMMARY

Gonorrhea is almost exclusively transmitted by sexual contact. Infection is most frequently seen in people under age 30 who have had several sex partners. The incubation period differs for men and women. Women more often have asymptomatic infection and complications. PPNG is a strain of *N. gonorrhoeae*

that is resistant to penicillin and other β-lactam antibiotics. PPNG is prevalent throughout the world. The current recommendation for antimicrobial therapy is ceftriaxone or one of several other oral antibiotics such as cefixime, ofloxacin, or ciprofloxacin.

Exposures and conditions associated with risk of acquiring gonorrhea, including PPNG, include unprotected sex, multiple sex partners, low socioeconomic status, inner city residence, illicit drug use, and single marital status. Prevention and control measures focus on health education, safer sex practices, partner notification, and treatment.

REFERENCES

1. Centers for Disease Control: 1989 sexually transmitted diseases guidelines, *MMWR* 38(S-8):vii-43, 1989.
2. Centers for Disease Control and Prevention: 1993 sexually transmitted disease guidelines, *MMWR* 42(RR-14):1-10, 47-67, 1993.
3. Centers for Disease Control and Prevention: CDC surveillance summaries, August 13, 1993, *MMWR* 42(SS-3), 1993.
4. Cheng DSF: Gonorrhea. In Parish LC, Gschnait F, editors: *Sexually transmitted diseases: a guide for clinicians.* New York, 1989, Springer-Verlag.
5. Elkins C, Sparling PF: Immunobiology of *N. gonorrhoeae.* In Quinn TC, editor: *Sexually transmitted diseases.* New York, 1992, Raven Press. (Gallin JI and Fauci AS (eds.): Advances in Host Defense Mechanisms Series:8).
6. Handsfield HH: *N. gonorrhoeae.* In Mandell GL, Douglas RG Jr, Bennett JE, editors: *Principals and practice of infectious diseases,* ed 3. New York, 1990, Churchill Livingstone.
7. Hook EW 3d, Handsfield HH: Gonococcal infections in the adult. In Holmes KK and others, editors: *Sexually transmitted diseases,* ed 2. New York, 1990, McGraw-Hill.
8. Knapp JS, Zenilman JM, Thompson SE: Gonorrhea. In Morse SA, Moreland AA, Thompson SE, editors: *Atlas of sexually transmitted diseases,* London, 1990, Gower Medical Publishing.
9. Mårdh P-A, Danielsson D: *N. gonorrhoeae.* In Holmes KK and others, editors: *Sexually transmitted diseases,* ed 2. New York, 1990, McGraw-Hill.
10. McCutchan JA: Gonococcal and chlamydial genital infection. In Braude AI, Davis CE, Fierer J, editors: *Infectious diseases and medical microbiology.* Philadelphia, 1986, Saunders.

11. Morse SA: Neisseria and Branhamella. In Braude AI, Davis CE, Fierer J, editors: *Infectious diseases and medical microbiology.* Philadelphia, 1986, Saunders.

12. Quinn TC, Cates W Jr: Epidemiology of sexually transmitted diseases in the 1990s. In Quinn TC, editor: *Sexually transmitted diseases.* New York, 1992, Raven Press. (Gallin JI, Fauci AS (eds.). Advances in Host Defense Mechanisms Series;8).

13. Schwarcz SK and others: Natural surveillance of antimicrobial resistance in *N. gonorrhoeae, JAMA* 264:1413-1417, 1990.

14. Sparling FP: Biology of *N. gonorrhoeae.* In Holmes KK and others, editors: *Sexually transmitted diseases,* ed 2. New York, 1990, McGraw-Hill.

SUGGESTED READINGS

Evangelista AT, Beilstein HR: 1993 Cumitech 4A: laboratory diagnosis of gonorrhea. Abramson C, editor. Washington, 1993, American Society for Microbiology.

Granato PA, Howard BJ, Deal CD: Neisseria. In Howard BJ and others, editors: *Clinical and pathogenic microbiology,* ed 2. St. Louis, 1994, Mosby.

Young H, Moyes A: Comparative evaluation of AccuProbe culture identification test for *N. gonorrhoeae* and other rapid methods, *J Clin Microbiol* 31:1996-1999, 1993.

Burn Patient with *Pseudomonas* Infection

CANDACE FRIEDMAN

CLINICAL PRESENTATION

While lighting a barbecue, 40-year-old Jane Williams caught her apron on fire. Fortunately, she was able to extinguish the flames, but she sustained a significant burn. When she was assessed in the emergency room, she was diagnosed with partial-thickness and full-thickness burns on her chest, abdomen, and arms that covered about 40% of her total body surface area (TBSA).

Ms. Williams received immediate care in the trauma section of the emergency room. The staff performed several invasive procedures, including insertion of intravascular lines and a urinary catheter. All invasive procedures were performed with aseptic technique to minimize the potential for infection. As soon as she was stable, Ms. Williams was transferred to the intensive care burn unit.

On Ms. Williams's sixth hospital day she developed a fever and hypotension. Her white blood cell count rose from 6,500 to 19,800 mm³. There was greenish drainage from her burn wounds, which were edematous at the margins. The burn wounds were cultured every 48 hours, starting at admission, and from day 4 the cultures grew 100,000 colony-forming units of *Pseudomonas aeruginosa* per gram of burn wound tissue. All blood cultures were negative.

Ms. Williams was treated in the burn unit with supportive care and topical silver sulfadiazine for 8 weeks. Her infection resolved and she was discharged home.

HOST-ENVIRONMENT INTERACTION

The Host

Burns remove an important anatomic protective barrier against infection by destroying skin integrity. A full-thickness burn strips the tissue of its blood supply through complete vascular occlusion, which renders the tissue nonviable. When, as in Ms. Williams's case, the skin barrier is absent and there is altered perfusion to the wound, the risk of infection is a major concern.

One factor associated with the risk of infection is the size of the burned area. Serious infections are not expected in persons with burns over less than 30% of TBSA. The incidence of infections in burned individuals also increases with age. There is a dramatic increase in the risk of infection for persons over age 60.[9] Both humoral and cellular defense mechanisms are modified after a significant burn, especially during the first few weeks. The phagocytic, chemotactic, and bactericidal abilities of white blood cells change. A depressed complement response and the development of anergy to common antigens is frequent in burn patients. This change in immune function permits proliferation of microbes on the wound and systemic invasion. Typically the decrease in host resistance after a burn is a more important determinant of the seriousness of infection than is the virulence of the causative organisms.[9] The status of the cell-mediated immune system may be a reliable predictor of the burned patient's clinical outcome.[4]

The patient's normal flora and the environment may harbor organisms that infect a burn. Most burn infections are endogenous, originating from the patient's own microbial flora. Burke and associates found that burns in approximately 80% of patients were colonized by microorganisms from the patient's own gastrointestinal tract.[1] In addition, increased gut permeability occurs early after burns. This correlates with the extent of burn injury and may result in bacterial translocation, increasing the risk of infection.[6]

Microbiologic environment

Approximately 20% of burn wounds are colonized by cross-contamination.[1] Most mortality secondary to infection results from organisms such as gram-negative opportunistic microbes, particularly *P. aeruginosa.*

P. aeruginosa is a gram-negative, aerobic, motile, straight rod-shaped bacterium prevalent in moist environments including those in hospitals. Most strains can grow with as little as one organic compound as a nutritional source. *P. aeruginosa* is a ubiquitous inhabitant of water, vegetation, and moist soil. It can be isolated from the gastrointestinal tract and stool of approximately 5% to 10% of healthy persons. It can also be found sporadically in moist areas of skin (e.g., axilla, groin), as well as the nose and throat.

P. aeruginosa rarely causes infection in immunologically competent individuals. However, this microorganism has several virulence factors, including endotoxins, proteases, and an extracellular slime, which may have particularly devastating effects in burn patients. *P. aeruginosa* proliferates in burn tissue because of the absence of a local blood supply. The avascular eschar is a favorable culture medium for the microorganism and serves as a staging area for the invasion of viable tissue.[2]

The use of antimicrobials presents a threat of superinfection with resistant microorganisms including enterococci,[7] *S. aureus*, particularly methicillin-resistant strains, and *Pseudomonas*. A particular species may be prevalent in a specific burn unit as a result of repeated use of topical or systemic antimicrobials.

Burn wound infection is distinguished from colonization by the finding of: 1) bacterial invasion of viable tissue in wound biopsy, 2) isolation of bacteria from blood, or 3) viral biopsy and a change in burn wound appearance or character or by clinical signs and symptoms and culture-documented bacteremia or biopsy.[3]

The physical environment

Ms. Williams was transferred to the burn center after immediate emergency care was provided. Burn centers or units usually consist of private rooms with individual handwashing facilities. Hands are washed before and after patient contact, and personnel use barrier techniques during patient care.

Ms. Williams received intravenous fluids to compensate for fluid shifting and enteral feedings to maintain good nutrition. Twice a day her wounds were cleansed with saline and coated with silver sulfadiazine. Every day she was placed on a plinth and immersed in the hydrotherapy tub for full body cleansing and removal of gross debris and loose skin. The burned areas on her arms were excised on her fourth hospital day and the underlying viable tissue was covered with autografts.

Fomites and environmental surfaces may play a role in transmission of microorganisms. These items include hydrotherapy tanks, mattresses, and plinths. Hydrotherapy tubs are used to remove tissue while the patient is immersed in a water bath. However, any microorganisms in the water may contaminate the wound.

The social environment

Ms. Williams was alert but anxious and overwhelmed by her sudden serious injury.

She would require many months of pain control and rehabilitation, and she was concerned about the potential for infection before her wounds were completely healed. She also worried about the time she would lose from work and how her family would adjust to any required changes. All of the burn care requirements and infection control principles were explained carefully to her family by the nursing staff. Staff members introduced Ms. Williams and her family to a community support group.

PREVENTION AND CONTROL

Prevention and control of infections in burn patients depend on maintaining the patient's normal flora and preventing contamination of the burn wound. Conservative systemic antimicrobial therapy, wound management—especially closure—and optimal unit design and procedures are important components of patient care.

Topical antimicrobials are used to decrease the bacterial load in the wound because systemic antimicrobials may not penetrate the avascular eschar. Systemic antimicrobials are avoided when possible in order to minimize the risk that the normal flora will be displaced by resistant microorganisms. Prophylactic broad-spectrum antibiotics are not routinely used for the same reason.

Topical antibiotic creams, ointments, and solutions such as silver sulfadiazine and silver nitrate are routinely used in burn centers to decrease the bacterial population in burns. Ms. Williams was initially treated with topical silver sulfadiazine cream.

The burn eschar is a hospitable medium for bacteria that may invade, colonize, and proliferate. The longer the wound remains open, the greater the risk of infection. Therefore, early cleaning and closure of wounds provides the best chance of minimizing infection risk and increasing survival. The burned tissue should

be removed and the underlying fascia covered with autografts or skin substitutes to reduce the size of the burn and limit the area available for bacterial growth. This approach has significantly reduced risk of infection and improved survival of severely burned adults.[9]

Infections common to other seriously ill patients, such as pneumonia and septicemia, may also occur in burned patients. Nurses must take meticulous care with all invasive devices, such as vascular lines, urinary catheters, tracheostomies, and other biomedical devices. Scrupulous attention to clean and sterile technique is crucial throughout the entire hospitalization of burned patients. Personnel in burn units typically wear scrub clothes. Gloves are worn during work with wounds and disposable plastic or other fluid resistant gowns are worn during procedures to decrease the potential for transmission of microorganisms. Masks are worn when the wound is exposed to decrease the potential for exposure to the microorganisms of the caregiver's respiratory secretions. Some burn specialists recommend that the heads of care providers be covered during contact with patients who are burned over 30% of TBSA.[10]

During outbreaks of infections in burn units, the epidemic microorganism has been recovered from up to 50% of the hands of health care staff. Since the major reservoir for these microorganisms is the skin surface of patients, hand washing is important to prevent cross-contamination. Hand-washing sinks must be readily available in patients' rooms, and staff should wash their hands routinely with an antimicrobial soap before and after patient contact.

Burn units are typically designed with private rooms and sinks that allow for the use of individual patient barrier technique, including hand washing. Access to the unit is limited to decrease traffic and visitors may be required to wear special garb.

Special care must be taken to prevent the

transmission of microorganisms by fomites such as hydrotherapy tanks. The filling hose, tank, agitator, trap, and drain of these tanks must be decontaminated regularly. Disinfectants such as sodium hypochlorite may be added to the water to reduce microbial load.[8] Staff wear long gloves and a clean plastic apron during hydrotherapy treatments to prevent transfer of microorganisms from the patient to themselves or the reverse. Because of these problems, immersion hydrotherapy is being replaced by showers or spray tables as the preferred method for burn wound cleaning and debridement in burn centers. Inanimate objects that cannot be adequately disinfected

should not be permitted in direct contact with the patient's wounds. Laminar airflow ventilation rooms and other specially designed enclosed areas are intended to decrease cross-contamination. However, data suggest that for burn patients, similar protection can be achieved using standard infection control practices.[5]

SUMMARY

Sepsis resulting from systemic infection remains the leading cause of death among hospitalized burn patients. Though the microbial flora may be temporarily reduced during

SUMMARY TABLE 12. Burn patient with *Pseudomonas* infection

Host-environment model	Case presentation	Factors that influence infectious process	Prevention and control
Host factors	40-year-old healthy woman 20% partial- and full-thickness burns	Patient's age Size and type of burn	Use topical antimicrobials for wound
Microbiologic factors	*Pseudomonas aeruginosa*	Contact transmission	Use aseptic techniques and barrier practices Avoid prophylactic broad spectrum antimicrobials Decrease size of wound
Physical environment	Burn unit	Open wounds and invasive devices	Assure optimal room design to support technique Disinfect appropriate equipment and fomites Use barrier techniques
Social environment	Skill of health provider in barrier precautions and aseptic technique	Culture or standards supporting appropriate technique	Enforce high standards for barrier precautions Educate patient and family

the burning, subsequent management must be meticulous if risk of infection is to be minimized. Risk of infection and associated mortality have decreased in some patient populations when aseptic techniques, strict protocols regarding care practices, and prompt medical management are used.[7] Ms. Williams developed a *Pseudomonas* infection in spite of the nursing staff's best efforts. This prolonged her hospital stay and required additional antimicrobials and costs. Fortunately, her infection responded to treatment and, once the infection cleared, she progressed along an expected care path and was discharged 2 months after admission.

REFERENCES

1. Burke JF, et al: The contribution of a bacterially isolated environment to the prevention of infection in seriously burned patients, *Ann Surg* 186:377, 1977.
2. Farmer JJ: Pseudomonas in the hospital, *Hosp Pract* 11:63, 1976.
3. Garner JS, et al: CDC definitions for nosocomial infections, *Am J Infect Control* 16:128, 1988.
4. Kravitz M: Immune consequences of burn injury. *AACN Clin Issues* 4:399-413, 1993.
5. May SR, DeClement FA: Effects of patient isolation techniques in burn treatment centers, *American Burn Association Proceedings* 14:60, 1982.
6. Ryan C, et al: Increased gut permeability early after burns correlates with the extent of burn injury, *Crit Care Med* 20:1508-1512, 1992.
7. Smith DJ, Thomson PD: Changing flora in burn and trauma units: historical perspective—experience in the United States, *J Burn Care Rehabil* 13:276, 1992.
8. Thomson PD, et al: A survey of burn hydrotherapy in the United States, *J Burn Care Rehabil* 11:151-155, 1990.
9. Tompkins RG, Burke JF: Infections of burn wounds. In Bennett JV, Brachman PS, editors: *Hospital infection,* ed 3. Boston, 1992, Little, Brown.
10. Weber JM, Tompkins DM. Improving survival: infection control and burns, *AACN Clin Issues* 4:414-423, 1993.

SUGGESTED READINGS

Arnow PM, et al: Control of methicillin-resistant *S. aureus* in a burn unit: role of nurse staffing, *J Trauma* 22:954, 1982.

Lee JJ, et al: Infection control in a burn center, *J Burn Care Rehabil* 11:575, 1990.

Luterman A, Dasco CC, Curreri PW: Infections in burn patients, *Am J Med* 81:45, 1986.

Marvin JA, Einfeldt LE: Infection control for the burn patient, *Nurs Clin North Am* 15:833, 1980.

Mayhall CG: Surgical infections including burns. In Wenzel RP, editor: *Prevention and control of nosocomial infections,* ed 2. Baltimore, 1993, Williams & Wilkins.

Murthy SK, et al: Oropharyngeal and fecal carriage of *P. aeruginosa* in hospital patients, *J Clin Microbiol* 27:35, 1989.

Tredget EE, et al: Epidemiology of infection with *P. aeruginosa* in burn patients: the role of hydrotherapy, *Clin Infect Dis* 15:941, 1992.

Herpetic Whitlow in a Critical Care Nurse

BARBARA R. MOONEY

CLINICAL PRESENTATION

Ruth Frank, a 31-year-old nurse working in the surgical intensive care unit (SICU), reported to the Occupational Health Service (OHS) with a very painful lesion on her left thumb. Ms. Frank was well known to the OHS, since she had periodic dermatitis on her hands caused by an allergic reaction to latex. She had no other health problems. She worked 12-hour shifts three nights each week in the SICU but was unable to work one night because of her painful thumb. The occupational health physician diagnosed herpetic whitlow and asked the occupational health nurse to investigate.

During the interview the health nurse determined that Ms. Frank, who is right-handed, would frequently suction patients' respiratory secretions without using a glove on her left hand because it exacerbated her dermatitis. Several years ago the infection control practitioner (ICP) recommended that the hospital purchase a suction cannula with a closed suction-controlling device; however, this safer cannula was frequently back-ordered. When it was unavailable, an open cannula was supplied that allowed contact of patient secretions with the health care provider's nondominant hand. Ms. Frank reported that 4 days previously she repeatedly suctioned Mr. Jones with the open device without wearing a glove. She thought she had washed her hands after completing each procedure. The skin on her left hand appeared irritated with splits in various areas that created portals of entry for

infecting organisms. The pain in her thumb was so severe that she was unable to wear a glove on that hand. She was restricted from direct patient care for 9 days until the lesion on her finger crusted and healed, after which she was reassigned to patient care in the SICU. She agreed to wear hypoallergenic gloves on both hands for all suctioning procedures.

HOST-ENVIRONMENT INTERACTION
The host

Herpes simplex virus (HSV) is distributed worldwide and susceptibility is universal. Humans are the only hosts for this virus.[1]

HSV enters the body at the point of contact with broken skin or mucous membranes. The primary infection can be quite painful and is often accompanied by systemic manifestations. After an incubation period of 2 to 7 days, the initial infection is commonly characterized by fever, malaise, and swollen glands. Lesions appear at the site of inoculation, or entry, of the virus. These lesions are vesicles filled with clear fluid on a reddened base, which crust and heal, usually without scarring, in about 3 to 10 days. Live virus is found in the clear fluid from the vesicle, the ulcerated skin beneath a broken vesicle, and sometimes in saliva or genital secretions.

After the acute clinical symptoms subside, the virus resides in nerve endings adjacent to the point of entry for the virus. As with all viruses in the family *Herpesviridae*, the body may not clear HSV after the primary infection. Initial infection is followed by latency and the potential for local recurrences. Stress and sun exposure can stimulate the virus to replicate and cause recurrent lesions. Periodic local recurrences of HSV lesions also occur with herpetic whitlows,[4] although more commonly with HSV type II than with type I. Persons with oral or genital HSV disease may excrete virus into saliva or genital secretions without any symptoms or vesicles. Periods of stress, such as illness or hospitalization, increase viral excretion. There may be continued pain or lack of sensation in the affected area after lesions are healed. This usually subsides over time but may occasionally last for months or years. In addition, newborn infants and individuals who are immunocompromised by an underlying disease or treatment are unable to suppress herpes simplex virus (HSV) efficiently. These individuals have much more severe and prolonged initial and recurrent disease, often with life-threatening complications.

The microbiologic environment

Herpetic whitlow is caused by HSV, a member of the virus family *Herpesviridae*. A double-stranded deoxyribonucleic acid (DNA) virus, HSV is differentiated into type I, which is most often associated with oral disease, and type II, which is usually associated with genital disease. Type differentiation is distinguishable only in the laboratory, not by site of infection, since either type can be found at either site. HSV type II may be associated with cervical and vulvar malignancy. Among adults, 70% to 90% may have antibodies against HSV type I. Seroprevalence for HSV type II averages 20% but may be as high as 60% in selected populations.

Transmission of HSV occurs when a virus-containing body substance, such as vesicular fluid, saliva, or genital secretions, comes into contact with nonintact skin or mucous membranes (the portal of entry) of a susceptible person. In addition, infected persons may transmit the virus to and cause infection at another site on their own bodies (e.g., self-inoculating an eye while rubbing it with a virus-contaminated hand). Both HSV Type I and Type II cause herpetic whitlow, which can be a primary infection, reactivation, or reinfection.[2-5]

The physical environment

In general, environmental factors play a minor role in transmission of HSV because direct contact with contaminated secretions is required for spread. In health care settings, personnel are at risk for acquisition of HSV and may be a source of the virus to others if appropriate barrier techniques are not followed during patient care. Fomites are a rare source for infection if an object is soiled with virus-laden secretions. Occupational herpetic whitlows occur most frequently when the health care worker's hand contacts the patient's virus-laden saliva during suctioning or mouth care or genital secretions during perineal care. The portal of entry in Ms. Franks's case was chapped, abraded, or nonintact skin on her hand or finger. Transmission of HSV leading to occupationally acquired herpetic whitlow has occurred in a variety of care settings, including intensive care units, and dental offices. Nurses, dental staff, and respiratory therapists are often affected. Primary herpes Type I infection has also been reported following mouth-to-mouth resuscitation.

HSV infections occur at any time throughout the year and do not appear to be seasonal.[1]

The social environment

Individuals in lower socioeconomic groups have a higher prevalence of HSV type II infection. HSV type I infection occurs equally in all socioeconomic levels.

Infection with HSV type I frequently occurs in childhood. Transmission of the virus can occur within families, in day-care centers, and in other settings where young children contact each other's secretions. As in Ms. Franks's case, transmission can occur in health care facilities when appropriate barriers are not used.

Sexual transmission is responsible for the spread of genital HSV, whether caused by type I or II. Prevalence is higher in persons with multiple sexual partners. Presence of genital ulcer disease can increase the risk for sexual transmission of other diseases, such as human immunodeficiency virus (HIV) and hepatitis B virus (HBV).

PREVENTION AND CONTROL

Spread of HSV infection may be prevented by using barriers or by preventing contact with contaminated secretions or lesions. Kissing should be avoided when oral lesions are present. Sexual contact and vaginal delivery should be avoided when genital lesions are present. Consistent use of condoms may prevent spread of genital disease, depending on the location of the lesions.

Barriers and appropriate techniques will prevent HSV spread in health care facilities.[6,8] In the 1960s and 1970s, occupational exposure of health care workers to HSV occurred during suctioning of oral secretions. Only one glove was used on the dominant hand during suctioning, and the ungloved nondominant hand controlled the suction. The design of suction catheters allowed direct contact of suctioned secretions with the finger controlling the suction on the nondominant hand. When this problem was identified, procedures were modified by most facilities to require a glove on each hand. Suction kits began to include two gloves rather than just one. In addition, some manufacturers instituted engineering controls by designing catheters with closed suction-controlling devices to eliminate exposure to suctioned secretions. Education of

employees in proper technique and use of safer devices became key elements in decreasing the risk of herpetic whitlow.

With these control measures in place, the incidence of herpetic whitlow among health care workers greatly decreased in the early 1980s. However, occasional instances of newly diagnosed herpetic whitlow still occur, and employees infected years ago may continue to have periodic recurrences. In addition, employees with active lesions may constitute a risk of transmission to patients if the patient is exposed to virus from an infected lesion.[6,8]

The occupational health nurse counseled Ms. Frank regarding prevention of self-inoculation of the virus to another site. Ms. Frank was instructed to refrain from direct patient care activities until the lesion had crusted. In the past, there has been controversy about whether to allow health care workers with herpetic whitlows to perform patient care wearing gloves. Some facilities have permitted staff to continue their duties. It has been speculated that not all gloves remain intact and that even small pinholes allow virus to pass through to the patient during care activities. Whether enough virus to cause infection can pass through to a patient is unknown. However, a glove may delay crusting and increase self-inoculation to another site on the same hand. In addition, the pain that occurs with the whitlow usually prohibits the employee from wearing a glove. Consequently, since patient care cannot be performed without covering the lesion, the employee usually has no choice but to refrain from patient care activities until the lesion is crusted. Ms. Frank was assigned to help the SICU nurse manager with administrative duties for the duration of the lesions, which included writing a standard for the unit specifying the importance of wearing gloves on both hands during suctioning.

The occupational health physician prescribed acyclovir for Ms. Frank's herpetic whitlow. This is an antiviral agent that can help the immune system suppress but not cure HSV. The acyclovir decreased Ms. Frank's symptoms, promoted healing and thereby decreased the length of time that she was unable to care for patients. Long-term, low-dose suppression therapy may decrease the frequency of recurrences.[7] However, acyclovir resistance has been reported in HSV.

The occupational health nurse and ICP scheduled time at a SICU staff meeting to discuss and reinforce the use of gloves during procedures. The unit manager ordered a supply of vinyl and hypoallergenic gloves for workers with latex allergies. In addition, the ICP reviewed with the occupational health staff the importance of counseling workers with dermatitis about the use of gloves, obtaining hypoallergenic gloves as needed and promoting practices and products to help heal the skin. Intact skin, handwashing, and use of

SUMMARY TABLE 13. Herpetic whitlow in a critical care nurse

Host-environment model	Case presentation	Factors that influence infectious process	Prevention and control
Host factors	31-year-old healthy woman	All humans suscep-tible No natural immunity Dermatitis on hands with periodic exac-erbations after pri-mary infection	No vaccine Promote intact skin to eliminate portal of entry
Microbiologic factors	Herpes simplex virus type I	Contact transmission: nonintact skin ex-posed to active her-pesvirus in pa-tient's saliva Virus not cleared from body after primary infection	Consider acyclovir treatment to pro-mote healing and decrease infective period
Physical environment	12-bed surgical inten-sive care unit in busy teaching hos-pital	Contact with saliva (any/all patients who may be shed-ding herpesvirus) Open suction catheter used when closed unavailable	Do not allow lesion to contact patients Do not provide direct patient care, even with gloves, until lesion is healed Wear glove on non-dominant hand while suctioning patient
Social environment	Nurse works 12-hour shifts three nights per week	Frequent lack of glove use during suctioning	Reinforce compliance with proper barrier techniques with all nursing personnel

gloves are the major defenses against contact transmission HSV. The ICP also contacted the hospital's purchasing department to ensure that a suction cannula with a closed suction system was always available to the hospital staff.

SUMMARY

Herpetic whitlow has been a well known risk to health care workers for decades. Since any person may be a source of HSV, control measures must be universally applied to all patients.

Handwashing, the cornerstone of infection control practice, has always caused some damage to the hands of health care workers who wash hands frequently. Recent governmental regulations and changes in infection prevention practices have greatly increased glove use. This has increased the numbers of persons who have dermatitis attributable to gloves. It has become increasingly difficult to maintain the integrity of the skin of health care workers' hands.

Because HSV infection is not curable, prevention is important. Work practice controls, engineering controls, and intact skin could eliminate or significantly reduce the risk for acquisition of herpetic whitlow.

REFERENCES

1. Benenson AS, ed. *Control of Communicable Diseases in Man*, 15th ed. Washington, DC: American Public Health Association; 1990;212-213.
2. Crane LR, Lerner AM. Herpetic whitlow: A manifestation of primary infection with herpes simplex virus type 1 or type 2. *J Infect Dis.* 1978;137:855-856.
3. Gill MJ, Arlette J, Buchan K. Herpes simplex virus infections of the hand: a profile of 79 cases. *Am J Med.* 1988;84:89-93.
4. Harburchak DR. Recurrent herpetic whitlow due to herpes simplex virus type 2. *Arch Intern Med.* 1978;138:1418-1419.
5. Hendricks AA, Shapiro EP. Primary herpes simplex infection following mouth-to-mouth resuscitation. *JAMA.* 1980;243:257-259.
6. Klotz RW. Herpetic whitlow: an occupational hazard. *AANA Journal.* 1990;58:8-13.
7. Schwandt NW, Mjos DP, Lubow RM. Acyclovir and the treatment of herpetic whitlow. *Oral Surg Oral Med Oral Pathol.* 1987;64:255-258.
8. Weisman E, Troncale JA. Herpetic whitlow: a case report. *J Fam Pract.* 1991;33:516-520.

SUGGESTED READINGS

Benenson AS, ed. *Control of Communicable Diseases in Man,* 15th ed. Washington, DC: American Public Health Association; 1990.

Henderson DK. Nosocomial herpesvirus infections. In: Mandel GL, Douglas RG, Bennett JE, ed. *Principles and Practice of Infectious Diseases,* 3rd ed. New York: Churchill Livingstone; 1990;2236-2237.

Perl TM, et al. Transmission of herpes simplex virus type 1 infection in an intensive care unit. *Ann Intern Med.* 1992;117:584-586.

Adolescent Female with *Chlamydia* Infection

LORRAINE M. HARKAVY

CLINICAL PRESENTATION

Jeanette Westin is a high-school senior. In an attempt to meet other students, she has joined a variety of school clubs. Recently she has become sexually active and has had sexual relations with three new partners. In the past several weeks she has noted a more frequent need to urinate and has begun to notice an increase in vaginal secretions and mucus. Jeanette was referred by the school nurse to a local sexually transmitted disease (STD) clinic. She was interviewed by a nurse practitioner who, after taking a social history, suspected an STD. Vaginal examination revealed mucopurulent cervicitis. When the nurse found pyuria by urinalysis but no growth on cultures, she became concerned that Jeanette also had acute urethral syndrome characterized by dysuria, frequency, and pyuria with negative culture. The nurse informed the clinic physician of her diagnosis, prescribed doxycycline, and instructed Jeanette to take it for 7 days. Specimens collected before treatment were positive for *Chlamydia trachomatis* and negative for *Neisseria gonorrhoeae*. The nurse also counseled Jeanette to instruct her sexual partners to seek care.

HOST-ENVIRONMENT INTERACTION
The host

Chlamydia trachomatis infection is the most common STD, causing about 50% of the cases of nongonococcal urethritis (NGU) in men.[2]

Risk is increased in the presence of *Neisseria gonorrhoeae*,[5] and sexual partners of those infected are at risk of more serious disease if early treatment is not implemented. Women are often asymptomatic. Consequently, they may not change their sexual habits or recognize the need for medical care, and may continue to transmit the organism to other sexual partners or their newborn or unborn children. In men, *Chlamydia* causes half of the cases of acute epididymitis, as well as postgonococcal urethritis (PGU). *Chlamydia* is also associated with proctitis, particularly in homosexual men, and Reiter's syndrome, a form of reactive arthritis which includes inflammation of the joints and other musculoskeletal lesions.

In women, *C. trachomatis* is one cause of bartholinitis, infection of the Bartholin gland duct. Mucopurulent endocervicitis is often unrecognized because there are no specific symptoms. Surveys have shown that as many as 70% of women with symptomless cervical infection may be infected with *Chlamydia*.[1] As with Jeanette, women may have acute urethral syndrome with dysuria, frequent urination, and pyuria but with no microorganisms in the urine. *Chlamydia* is also responsible for much of the pelvic inflammatory disease (PID) in the United States. Although the exact incidence is unknown, a large proportion of women with cervicitis develop endometritis. Salpingitis leads to scarring of the fallopian tubes and ectopic pregnancy, ovarian infection, and infertility. *Chlamydia* is one cause of Fitz-Hugh-

Curtis syndrome, which is characterized by acute inflammation of the liver and adjacent peritoneum, and fibrous adhesions of the liver and diaphragm. Women with cervical chlamydial infection at the time of elective abortion are at risk for pelvic infections after the procedure.

Considerable controversy exists regarding the effect of *Chlamydia* on outcome of pregnancy. Studies of the association between *Chlamydia* infections and increase in premature rupture of membranes (PROM), premature labor, stillbirth, spontaneous abortion, and neonatal death are inconclusive. The inconsistent findings of these studies may be the result of varied study designs, timing of the study in the course of pregnancy, lack of matching controls, or presence of other confounding organisms.

Newborns acquire *Chlamydia* during passage through the birth canal from mothers who are harboring the organism. Newborns with chlamydial conjunctivitis may not develop symptoms for as long as 5 to 21 days. Conjunctival redness and swelling may occur. The disease is usually self-limiting with resolution within weeks to months even without treatment. However, there have been reports of persistent infection with resultant corneal scarring. As many as 35% to 50% of newborns of infected women develop mucopurulent conjunctivitis, and 11% to 20% develop pneumonia.[4] Chlamydial pneumonia in the newborn is serious. Disease in these infants is characterized by bilateral rales and lung infiltrates, congestion, staccato cough, absence of fever, eosinophilia, and failure to gain weight. (See Clinical Study 19).

Although the infected mother develops immunoglobulin G (IgG) antibodies, these do not prevent reinfection in the mother or infection in the neonate. Secretory IgA, a neutralizing antibody, reduces shedding of the organism and may account for decreased infection after repeated exposure. The role of cellular immunity is undefined but is likely to be important, since *Chlamydia trachomatis* is an intracellular organism.

The microbiologic environment

The order *Chlamydiales* is made up of the *Chlamydiaceae* family, of which there are three species: *C. trachomatis*, *C. psittaci*, and *C. pneumoniae*. With one exception (*C. psittaci*, which causes psittacosis in birds and humans), *Chlamydiae* causes disease in humans only. Chlamydiae are classified as bacteria but share a number of properties with viruses. Chlamydiae, like viruses, are obligate intracellular microbes and can grow only in the host cell. Like bacteria, however, chlamydiae contain both deoxyribonucleic acid (DNA) and ribonucleic acid (RNA), divide by binary fission, and have cell walls similar to those of gram-negative bacteria.[2]

Before chlamydiae grow, they must be taken up by a host cell. The chlamydiae replicate inside the host cells, forming elementary bodies (EBs) that remain within the cell during their entire growth cycle of 48 to 72 hours. When there is a predominance of EBs, the metabolically active form of the organism, the inclusion membrane bursts and the infectious EBs are released into the host cell cytoplasm, causing host cell rupture and release of the infectious EBs.

More than a dozen serotypes (A, B, Ba, C to K, L1 to L3) of chlamydiae are capable of causing disease. STD is usually caused by serotypes D to K. Serotypes L1 to L3 cause lymphogranuloma venereum (LGV), another STD characterized by generalized systemic symptoms, anogenital lesions, lymphadenopathy, and destruction of perineal tissue. LGV is less common in the United States than in other parts of the world.

Cytology, serology, culture, and detection of antigen may all be used to establish a diagnosis of chlamydial infection. Cytology using the Giemsa stain or fluorescent antibody staining techniques to detect inclusions that are specific for chlamydiae infections, are rapid diagnostic tests but identify only about 20% of cervical infections.[6] Enzyme-linked immunosorbent assay (ELISA) and the direct fluorescent monoclonal antibody staining detect chlamydial antigen. Both these tests are highly specific and sensitive and can be completed in hours. They are often used because they provide rapid results at low cost. Both tests have a 3% to 5% false-positive rate that may lead to misdiagnosis if used to test individuals from populations with low prevalence of the disease. Therefore, these tests should not be used for screening in low-prevalence populations.

Culture is the standard of accuracy, but optimal results depend on proper collection of appropriate specimen, prompt transport, refrigerated storage if necessary, correct transport media, and careful laboratory techniques. It is imperative that the specimen contain cellular material for the organism (an obligate intracellular microbe) to be recovered. Wood sticks or swabs used to collect the specimen interfere with isolation of the organism and must be removed from the specimen container. Chlamydiae require a susceptible tissue culture cell line to reproduce. A minimum of 24 to 72 hours is required for the organism to grow. After that the culture is stained with iodine or Giemsa and is examined microscopically for inclusion bodies. Presumptive diagnosis is appropriate in some instances, particularly if the patient presents with urethritis, if culture and Gram stain have excluded gonococcal infections.

The physical environment

The physical environment does not play a significant role in sexually transmitted chlamydial infections. The infection is not seasonal or geographic but occurs at any time of the year and is widespread throughout the United States and the world.

The social environment

The epidemiology of chlamydial infection is similar to that of other STDs. As with Jeanette, young, unmarried, sexually active persons with multiple, new, or infected sex partners are at risk for acquiring *Chlamydia*. Infection is also associated with low socioeconomic status, presence of gonorrhea, and the use of oral contraception.

The social and psychologic implications of this disease are exceeded only by the physical complications. *Chlamydia* is the most common cause of the more than 1 million cases of PID diagnosed and treated each year. Many of these infections result in infertility or hospitalization. Prevention of *Chlamydia* infections would reduce these serious consequences.

PREVENTION AND CONTROL

The objectives of the U.S. government's national strategy for improving the health of its citizens call for the reduction of *Chlamydia* infections and PID.[7]

The control of STDs requires open discussions about health and sexual attitudes and behaviors and involves schools, health professionals, and the media. Community-based educational programs for sexually active persons should review the epidemiology of chlamydial disease, implications for the neonate, and the natural history of infection, including the frequency of asymptomatic infections. The benefits of abstinence, monogamous relationships, use of barrier methods during sexual activity and regular and appropriate gynecologic examinations for women should be emphasized.

Treatment of all sexual partners is essential. Persons identified with gonococcal infections should also be treated concomitantly for *Chlamydia* (see Clinical Study 11). Persons seen in STD clinics may be lost to follow-up, especially if they are asymptomatic. Therefore, treatment of suspected infections at the initial visit is a useful strategy.

Optimal communication between the patient and the health care provider is imperative. It includes patient education in a language and at a level of literacy that the patient or family members are able to understand. The Centers for Disease Control (CDC) publication *Chlamydia trachomatis* Infections: Policy Guidelines for Prevention and Control,[2] recommends important education and screening topics.

The CDC recommends *Chlamydia* screening for

1. Asymptomatic persons who attend clinics for STD
2. Persons who attend high-risk health care facilities (e.g., adolescent and family planning clinics)
3. Sexually active adolescents and young adults

CDC EDUCATION TOPICS TO PREVENT *CHLAMYDIA TRACHOMATIS* INFECTIONS[2]

1. Instructions for taking medication, including the dosage, timing, and length of the regimen. Patients must clearly understand that they must continue to take medication according to schedule despite abatement of symptoms.
2. Advice regarding follow-up for side effects or the difficulty with medication, continued or worsened symptoms, and test of cure, if indicated.
3. Suggestion to abstain from sexual activity until treatment is completed by both patient and partner. If this is not possible, patients should be encouraged to use condoms until treatment is completed.
4. Suggestion to cease sexual activity immediately if the same or other STD symptoms recur and to return to the practitioner or clinic with the steady sex partner.
5. Suggestion to use barrier methods regularly, particularly condoms, to prevent chlamydial infection and other STDs.

---

4. Those of lower socioeconomic status
5. Those with multiple sex partners
6. Those with a history of other STDs

The American College of Obstetrics and Gynecology recommends that unmarried pregnant women and women who start their prenatal care late should also be screened.[2] Screening should take place at the initial prenatal visit and in the third trimester.[3]

Early detection and appropriate treatment result in successful cure in 95% of patients. Tetracycline or doxycycline can be used to treat chlamydial infections. A 7-day regimen is recommended.[4] In pregnant women, erythromycin is the drug of choice. Erythromycin may cause gastrointestinal disturbance, requiring dosage reduction and extension of therapy. The ideal drug would be one that could be given in a single dose that would reduce the number of treatment failures that may occur in noncompliant populations. Other drugs being evaluated to treat *Chlamydia* are azithromycin, rifabutin (a rifamycin derivative), clarithromycin, and amoxicillin and ampicillin esters.

Neonatal chlamydial infection is best prevented by appropriately treating the mother. It is still recommended that all neonates receive a prophylactic agent into the eyes to prevent both chlamydial and gonococcal ophthalmia neonatorum (see Clinical Study 19). Unwashed hands of health care workers may spread neonatal eye infections in the nursery.

SUMMARY

C. trachomatis is the most common sexually transmitted bacterial pathogen in the United States and possibly worldwide. Although the organism was identified in the early 1900s as the cause of trachoma, a serious eye infection, only in the past 15 years was *Chlamydia* recognized as a common pathogen causing a variety of infections.

The sexual revolution may have contributed to spread of this organism to large numbers of sexually active teenagers and adults. The high

SUMMARY TABLE 14. Adolescent female with *Chlamydia* infection

Host-environment model	Case presentation	Factors that influence infectious process	Prevention and control
Host factors	Adolescent female	Universal susceptibility No immunity	No vaccine
Microbiologic factors	*Chlamydia trachomatis*	Direct transmission during sexual activity	Screen high-risk persons Treat sexual partners
Physical environment	Not applicable	Not applicable	Not applicable
Social environment	Sexually active	Multiple sex partners	Provide universal access to care Counsel Educate about sexual transmission Notify sexual partners Encourage use of barrier devices

frequency of asymptomatic infection results in large numbers of untreated persons who are reservoirs of the organism and if female, are at risk of infertility.

The annual financial burden of chlamydial disease has been reported to be more than $2 billion.[8] The most expensive consequences of chlamydial infections are the cost of managing women with PID and its complications and infants with chlamydial pneumonia, many of whom must be hospitalized.

REFERENCES

1. Cates W, Wasserheit JN. Genital chlamydial infections: epidemiology and reproductive sequelae. *Am J Obstet Gynecol.* 1991;164(6):1771-1781.
2. Centers for Disease Control: *Chlamydia trachomatis* infections: policy guidelines for prevention and control. *MMWR* 1985;34(3S):53S-74S.
3. Marecki MA. *Chlamydia trachomatis:* a developing perinatal problem. *J Perinat Neonat Nurs.* 1988;1(4):1-11.
4. Meriwether CD, Evans MI, Sokol RJ. *Chlamydia trachomatis:* a practical obstetric/gynecologic management approach. *Int J Gynaecol Obstet.* 1986;24:407-415.
5. Reeve P, ed. *Chlamydial Infections.* New York, NY: Springer-Verlag; 1987.
6. Sweet RL, Gibbs RS. *Infectious Diseases of the Female Genital Tract,* 2nd ed. Baltimore, MD: Williams & Wilkins; 1990.
7. U.S. Department of Health and Human Services. *Healthy People 2000.* Washington, DC: Superintendent of Documents, United States Government Printing Office; 1990.
8. Washington AE, Johnson RE, Sander LL. *Chlamydia trachomatis* infections in the United States: what are they costing us? *JAMA.* 1987;257:2070-2072.

SUGGESTED READINGS

Faro S. *Chlamydia trachomatis:* female pelvic infections. *Am J Obstet Gynecol.* 1991;164(6):1767-1770.
Hammerschlag MR. Chlamydial infections. *J Pediatr.* 1989;114(5):727-734.
Hossain A. *Chlamydia trachomatis* infections. *Int J Gynaecol Obstet.* 1989;29:107-115.
Schacter J. Breaking the chain of chlamydial infection. *Contemp Obstet Gynecol.* 1987;32:146-159.
Winkler B. Needed: a program to control chlamydial infections. *Contemp Obstet Gynecol.* 1987;32:30-40.

Rotavirus in a Day-Care Center

ARLENE M. BUTZ

CLINICAL PRESENTATION

Jimmy Markam is an 8-month-old boy who attends a day-care center 3 days a week in a large city in Maryland. At the center Jimmy is in a room with nine other infants who are cared for by four staff members. On January 12 Jimmy developed watery profuse diarrhea, vomiting, and a low-grade fever during the course of 1 day. He did not have a runny nose, cough, difficult breathing, or sneezing. It was the policy of the day-care center to exclude children with diarrhea, consequently his parents were asked to keep him home until the diarrhea subsided and he had been examined by a physician.

Jimmy was examined by a pediatrician, who diagnosed rotavirus gastroenteritis by use of an enzyme-linked immunosorbent assay (ELISA) test. He had not had any serious disease, hospitalizations, or allergies. Jimmy was cared for at home by his parents for 3 days, during which the diarrhea subsided. He then returned to the day-care center. By the end of the week, five other infants in the same day-care room had been excluded from the center because of diarrhea and fever. One staff member was absent for 3 days with a mild diarrheal illness.

HOST-ENVIRONMENT INTERACTION
The host

The major host factor associated with rotavirus infection is age. The very young and the elderly, whose immune systems are either immature or compromised are particularly susceptible. Rotavirus gastroenteritis is one of the most common childhood illnesses throughout the world and is a leading cause of infant mortality in many countries. Rotavirus gastroenteritis has a predisposition for children 6 weeks to 5 months of age and is the cause of diarrhea in approximately one half of infants and young children hospitalized with diarrhea. Almost all children are infected with rotavirus during their first 4 years of life.[3]

Rotavirus infection in children usually presents with profuse diarrhea, often preceded or accompanied by vomiting; low-grade fever; and at times, respiratory illness. In severe cases of rotavirus infection, dehydration and acidosis can lead to renal collapse and death. The staff member with diarrheal disease reported the typical scenario of adult rotavirus infection, which is asymptomatic or minor illness. There is no known genetic predisposition for increased risk of rotavirus infection. Currently there is no vaccine available, but several are under development.

The microbiologic environment

Rotavirus is a member of the Reoviridae family of animal viruses, which contain segmented double-stranded ribonucleic acid (RNA). Members of the genus *Reovirus* possess an outer protein shell and high molecular weight. Three serotypes of the *Reovirus* genus, including rotavirus, infect humans. Most rotaviruses known to infect humans and animals share a common group antigen and are termed group A rotaviruses. This group contains at least six serotypes of human rotaviruses. The ingestion of relatively small numbers of infectious rotavirus particles can result in infection and symptoms.

Rotavirus is usually transmitted by the fecal-oral route. Because rotavirus has been reported to survive on hands after contamination (57% of subjects up to 20 minutes and 43% of subjects up to 60 minutes[2]), the other five infants who subsequently contracted diarrhea most likely became infected by transmission from the staff or the environment. For example, transfer of infectious rotavirus could have occurred from infected hands of staff (while changing Jimmy's diapers) or by sharing objects that Jimmy handled.

The other infants probably became infected before or during the day that Jimmy was symptomatic. The incubation period is about 24 to 48 hours. As with Jimmy, diarrhea of 5 to 8 days' duration is frequently accompanied by vomiting or fever. Fecal shedding of virus usually occurs for 5 to 7 days and is greatly decreased or absent after day 8.

ELISA is the preferred diagnostic test. Because all strains of rotavirus produce clinical illness, it is not necessary to determine specific viral serotype or subgroup of rotavirus except for epidemiologic purposes.

The physical environment

Several environmental factors are associated with the transmission of diarrheal disease in day-care centers. Temperature, season, water, air, and type of work and play surfaces all have a role. In temperate regions, including Jimmy's hometown, Baltimore, outbreaks of rotavirus gastroenteritis usually occur in colder and drier months of the year. A dry atmosphere in combination with lower air temperature is the best environment for rotavirus outbreaks. This was the case in the January outbreak in Jimmy's day-care center. Rotavirus is associated with the winter season. However, rotavirus is not simply a winter disease in the United States. It appears in the fall in the Southwest and in the winter and spring in the Northwest.[3] Infection is rare in the summer.

Water can act as a vehicle for transmission of gastroenteritis. Rotaviruses can retain their infectivity for several days in a water environment,[4] such as the sink handles at the diaper changing station in Jimmy's day-care center. Some data imply that rotaviruses may also be spread by air. During many nosocomial outbreaks of rotavirus gastroenteritis, patients report symptoms of upper respiratory tract infection before the symptoms of diarrhea. Jimmy had a runny nose that was unnoticed before he developed diarrhea. It has been suggested that respiratory symptoms may result from inhalation and replication of the virus in the respiratory tract.[1] However, the association of respiratory symptoms and rotavirus infection may be coincidental.

The virus may have been transmitted to the other infants by contaminated fomites or surfaces. Rotaviruses can remain stable in feces for months at room temperature. Ansari et al.[1] reported that rotaviruses can remain viable on inanimate surfaces for several days in dried surfaces. This may have contributed to the infection of five other infants in the same room. Rotaviruses can also survive on plastic, glass, and stainless steel for more than 10 days at room temperature at low or medium relative humidity.

Day-care centers are a high-risk site for the transmission of rotavirus infections. In such settings, children have been observed to put toys and other objects in their mouths every 2 to 3 minutes and pass the moist object to another child.[5] The contamination of inanimate objects and surfaces, including toys, diaper-changing tables, toilet seats, and diaper pails, can occur either directly by contact with the infected feces or indirectly through virus-containing aerosols or contact with contaminated objects or hands.

The social environment

Agents such as rotavirus and other organisms spread by the fecal-oral route are readily transmitted in crowded environments such as day-care centers, nursing homes, and conditions where people live closely together. In such situations, personal hygiene and environmental sanitation are very important but difficult to maintain. Staff are often busy or do not appreciate the importance of strict hygiene and attention to the environment, and many children and elderly persons have suboptimal personal hygiene.

PREVENTION AND CONTROL

Prevention and control strategies are aimed at decreasing the fecal-oral route of transmission. Hands of staff, contaminated directly from infected feces or indirectly via surfaces or objects, were probably the most important vehicle of the transmission of rotavirus in this day-care center. Handwashing and cleaning and disinfection of the environment are the two most important prevention strategies.

Strict handwashing, the mechanical removal of infectious agents from the hands, was instituted in the day-care center after the diarrhea outbreak. Continual education of day-care staff regarding the importance of correct sanitation procedures and frequency of handwashing was necessary to maintain adequate levels of cleanliness in the infant room. Staff were taught to wash their hands before food and formula preparation, before feeding an infant, after using the bathroom or diapering an infant, and when visible contamination or soiling of their hands occurred. Disposable hand towels and gloves were provided for staff in the infant room to use during the outbreak of diarrhea. For children aged 2 years

and older, the staff implemented a handwashing training program.

The staff established more thorough and consistent guidelines for cleaning and disinfection of environmental surfaces and fomites. They were instructed to use standard household cleaning products for most environmental surfaces. Locations targeted for extra cleaning and disinfection included moist surfaces, such as food preparation and consumption areas, diaper-changing surfaces, toilets, water fountains, toys, and telephone receivers.

The diaper-changing area was considered a possible source of rotavirus contamination. Therefore the following policy was instituted in the day-care center: (1) a specified diaper-changing area would be separated from the general play area; (2) when changing a soiled diaper, disposable gloves would be used; (3) disposable diapers would be used until the diarrheal outbreak subsided and considered as a permanent policy; (4) after each use, the diaper-changing surface would be wiped clean with a detergent solution or soap and water and allowed to dry; (5) diapers would be disposed in a covered container lined with a plastic bag; and (6) the staff would wash their hands after gloves were removed. Infants were provided with washable toys. The toys were cleaned with dishwashing detergent and water, then rinsed in a dilute bleach solution followed by water at the end of each day.[5]

Rotavirus vaccines would be an effective preventive measure. Three rotavirus vaccines have been developed and are undergoing safety and effectiveness testing.

SUMMARY

Rotavirus infection is primarily a disease affecting the very young and elderly. Almost every child is infected with rotavirus during the first 4 years of life. Ingestion of a relatively small number of infectious rotavirus particles can result in infection. The mode of transmis-

SUMMARY TABLE 15. Rotavirus in a day-care center

Host-environment model	Case presentation	Factors that influence infectious process	Prevention and control
Host factors	8-month-old healthy boy	Immature immunity	Vaccine not available
Microbiologic factors	Rotavirus	Fecal-oral contamination Direct or indirect contact	Antiviral agents not available
Physical environment	Day-care center	Crowded conditions Frequent contact between children and staff	Clean and disinfect surfaces and hands Establish separate diapering/toileting areas Use washable toys Segregate infected child
Social environment	Young children closely interacting	Increased hand-to-mouth activity Play in proximity to others Shared toys and other fomites Caregivers and children may not use adequate handwashing techniques	Develop and implement guidelines for diapering, hygiene, and sanitation Educate children and staff Monitor compliance Establish policy to exclude children with diarrhea

sion is primarily fecal-oral, with an incubation period of 24 to 48 hours. However, the virus is usually shed in the feces of an infected child for 5 to 7 days.

Factors associated with transmission include temperature, season, relative humidity, and sanitation. Rotaviruses can remain stable on inanimate surfaces for several days; thus, these surfaces may be a vehicle for transmission.

Prevention and control strategies are aimed at interrupting the fecal-oral route of transmission. Handwashing and cleaning and disinfection of the environment are the two most important strategies for preventing the transmission of rotavirus. High-risk areas for trans-

mission of rotavirus include areas of food preparation, food consumption, diapering, and toileting. Rotavirus vaccines are undergoing safety and effectiveness testing and are not yet available for routine use. Rotavirus vaccines may eventually be the best control measure.

REFERENCES

1. Ansari SA, Springthorpe VS, Sattar SA. Survival and vehicular spread of human rotaviruses; possible relation to seasonality of outbreaks. *Rev Infect Dis.* 1991;13:448-461.
2. Ansari SA, et al. Rotavirus survival on human hands and transfer of infectious virus to animate and nonporous inanimate surfaces. *J Clin Microbiol.* 1988; 26:1513-1518.

3. Ho M, et al. Rotavirus as a cause of diarrheal morbidity in the United States. *J Infect Dis.* 1988; 158:1112-1116.

4. Pancorbo OC, et al. Infectivity and antigenicity reduction rates of human rotavirus strain Wa in fresh waters. *Appl Environ Microbiol.* 1987;53:1803-1811.

5. Yamauchi T. Guidelines for attendees and personnel. In Donowitz LG. *Infection Control in the Child Care Center and Preschool.* Baltimore, MD: Williams & Wilkins; 1991.

SUGGESTED READINGS

Butz A, et al. Occurrence of infectious symptoms in children in day care homes. *Am J Infect Control.* 1990;18:347-353.

Donowitz LG. *Infection Control in the Child Care Center and Preschool.* Baltimore, MD: Williams & Wilkins; 1991.

Holaday B, et al. Patterns of fecal coliform contamination in day-care center. *Public Health Nurs.* 1990;7:224-228.

Van RA, et al. The effect of diaper type and overclothing on fecal contamination in day-care centers. *JAMA.* 1991;265:1840-1844.

Measles (Rubeola) in an Immunized Child

EMILY RHINEHART

CLINICAL PRESENTATION

Rena Monroe, a previously healthy 8-year-old girl, came to the Children's Health Clinic on April 15. Her mother reported that she had had a cough, runny nose, and fever for 3 days. On the day she came to the clinic, Rena had a generalized, erythematous maculopapular rash that began on her face and was spreading to her trunk and extremities. Physical examination revealed moderate conjunctivitis and very small, flat, gray spots on her posterior pharynx and buccal mucosa. The rash and spots prompted the physician to suspect measles (rubeola). Even though Rena reportedly had received all the recommended childhood immunizations and measles would not be expected in an 8-year-old immunized child, the physician included measles in the differential diagnosis. The clinic staff had received reports of a measles outbreak at a nearby college from the local public health department and were aware that measles was in the community. Rena's mother reported that a student from the college had provided child care for Rena and her younger brother about 2 weeks before Rena became ill.

The physician sent a nasopharyngeal aspirate from Rena to the virology laboratory at a nearby university hospital for direct immunofluoresence examination (IFA) for measles antigen.[14] The positive results received the next day confirmed the presence of measles. Serum sent to the state laboratory for antibody testing was also reported as positive several days later.[11]

Since Rena was not acutely ill, she was sent home. Her mother was instructed to take her temperature every 4 hours and administer acetaminophen if her temperature was greater than 99.5° F (37.5° C) orally. The nurses told Mrs. Monroe that Rena's symptoms should subside within 5 to 7 days as her temperature returned to normal and her rash faded. She was instructed to have Rena rest in the house until then and stay away from others who may be susceptible to measles, particularly infants under 15 months of age and children who had not been immunized. Rena's 6-year-old brother, Edward, already exposed to her and the college student, had also received measles vaccine. The nurses instructed Rena's mother to observe Edward and call the pediatrician if he developed a fever or a rash similar to his sister's. Rena spent the next week resting at home and returned to school the following week. Edward did not develop measles.

HOST-ENVIRONMENT INTERACTION
The host

Measles is a very common childhood disease that occurs in every country of the world. In the United States it has been controlled by widespread immunization with measles vaccine. However, outbreaks occur.[4-8,10] Most of the outbreaks involve infants and preschool-age children in urban areas who have not been immunized, school-age children (5- to 19-year-olds), and post–school-age young adults (>20-year-olds), with many cases occurring in college students. Epidemics are more common in countries where immunization is limited or sporadic.

As in Rena's case, measles usually causes a febrile illness. The prodromal hallmarks are malaise, cough, coryza, and conjunctivitis accompanied by a confluent morbilliform rash.[11] The rash usually appears about 14 days following infection and 2 to 4 days after the onset of the prodromal symptoms. It typically lasts 5 to 7 days. The patient is infectious during the prodrome and the first few days of the rash, generally 4 days before to 4 days after the onset of the rash.[1,15] The observation of bluish to gray Koplik's spots in the posterior pharynx is considered confirmatory, although many younger physicians and nurses have not seen measles and may not recognize these lesions. Koplik's spots, which do not occur in all patients, are present for a short period at the end of the prodrome, just before onset of the rash, and may remain for 1 to 2 days after onset of rash.[16] Measles may be accompanied by otitis media or bronchopneumonia or both.[4] In about 1 of every 1000 cases, the infection is complicated by pneumonia or encephalitis, which may result in death or permanent neurologic sequelae depending on the child's age.[13] Children under age 5 and adults are at greatest risk for complications and death.[11]

In other nations, infantile measles is a significant public health problem and is often associated with severe diarrhea and malnutrition.[15] In these countries, a significant number of persons who survive the first month after measles die the following year. Fatal cases among infants were also reported in the most recent U.S. outbreaks.[4-8,10]

The microbiologic environment

Measles is caused by an enveloped ribonucleic acid (RNA) virus of the paramyxovirus family.[11] For rapid diagnosis the organism may be detected in nasal secretions by IFA, which detects viral antigen.[14] Acute or acute and convalescent sera may be tested for measles antibody to verify diagnosis.[11] If individuals have Koplik's spots, laboratory confirmation is not considered necessary.

Measles, considered to be one of the most contagious communicable infectious diseases, is transmitted by droplets as well as airborne droplet nuclei. The virus is sensitive to strong light and drying conditions but survives very well in aerosolized droplets.[12,14] The virus is excreted from the respiratory tract of the infected individual for 1 to 2 days before onset of symptoms and until 4 days after onset of rash. The measles virus may travel 3 to 4 feet in large respiratory droplets and enter the respiratory tract of a susceptible individual or contaminate a fomite that is subsequently placed in the mouth of a young child. The virus may also be carried many feet in air currents via droplet nuclei and be inhaled by a susceptible person.

Incidence of infection is very high in exposed susceptible persons, which results in epidemics, usually in the winter and spring. Once a susceptible individual is exposed, the incubation period may last 8 to 21 days but is most often 10 to 14 days.[11] Measles does not have a long-term infectious carrier state.[6]

The physical environment

Because measles is extremely contagious and transmitted by respiratory droplets and airborne droplet nuclei, it is easy to appreciate why outbreaks occur. In the United States, outbreaks on college campuses occurred in exposed students living in dormitories.[5,10] A student with mild measles symptoms, resting in his or her dormitory room, might expose susceptible students during the incubation period and before measles is recognized with the onset of rash. In areas with depressed socioeconomic conditions, crowded living situations with poor ventilation frequently lead to epidemics among nonimmunized children.

Transmission to Rena may have occurred by droplet spread of the virus when her neighbor, a 20-year-old college student, came to baby-sit during spring break. When Rena's mother called the young woman to ask if she had been ill, the college student indicated she had had a mild febrile illness and a rash several days after being at the Monroe's home.

The social environment

Rena lives in a suburb near the state university. Although most public school systems require proof of childhood immunization before entrance, some colleges do not. Recent U.S. outbreaks have resulted in revision of immunization recommendations as it became clear that a single dose of vaccine at age 15 months may not provide lifelong immunity.[2,6] Both the American Academy of Pediatrics (AAP) and the Centers for Disease Control and Prevention (CDC) now recommend initial immunization at 15 months followed by a second dose at 4 to 6 years of age (CDC) or 12 to 14 years of age (AAP). These recommendations were not in place when Rena's baby-sitter was in public school, and her college did not require a second immunization before entry.

PREVENTION AND CONTROL

The primary strategy for prevention of measles is to minimize the number of susceptible persons by immunizing as large a portion of the population as possible. Before the introduction of the first measles vaccines in the United States in the 1960s, most people acquired natural infection and lifelong immunity during childhood. Consequently, the likelihood of natural immunity increases with age, and it is assumed that persons born before 1957 are naturally immune. However, clinical assessment of persons in this age group should include questions regarding measles immunity to identify individuals who have not had the disease and have not been immunized.

Today vaccine is used to provide immunity and eliminate complications from the disease.

Between 1961 and 1979 several measles vaccines were used in the United States. These vaccines varied by type (live, killed, attenuated) as well as by recommendations for timing of administration by age. In 1971 a trivalent vaccine containing measles, mumps, and rubella vaccines (MMR) was introduced and recommended for administration at 1 year of age. In 1976, after a number of studies to determine the optimal age for measles immunization, the AAP again changed its recommendation for age of immunization to 15 months. This timing seems to result in maximum efficacy, with 87% to 99% of recipients having detectable antibody following immunization, versus 79% to 89% when vaccine was administered at 12 months of age. The lower response rate in those vaccinated at a younger age may be caused by interference from maternally acquired antibodies that are circulating in the younger infants.[16] However, administration of measles vaccine to younger infants (6 to 15 months old) is recommended if there is an outbreak and they have been exposed. If infants less than 15 months of age are immunized to protect them during an outbreak, they should be reimmunized at 15 months and later, consistent with the routine immunization schedule.[2]

In the 1970s, vaccine manufacturers became aware that if the measles vaccine was not refrigerated, its effectiveness was diminished. This led to the addition of stabilizing agents in 1979.[16]

The measles outbreaks in the late 1980s and early 1990s struck a significant number of school-age and post–school-age individuals who had been vaccinated in the 1970s. Experts now believe that the cases among these age groups were caused by timing of administration (at 12 months of age or younger) or receipt of a vaccine that was not stored or handled properly before 1979. Some cases may have been the result of lack of an individual response to the immunization, but it is not believed that protection waned from a successful primary immunization.[7]

Although Rena received the measles vaccine as recommended, she apparently did not develop immunity. The apparent lack of response in Rena's case may have been caused by failure of her immune system to respond or improper handling of the vaccine, which compromised its effectiveness.

Occupational health services in many hospitals and other health care settings have policies to ensure the immunity of health care workers. In many organizations health care workers who were born after 1957 must demonstrate immunity by providing documentation of a physician-diagnosed case of measles, positive antibody titer, or two immunizations.[6]

Prevention of measles transmission in health care facilities requires (1) identification of those who either have active illness or are known to be susceptible and have been exposed to measles; (2) physically separating them in single rooms provided with negative-pressure, unrecirculated air; and (3) ensuring that staff who care for these patients are immune.[3] Those who enter the room of a patient with measles should be immune.[12] Recognizing that immunity is widespread among health care providers and that masks may allow some exposure to airborne droplet nuclei, it is more prudent to rely on immunity as a protective measure. Once exposed, a susceptible health care worker should be restricted from work until the incubation period has passed.

Since measles may be airborne, proper air handling is essential to prevent transmission.[17] In the clinic, Rena was placed in a single room with ventilation which ensured that air from the room did not flow out to the hallway or other spaces (negative pressure) and was exhausted directly to the outside of the building rather than recirculated through the clinic. If she had been admitted to the hospital, she would have been placed in a single room with the same type of air-handling system.

Control of measles epidemics requires community action. In the face of confirmed measles in a student, school officials would review health records to confirm immunity of the other students and staff. Those students whose immunity could not be confirmed would be excluded from attendance for the duration of the incubation period.

When exposure is recognized early, individuals at risk may be protected if immunized within 72 hours of exposure. If more than 72 hours have elapsed since initial exposure, immune serum globulin (ISG) may prevent or modify the disease.[1,6] However, those receiving vaccine or ISG after exposure must be considered potentially infectious consistent with the incubation period.

The AAP recommends administration of measles vaccine to exposed infants between 6 and 15 months of age. The vaccine must be readministered at 15 months of age if infection does not occur.[2]

SUMMARY

Measles is a highly contagious viral illness that occurs in isolated cases or large outbreaks. Periodic epidemics occur in nations where childhood immunization may not be widely available. Although measles is usually a mild illness in older children, serious neurologic sequelae can occur, and there may be significant mortality in infants. Control of measles in the United States has depended on mandatory immunization for children entering elementary school. Problems with efficacy related to timing of administration and vaccine handling have occurred in the past 30 years. These factors have led to a lack of immunity in some immunized persons born between 1959 and 1979. Outbreaks among college students in the late 1980s and early 1990s were a result of ineffective immunization during childhood or

SUMMARY TABLE 16. Measles (Rubeola) in an immunized child

Host-environment model	Case presentation	Factors that influence infectious process	Prevention and control
Host factors	8-year-old healthy girl	Received MMR vaccine at 15 months Apparent vaccine failure, or never received it College student vaccine status unknown	Effective vaccine available (MMR) Check vaccine preparation for appropriate storage Review child's immune status Fully immunize college students and children Follow recommendations for immunization during outbreaks
Microbiologic factors	Rubeola virus	Highly contagious; all humans susceptible Transmitted through droplets and droplet nuclei	Treat symptoms No antimicrobial therapy available Isolate infected persons
Physical environment	Community-acquired infection; home environment	Close contact with infected baby-sitter Airborne transmission likely No special ventilation in home	Isolate infected person during communicable period
Social environment	College setting	Crowded living in dormitories Lack of policy to immunize students fully	Implement college policy to ensure appropriate immunizations for measles Require compliance Educate parents and young people

waning immunity and prompted addition of a second dose of vaccine to the routine immunization regimen.

The prevention and control of measles in health care facilities relies on identification of infected persons at the time of initial assessment, separation of potentially infectious patients with special precautions and airborne handling systems, and immunity among health care providers and the community.

REFERENCES

1. American Academy of Pediatrics: *Report of the Committee on Infectious Diseases*, 23rd ed. Elk Grove Village, IL: American Academy of Pediatrics; 1994.
2. American Academy of Pediatrics Committee on Infec-

tious Disease. Measles: reassessment of current immunization policy. *Pediatrics* 84(6):1110-1113, 1989.

3. Atkinson WL, et al. Transmission of measles in medical settings—United States, 1985-1989. *Am J Med.* 1991;91 (suppl3b): 320S-324S.

4. Centers for Disease Control. Measles outbreak—Los Angeles County, California. *MMWR* 1988;38(4): 49-52, 57.

5. Centers for Disease Control. Measles—United States: first 26 weeks, 1989. *MMWR* 1989;38(50):863-866, 871-872.

6. Centers for Disease Control. Measles prevention: recommendations of the Immunization Practices Advisory Committe. *MMWR.* 1989;38(S9):1-18.

7. Centers for Disease Control: Measles prevention: supplementary statement. *MMWR* 38(1):11-14, 1989.

8. Centers for Disease Control. Measles outbreak—Chicago. *MMWR.* 1989;38(34):591-592.

9. Centers for Disease Control. Measles—United States, 1988. *MMWR.* 1989;38(35):601-605.

10. Centers for Disease Control. Measles—United States, 1989, and first 20 weeks, 1990. *MMWR.* 1990; 39(21):353-355, 361-363.

11. Cherry J. Measles. In Feigan R, Cherry J, eds. *Textbook of Pediatric Infectious Diseases,* 3rd ed. Philadelphia, PA: W. B. Saunders; 1992.

12. Garner J, Simmons BP: Guidelines for isolation precautions in hospitals. *Infect Control.* 1983;4:245-325.

13. Gershon A. Measles virus (rubeola). In Mandell G, Douglas RG, Bennett J, eds. *Principles and Practices of Infectious Diseases,* 3rd ed. New York, NY: John Wiley & Sons; 1990.

14. Minnich LL, Goodenough F, Ray CG. Use of Immunofluorescence to identify measles virus infections. *J Clin Microbiol.* 1991;29(6):1148-1150.

15. Orenstein WA, Markowitz LE, Hinman AR. Measles. In Last JM, Wallace RB, eds. *Public Health and Preventive Medicine,* 13th ed. Norwalk, CT: Appleton & Lange: 1992.

16. Preblud SR, Katz SL. Measles vaccine. In Plotkin S, Mortimer E, eds. *Vaccines.* Philadelphia, PA: W.B. Saunders; 1992.

17. Rhinehart E, LeClair J. The physical environment. In Berg R, ed. *The Association for Practitioners in Infection Control Curriculum,* vol. 111. Dubuque IA: Kendall Hunt; 1988.

Kidney Transplant Patient with Staphylococcal Sepsis

MARILYN SCHOENTHAL

CLINICAL PRESENTATION

Mary Conklin is a 30-year-old woman who had a renal transplant as a consequence of end-stage renal disease (ESRD). At age 10, she was diagnosed with type I juvenile diabetes. At that time her kidneys were functioning well, but over the past 5 years, she developed progressive renal failure and for the past 2 years had been hemodialyzed three times per week as an outpatient. Her diabetes was controlled with 60 units of NPH insulin administered every morning.

After the transplant surgery, Ms. Conklin's initial postoperative course was uneventful. The transplanted kidney was producing urine, and her serum creatinine and serum urea nitrogen were decreasing. At the time of surgery Ms. Conklin was started on the routine renal transplant protocol, which included prophylactic cefazolin every 8 hours for 48 hours, methylprednisolone to be changed to prednisone, cyclosporine, and azathioprine. She was transferred from the surgical intensive care unit (SICU) to the surgical inpatient floor on the second postoperative day. A central venous catheter was left in place because of her extremely poor peripheral access and high output failure, which required large volumes of intravenous (IV) fluid replacement.

On the fifth postoperative day, Ms. Conklin suddenly developed shaking chills with fever, hypotension, and tachycardia. Her white blood cell profile with differential that morn-ing showed a dramatic rise in bands (immature white cells) indicating infection. Ms. Conklin was readmitted to the SICU with a diagnosis of probable sepsis.

Ms. Conklin's symptoms were those typically associated with bacteremia, but identification of the primary source of her infection was a challenge. Her surgical wound was free of swelling and tenderness. Urine obtained from the indwelling urinary catheter was clear, dilute, and light amber in color. The urine cell count did not indicate infection. She was unable to produce a sputum specimen. A chest radiograph showed clear lung fields. Several blood cultures were drawn. The original central catheter tip was removed via aseptic technique, cut into distal and proximal segments, and sent for culture by the semiquantitative method.[8] The external site of the central line was slightly reddened but free of drainage. Ms. Conklin was given three antibiotics to achieve broad-spectrum coverage: vancomycin, tobramycin, and metronidazole. The original catheter tip and a blood culture were positive for *Staphylococcus aureus* sensitive to methicillin. Ms. Conklin continued receiving vancomycin because she was allergic to penicillin.

HOST-ENVIRONMENT INTERACTION
The host

Ms. Conklin had host-related risk factors for infection typically seen in patients who develop sepsis after surgery. She was a long-term type 1 diabetic with ESRD and chronic anemia secondary to renal failure. The chemotherapeutic agents administered to prevent her reaction to antigens in the donor organ also severely compromised her immune system. One of these agents, cyclosporine, prevents T lymphocytes from attacking the transplanted organ. Azathioprine impairs the function of B lymphocytes (B cells) and cytotoxic T cells. Corticosteroids also block the immune response.[1] By compromising the immune system, these agents place the transplant recipient at very high risk for posttransplant nosocomial infection. Many renal transplant recipients develop infection, which is the leading cause of death among this group.[13]

The microbiologic environment

S. aureus is a gram-positive organism that typically inhabits human skin and mucous membranes, particularly the anterior nares.[7] The organism is nonmotile and does not form spores. It is one of the most frequently identified gram-positive organisms in sepsis.[9] The most common sites of *S. aureus* infections are skin (cellulitis, surgical wounds, IV sites) and the bloodstream. Staphylococcal endocarditis, meningitis, osteomyelitis, and pneumonia also occur both in the community and in health care settings. Although *S. aureus* can be airborne for short distances, direct contact is the most usual mode of transmission.

Some staphylococci produce an extra cellular material (slime) that enables them to adhere to implanted devices (valves, joints) and catheters. This may have contributed to Ms. Conklin's sepsis.[15] Some strains of *S. aureus* produce an enterotoxin that can produce food poisoning if ingested (see Clinical Study 2). A similar toxin elaborated by staphylococci produces toxic shock syndrome (TSS) (see Chapter 10).[10] *S. aureus* continues to be one of the major causes of nosocomial infections in both immunocompromised and immunocompetent hosts.

Staphylococci grow readily on blood agar within a day. *S. aureus* is differentiated by the production of the enzyme coagulase, which confers the ability to clot plasma; thus the designation coagulase-positive staphylococci. During outbreaks or clusters of infection, it is often desirable to differentiate strains of *S. aureus*. Techniques used for typing strains include antimicrobial susceptibility testing, plasmid and DNA fragment profiles, serotyping, and bacteriophage typing. The most established of the techniques is bacteriophage (phage) typing, which has been in use since the early 1950s. Phage typing establishes the relatedness of isolates or strains of *S. aureus* according to their susceptibility to lysis by certain strains of viruses that infect bacteria. These viruses are called bacteriophages. Identical or very similar patterns of phage susceptibility indicate that the strains are closely related. Unfortunately, however, many strains of *S. aureus* are not susceptible to any of the available bacteriophages and are therefore nontypable by this system.[7]

Strains of both *S. aureus* and coagulase-negative staphylococci such as *Staphylococcus epidermidis* which are resistant to multiple antimicrobial agents are becoming increasingly common in hospitals, the community (see Clinical Study 5) and other care facilities.

The physical environment

Several factors related to the physical environment may have contributed to Ms. Conklin's central line infection. The catheter was left in place for 5 days. The longer a catheter remains in place, the more likely it is to become colonized. Multiple IV fluid bags were used over the course of several days to replace intravascular volume lost during high urine output renal failure. Pathogens may be introduced during IV bag changes or from open stopcock ports, tubing changes, and line site care (see Chapter 5). A transparent occlusive dressing remained in place for 2 days before the onset of symptoms. In this particular hospital, transparent occlusive dressings may remain in place for up to 7 days. Some evidence shows that transparent dressings may increase the numbers of organisms colonizing the insertion site and risk of infection.[4] Ms. Conklin's own skin flora could have included *S. aureus* and been the source of the organism causing the infection.

S. aureus is ubiquitous in and out of hospitals and long-term care facilities. Inadequate handwashing has been cited repeatedly, often by default, as responsible for patient-to-patient transfer of strains in outbreaks. Even the use of gloves has not consistently prevented the transfer of this organism.[5]

The social environment

The social environment of the immune compromised patient receiving technically complex care can influence the care and its outcomes. Ms. Conklin is married and lives with a very supportive husband in a home in the country. She is well informed about her diabetes and renal disease. She administers her own insulin every morning and regularly tests her blood glucose. Before her surgery, she was hemodialyzed three times per week as an outpatient in a local facility. Ms. Conklin maintains her optimal weight of 52 kg following an 1800 calorie American Diabetes Association (ADA) diet.

Ms. Conklin and her husband met with several kidney transplant patients being followed as outpatients by the transplant team. Ms. Conklin received information describing the medication she would receive after surgery and the adjustments in her daily insulin dose that might be necessary to compensate for the effects of corticosteroid therapy, which can alter serum glucose levels. She was aware that she would be immunocompromised after her surgery and would need to minimize social interactions that would put her at risk for infection. Crowds and friends or family members having an infection and some household pets (e.g., cats and associated toxoplasmosis) were to be avoided. The importance of personal hygiene and handwashing practices were reviewed.

During Ms. Conklin's hospitalization her central line was inserted and maintained by staff who carefully followed appropriate aseptic techniques. Her infection occurred despite conscientious management of many aspects of her social environment.

PREVENTION AND CONTROL

Ms. Conklin was a compromised host at risk for developing bacteremia after surgery because of her long-term diabetes, ESRD, and immunosuppression. Staff, other patients, and the patient herself may have been sources of *S. aureus.* Careful and consistent use of barrier techniques, particularly handwashing and glove use, must be practiced by the nursing staff if transmission of *S. aureus* from human hands and nares is to be prevented.

Catheter-related bacteremias should be verified by culture of blood obtained from peripheral sites and from the catheter using a semiquantitative technique.[3,8] Duration of insertion of intravascular lines, including central venous catheters, is directly associated with line colonization and bacteremia. Catheter-related infections involving central lines should be treated with antibiotics and/or catheter removal. It is essential to determine whether the bacteremia is strictly catheter related or if there is an underlying endocarditis or other focus of infection. The type and duration of the antibiotic therapy must be adequate for the type of infection.

Polyvinyl chloride catheters have been associated with increased risk of catheter colonization. Most intravascular catheters are made of Teflon or polyurethane.[15] Technologic advances in catheter materials may provide catheters with smoother surfaces that will prevent the adherence of bacteria to the catheter walls and thrombus formation, both of which potentiate infection.[9]

Handwashing behavior is very difficult to change. Nurses may believe they wash hands more frequently than they really do.[14] Efforts to improve handwashing frequency and effectiveness can be directed toward changing behavior or improving products.[6]

Several studies have assessed the use of transparent dressing materials. Transparent dressings allow convenient site inspection, form an occlusive barrier, and decrease nursing time required for catheter care. However,

SUMMARY TABLE 17. Kidney transplant patient with staphylococcal sepsis

Host-environment model	Case presentation	Factors that influence infectious process	Prevention and control
Host factors	30-year-old woman Juvenile-onset diabetes mellitus ESRD Postoperative cadaver kidney transplant	Diabetes Anemia surgery Immunosuppression	Control diabetes and anemia and maximize renal status prior to surgery Monitor surgical incision Observe for signs/ symptoms indicating infection No vaccine
Microbiologic factors	*Staphylococcus aureus*	Slime may enhance adherence to catheter	Use appropriate antimicrobial prophylaxis
Physical environment	Surgical intensive care unit	Care providers may be sources of microorganisms Central venous catheter in place 5 days Appropriate IV fluid system maintenance	Use private room, barrier techniques, handwashing, aseptic technique during catheter placement, meticulous line care Remove intravascular catheters as soon as possible
Social environment	Appropriate care enhanced immune competence and minimized risk of exposure from diabetes, pets, hygiene, social interactions	Careful personal hygiene Good barrier techniques and aseptic practices	Review personal hygiene practices Require compliance of staff, spouse, and visitors with handwashing practices and barrier techniques

inadequate moisture vapor permeability may increase skin colonization[4] above that of a dry gauze dressing.[2] Dressings with increased permeability and some containing antimicrobials are being developed.

SUMMARY

The high morbidity, mortality, and cost associated with bloodstream infections prompt emphasis on prevention and control. In one study, 4.5 of every 1000 patients admitted to the hospital developed nosocomial *S. aureus* bloodstream infection. Mortality associated with *S. aureus* ranges from 24% to 49%.[12] Early recognition and aggressive treatment are important.

Gram-positive organisms account for approximately one third of all cases of septic shock.[11] The pathophysiologic alterations associated with septic shock are caused by the activation of extremely destructive multiple pathways and include multisystem organ failure. Current research is examining how these pathways can be interrupted.

REFERENCES

1. Blanford NL. Renal transplantation: a case study of the ideal. *Crit Care Nurs.* 1993;13(1):46-55.
2. Conly JM, Grieves K, Peters B. A prospective, randomized study comparing transparent and dry gauze dressings for central venous catheters. *J Infect Dis.* 1989;159(2):310-319.
3. Elliott TSJ. Intravascular-device infections. *J Med Microbiol.* 1989;27:161-167.
4. Hoffman KK, et al. Transparent polyurethane film as an intravenous catheter dressing. *JAMA.* 1992;267:2072-2076.
5. Larson E: Hand-washing: it's essential even when you use gloves. *Am J Nurs.* 1989;89:934-939.
6. Larson E. Skin cleansing. In Wenzel RP ed. *Prevention and Control of Nosocomial Infections,* 2nd ed. Baltimore, MD: Williams & Wilkins; 1993;450-459.
7. Lennette EH, et al. *Manual of Clinical Microbiology,* 4th ed. Washington, DC: American Society for Microbiology; 1985;145-151.
8. Maki DG, Weise CE, Sarafin HW. A semiquantitative culture method for identifying intravenous-catheter-related infection. *N Engl J Med.* 1977;296:1305-1309.
9. Pittet D. Nosocomial bloodstream infections. In Wenzel RP, ed. Prevention and Control of Nosocomial Infections, 2nd ed. Baltimore, MD: Williams & Wilkins; 1993; 512-555.
10. Reingold AL. Toxic Shock Syndrome: an update. *Am J Ob Gyn.* 1991;165(4):1236-1239.
11. Rice V. Shock, a clinical syndrome: an update. Part I. *Crit Care Nurs.* 1991;11(4):20-27.
12. Roberts FJ, Geere IW, Coldman A. A 3-year study of positive blood cultures, with emphasis on prognosis. *Rev Infect Dis.* 1991;13:34-46.
13. Rubin RH, Tolkoff-Rubin NE. Opportunistic infections in renal allograft recipients. *Transplant Proc.* 1988; 20:12-18.
14. Simmons B, et al. The role of hand-washing in prevention of endemic intensive care unit infections. *Infect Control Hosp Epidemiol.* 1990;11:589-594.
15. Widmer AF. IV-related infections. In Wenzel RP, ed. *Prevention and Control of Nosocomial Infections,* 2nd ed. Baltimore, MD: Williams & Wilkins; 1993;556-579.

Influenza in an Elderly Resident of a Nursing Home

PATRICIA J. CHECKO

CLINICAL PRESENTATION

Mabel Tingley is an 87-year-old resident of a 200-bed long-term care facility (LTCF) in Kansas. She is an alert, ambulatory patient who lived independently until 3 months previously, when she sustained a hip fracture in a fall in her home. At the LTCF she shares a room with three other elderly women. Two days after her daughter and grandchildren visited her in early December, Mrs. Tingley had abrupt onset of fever (38.8° C, or 102° F), chills, headache, myalgia, and fatigue. Over the next few days she developed a sore throat, coryza, and a nonproductive cough. She was seen on day 3 by her physician, who considered influenza a possible diagnosis and obtained a throat swab to be sent to the state laboratory for viral culture.

By the end of the week several other residents had influenza-like illness, including Mrs. Tingley's roommate, Sarah Forbes, a 75-year-old woman with congestive heart failure (CHF) and insulin-dependent diabetes. Two staff members were also absent, reporting acute febrile respiratory illness.

The laboratory isolated influenza A (H3N2) from the nasopharyngeal specimens from Mrs. Tingley and two other residents. By the time the report was available, 21 residents in four wings of the facility had influenza-like illness. Nursing home physicians ordered amantadine preventive therapy for the remaining residents. Residents were monitored three times each day for signs and symptoms of amantadine toxicity.

Influenza vaccine had been administered by the deltoid route to 110, or 55%, of the residents during November. Both Mrs. Tingley and Ms. Forbes received the vaccine. Mrs. Tingley had respiratory symptoms and malaise for 7 days. Ms. Forbes developed pneumonia and was transferred to an acute care facility where she died 9 days later. By the end of the epidemic influenza-like illness occurred among 10 (9%) of the vaccinated residents and 18 of the 90 (20%) unvaccinated residents.

HOST-ENVIRONMENT INTERACTION
The host

Host factors associated with influenza include age and previous exposure to the specific or related subtype. Age-specific incidence during an epidemic is associated with existing immunity to related strains and the amount of exposure. As a result, incidence is often highest in school-age children, who are less likely to have acquired immunity from previous exposure. The elderly and persons with underlying cardiovascular, pulmonary, metabolic, or renal disease are at increased risk for excess mortality and morbidity from influenza. Attack rates of 60% and case fatality rates of 30% have been reported in nursing homes, where large numbers of high-risk people live in a communal setting. Two types of complications occur: primary influenza viral pneumonia and secondary bacterial pneumonia. During epidemics, high-risk persons may require hospitalization two to five times more often than the general population, depending on the age group.[6]

In the United States, more than 10,000 excess deaths were attributed to influenza during each of seven different epidemics from 1977 to 1988, with more than 40,000 each for two of these epidemics. Approximately 80% to 90% of the pneumonia and influenza deaths occurred among persons over 65 years of age.[6]

The microbiologic environment

Influenza viruses (types A, B, and C) are the only members of the *Orthomyxoviridae* family, and all have the same structural and morphologic characteristics. These single-stranded ribonucleic acid (RNA) viruses have two major antigens, hemagglutinin (HA) and neuraminidase (NA). Three major HA and two NA antigenic subtypes have been identified. The epidemiologic history and antigenic type form the basis of classification of the virus. The designation specifies the virus type, geographic area, and year of first isolation and HA/NA type (e.g., influenza A/Shanghai/11/87 [H3N2]).

Frequent point mutations in the HA and NA genes of a specific influenza strain cause slight modifications of the virus year by year (antigenic drift). These minor changes are responsible for annual epidemics and regional outbreaks of influenza. Antigenic shift occurs when genetic reassortment produces a new virus to which few members of the population have immunity. There antigenic shifts occur only with influenza A and are responsible for worldwide epidemics called pandemics. The most recent pandemics occurred in 1957 and 1968.

The predominant mode of transmission is via small particle aerosols. Direct contact with droplets can also transmit the virus. Large amounts of virus are present in the respiratory secretions of infected persons; consequently, one infected person can transmit virus to many susceptible people through sneezing, coughing, or talking.

The virus can survive in dried mucus for several hours and on environmental surfaces for 1 to 2 days, providing an opportunity for hand contamination and transmission.[3,4]

The incubation period is very short, usually 1 to 3 days. Persons are most infectious before onset of symptoms. Adults may shed virus up to 5 days after onset and children up to 7 days. In a closed environment such as a nursing home, large numbers of persons can become infected in a few days, before an outbreak is recognized.

Laboratory confirmation of the diagnosis requires isolation of influenza virus from pharyngeal or nasal secretions or washings or identification of viral antigen in nasopharyngeal cells by enzyme-linked immunosorbent assay (ELISA) or fluorescent antibody (FA) tests. Specimens must be collected within 3 days after onset of illness. Serologic diagnosis requires collection of acute and convalescent sera and is of less value as a means of rapidly identifying influenza activity in a population. Although the diagnosis is often made on clinical and epidemiologic grounds, distinguishing influenza A outbreaks from those caused by influenza B or another respiratory virus is essential to determine if amantadine prophylaxis and treatment (effective only against influenza type A) are indicated and to identify and report regional influenza activity. About 59 laboratories in the United States participate in the World Health Organization's global influenza surveillance network.[5]

The physical environment

Closed populations such as those in LTCFs provide an ideal setting for the spread of influenza. Advanced age, underlying disease, the need for intensive hands on care, and communal activities all facilitate transmission of the virus once introduced from the community by employees or visitors.

Influenza is seasonal. In the United States influenza activity usually peaks between late

December and early March. Consistent with this seasonality, survival of the virus in aerosols is enhanced by low relative humidities such as those in temperate zone winters.

The social environment

Activities within the LTCF setting are conducive to the acquisition and transmission of the virus. Group activities are an important part of nursing home life, and residents are encouraged to participate. Ambulatory residents, like Mrs. Tingley and Ms. Forbes, often eat in a communal dining room and participate in group physical and occupational therapy sessions as well as recreational activities. The elderly individual may also require intensive direct care ranging from assistance with activities of daily living to total care for those with poor physical function. All of these activities facilitate influenza transmission.

PREVENTION AND CONTROL

Control of influenza is based primarily on prevention by immunization and chemoprophylaxis. The most effective measure for reducing risk of influenza is vaccination of high-risk persons each year before the influenza season begins. The influenza vaccine is an inactivated vaccine that incorporates three virus strains believed likely to circulate in the United States during the coming winter. Annual immunization is recommended for persons over 65, those with chronic medical problems, and specifically for nursing home residents. Health care personnel who have contact with high-risk persons and employees of nursing homes and chronic care facilities should also be immunized.[6]

Immunization protects 70% to 80% of healthy young adults when the vaccine strains match the prevalent wild strains. Although the vaccine is less efficacious in the elderly and mortality among immunized elderly nursing home residents can occur,[8,11] several studies have determined that the vaccine can reduce the incidence, severity, and duration of clinical influenza in these residents.[1,2] Only 55% of residents were immunized at Mrs. Tingley's LTCF. Studies suggest that vaccination rates of 70% to 80% of susceptible individuals is necessary to produce immunity widespread enough to interrupt transmission of the virus and reduce the risk of outbreaks.[10]

Amantadine hydrochloride and rimantadine hydrochloride are antiviral agents with specific activity against influenza A. Only amantadine is licensed in the United States. Chemoprophylaxis is 70% to 90% effective in preventing illness caused by influenza A. When outbreaks occur in a nursing home or other institution with high-risk persons, chemoprophylaxis should be started as early as possible to reduce transmission. Nursing homes need to have a contingency plan to ensure rapid administration of amantadine to residents and employees that should include pre-approved medication orders and protocols to obtain physician orders quickly. When used for outbreak control, amantadine should be given to all LTCF residents regardless of their vaccination status and should be offered to all unvaccinated staff who provide direct patient care.[5]

Influenza is often described as transmitted by the airborne route. It is accepted that controlled airflow that directs air from infected person(s) away from others is important to prevent transmission of airborne microorganisms; nonetheless, airflow control precautions are typically not specified as part of influenza control strategies for either long term or acute care.[7,12]

Additional infection control practices to contain the nosocomial spread of influenza should focus on early identification and cohorting of infected patients. In this case, the staff caring for Mrs. Tingley, Ms. Forbes, and other residents with influenza were cohorted and visitors restricted. Careful handwashing, use of barrier precautions when handling body substances and precautions to control respiratory secretions have been suggested as important elements of disease control.

SUMMARY

Influenza is a highly contagious respiratory infection that is responsible for significant morbidity and mortality among the elderly. Outbreaks in LTCFs are common, severe, typically explosive, and likely to occur as an annual event. Person-to-person spread occurs through small-particle aerosol transmission with an incubation period of 1 to 5 days. Respiratory shedding typically persists for 3 to 5 days.

Factors associated with transmission and infection include lack of immunity to the specific infecting virus, seasonality, and institutional settings such as schools, hospitals, and LTCFs that often include large numbers of susceptible individuals.

Prevention and control strategies are aimed at primary prevention by annual vaccination. Although some concern exists regarding the

SUMMARY TABLE 18. **Influenza in an elderly resident of a nursing home**

Host-environment model	Case presentation	Factors that influence infectious process	Prevention and control
Host factors	Woman over 65 years of age	Chronic disorders (pulmonary, cardiovascular) Waning immunity	Annual vaccination; vaccinate all residents and staff between mid-October and mid-November
Microbiologic factors	Influenza A and B	Airborne route, primarily droplet nuclei (small-particle aerosol) Direct contact via hands	Amantadine hydrochloride prophylaxis
Physical environment	Long-term care facility	Crowded conditions; frequent contact between residents, staff, and visitors	Cohort all potentially infected (exposed) residents Restrict admissions during an outbreak Cohort personnel and residents
Social environment	Elderly, chronically ill residents closely interacting	Communal living with group activities Intensive hands-on care for many aspects of daily living Community interface with staff and visitors	Develop plan to contain an outbreak Include preauthorized consent for vaccination and/or chemoprophylaxis Restrict visitors and/or group activities

relative decrease in the efficacy of the influenza vaccine with increasing age of the immunized population, studies substantiate its effectiveness in reducing the incidence, severity, duration, and mortality associated with influenza in the elderly and particularly those in group or institutional settings. It is recommended for all LTCF residents and caregivers. An annual vaccination program and effective surveillance to detect influenza outbreaks are critical components of infection prevention and control. Specific definitions for surveillance of influenza-like illness have been proposed.[9] Amantadine prophylaxis may be an effective adjunct to vaccination during an outbreak of influenza A. When amantadine is given, patients should be closely monitored for side effects.

Other measures recommended during an outbreak of influenza include cohorting residents and staff, restricting admissions and visitors, emphasizing the importance of appropriately handling body substances, and implementing airborne disease precautions for all symptomatic residents.

REFERENCES

1. Arden NH, et al. The roles of vaccination and amantadine prophylaxis in controlling an outbreak of influenza A (H3N2) in a nursing home. *Arch Intern Med.* 1988; 148: 865-868.
2. Baker WH, Mullolly JP. Influenza vaccination of elderly persons: reduction in pneumonia and influenza hospitalization and deaths. *JAMA.* 1980;244:2547-2549.
3. Bean B, et al. Survival of influenza viruses on environmental surfaces. *J Infect Dis.* 1982;146:47-51.
4. Benenson AS, ed. *Control of Communicable Diseases in Man.* 15 ed. Washington, DC; American Public Health Association, 1990.
5. Centers for Disease Control and Prevention. Influenza surveillance, United States, 1991-92. In CDC Surveillance Summaries, September 4, 1992. *MMWR* 1992; 41(SS-5):35-43.
6. Centers for Disease Control. Prevention and control of influenza: recommendation of the Immunization Practices Advisory Committee. *MMWR.* 1992;41(RR-9):1-16.
7. Garner JS, Hierholzer WJ. Controversies in isolation policies and practices. In Wenzel RP. *Prevention and Control of Nosocomial Infections,* 2nd ed. Williams and Wilkins; Baltimore; 1993:70-81.
8. Gross PA, et al. Association of influenza immunization with reduction in mortality in the elderly population: a prospective study. *Arch Intern Med.* 1988;148:562-565.
9. McGeer A, et al. Definitions of infection for surveillance in long-term care facilities. *Am J Infect Control.* 1991;19:1-7.
10. Patriarca PA, et al. Risk factors for outbreaks of influenza in nursing homes: a case-control study. *Am J Epidemiol.* 1986;124:114-119.
11. Saah AF, et al. Influenza vaccine and pneumonia mortality in a nursing home population. *Arch Intern Med.* 1986;146:2353-2357.
12. Valenti WM. Selected viruses of nosocomial importance. In Bennett JV, Brachman PS. *Hospital Infections.* 3rd ed. Little Brown: Boston; 1992:729-821.

SUGGESTED READINGS

Betts RF, Douglas RG Jr. Influenza virus. In Mandell GL, Douglas RG Jr, Bennett JE, eds. *Principles and Practice of Infectious Disease,* 3rd ed. New York, NY: Churchill Livingstone; 1990; 1306-1322.

Cartter ML, et al. Influenza outbreaks in nursing homes: how effective is influenza vaccine in the institutionalized elderly? *Infect Control Hosp Epidemiol.* 1990;11: 473-478.

Centers for Disease Control. *Managing an Influenza Vaccination Program in the Nursing Home.* Atlanta: United States Department of Health and Human Services, Public Health Service, Centers for Disease Control; 1987.

Centers for Disease Control and Prevention. Prevention and control of influenza: recommendations of the Immunizations Practices Advisory Committee. *MMWR* 1992;41(RR-9):1-16.

Gravenstein S, Miller BA, Drinks P. Prevention and control of influenza A outbreaks in long-term care facilities. *Infect Control Hosp Epidemiol.* 1992;13:49-54.

Chlamydia Trachomatis Conjunctivitis and Pneumonia in Two Infants

LINDA G. TIETJEN
BETH HEWITT STOVER

CLINICAL PRESENTATION

Two mothers, Ellen Graham and Jeanne Simmons, delivered their infants at the same large, urban university hospital. Both infants became ill and returned to the pediatric clinic for care.

Case I

Laurie Graham is a 1-week-old girl who was a 5-pound, 37-week gestation neonate born to a 17-year-old single mother and delivered vaginally. Laurie received topical silver nitrate at birth for prevention of gonococcal ophthalmia neonatorum and was discharged from the hospital after a 72-hour stay.

At 6 days of age, Laurie developed mild nasal congestion and watery discharge from the right eye. The next day, both eyes were swollen and the drainage was mucopurulent. On day 7, she was seen in the neonatal follow-up clinic at the hospital where she was born. The nursing assessment revealed infection of the conjunctiva, marked edema of the eyelids, and purulent drainage from both eyes. Her mother told the nurse that both eyes were crusted when Laurie had awakened in the morning. Laurie was afebrile, and her white blood count (WBC) was 12,600/mm.[3] Her lungs were clear to auscultation, and no respiratory distress was noted. A smear of the eye discharge was sent to the laboratory for polymerase chain reaction (PCR) testing; it was positive, confirming the presence of chlamydia. The infant was placed on a 14-day course of oral erythromycin. Laurie's mother was referred to and seen in the gynecology clinic that day and, after examination and laboratory testing, she was also treated. These infections were reported to the county health department sexually transmitted disease (STD) clinic who will contact Laurie's mother and attempt to identify, evaluate, and treat her sexual partner(s).

Case II

Sally Simmons, a 35-day-old girl, was brought to the pediatric medical clinic of the same hospital because of a 1-week history of nasal congestion and 2 days of coughing and rapid breathing. Sally was a 6-pound 10 ounce term infant delivered vaginally. She received ocular prophylaxis with erythromycin ophthalmic ointment at birth. Her mother was single and 22 years old.

Sally was examined by the clinic physician. Her physical examination revealed nasal congestion, tachypnea, a paroxysmal staccato cough, and rales, but no fever. Her liver and spleen were palpable on physical examination. Sally's chest radiograph showed bilateral patchy infiltrates with hyperinflation. An ear examination revealed otitis media. Sally's WBC was 13,200/mm^3, and she had eosinophilia. *Chlamydia trachomatis* pneumonia was considered. A nasopharyngeal aspirate obtained by nasal washing and serum were sent to the clinic's laboratory for chlamydia testing. Within 12 hours, direct immunofluorescent stain using monocolonal antibody detected the presence of elementary bodies (EBs) in the aspirate and confirmed the diagnosis of chlamydia. Three days later, a reference laboratory reported that the serologic test for *C. trachomatis* immunoglobulin M (lgM) was positive, with a titer of 1:64.

HOST-ENVIRONMENT INTERACTION
The host

C. trachomatis is sexually transmitted. Perinatal acquisition occurs as the neonate passes through the mother's infected cervix during delivery. Humans have no natural immunity, and the immune response does not provide complete protection against subsequent infection. Maternal antibody does not protect infants from developing an infection with *C. trachomatis.*[1,2]

In the United States and Europe, *C. trachomatis* conjunctivitis is more common than gonococcal ophthalmia neonatorum. *C. trachomatis* is associated with more than 4 million infections annually in the United States.[5] Up to 40% of men with nongonococcal urethritis (NGU) are infected with *C. trachomatis,* and a large percentage of women contacts of these men harbor *C. trachomatis.* As many as 10% of sexually active women may have asymptomatic chlamydia infection. Chlamydia is reported to be found in up to 50% of sexually active adolescent girls seeking care for symptoms of pelvic inflammatory disease (PID).

Between 60% and 70% of neonates born to infected mothers acquire *C. trachomatis* at delivery.[1,5] Laurie and Sally were both at risk for acquiring chlamydia infection during birth because their mothers had asymptomatic chlamydial endocervical infection. Many infants born to mothers with chlamydia develop

conjunctivitis, as Laurie did. Others, like Sally, develop pneumonitis.

After passage through an infected birth canal, *C. trachomatis* invades the mucous membranes in the eyes, nose, and/or oral cavity of the neonate. Inclusion conjunctivitis and pneumonia may develop. Nasal congestion, injection of the sclera, edema of the eyelids, and mucopurulent drainage are the usual symptoms of chlamydia conjunctivitis. Unilateral eye involvement may occur; however, infection is usually bilateral. Neonatal inclusion conjunctivitis may occur from the first few days of life up to 3 weeks of age. The average incubation period is 1 week.

Chlamydial pneumonia usually becomes apparent in the fourth through the twelfth weeks of life.[3,8,11] When pneumonia develops, the most common manifestations are a persistent cough, rales, and wheezing. Fever is usually absent. Radiographic findings show hyperexpansion of the lungs with bilateral interstitial infiltrates.[14] Chronic pulmonary disease may appear. The WBC is usually within a normal range but with an increase in eosinophils.

The microbiologic environment

C. trachomatis is an obligate intracellular bacterial parasite. Chlamydia depend on host cells for energy. The organism has both ribonucleic acid (RNA) and deoxyribonucleic acid (DNA) and produces iodine-staining cytoplasmic inclusions. The chlamydia attaches itself to the surface of the host cell, becomes phagocytized, and reorganizes inside the host cell into an inclusion body. Replication proceeds for 48 to 72 hours, after which infectious chlamydia elements are released and another infectious cycle begins.

Transmission of *C. trachomatis* occurs via contact with infectious secretions. Sexual contact and contact during the perinatal period are the most common transmission routes. Microorganisms are transmitted to the neonate by direct contact between the infected mother's cervical secretions and the infant's mucous membranes during passage through the endocervical canal. Several sites in the infant can be inoculated independently during the birth process.[8,13,14] Infants whose mothers have *C. trachomatis* cervical infection at the time of birth are at 1% to 16% risk of pneumonia and at 15% to 37% risk of conjunctivitis.[8] Postnatally, an infant may aspirate secretions with its first breaths. Aspiration may lead to colonization of the upper respiratory tract. Infants delivered by cesarean section can be exposed if the membranes rupture spontaneously before delivery. Infants born to mothers with premature rupture of membranes appear to develop infections earlier.[9]

Once *C. trachomatis* is transmitted to the infant, it infects and disrupts the epithelial surfaces of the nasopharynx and airway, producing localized infection of the mucous membranes. However, the organism does not invade or destroy deep tissue or produce exotoxins.[9] If ocular infection is not treated, conjunctivitis may persist for months. Clinical symptoms in the untreated infant with pneumonia may last for several weeks, with the infant exhibiting inspiratory rales and radiographic signs for months.[1,2,6,8]

Laboratory diagnosis can be achieved by several methods. DNA gene probes and cell culture are useful in diagnosis of *C. trachomatis* infection. Once organisms have grown and intracytoplasmic inclusions are produced, direct visualization with monoclonal fluorescein-labeled antibody for *C. trachomatis* can be used for species-specific identification. Although cell culture has a sensitivity of 70% to 90% and specificity reaches nearly 100%, its major disadvantage is that it takes 3 to 7 days to obtain results. Nonculture techniques for detecting *C. trachomatis* are being developed. These include the direct fluorescent antibody tests (DFA), enzyme linked immunoassay tests (EIA/ELISA), nucleic acid hybridization tests (DNA probe), and gene amplification using the PCR tests. Total processing times for these newer laboratory techniques vary from 30 minutes to 4 hours. ELISA is neither as sensitive nor as specific as the DFA monoclonal antibody test method. The specificity for nonculture tests is reported to be as high as 99%; however, false-positive results in groups of patients with a low prevalence of chlamydia infection have been reported.[5] Most studies of nonculture tests have been performed using endocervical secretions. The data on the performance of these tests with conjunctival and nasopharyngeal specimens are limited.[5]

The physical environment

Although transmission of chlamydia occurs most often via the sexual and perinatal routes, infection following use of ophthalmologic equipment contaminated with chlamydia has been reported.[17] Since chlamydia is transmitted by contact with infectious secretions, nosocomial transmission of chlamydia to other infants or staff via contact may be possible but is rarely reported.[7] General infection prevention precautions such as adequate space between infants, careful and consistent handwashing and gloving techniques, and infant-specific use of instruments help minimize transmission in this setting. Nurses and other clinicians caring for patients with chlamydia infections should emphasize the importance of using good hygiene in the home to prevent contact transmission.

The social environment

Chlamydia is the agent of the most common sexually transmitted disease (STD) in the United States.[4,5] It is most prevalent among adolescent sexually active girls, individuals of low socioeconomic status, African Americans, and inner-city dwellers. (See Clinical Study 14). As much as 35% to 50% of nongonococcal cervicitis is associated with chlamydia; 8% to

30% of women with chlamydial infection have salpingitis and are at increased risk for postpartum endometritis.

Infants born to sexually active adolescents having multiple sexual partners are at high risk for neonatal *C. trachomatis*. Based on a conservative estimate of 5% of the U.S. population having *C. trachomatis* genital infection, the estimated incidence of chlamydia pneumonia in infants is 5 to 10 cases per 1,000 live births, and of chlamydia conjunctivitis, 18 to 25 cases per 1,000 live births.[9] These two preventable neonatal infections contribute significantly to health care costs.

Lack of education about STDs, promiscuity, failure to admit that one is at risk, and poor access to health care contribute to the incidence of chlamydia infection. Young sexually active couples frequently fail to use barrier contraception and infection prevention measures and may not recognize that they are at risk of acquiring an STD. Because of asymptomatic disease, some are not aware that they have chlamydia infection, as in the case of Laurie's and Sally's mothers. Many infected persons are asymptomatic and go untreated for months. During this time, these individuals unknowingly infect their sexual partner(s) or their infant(s).[5]

PREVENTION AND CONTROL

No vaccination is available to prevent *C. trachomatis*. Since this infection is principally an STD, preventive measures taken by sexually active individuals can help reduce the incidence of genital infections and subsequent neonatal infections. Minimizing the number of sexual partners and avoiding unprotected sex are effective measures for preventing sexual transmission. A reduction in risk of *C. trachomatis* has been noted among high-risk women who use barrier contraceptives and spermicides.[10,12] Providing education at the time of medical care, selectively using

diagnostic tests during routine gynecologic examinations and at prenatal examinations, treating infected individuals, identifying and treating exposed sexual partner(s), and reculturing after treatment may further reduce the incidence of *C. trachomatis* infections.

Pregnant women at risk for chlamydia should be screened during pregnancy to prevent maternal complications and neonatal infections. Sally's and Laurie's mothers were not screened prenatally or during pregnancy. It is important to identify and treat pregnant women with *C. trachomatis* infection. Screening during the first trimester of pregnancy followed by treatment can prevent complications during pregnancy. Additionally, screening during the third trimester followed by treatment may prevent neonatal disease. Evaluation and treatment of the infected pregnant woman's sex partners is necessary to prevent reinfection.

To prevent pneumonia caused by *C. trachomatis* in infants, the mother with a chlamydial genital infection and her partner(s) must be treated before delivery. Both she and her partner(s) should be educated about methods to prevent recurrent infections (e.g., use of a condom during intercourse if unsure of partner's health status and/or limiting the number of sex partners) and the importance of treatment compliance and then reculturing after treatment to ensure a cure.

Noncompliance with treatment and/or reinfection can lead to exposure of infants such as Laurie and Sally at birth. Therefore, health care providers must ensure that infected women understand why they need to be treated and how to take the medicine. The women also need to understand the importance of completing the treatment course and returning for follow-up evaluation. For example, if Laurie's and Sally's mothers had been cultured during pregnancy and adequately treated before labor and delivery, the infants might not have developed disease.

In settings of low prevalence or limited resources, where testing for chlamydia is not usually done, women and men with positive gonorrhea cultures or clinical signs of an infectious cervicitis should be treated for *C. trachomatis*.[15] Doxycycline or azithromycin are the antibiotics of choice.[5] These antibiotics are contraindicated during pregnancy when erythromycin is the drug of choice.[5] Ofloxacin or sulfisoxazole are alternative antibiotics for chlamydia infections. However, ofloxacin is not recommended for adolescents under 17 years or for pregnant women. Sulfisoxazole is less effective than other antimicrobials.

Although the efficacy of topical antimicrobials in newborns has not been established, prophylactic treatment using erythromycin ophthalmic ointment, tetracycline ophthalmic ointment, or silver nitrate aqueous solution

SUMMARY TABLE 19. *Chlamydia trachomatis* **conjunctivitis and pneumonia in two infants**

Host-environment model	Case presentation	Factors that influence infectious process	Prevention and control
Host factors	Case I: 7-day-old girl, 37-week gestation Case II: 35-day-old girl	Maternal antibodies do not protect infant	No vaccine available; identify infection
Microbiologic factors	*Chlamydia trachomatis* of immunotypes D to K	Sexual transmission or inoculation of eyes or mucous membranes during passage through birth canal Highly transmissible	Use ophthalmic prophylaxis with tetracycline or erythromycin ointment (may not prevent conjunctivitis or pneumonia) Treat infected mother and sexual contacts
Physical environment	Passage through infected endocervical birth canal Possible direct contact with infected eye drainage to mucous membrane	Maternal cervical infection at time of infant's birth Other susceptible hosts having direct contact with infectious secretions, then transmission via contact with mucous membranes	Use appropriate hygiene Diagnose and treat high-risk pregnant females Use barrier precautions for contact with infant(s) Disinfect/sterilize instruments and other objects having contact with infectious secretions

Continued.

SUMMARY TABLE 19. *Chlamydia trachomatis* conjunctivitis and pneumonia in two infants — cont'd

Host-environment model	Case presentation	Factors that influence infectious process	Prevention and control
Social environment	Young sexually active single mother having untreated cervical infection	Mother not identified as infected	Educate sexually active persons regarding infection risks for themselves and infants Identify and culture at-risk mothers Administer prophylaxis at birth to infants of mothers at risk or identified as having *C. trachomatis* Avoid sexual contact with infected individuals Report cases of maternal/infant infection to health department for epidemiologic follow-up Educate parents and health care workers to prevent transmission Encourage compliance with treatment regimen

may be beneficial in the prevention of chlamydial conjunctivitis. It is recommended that ophthalmic prophylaxis be applied within 1 hour of birth.[4,13] Topical treatment does not eliminate nasopharyngeal carriage or pulmonary infection. When conjunctivitis occurs or chlamydial pneumonitis is diagnosed, oral erythromycin is prescribed. If erythromycin is not tolerated, sulfonamides may be given. Infants born to mothers who have chlamydia cervicitis should be treated with oral erythromycin for 10 to 14 days.[8]

SUMMARY

Prevention of neonatal infection requires prevention of maternal infection. Universal or selective screening to identify and treat pregnant women, their sexual partners, and infected asymptomatic infants will most efficiently identify infected individuals and reduce the number of infants hospitalized with chlamydial infection.[9,16] Infants born to high-risk mothers should receive appropriate medical therapy and follow-up care. As more health care providers are made aware that chlamydial pneumonia and conjunctivitis can be prevented by appropriately diagnosing and treating infected mothers before delivery, the morbidity and costs of these infections to the health care system should decrease.

ELISA, direct fluorescent staining using monoclonal antibody, gene probe methods, and PCR test methods can be useful in providing rapid identification of chlamydia genital tract infection during pregnancy. Prompt diagnosis and treatment of the infected pregnant or parturient woman and her infant are important in the prevention of neonatal chlamydial conjunctivitis and pneumonia.

Young sexually active persons need education regarding infection risks to themselves, their partners, and their offspring. This education should include review of the importance of prevention and control measures, such as sexual abstinence, use of condoms and spermicides. Emphasis should also be placed on prompt medical intervention when any sign of genital infection occurs. Education should stress the importance of compliance with antimicrobial treatment regimens.

Diagnosis and treatment of a pregnant woman before delivery may be impossible if resources are limited. Even if therapy is prescribed, it may be ineffective if the patient cannot afford it or is noncompliant or if the sexual partner does not receive treatment. Untreated symptomatic or asymptomatic infection can lead to long-term complications, including infertility, ectopic pregnancy, and possibly spontaneous abortion.

In men, common presentations of chlamydial infection are urethritis, epididymitis, proctitis, and proctocolitis. *C. trachomatis* in sexually active women most often occurs as cervical infection, mucopurulent cervicitis, acute salpingitis, endometritis, or dysuria-pyuria urethral syndrome. The social impact of *C. trachomatis* infection on young sexually active men and women can be significant. Reduction of chlamydia-associated morbidity is a significant challenge to the United States and international health organizations. Improved education strategies and alteration of sexual practices by those at risk of infection are needed for the prevention and control of chlamydial infection.

REFERENCES

1. Alexander ER, Harrison HR. Role of *Chlamydia trachomatis* in perinatal infection. *Rev Infect Dis.* 1983;5:713-719.
2. Beem MD, Saxon EM. Respiratory tract colonization and a distinctive pneumonia syndrome in infants infected with *Chlamydia trachomatis. N Engl J Med.* 1977;296:306-310.
3. Behrman RE, et al, eds. *Nelson Textbook of Pediatrics,* 14th ed. Philadelphia: W.B. Saunders; 1992.
4. Bowie WR, Holmes KK. *Chlamydia trachomatis.* In Mandell GL, Douglas RG Jr, Bennett JE eds. *Principles and Practice of Infectious Diseases,* 3rd ed. New York, NY: Churchill Livingstone; 1990.
5. Centers for Disease Control and Prevention. Recommendations for the prevention and management of *Chlamydia trachomatis* infections, 1993. *MMWR.* 1993; 42(RR-12):1-39.
6. Chirgwin K, Hammerschlag MR. Chlamydia pneumonia. In Feigin RD, Cherry JD, eds. *Textbook of Pediatric Infectious Diseases,* 3rd ed. Philadelphia, PA: W.B. Saunders; 1992.
7. Garner JS, Simmons BP. Guidelines for isolation precautions in hospitals. *Infect Control.* 1983;4 (suppl): 316-349.
8. Gutman L. Chlamydial infections. In Feigin RD, Cherry JD, eds: *Textbook of Pediatric Infectious Diseases,* 3rd ed. Philadelphia, PA: W. B. Saunders; 1992.
9. Holmes KK, ed. *Sexually Transmitted Diseases,* 2nd ed. New York, NY: McGraw-Hill; 1990.
10. Louv WC, et al. A clinical trial of nonoxynol-9 for preventing gonococcal and chlamydial infections. *J Infect Dis.* 1988;158:518-523.
11. Mustafa MM, McCracken GH. Perinatal bacterial diseases. In Feigin RD, Cherry JD, eds. *Textbook of Pediatric Infectious Diseases,* 3rd ed. Philadelphia, PA: W. B. Saunders; 1992.
12. Niruthisard S, Roddy RE, Chutivongse S. Use of nonoxynol-9 and reduction in rate of gonococcal and chlamydial cervical infections. *Lancet.* 1992;339:1371-1375.

13. Peter G, et al, eds. *Report of the Committee on Infectious Diseases*, 23rd ed. Elk Grove Village, IL: American Academy of Pediatrics; 1994.

14. Schacter J, Grossman M. Chlamydia. In Remington JG, Klein JO, eds: *Infectious Diseases of the Fetus and Newborn*, 3rd ed. Philadelphia, PA: W. B. Saunders; 1990.

15. Scott JR, et al, eds. *Danforth's Obstetrics and Gynecology*, 6th ed. Philadelphia, PA: J. B. Lippincott; 1990.

16. Weinstock HS. *Chlamydia trachomatis* infection in women: a need for universal screening in high prevalence populations? *Am J Epidemiol.* 1992;135:41-47.

17. Wilfert C, Gutman L. Chlamydia infections. In Feigin RD, Cherry JD, eds. *Textbook of Pediatric Infectious Diseases*, 3rd ed. Philadelphia, PA: W. B. Saunders; 1992.

SUGGESTED READINGS

Feigin RD, Cherry JD, eds. *Textbook of Pediatric Infectious Diseases*, 3rd ed. Philadelphia, PA: W. B. Saunders; 1992.

Marlow DR, Redding BA. *Textbook of Pediatric Nursing*, 6th ed. Philadelphia, PA: W. B. Saunders; 1988.

Community-Acquired Aspergillosis in a Cancer Patient

MARIE C. TSIVITIS

CLINICAL PRESENTATION

Lenore Gage is a 32-year-old woman diagnosed with leukemia one year ago. She received intensive chemotherapy followed by a matched bone marrow transplant (BMT) from her younger sister six months ago. Ms. Gage had multiple bacterial and mucocutaneous yeast infections during her hospitalization but recovered from all infections following aggressive antimicrobial therapy. She was discharged from the hospital four weeks ago. Ms. Gage also has a history of seasonal allergic rhinitis with occasional mild asthma attacks.

Ms. Gage has not returned to her work in a local antique shop because of persistent anemia and some neutropenia. To stay occupied, she takes daily walks in the woods behind her parents' home and has begun cleaning out the attic after rain from a leak in the roof ruined some of the items stored there. While she cleans, she ties a bandanna loosely over her nose and mouth to reduce the amount of dust she inhales.

Several weeks after her discharge from the hospital, Ms. Gage returned to the cancer center for a scheduled visit. She told the treatment team that she was having some fatigue and shortness of breath, which she attributed to being out of shape. The nurse noted that she had a temperature of 38.4° C (101° F), nonproductive cough, and some congestion. These symptoms had started in the last few days. Ms. Gage's physician interviewed and examined her. He found her breath sounds clear except for some upper airway rhonchi with expiratory wheezing. He ordered a chest x-ray, which did not show any infiltrates indicating a pneumonia or invasive disease. The physician then ordered that expectorated and induced sputum be sent for bacterial and fungal stains and cultures. Ms. Gage was unable to produce expectorated sputum, but two induced sputum specimens revealed septate hyphae. Cultures subsequently grew fungi that were later identified as *Aspergillus fumigatus*. Ms. Gage was diagnosed with aspergillosis.

HOST-ENVIRONMENT INTERACTION
The host

Aspergillus is a ubiquitous organism that rarely causes disease in healthy, immune-competent individuals, who are protected from infection by the phagocytic cells of the immune system, including neutrophils, monocytes and macrophages. Neutropenic individuals, such as those undergoing immunosuppressive therapy for cancer, particularly hematologic malignancy or transplantation, and those with end-stage HIV disease, are at risk for developing invasive disease from *Aspergillus*. The duration of neutropenia appears to be the strongest predictor of subsequent development of invasive aspergillosis.[11] Other risk factors associated with the development of invasive *Aspergillus* infection include intense or prolonged use of broad-spectrum antibiotics that eliminate bacteria that compete with *Aspergillus* for nutrients and that allow for fungal overgrowth. Extensive corticosteroid use, severe diabetes mellitus, and chronic lung disease also predispose to aspergillosis.[5]

Aspergillosis describes several disorders, including allergic bronchopulmonary aspergillosis, local *Aspergillus* infection, and invasive disease. Allergic bronchopulmonary aspergillosis most often affects the patient with preexisting asthma. The patient may have worsening respiratory complaints and report expectorating mucus plugs during coughing. The chest x-ray film may show fleeting pulmonary infiltrates due to bronchial plugging and bronchiectasis. Ms. Gage's diagnosis was made from her history and symptoms and verified by sputum stains. In some cases, *Aspergillus* is not recovered from any cultures prior to death despite suspicion of a fungal infection, and infection is identified only by post-mortem examination.

The most serious form of aspergillosis is infection with tissue invasion, which may disseminate to systemic disease. This illness presents as an acute pneumonia with variable symptoms including fever, chest pain, pulmonary infiltrates, and pleural involvement. Chest radiograph may reveal lobar or patchy focal infiltrates. Sometimes the chest film will look normal until just before death. Pulmonary infiltrates may progress to cavitation, especially if bone marrow function returns. Disease may involve the vasculature of the lungs and may invade the heart and other organs. Once the disease has reached this stage, it may overwhelm all host defenses and be fatal. Some diagnostic procedures to detect aspergillosis include invasive techniques such as percutaneous needle biopsy, bronchoscopy and open lung biopsy. Fortunately, Ms. Gage's sputum specimens were positive for *Aspergillus* and she was spared invasive procedures. Her diagnosis of allergic pulmonary aspergillosis was reached before the disease became invasive and much more difficult to treat.[4]

The microbiologic environment

Aspergillus is a common saprophytic mold found in most parts of the world. The spores of this mycelial fungus are ubiquitous in the environment. Although over 300 species exist, only a few are regularly associated with human disease. Each of these can produce any of the three disease states. The most frequent pathogen is *A. fumigatus*. *A. flavus* is the second most common pathogen but a more common environmental contaminant. Both species can cause serious, often life-threatening disease in immunocompromised hosts.[11]

Classification of the species is based on color and microscopic appearance of the spore-bearing, club-shaped extensions. Most clinical laboratories are equipped to identify the two most common forms but may identify the genus only (*Aspergillus*). *Aspergillus* grows at relatively high temperatures, 45° C (113° F) and above, and can commonly be found in decaying vegetation and natural construction materials. Its spores (conidia) are small (2.5 to 3.0 μm) and are easily suspended in air. When inhaled, these spores may inoculate the paranasal sinuses and may even reach the alveoli of the lungs. Airborne spores may also enter other body sites, such as surgical or traumatic wounds, that are exposed to the contaminated environment.

Disease occurs in only a minority of individuals after inhalation and colonization of the lungs. Rates of colonization vary widely, ranging from 7% of patients with COPD[3] to 57% of patients with cystic fibrosis.[6] In one study 67% of patients with AIDS were colonized.[8,10] The incidence of colonization probably varies by specific environmental and geographic factors.

The physical environment

It is difficult to control the physical environment of the immunocompromised host, and exposure to *Aspergillus* may occur in a variety of settings. Hospital and other institutional outbreaks have been associated with renovation and construction that contaminate the air in patient environments[1,2,7,9] (see Clinical Study 10). Ventilation with unfiltered outdoor air and construction in the springtime, especially after rain, have also been associated with an increase in *Aspergillus* colonization and infection.[1]

It is also difficult to assess and control contamination in nontreatment environments. Following her BMT, Ms. Gage was told to avoid dusty and moldy environments until her immune status returned to normal. However, she did not follow these instructions because she did not fully understand the risks. Although she knew her attic was dusty, she did not realize that after rain leaked through the roof, mold spores present in the dust would germinate and release additional spores into the air. Ms. Gage thought that the use of a cloth scarf would prevent inhalation of dust and organisms in the attic. She also did not associate the rain-soaked springtime woods with molds and spores and therefore did not consider it a hazardous environment. Patient and family education are important in preventing these exposures.

The social environment

The living and working conditions of individuals at risk for developing aspergillosis may be sources of additional reservoirs of spores. For example, high-risk immunosuppressed individuals who work with soil, construction materials, or decaying vegetation, such as trees or dried flowers, may be adversely affected despite the best efforts of the health care providers.

Through her leisure activities, Ms. Gage inadvertently exposed herself to several sources of *Aspergillus* spores, including the rain-soaked dusty attic, the rain-soaked woods where she took her daily walks, and the construction sites she passed on her way to the treatment center.

PREVENTION AND CONTROL

Prevention of aspergillosis includes two primary strategies: preventing colonization and preventing disease. The first strategy is to protect the host from exposure to *Aspergillus* found in specific high-risk environments. For example, in a hospital setting it is advisable to relocate susceptible patients prior to major disruption of ceilings and walls and during renovation and construction.

It is important for immune-compromised patients to avoid sources of *Aspergillus* spores in the community. Ms. Gage used a cloth bandanna to reduce the inhalation of spores, but this was an ineffective filter for mold spores. She should have been advised against walking in wooded areas, where spores are abundant.

When active disease has been diagnosed, treatment invariably requires antifungal agents with or without concomitant surgery to remove accumulations of fungus seen in aspergilloma and local infections (*i.e.*, fungus balls in the lung, eye, bone). In cases of allergic aspergillosis, desensitization may reduce symptoms. The treatment of choice for invasive infection is amphotericin B, sometimes with flucytocine.[4] Amphotericin B is given intravenously for several weeks. Only one other antifungal agent—itraconazole, an oral agent— has demonstrated any in vitro or in vivo success. Although Ms. Gage was diagnosed with allergic pulmonary aspergillosis, because of her immunosuppression she was at very high risk for developing invasive pulmonary disease. She was treated aggressively to prevent invasive disease with two weeks of amphotericin B and discharged to her home on itraconazole.

It is essential to inform patients and their families about appropriate precautions to prevent colonization with new organisms and how to recognize and avoid risky environments (e.g., moldy, damp, warm contaminated environments). Equally important, patients must comply with prophylactic treatments and maintain optimal health during periods of risk, with good nutrition, adequate rest, and other efforts.

Ms. Gage and her family were advised to seal the door to the attic until her white blood cell count returned to a safe range. After an instruction and discussion, Ms. Gage volunteered not to broom-sweep any dusty areas or otherwise create (or enter) dusty environments during her at-risk period. In addition, for the next few months, she agreed to take walks on the beach, away from naturally decaying vegetation, and to avoid construction areas, including the area near the back entrance of the clinic, recently closed because of concern over the risk of exposing patients to active demolition across the street.

SUMMARY TABLE 20.   Community-acquired aspergillosis in a cancer patient

Host-environment model	Case presentation	Factors that influence infectious process	Prevention and control
Host factors	Cancer patient, immunocompromised, with recent bone marrow transplant	Impaired immunity from chemotherapy, corticosteroids, irradiation, underlying disease, neoplasia, malnutrition	Support host immunity
Microbiologic factors	*Aspergillus fumigatus* mold spores	Spores inhaled Colonization of upper respiratory tract may proceed to deep/systemic infection	Treat with amphotericin B or other antifungal agent for serious infection
Physical environment	Spore-laden dust in attic and woods	Dust becomes airborne when renovation, construction or natural events disrupt inner walls, suspended ceiling tiles, or other reservoirs of mold	Seal off or eliminate sources with airtight barriers Use HEPA filters to reduce bioburden Avoid active construction sites
Social environment	Cleaning attic Walking in woods Activities near active construction sites	Chemotherapy given in building next to dusty environment; springtime rain has reactivated mold in woods and attic	Be aware of potential sources of mold Educate susceptible persons and others to recognize and avoid risk

SUMMARY

Aspergillosis is a potentially devastating infectious fungal complication in certain immunocompromised patients. The ecology and epidemiology of *Aspergillus* make it an extremely challenging microbial adversary. Strategies to prevent the development of disease depend upon multidimensional approaches to prevent colonization of hosts before and during their periods of greatest susceptibility and to use environmental control measures to minimize the aerosolized spores that enter the susceptible host's immediate environment. An antifungal agent is sometimes administered to prevent disease. Diagnosis is difficult and complicated by other conditions in these hosts including concurrent infections and the relative difficulty of recovering *Aspergillus* from routine clinical specimens. Once the diagnosis is made, prompt and aggressive treatment is crucial to the survival of high-risk hosts.

REFERENCES

1. Arnow PM, et al. Endemic and epidemic aspergillosis associated with in-hospital replication of aspergillus organisms. *J Inf Dis.* 1991; 164:998-1002.
2. Arnow PM, et al. Pulmonary aspergillosis during hospital renovation. *Am Rev Respir Dis.* 1978;118:49-53.
3. Henderson AH, English MP, Vecht RJ. Pulmonary aspergillosis: a survey of its occurrence in patients with chronic lung disease and a discussion of the significance of diagnostic tests. *Thorax.* 1968;23:513-518.
4. Holmberg K, Meyer RD. *Diagnosis and Therapy of Systemic Fungal Infections. New York,* NY: Raven Press; 1989.
5. Karan GH, Griffin FM. Invasive pulmonary aspergillosis in nonimmunocompromised, nonneutropenic hosts. *Rev Infect Dis.* 1986;8:357-363.
6. Nelson LA, Callerame ML, Schwertz RH. Aspergillosis and atopy in cystic fibrosis. *Am Rev Respir Dis.* 1979; 120:863-873.
7. Opal SM, et al. Efficacy of infection control measures during a nosocomial outbreak of disseminated aspergillosis associated with hospital construction. *J Infect Dis.* 1986;153:634-637.
8. Purcell KJ, Telzac EE, Armstrong D. Aspergillus species colonization and invasive disease in patients with AIDS. *Clin Infect Dis.* 1992;14:141-148.
9. Sarubbi FA, et al. Increased recovery of *Aspergillus flavus* from respiratory specimens during hospital construction. *Am Rev Respir Dis.* 1982;125:33-38.
10. Staib F, Seibold M, Grosse G. Aspergillus findings in AIDS patients suffering from cryptococcosis. *Mycoses.* 1989;32:516-523.
11. Warnock DW, Richardson MD. *Fungal Infections in the Compromised Host,* 2nd ed. New York, NY: John Wiley & Sons; 1991.

SUGGESTED READINGS

Pepys J, et al. Clinical and immunologic significance of aspergillus fumigatus in the sputum. *Am Rev Respir Dis.* 1959;80:167-180.

Rhame FS, et al. Extrinsic risk factors for pneumonia in the patient at high risk of infection. *Am J Med.* 1984; 76(5A):42-52.

Schimpff SC, et al. *Eradication of an Environmental Source of Aspergillus in a Cancer Center.* Presented at the Sixteenth Interscience Conference on Antimicrobial Agents and Chemotherapy. Abstract 330. October, 1976; Chicago, IL.

Schmitt HJ, et al. *Aspergillus* species from hospital air and from patients. *Mycoses.* 1991; 33:539-541.

Giardia in a Traveler

WENDY A. CRONIN

CLINICAL PRESENTATION

Mary Finn is a 25-year-old healthy, active woman. She and two friends took a 3-week vacation in Asia, where they visited several countries. Following the directions given them by their local health department, they were careful to avoid eating salads and drinking tap water or drinks served with ice. The last night of their vacation, she enjoyed an ice cream dessert at a hotel. Two weeks after she returned home, she developed mild diarrhea, gastric discomfort, and flatulence that lasted for several days. She had no fever. Ms. Finn visited her physician. Her stool culture and microscopic examination for ova and parasites were negative for enteric pathogens, and no treatment was given. After a few days the symptoms subsided. However, the next week her symptoms returned and again subsided. After a month of intermittent symptoms and weight loss of 8 pounds, Ms. Finn went back to her physician. The physician again requested a stool sample to culture and test for ova and parasites. He also asked Ms. Finn to bring stool specimens for the next 2 days to the laboratory for additional ova and parasite tests. The stool cultures were again negative for enteric pathogens. The first two specimens were also negative for ova and parasites. However, *Giardia lamblia* cysts were seen in the third stool specimen. Ms. Finn's condition was diagnosed as giardiasis and treated orally with metronidazole. Her symptoms did not return.

HOST-ENVIRONMENT INTERACTION
The host

Giardiasis is the most frequently reported parasitic disease. *Giardia* is transmitted by the fecal-oral route. The patient's history often includes travel and drinking inadequately treated surface water.[9] *G. lamblia* is endemic where people live in poverty with poor sanitation and personal hygiene. In these settings, *G. lamblia* is one of the first enteric pathogens to infect infants. Peak prevalence may reach 15% to 20% in children less than 10 years of age.[8] A low gastric pH probably provides some protection against infection, and children who have relatively alkaline gastric secretions as a consequence of malnourishment are more likely to be infected.[2] In the United States, campers who drink untreated surface water, persons who practice poor fecal-oral hygiene, children in day-care centers, sexually active homosexual men, persons who are institutionalized, and individuals who are immunoglobulin A (IgA) deficient are also at risk of infection. In day-care centers, as many as 50% of children less than 3 years of age may be infected.[8] These children are frequently symptomatic and have been shown to spread infection to the community.[8] Children in day care may asymptomatically carry infectious giardial cysts for up to 6 months.[16]

Immune protection against giardiasis involves both humoral and cellular systems. Specific antibodies to both the trophozoite (free-living) and cyst stages enhance ingestion by macrophages.[8,18] Evidence suggests that acquired immunity provides partial protection against reinfection. People who reside in endemic areas are less susceptible to infection than visitors, and children appear to be more susceptible than adults.[7,8] Human milk has been found to contain antigiardial antibodies and appears to provide nursing infants with some protection against infection.[8] People with acquired immunodeficiency syndrome (AIDS) demonstrate impaired immune response to the parasite but usually do not exhibit more severe illness.[10]

Giardiasis is asymptomatic in 39% of infected children and 76% of infected adults.[20] The most common symptoms include diarrhea, abdominal cramps, nausea, sulfuric belching, and flatulence. As in Ms. Finn's case, diarrhea is usually intermittent. Diarrhea varies in severity and may be explosive, with frequent watery stools, or involve only a few loose stools. Each episode lasts 5 to 10 days, alternating with constipation or normal stool. Occasionally, giardiasis is accompanied by fever, vomiting, and abdominal distention. Although most cases resolve spontaneously within a few weeks, weight loss of at least 10 pounds occurs in 50% of patients.[8] Blood and mucus in the stool are extremely rare, as are white blood cells or pus. The absence of these signs may help to differentiate giardiasis from invasive bacterial diarrhea caused by *Shigella*, *Escherichia coli*, *Salmonella*, amebae, and ulcerative colitis.[18]

Chronic giardiasis may follow initial infection; in one study, as many as 58% of symptomatic patients developed chronic infection.[3] Patients with chronic infection experience extreme malaise. Diarrhea is less severe than in acute illness, but stools are greasy and foul smelling. Abdominal burning, nausea, and anorexia may occur. Intestinal biopsy may reveal visible changes in the upper intestinal mucosa, and malabsorption results in decreased absorption of vitamins A and B$_{12}$, fat, and carbohydrates.[8,18] In infants and children, chronic infection is associated with growth retardation.[18]

The microbiologic environment

Among the several species of *Giardia*, *G. lamblia* is most frequently associated with human infection. *G. lamblia*, a flagellated protozoan, infects the upper bowel, where it is found as both trophozoite and thick-walled oval cysts. After ingestion, the cyst incubates for 1 or 2 weeks in the upper bowel, where it evolves to become two trophozoites. Ingestion of only 10 to 25 cysts is enough to cause infection.[19] The trophozoite is pear shaped and has a characteristic facelike appearance. Four pairs of flagella provide motility. Attachment to the intestinal mucosa is aided by the presence of a large ventral adhesive disk. Multiplication occurs by binary fission of the trophozoite. The trophozoites then encyst in the intestine by a mechanism that is not fully understood. These new cysts either mature and divide to form more trophozoites or are passed in the stool.

Diagnosis is usually made by observation of cysts in stool specimens. Trophozoites can be found in biopsy specimens of the jejunum and duodenum, but unlike the cyst form, they are rarely seen in stool specimens. Stool examination may be negative at the time of onset of symptoms, since new cysts have not yet formed. This was the case when Ms. Finn first visited her physician. Some patients pass cysts intermittently or in low numbers, so stool samples should be obtained every 2 days for a total of three or four samples.[14] Stools are examined for cysts either directly in saline or after concentration in formol ether or zinc sulfate and staining with iron hematoxylin eosin or iodine. In the acute phase of illness, motile trophozoites are infrequently seen in direct saline suspensions.

If no cysts are observed, diagnosis can be made by duodenal aspirate or biopsy, which may demonstrate presence of trophozoites. Alternatively, a less invasive technique, the *string test* (Enterotest, Hedeco Co., Palo Alto, Calif.) can be used. This test requires that the patient swallow a gelatin capsule attached to a nylon line that is long enough to pass into the upper small intestine. After several hours, the line is removed via the mouth, and the adherent mucus is viewed through a microscope for evidence of trophozoites. Finally, small amounts of giardial antigen can be detected by enzyme-linked immunosorbent assay (ELISA) and counterimmunoelectrophoresis testing. These tests have only recently become widely available but will probably be used increasingly for diagnosis of *G. lamblia* infection in the future. Serologic testing for antigiardial antibodies is sometimes used to survey prevalence of infection, such as during outbreaks.

The physical environment

Giardiasis is found worldwide.[18] Infection is usually transmitted via contaminated water. Cysts can survive in cold and tepid water for 1 to 3 months.[18] Where giardiasis is endemic and sanitation systems are limited, *G. lamblia* is typically transmitted via fecally contaminated water, including tap water. Ice cream has been shown to be a vehicle for infection, and this was the likely source of Ms. Finn's infection.[4] In addition, salads and fruits without a removable peel may be contaminated during preparation by cyst carriers or as a consequence of use of fecal material as fertilizer that transmits the parasite.

In the United States the most common source of giardiasis is surface water processed through faulty purification systems (e.g., inadequate filtration with or without inadequate chlorination).[6,8] Hikers have become infected by drinking untreated water from streams or lakes. *G. lamblia* is carried by mammals other than humans, and in at least one case, the water was contaminated by infected beavers.[8]

The disease was subsequently dubbed "beaver fever" in some backpacking circles.

The social environment

Fecal contamination of drinking water is the most common source of infection in all countries. Lack of handwashing after defecation and before handling food provides yet another source of infection. In the United States, spread from persons with inadequate or poor hygiene is the second most common route of transmission. Crowded conditions and lack of handwashing after defecation or diaper changes can increase the risk of infection for children in day-care centers and inmates in correctional or mental institutions.[1] Anal sex also contributes to person-to-person spread of fecal pathogens.

PREVENTION AND CONTROL

Prevention of giardiasis requires proper handling of surface water, adequate sanitation systems, and proper hygiene to prevent person-to-person transmission and contamination of food. Chlorination alone should destroy *G. lamblia* cysts, but variations in water temperature, pH, clarity, and contact time can alter the effectiveness of chlorine.[8] Therefore, chlorination should be supplemented with flocculation (formation of particle aggregates from suspension), sedimentation, and filtration. In the United States, where giardiasis is on the increase, the 1989 Safe Water Drinking Act identifies control of *G. lamblia* in community water supplies as a priority.[15]

Persons traveling to countries where giardiasis is endemic or camping in wilderness areas should boil drinking water for 20 minutes.[17,22] Where boiling is impossible chemical disinfection can be used although it is not as effective.[17] Two percent tincture of iodine (0.5 ml/L for 30 min), a solution of saturated crystalline iodine (12.5 ml/L for 15 min), halazone (5 tablets/L for 30 min), for other chlorine and iodine products may be used.[11,12] Chemical disinfection is most reliable when water is visibly clear and 20° to 25° C (68° to 77° F). In addition, those traveling to endemic areas, as Ms. Finn did, should avoid drinks with ice, desserts served with ice, and ice cream, even in hotels and restaurants where the environment appears to be clean and safe.[4] When traveling, a good rule of thumb is, "If you can't cook it or peel it, don't eat it." Travelers should drink bottled beverages, boiled teas or coffee, completely cooked foods, and fruits or vegetables that can be peeled.

Handwashing is the most effective way to prevent person-to-person spread of infection. Handwashing should be practiced after defecation, before eating, and before and after diaper changes and other possible contact with fecal material. Food handlers should take care to wash hands before preparing and serving food. Public health professionals can effectively reduce risk with enteric pathogen infec-

SUMMARY TABLE 21. *Giardia* in a traveler

Host-environment model	Case presentation	Factors that influence infectious process	Prevention and control
Host factors	25-year-old healthy woman	Susceptibility universal although antigiardial antibodies may slightly reduce risk Malnutrition appears to increase risk	No vaccine Adequate nutrition
Microbiologic factors	*Giardia lamblia* (protozoan)	Fecal-oral contamination, contact and common vehicle transmission	Treat with quinacrine hydrochloride or metronidazole
Physical environment	Travel to an endemic area	Contaminated food Contaminated water supply	Eat only cooked foods and fruits that can be peeled Boil or chemically disinfect drinking water
Social environment	Poverty Lack of health education	Poor fecal-oral hygiene Fecal contamination of water	Educate about handwashing after defecation and before handling food Provide filtered, chlorinated water supply Provide adequate sanitation system

tion by encouraging handwashing with soap and water.[5,13]

There are several effective treatments for giardiasis. All frequently produce side effects and should be used carefully. The drug of choice is quinacrine hydrochloride. Treatment with quinacrine is associated with a 90% to 95% likelihood of cure.[18] Although not approved for use in the United States, a second effective treatment is metronidazole, which is 80% to 95% successful.[8] A third drug, furazolidone is less effective in adults than quinacrine or metronidazole but may be desirable for treatment of children because it is available in a pleasant-tasting liquid suspension.[18] Finally, although not available in the United States, a single dose of tinidazole has been shown to be effective in 90% of cases and is frequently used outside the United States.[21]

SUMMARY

G. lamblia is the most common intestinal parasite worldwide. Humans become infected after drinking water or eating food that has been contaminated with the cyst form of the parasite and occasionally by person-to-person contact. Ingesting only a few cysts can result in infection. Diagnosis of giardiasis should be considered in any person with prolonged diarrhea or malabsorption, especially if there is a history of recent travel to a foreign country, wilderness camping, a child in day care, or anal sexual contact. To diagnose giardiasis, the physician or nurse should be backed by well-trained laboratory staff who can identify cysts and trophozoites in stool or biopsy specimens. Quinacrine hydrochloride, if available, or metronidazole are the drugs of choice for treatment of *G. lamblia* infection.

Prevention and control of giardiasis requires a safe water supply, effective sanitation systems, and good personal hygiene, particularly handwashing after defecation and before handling food. Travelers to underdeveloped parts of the world and wilderness campers should avoid drinking water that has not been boiled or otherwise disinfected. Public health education can help to reduce the spread of fecal pathogens by reinforcing good hygiene.

REFERENCES

1. Black RE, et al. Handwashing to prevent diarrhea in day care centers. *Am J Epidemiol.* 1981;113:445-451.
2. Burke JA: Giardiasis in childhood. *Am J Dis Child.* 1975; 129:1304.
3. Chester AC, et al. Giardiasis as a chornic disease. *Digest Dis Sci,* 1985; 30:315-218.
4. DeLalla F, et al. Outbreak of *Entamoeba histolytica* and *Giardia lamblia* infections in travelers returning from the tropics. *Infection.* 1992; 21:78-82.
5. Feachem RG. Interventions for the control of diarrheal diseases among young children: promotion of personal and domestic hygiene. *Bull World Health Organ.* 1984;62:467-475.
6. Fraser GG, Cooke MB. Endemic giardiasis and municipal water supply. *Am J Public Health.* 1991; 81(6):760-762.
7. Gilman RH, Brown KH, Visbesvara GS, et al. Epidemiology and serology of *Giardia lamblia* in a developing country: Bangladesh. *Trans R Soc Trop Med Hyg.* 1985;79:469-473.
8. Hill DR. *Giardia lamblia.* In Mandell GL, Douglas RG and Bennett JE, eds. *Principles and Practice of Infection Diseases,* 3rd ed. New York, NY: Churchill Livingstone; 1992;2110-2114.
9. Isaac-Renton JL, Philion JJ. Factors associated with acquiring giardiasis in British Columbia residents. *Can J Public Health.* 1992;83:155-158.
10. Janoff EN, Smith PD, Blaser MJ. Acute antibody responses to *Giardia lamblia* are depressed in patients with AIDS. *J Infect Dis.* 1988;157:798-804.
11. Jarroll EL, Bingham AK, Meyer EA. *Giardia* cyst destruction: effectiveness of six small-quantity water disinfection methods. *Am J Trop Med Hyg.* 1980;29:8-11.
12. Kahn FH, Visscher BR. Water disinfection in the wilderness: a simple, effective method of iodination. *West J Med.* 1975;122:450-453.
13. Khan MU. Interruption of shigellosis by handwashing. *Trans R Soc Trop Med Hyg.* 1982;76:164-168.
14. Naik SR, Rau NR, Vinayak VK. A comparative evaluation of three stool samples, jejunal aspirate and jejunal mucosal impression smears in the diagnosis of giardiasis. *Ann Trop Med Parasitol.* 1978;72:491-492.
15. National Primary Drinking Water Regulations: Filtration, Disinfection, Turbidity, *Giardia Lamblia,* Viruses, Legionella and Heterotrophic Bacteria. Final rule,

Federal Register, 40 CFR (parts 141 and 142). June 29, 1989;54:27486-541.

16. Pickering LK, et al. Occurrence of *Giardia lamblia* in children in day care centers. *J Pediatr.* 1984;104:522-526.

17. Potts JF, Setners PA. Vacation diarrhea: how should it be managed? *Postgrad Med.* 1990;88(1):83-90.

18. Reisberg B: Amebiasis and giardiasis. In Youmans GP, ed. *The Biologic and Clinical Basis of Infectious Diseases,* 3rd ed. Philadelphia, PA: W. B. Saunders; 1986; 533-537.

19. Rendtorff RC, Holt CJ. The experimental transmission of human intestinal protozoan parasites. IV. Attempts to transmit *Entamoeba coli* and *Giardia lamblia* by water. *Am J Hyg.* 1954;60:327-328.

20. Rose JB, Haas CN, Regli S. Risk assessment and control of waterborne giardiasis. *Am J Public Health.* 1991:81: 709-713.

21. Speelman P. Single-dose tinidazole for the treatment of giardiasis. *Antimicrob Agents Chemother.* 1985;27: 227-229.

22. Tietjen L, Cronin W, McIntosh N. High-level disinfection. In *Infection Prevention for Family Planning Service Programs.* Durant, OK: Essential Medical Information Systems; 1992;74-75.

Clostridium Difficile in a Nursing Home Resident

JEAN M. POTTINGER

CLINICAL PRESENTATION

Elaine Smith, aged 80, has resided at Valley Long Term Care Center for 2 years. She shares a room and bathroom with two other residents. One roommate provides her own care, and the other requires total nursing care. One month ago, Mrs. Smith was hospitalized for a left-sided cerebrovascular accident (CVA). During her hospital stay she developed pneumonia and a urinary tract infection (UTI). Mrs. Smith returned to Valley Long Term Care Center 2 weeks ago. She is frequently confused but is oriented to self and recognizes her family. She is unable to walk and requires help to stand and transfer from the bed to a chair. Because of her limited mobility she uses a commode. A urinary catheter inserted while she was in the hospital is still in place.

Mrs. Smith completed a course of oral antibiotics at the long-term care center for treatment of the pneumonia and UTI. Ten days after her transfer back to the center, she started having watery, foul-smelling diarrhea. A cytotoxin test on a stool specimen was positive for *Clostridium difficile*. One of Mrs. Smith's roommates and two residents in nearby rooms, all of whom had recently been treated with antibiotics, also developed diarrhea. Health care workers at the center denied having any episodes of diarrhea.

HOST-ENVIRONMENT INTERACTION
The host

Nosocomial diarrhea in acute and long-term care facilities is most often associated with the overgrowth of toxicogenic strains of *C. difficile*. The infection is confined to the colon and ranges from asymptomatic colonization to severe, potentially fatal colitis. Diarrhea, the most common symptom of *C. difficile* infection, varies from mild and self-limiting to severe, with as many as 20 to 30 watery, green, foul-smelling stools per day. The diarrhea may be accompanied by fever, abdominal cramps, and leukocytosis; the stools also may contain blood and leukocytes.[1,5,9]

Antibiotics and chemotherapeutic agents have been implicated as the primary risk factors for infections caused by this organism. The antibiotics most often associated with *C. difficile* disease are those with broad antimicrobial activity, such as ampicillin, clindamycin, and cephalosporins. However, almost all antibiotics and all routes of administration have been implicated. No dose-response relationship has been detected.[2,11]

Other risk factors include long hospitalization, antecedent infection, stay in an intensive care unit (ICU) and colonization with the organism. Lengthy hospitalization and ICU admission may reflect more severe underlying disease and provide increased opportunity for exposure. Gastrointestinal (GI) stimulants, antacids, stool softeners, enemas, and nasogastric intubation increase the risk of infection by altering the normal GI flora.[3,4,10]

Age is a factor in this disease for reasons that are not apparent. For example, up to 75% of infants are colonized with *C. difficile* but do not develop colitis. Children rarely develop *C. difficile* infection even with frequent antibiotic administration. The organism is carried in the GI tract of 3% to 5% of adults.[1,5] Older adults are far more susceptible, and severity of disease increases with age.[1,5,9,10]

The microbiologic environment

C. difficile is an obligate anaerobic, gram-positive, spore-forming bacillus that is widespread in nature in hay, sand, and soil. It has also been found in the stool of animals, but animals have not been shown to be important in transmitting the organism to humans.

The presence of *C. difficile* alone does not result in disease. Disease occurs when the organism is present and the normal flora of the bowel is disturbed. *C. difficile* produces spores that enable it to survive during antibiotic administration. The spores revert to vegetative forms when the antibiotic levels in the colon are low.

Colitis associated with antibiotics was recognized in the 1950s. In the late 1970s the toxin produced by *C. difficile* was identified as the causative agent. *C. difficile* disease is mediated by two toxins, designated A and B. These toxins cause hemorrhage and cellular damage in the colon that disrupt cell membranes and protein synthesis and result in fluid accumulation in the intestines. A motility-altering factor also causes diarrhea by stimulating muscle contractions. No evidence exists that *C. difficile* invades the tissue of the colon.

Endoscopic examination reveals erythema, friability, hyperemia, or frank hemorrhage of the colon wall. A more severe form of the disease is pseudomembranous colitis, in which yellow-white plaques of fibrin, mucus, necrotic epithelial cells, and leukocytes adhere to the inflamed colon and coalesce to produce the classic pseudomembrane. Complications of *C. difficile* infection include dehydration, electrolyte imbalance, colon perforation, and toxic megacolon.[1,5,9]

Diagnosis can also be made by culturing *C. difficile* from the stool on selective media. The presence of *C. difficile* in the stool is not diagnostic and must be correlated with the patient's clinical picture. Diagnosis also can be made by detecting toxin A or B or both from a stool sample. Methods of toxin detection include tissue culture assay, latex agglutination, and rapid enzyme-linked immunosorbent assay (ELISA).

The patient may carry *C. difficile* in the GI tract or acquire it after admission to a health care facility. When *C. difficile* is transmitted to a new host, it appears to be transmitted primarily from person to person. The organism has been cultured from the hands of hospital personnel caring for patients with infections.[7] It has been proposed that these organisms can be transmitted to patients by transient carriage of the organism on the hands of health care workers.[6,9]

The average period between hospital admission and *C. difficile* carriage is 12 days, with diarrhea often beginning 2 days later. Diarrhea can occur as long as 30 days after the antibiotic is discontinued. A person can carry detectable levels of *C. difficile* in the GI tract for up to 6 months after the infection is treated and the symptoms resolved. Relapses may occur during that period, with or without antibiotic therapy.[8,9]

The physical environment

The environment around a patient with either asymptomatic carriage of *C. difficile* or diarrhea may be heavily contaminated with the organism. *C. difficile* has been found on beds, side rails, linen, over-bed tables, night stands, commodes, and bathroom surfaces. The significance of this environmental contamination is not clear, but since spores can persist indefinitely in the environment, fomites may serve as a reservoir.[8,9] Although disinfecting the environment with a hypochlorite solution reduces environmental contamination with *C. difficile*,[7] further study is needed to determine the effect of environmental disinfection on transmission of *C. difficile*. Little evidence exists that implicates organisms from the environment as the source of *C. difficile* infections.

The social environment

Long-term care facilities have unique characteristics that increase the potential for transmitting organisms. The facility must provide medical care, a homelike residence, and social activities. It is a semiclosed environment with common washing and dining facilities. Social and group activities result in frequent resident interactions and more opportunity for direct contact between individuals than the acute hospital setting. Because a limited number of employees care for many residents, the lack of adequate staff may compromise sanitation expediting transfer of the organism.

Most residents are elderly, with multiple chronic underlying diseases. Patients are frequently transferred to and from hospitals, providing occasion for the exchange of resistant organisms. In addition, the semicontinent ambulatory resident may contaminate the environment with body fluids and unwashed hands.

PREVENTION AND CONTROL

C. difficile is presumed to be transmitted by direct contact. The organism has been cultured from the hands of health care workers, and several outbreaks have epidemiologically implicated person-to-person spread.[2,7,8] An important strategy to reduce transmission of *C. difficile* is to practice consistent handwashing between patient contacts and use gloves when handling body substances such as feces.[6] Regular use of barrier precautions should be integrated into routine patient care practices. Patients who have diarrhea should be placed in a private room with their own bathroom or commode.

Because the environment may be a reservoir, cleaning all patient care areas is important. Possible environmental sources, such as shared bathrooms, commodes, elevated toilet seats, and thermometers, should be cleaned and disinfected after each patient use.

Antibiotic restriction is a useful adjunctive procedure for decreasing the likelihood of symptomatic disease. Controlling antibiotic use, careful selection of broad-spectrum antibiotics, and using a minimum number of antibiotics per patient have been recommended to control outbreaks of *C. difficile*.[2,3,9]

At the long-term care center, the nurse manager held a special staff meeting of the personnel who cared for the patients on Mrs. Smith's unit. He emphasized handwashing after all direct contact with Mrs. Smith and other patients. Nurses and aides were reminded to wear gloves for all contact with feces, bedpans, commodes, and toilets. Mrs. Smith was temporarily placed in the same room with the two other residents who were infected with *C. difficile*, and each patient was assigned her own commode. The patients with diagnosed infections were treated with metronidazole for 10 days. All patient rooms and bathrooms were thoroughly cleaned and scrubbed. Mrs. Smith's diarrhea subsided after treatment, but she continued to be an asymptomatic carrier.

Education programs were presented for all the long-term care staff and for residents and their family members. The programs emphasized general hygiene and handwashing after using the bathroom. In addition to these efforts, the medical director reviewed all antibiotics prescribed for residents. Antibiotic therapy was restricted to those patients with documented infections.

SUMMARY

At one time, antibiotic-associated diarrhea was generally assumed to be noninfectious.

SUMMARY TABLE 22. *Clostridium difficile* in a nursing home resident

Host-environment model	Case presentation	Factors that influence infectious process	Prevention and control
Host factors	80-year-old woman with CVA Recent infections	Age Antibiotic therapy for for pneumonia and UTI Recent hospitalization	No vaccine
Microbiologic factors	*Clostridium difficile*	Person-to-person transmission	Wear gloves for contact with feces and toilet Practice consistent handwashing Restrict antibiotic use
Physical environment	Resident of long-term care facility Foley catheter	Community bathrooms Residents who are incontinent	Remove urinary catheter Use thorough cleaning and disinfection practices
Social environment	Semienclosed environment Crowding Social activities	Close contact with other residents Possible asymptomatic carriers	Educate about hygiene and handwashing

Although noninfectious causes of diarrhea do occur in health care settings, *C. difficile* is a significant nosocomial pathogen.

C. difficile appears to be transmitted by direct contact. Persons can be asymptomatically colonized with *C. difficile* and susceptible to disease when the normal flora of the bowel is disrupted by antibiotic therapy. Older adults are most susceptible to infection.

Prevention and control strategies consist of handwashing, wearing gloves for all contact with feces, and cleaning patient rooms and bathrooms. Restricting the use of antibiotics may also prevent *C. difficile* disease.

REFERENCES

1. Bartlett JG. *Clostridium difficile*: clinical considerations. *Rev Infect Dis.* 1990;12(suppl 2):S243-S251.
2. Bentley DW. *Clostridium difficile*–associated disease in long-term care facilities. *Infect Control Hosp Epidemiol.* 1990;11:434-438.
3. Brown E, Talbot GH, Axelrod P, Provencher M, Hoegg C. Risk factors for *Clostridium difficile* toxin-associated diarrhea. *Infect Control Hosp Epidemiol.* 1990;11:283-290.
4. Carpenter DR, Zielinski DA. How do you treat—and control—*C. difficile* infection? *Am J Nurs.* 1992;92(9):22-24.
5. Fekety R, Shah AB. Diagnosis and treatment of *Clostridium difficile* colitis. *JAMA.* 1993;269:71-75.
6. Johnson S, Gerding DN, Olson MM, Weiler MD, Hughes RA, Clabots CR, Peterson LR. Prospective, controlled study of vinyl glove use to interrupt *Clostridium difficile* nosocomial transmission. *Am J Med.* 1990;88:137-140.
7. Kaatz GW, et al. Acquisition of *Clostridium difficile* from the hospital environment. *Am J Epidemiol* 1988;127:1289-1294.
8. McFarland LV, Mulligan ME, Kwok RY, Stamm WE. Nosocomial acquisition of *Clostridium difficile* infection. *N Engl J Med.* 1989;320:204-210.
9. McFarland LV, Stamm WE. Review of *Clostridium difficile*–associated diseases. *Am J Infect Control.* 1986;14:99-109.
10. McFarland LV, Surawicz CM, Stamm WE. Risk factors for *Clostridium difficile* carriage and *C. difficile*–

associated diarrhea in a cohort of hospitalized patients. *J Infect Dis*. 1990;162:678-684.

11. Rowland M. When drug therapy causes diarrhea. *RN*. 1989;52(12):32-35.

SUGGESTED READINGS

Lynch P, Jackson MM, Cummings MJ, Stamm WE. Rethinking the role of isolation practices in the prevention of nosocomial infections. *Ann Intern Med*. 1987;107:243-246.

Smith PW, Rusnak PG. APIC guidelines for infection prevention and control in the long-term care facility. *Am J Infect Control*. 1991;19:198-215.

Swapan KN, et al. A sustained outbreak of *Clostridium difficile* in a general hospital: persistence of a toxigenic clone in four units. *Infect Control Hosp Epidemiol*. 1994; 25:6:382-389.

Infection in a Child with Hydrocephalus and a Ventricular Shunt

CANDACE FRIEDMAN

CLINICAL PRESENTATION

Six-week-old Megan Allen was admitted to the hospital with a temperature of 38.6° C (101.5° F). Her mother reported that Megan had had no obvious problems during the previous month. She had been eating well and appeared normal. However, in the past 48 hours she had been vomiting and become lethargic. A ventriculoperitoneal (VP) shunt was placed just after Megan's birth to control hydrocephalus. Although there was no evidence of local inflammation, the emergency room physician suspected a blocked shunt as the source of her symptoms.

On admission to the hospital the physician obtained a cerebrospinal fluid (CSF) sample for culture from the shunt reservoir, and Megan was empirically treated with intravenous vancomycin hydrochloride. The microbiology laboratory reported clusters of gram-positive cocci in the CSF culture 24 hours after admission. The cocci were later identified as coagulase-negative staphylococci (CNS).

Megan's medical team discussed the various medical and surgical therapies for shunt infection. They decided to externalize her shunt and continue vancomycin. However, Megan's infection did not resolve with therapy. The surgeon removed the shunt and Megan continued to take systemic antibiotics for 14 days. Eventually the shunt was replaced. Megan's health returned to normal and she was sent home.

HOST-ENVIRONMENT INTERACTION
The host

The use of extracranial shunting for the management of noncommunicating hydrocephalus began in 1949. Steady improvements in shunting devices have been associated with a progressive decline in shunt-related complications and have made extracranial shunting the procedure of choice.

Infection and malfunction are the most common complications of CSF shunts. A 1989 review of several outcome studies of CSF shunts reported that the overall incidence of infection ranged from none to 38% during the first year of placement.[12] This wide variation may be the result of a number of factors, including variation in the types of infections, the number of patients studied, the number of operative procedures performed, and the duration of the follow-up.

Host factors associated with risk of shunt infection are age, underlying skin disorders, and a history of recent shunt infections. Additional risk factors include the type of catheter and the surgeon's experience, including operation time.[8] Factors such as underlying disease, entry into the central nervous system for diagnostic purposes, prior meningitis, and type of hydrocephalus have not been associated with increased infection risk.[14]

Patients with infected ventricular shunts have various clinical presentations. Some have a toxic course with persistent fevers, anemia, and splenomegaly. More frequently, as with Megan, there is a nonspecific course of fever, nausea, vomiting, malaise, or other signs of increased intracranial pressure. The incidence of infection in infants less than six months old is 2.5 times higher than for older children.[11]

Infections associated with ventricular shunts are primarily caused by CNS,[1] which account for approximately half of all shunt infections.[13] Gram-negative enteric microorganisms are associated with up to 20% of infections.[9]

Microorganism

CNS are aerobic gram-positive organisms. *Staphylococcus epidermidis*, the most frequently isolated species of CNS, does not produce co-agulase, an enzyme that clots blood plasma and that distinguishes *Staphylococcus aureus* from CNS. Some species of CNS produce an extracellular exudate called slime that may increase the microbe's ability to adhere to smooth surfaces, such as that of a shunt. This slime is an important factor in the establishment and persistence of CNS on foreign bodies. The slime may also inhibit or protect against the action of lysozymes released by cells of the immune system.[6]

CNS are part of the bacterial flora of normal skin. For years they were considered harmless commensals. They are now known to be major nosocomial pathogens. Perhaps the most important factor related to the increasing number of infections caused by this organism is the presence of an indwelling medical device, such as a ventricular shunt, in the host. The principal mode of introduction of this microorganism is through direct perioperative inoculation of shunt surfaces.[6]

The interval between surgery and onset of shunt infection is largely a function of the characteristics of the infecting microorganism. Of shunt infections, 70% occur within 2 months after surgery.[15] Infections due to *S. aureus* typically occur within the first 2 post-operative months. Infections caused by CNS are more indolent and may occur many months or even a year later. Megan's infection with *S. epidermidis* occurred 6 weeks after the shunt was inserted.

Physical environment

Since most shunt infections occur soon after surgery, it is likely that the infecting microbes are introduced at the time of surgery through intraoperative shunt contamination or during manipulation of the shunt in the patient care unit. A study of 289 patients failed to show any relationship between the risk of infection and underlying disease, type of shunt, presence or absence of a valve, or type of valve.[15]

The use of implanted materials always presents risk of infection. Indwelling foreign bodies, such as central nervous system shunts, reduce the bacterial inoculum required to establish an infection. This reduction may result from physical changes in the structure of the prosthetic material after transplantation[7] or an adverse effect on local immune function.[5] The body's inability to eradicate bacterial inocula on a shunt surface may be related to two factors, the inability of the white blood cell to attach to the shunt surface and its impaired intracellular killing of ingested bacteria.[4] New simplified shunt systems have been designed to eliminate recesses where bacteria can multiply.

No single treatment is universally accepted for shunt infections.[9] Systemic antimicrobial treatment of these infections is usually unsuccessful unless combined with intraventricular antibiotics or shunt removal. Megan's infection did not resolve with initial antimicrobial therapy. Her shunt was removed and replaced after 2 weeks of successful therapy.

Social environment

Meticulous aseptic surgical technique and wound care are instrumental in the reduction of risk of shunt infections. The surgeon's experience and technique and the duration of surgery also influence infection risk.[6,8,14] Experienced surgeons and standardized procedures have lowered infection rates. Any entry into the spinal fluid, for either diagnostic or therapeutic reasons, must be performed under strict aseptic conditions. The use of noninvasive techniques for assessing shunt function has helped decrease infection risk.

PREVENTION AND CONTROL

Shunt infections are due to either introduction of microorganisms at the time of surgery or contamination of the system during manipulations after surgery. These two areas are the focus of prevention efforts.

The operative site is a potential reservoir of microorganisms. In one study of shunt insertions and revisions, CNS were recovered from cultures of the operative site before closure in 58 of 100 procedures.[1] In 55% of these patients, the same microorganism was present as normal flora on the patient's skin before the operation. Of nine patients whose shunts became infected, seven infections were caused by the microbe found at the time of surgery. Since normal skin flora play an important role in shunt infections, strict asepsis during placement is extremely important. Proper preparation of the skin site with an antimicrobial agent such as povidone iodine and adherence to proper aseptic procedures are imperative.

Questions have been raised regarding the advantages and disadvantages of anteriorly versus posteriorly placed shunts relative to infection risks. A recent report found no difference between the two.[2] On the other hand, the surgeon's experience and technique do contribute to the incidence of infections. Nelson[10] reported that surgeons who performed a greater number of shunts per year were associated with a lower risk of infection.

The use of prophylactic antimicrobial agents in the perioperative period is controversial. Data are conflicting, and few controlled, comparative studies have been reported.[3] More study is needed regarding the efficacy of prophylactic antibiotics in reducing the inci-

SUMMARY TABLE 23. Infection in a child with hydrocephalus and a ventricular shunt

Host-environment model	Case presentation	Factors that influence infectious process	Prevention and control
Host factors	One-month-old infant with hydrocephalus	Young age	
Microbiologic factors	Coagulase negative staphylococci	Ability to attach to foreign body	Antimicrobial prophylaxis and skin disinfection at time of surgery
Physical environment	Home care	Foreign body	Meticulous insertion technique Consistent barrier techniques
Social environment	Evaluation of variables associated with shunt infection	Skill and experience of surgeon Selection of therapy	Skill of surgeon Compliance with aseptic technique during manipulation

dence of postoperative shunt infections in infants such as Megan.

With a VP shunt, CSF is diverted through a polyethylene tube that exits the skull, transverses the subcutaneous tissue of the neck and thorax and enters the anterior peritoneal cavity. The shunt system sometimes contains a subcutaneous reservoir that provides small-needle access to CSF and a valve that maintains a minimum intraventricular pressure. This reservoir allows access for pressure measurements, testing patency, and sampling of CSF. Stringent aseptic technique must be maintained when the reservoir is entered to prevent contamination of the CSF.

SUMMARY

Central nervous system prosthetic devices are used to divert CSF into a body cavity for elimination in patients with hydrocephalus. CSF can be shunted from the lateral ventricle of the brain to the superior vena cava, right atrium, pleural cavity, or peritoneum. Extracranial shunting to the peritoneum is the procedure of choice.

There has been a general decrease in the incidence of central nervous system shunt infections in recent years, probably as a result of better techniques, standardization of procedures and improved materials from which shunts are constructed.[14] However, shunt infections are still a major complication of this therapy for hydrocephalus, and proper management of this device is important.

REFERENCES

1. Bayston R, Lari J. A study of the sources of infection in colonized shunts. *Dev Med Child Neurol.* 1974;16 (S32):16.
2. Bierbrauer KS, et al. A prospective, randomized study of shunt function and infections as a function of shunt placement. *Pediatr Neurosurg.* 1990-1991;16:287.
3. Bisno AL. Infections of central nervous system shunts. In Bisno, AL, Waldvogel, FA, eds. *Infections Associated with Indwelling Medical Devices.* Washington, DC: ASM; 1989.
4. Borges LF. Cerebrospinal fluid shunts interfer with host defenses. *Neurosurg.* 1982;10:55.
5. Chapman PH. Hydrocephalus in childhood. In Youmans JR, ed. *Neurological Surgery.* Philadelphia PA: W.B. Saunders; 1990.
6. Fan-Havard P, Nahata MC. Treatment and prevention of infections of cerebrospinal fluid shunts. *Clin Pharm.* 1987;6:866.
7. Guevara JA, et al. Bacterial adhesion to cerebrospinal fluid shunts. *J Neurosurg.* 1987;67:438.
8. Kestle JR, et al. A concerted effort to prevent shunt infection. *Childs Nerv Syst.* 1993;9:163.
9. Klein DM: Shunt infections. In Scott RM, editor: *Hydrocephalus.* Baltimore, MD: Williams & Wilkins; 1990:3.
10. Nelson JD. Cerebrospinal fluid shunt infections. *Pediatr Infect Dis.* 1984;3:S30-S32.
11. Pople IK, Bayston R, Hayward RD. Infection of cerebrospinal fluid shunts in infants: a study of etiological factors. *J Neurosurg.* 1992;77:29.
12. Quigley MR, Reigel DH, Kortyna R. Cerebrospinal fluid shunt infections. *Pediatr Neurosci.* 1989;15:111-120.
13. Renier D, et al. Factors causing acute shunt infection: computer analysis of 1174 patients. *J Neurosurg.* 1984;61:1072.
14. Saravolatz LD. Infection in implantable prosthetic devices. In Wenzel RP, ed. *Prevention and Control of Nosocomial Infections,* ed 2. Baltimore, MD: Williams & Wilkins; 1993.
15. Schoenbaum SC, Gardner P, Shillito J. Infections of cerebrospinal fluid shunts: epidemiology, clinical manifestations, and therapy. *J Infect Dis.* 1975;131:543.

SUGGESTED READINGS

Blomstedt GC. Infections in neurosurgery: a retrospective study of 1143 patients and 1517 operations. *Acta Neurochir.* 1985;78:81-90.
Choux, M et al. Shunt implantation: reducing the incidence of shunt infection. *J Neurosurg.* 1992;77:875.
McLaurin RL, Frame PT. Treatment of infections of cerebrospinal fluid shunts. *Rev Infect Dis.* 1987;9:595.
Ratcheson RA, Ommaya AK. Experience with the subcutaneous cerebrospinal fluid reservoir: preliminary report of 60 cases. *N Engl J Med.* 1968;279:1025.
Reingold AL, Broome CV. Nosocomial central nervous system infections. In Bennett JV, Brachman PS, eds. *Hospital infection,* ed 3. Boston, MA: Little, Brown; 1992.
Stephens JL, Peacock JE. Uncommon infections: eye and central nervous system. In Wenzel RP, ed. *Prevention and Control of Nosocomial Infections,* ed 2. Baltimore, MD: Williams & Wilkins; 1993.

Proteus Mirabilis Urinary Tract Infection in an Elderly Person at Home

T. GRACE EMORI

CLINICAL PRESENTATION

Lester Simpson is an elderly widower with moderately debilitating Parkinson's disease and insulin-dependent diabetes mellitus. He was discharged from the hospital 3 weeks ago after surgical repair of a fractured femur. He was injured when he fell in the bathroom of his daughter's home, where he lives. Mr. Simpson's physician ordered home health care for him. The aide from the home care agency, who comes for 2 hours every weekday, assists Mr. Simpson with gait training and the care of his indwelling urinary catheter and monitors his blood sugar. The daughter and son-in-law, who work full time away from the home, hired a neighbor to provide custodial care during the day. The rest of the time the family provides assistance.

Mr. Simpson was discharged from the hospital with an indwelling urinary catheter for urinary incontinence. Last week his urine became foul smelling and appeared cloudy, and he became disoriented, although his temperature did not increase from the usual 37° C (98.6° F). The daughter called his physician, who asked the registered nurse from the home care agency to see Mr. Simpson and take a urine specimen to the laboratory for urinalysis and culture. The urine was loaded with polymorphonuclear cells. The physician prescribed ampicillin for 10 days. The next day the laboratory reported more than 100,000 organisms/ml of a gram-negative rod-shaped organism, later identified as a pure culture of *Proteus mirabilis*. Mr. Simpson completed his regimen of ampicillin, and his urinary tract infection (UTI) resolved.

HOST-ENVIRONMENT INTERACTION
The host

The manifestations of UTIs vary from asymptomatic bacteriuria, which is microbial colonization of the urinary tract without symptoms, to severe damage to the kidneys.[7] Some UTIs resolve spontaneously, and others result in renal failure. Blockages of the urinary tract from congenital or acquired structural or neurologic lesions, enlarged prostate, and renal stones are common causes of UTIs. Sexual intercourse is frequently associated with UTI in women. An indwelling urinary catheter compounds the risk of a UTI because it can act as an obstruction, a channel for microorganisms to ascend into the bladder, a foreign body, and an irritant (see Chapter 5).[11] The four most important factors associated with increased risk of developing a UTI when an indwelling urinary catheter is present are (1) gender (female), (2) duration of catheterization, (3) absence of systemic antibiotics, and (4) inadequate care of the catheter.[10] Many localized symptoms of a UTI, such as dysuria, urgency, and frequency of urination, cannot be detected in a catheterized patient. However, the patient's urine may show evidence of infection, such as foul smell and cloudiness, and the patient may develop fever, back pain, or change in mentation. Data from a number of studies reported that bloodstream infections secondary to UTI are rare (1% to 4%), but when they occur, 13% to 30% of the patients die.[10]

The microbiologic environment

P. mirabilis is a member of the *Enterobacteriaceae* family. Three recognized *Proteus* species (sp.)—*P. mirabilis, P. penneri,* and *P. vulgaris*—are known human pathogens and are normally found in the gastrointestinal tract.[3] A striking characteristic of *Proteus* sp. that facilitates laboratory identification of the organism is the hundreds of flagella on each cell that give it extraordinary ability to swarm on moist agar media.

Proteus sp. can cause infections at all sites, including wounds, lungs, and the bloodstream. In nosocomial infections, they are most frequently isolated from the urinary tract. *P. mirabilis* accounted for almost 5% of the microorganisms in UTIs reported to the National Nosocomial Infections Surveillance (NNIS) system in 1986 to 1989.[9]

The *P. mirabilis* found in Mr. Simpson's urine most likely entered his bladder along the outside of the catheter (periurethral space) and/or through the catheter (intraluminal space). Less often, pathogens enter the urinary tract through the bloodstream.

Ampicillin is the drug of choice to treat most infections caused by *P. mirabilis*. Aminoglycosides and cephalosporins are among the alternative drugs. Although *P. mirabilis* is relatively susceptible to commonly used antimicrobial agents, some strains have become resistant. The *Proteus* sp. that are resistant to select aminoglycosides require the use of amikacin, the newer β-lactam antibiotics, or the newer quinolones.

The physical environment

UTI is the most common nosocomial infection. In the health care setting the most important risk factor for developing a UTI is the presence of an indwelling urinary catheter. For example, in respiratory intensive care units the incidence of UTI is six times higher among catheterized patients than among noncatheterized patients.[5] Prolonged catheterization (i.e., more than 30 days) is associated with UTI in virtually all patients.[12] The incidence of bacteriuria among catheterized patients is 10% to 12% per catheterized day.[13] Most UTIs resolve spontaneously when the urinary catheter is removed. However, UTIs are difficult to treat successfully as long as the catheter is in place, and resistant microorganisms are likely to become predominant if treatment is chronic or repeated. In general, asymptomatic bacteriuria should not be treated as long as the catheter remains.[7]

Many opportunities for contamination of the urinary catheter and drainage system arise, especially in long-term care. The urine collection bag must be opened and emptied at least twice a day, and if a leg bag is ordered, as in Mr. Simpson's case, the catheter and drainage tubing must be disconnected to attach the catheter to a leg bag. Mr. Simpson's caregivers tried to keep the leg bag clean, but since it was reused, it was not sterile. The catheter was irrigated with sterile water, but the irrigating equipment was reused after cleaning with soap and tap water. At the time of the infection, Mr. Simpson's catheter had not been changed since his discharge from the hospital.

A positive urine culture may mean bacteria are growing in the urine or are lodged on the intraluminal surface of the catheter in a biofilm, which consists of sheets of organisms that coat the catheter.[10] Proteins and urinary salts are subsequently embedded in this biofilm, leading to encrustation of the catheter surfaces, which can obstruct the flow of the urine through the catheter. Urease-producing bacteria, especially *P. mirabilis,* promote alkalization of the urine, which leads to crystal formation and further encrustation.

The social environment

Mr. Simpson depends on those who provide his care to use aseptic technique when handling his catheter and the drainage system. The home care agency has a written policy on catheter care techniques to prevent UTI when a catheter is in place; the techniques are discussed periodically at mandatory in-service classes for the staff. The home care nurse has instructed Mr. Simpson's family and the custodial caregiver in basic patient care techniques such as handwashing and care of the urinary catheter and drainage bag. She also frequently reinforces the importance of good catheter management to the home care aide.

PREVENTION AND CONTROL

The single most important measure to prevent nosocomial UTI is to avoid the use of the urinary catheter. If a urinary catheter must be used, it should be removed as early as possible. Urinary catheters should never be used solely for the convenience of caregivers.[14] Because localized symptoms may go undetected in a catheterized patient, caregivers should have a high level of suspicion if the urine or the patient shows evidence of infection. The cause of Mr. Simpson's urinary incontinence should be determined by examining both physical and emotional factors. If his incontinence is persistent, an external condom catheter, which may be associated with a lower risk of UTI, should be considered.[4] When an external condom catheter is used, special attention must be given to care of the skin around the penis and the urethra, since excoriation and ulceration are possible. If an indwelling urinary catheter must be used, the goal is to prevent microorganisms from entering the bladder through the intraluminal and periure-

thral spaces. The sterile closed-drainage system is effective in preventing organisms from contaminating the intraluminal space.[6] Aseptic technique is used when the drainage system must be opened to drain urine from the collection bag through the outlet port or to separate the catheter-drainage tubing junction to irrigate the bladder or attach the leg bag. Whenever leg bags are used to facilitate ambulation, the sterility of the catheter system is compromised. Although leg bags cannot be kept sterile, they should be kept clean with frequent decontamination. A recent study demonstrated that leg and drainage bags can be used safely for 4 weeks if they are decontaminated daily with a diluted bleach rinse solution.[1]

Management of long-term urinary catheters in the home poses some difficult challenges, and no solution is ideal. In the home setting the equipment and supplies available to provide optimal care for the person with an indwelling urinary catheter may be limited compared with those in the hospital, and the caregivers may have less training in aseptic technique. This may have been the case with Mr. Simpson's caregivers. It is also difficult to maintain a consistently high level of daily care. The efficacy of intensive perineal care and routine changing of catheters has not been demonstrated. However, when the patient is bathed, the perineal area should be cleaned as a part of routine hygienic care. The optimal frequency for changing the catheter and the drainage system is probably person-specific, such as when flow diminishes because of catheter encrustation and obstruction.

Intermittent urethral catheterization has been used successfully as an alternative to indwelling urinary catheterization, but no controlled trials have compared intermittent catheterization with long-term indwelling urinary catheterization for preventing UTI in these conditions.[2,8]

Various innovative catheter and drainage systems intended to prevent UTIs have been

SUMMARY TABLE 24.   *Proteus mirabilis* urinary tract infection in an elderly person at home

Host-environment model	Case presentation	Factors that influence infectious process	Prevention and control
Host factors	Elderly man with chronic disease Recently discharged from the hospital after surgical repair of hip fracture	Long duration of in-dwelling urinary catheter	Assess reason for persistent incon-tinence Use indwelling uri-nary catheter only when absolutely necessary Remove as early as possible
Microbiologic factors	More than 100,000 colonies/ml *Proteus mirabilis* cultured from urine	Urease-producing *Proteus mirabilis* promotes alkalin-ization of urine, which leads to crystal formation, encrustation, and possible obstruction of catheter	Treat *P. mirabilis* infec-tion with antimi-crobial therapy; (treatment may not be effective when indwelling urinary catheter is left in place)
Physical environment	At home	Closed-drainage sys-tem is opened fre-quently to drain urine, irrigate cath-eter, and attach the leg bag Difficult to maintain aseptic technique for prolonged cath-eterization in the home where sup-plies not always readily available or easily cleaned or sterilized	Protect intraluminal and periurethral spaces from con-tamination by keeping system closed and drain-age port and cath-eter tubing junction clean Maintain supplies for home care
Social environment	Home health aide provides periodic care each week Neighbor provides custodial care dur-ing day Daughter and son-in-law care for patient rest of time Consistency of care a challenge	Patient depends on his caregivers to manage indwelling urinary catheter to minimize risk of a UTI Those who provide direct care have little or no training in aseptic technique	Retrain and remind caregivers of im-portance of using clean technique when handling pa-tient's catheter and drainage system

tested. These include incorporating antimicrobial substances into the catheter at manufacture, drainage bag disinfectants, and one-way valves to prevent reflux from the drainage bag. Unfortunately, the efficacy of these systems has not been impressive. Although systemic antibiotic prophylaxis prevents short-term urinary catheter–associated UTIs, cost and risk of adverse reactions (including emergence of resistance) outweigh its benefit.

SUMMARY

Indwelling urinary catheter–associated UTI is the most common nosocomial infection. Microorganisms enter the urinary tract primarily along the intraluminal and periurethral routes. Sterile closed-drainage systems prevent UTIs. However, if the catheter is in place longer than 30 days, a UTI is almost inevitable. Maintaining a closed-drainage system free of contamination is difficult in the long-term care and home settings. The patient should be observed frequently for evidence of a UTI or obstruction of the drainage system. Indwelling urinary catheters should not be used unless their use is clearly indicated, and they should be removed as early as possible. If an indwelling urinary catheter must be used, caregivers should use aseptic technique when handling the catheter and drainage system to minimize the contamination of the system. Alternative methods of bladder drainage, such as intermittent catheterization and condom catheters, are options that should be used when possible.

REFERENCES

1. Dille CA, Kirchhoff KT, Sullivan JJ, Larson E. Increasing the wearing time of vinyl urinary drainage bags by decontamination with bleach. *Arch Phys Med Rehabil.* 1993;74:431-437.
2. Diokno AC, Sonda LP, Hollander JB, Lapides J. Fate of patients started on clean intermittent self-catheterization therapy 10 years ago. *J Urol.* 1983;129:1120-1122.
3. Farmer JJ III et al. Biochemical identification of new species and biogroups of *Enterobacteriaceae* isolated from clinical specimens. *J Clin Microbiol.* 1985;21:26-76.
4. Hirsh DD, Fainstein V, Musher DM. Do condom catheter collecting systems cause urinary tract infection? *JAMA.* 1979;242(4):340-341.
5. Jarvis WR, Edwards JR, Culver DH, et al. Nosocomial infection rates in adult and pediatric intensive care units in the United States. *Am J Med.* 1991;91:(3B):185S-191S.
6. Kunin CM, McCormick RC. Prevention of catheter-induced urinary tract infections by sterile closed drainage. *N Engl J Med.* 1966;274:1155-1162.
7. Kunin CM. *Detection, Prevention and Management of Urinary Tract Infections,* 2nd ed. Philadelphia, PA: Lea & Febiger; 1974;4-6.
8. Lapides J, Diokno AC, Gould FR, Lowe BS. Further observations on self-catheterization. *J Urol.* 1976;116:169-171.
9. Schaberg DR, Culver DH, Gaynes RP. Major trends in microbial etiology of nosocomial infection. *Am J Med.* 1991;91(3B):72S-75S.
10. Stamm WE. Catheter-associated urinary tract infections: epidemiology, pathogenesis, and prevention. *Am J Med.* 1991;91(3B):65S-71S.
11. Stamm WE. Urinary tract infections. In Gorbach SL, Bartlett JG, Blacklow NR, eds. *Infectious Diseases.* Philadelphia, PA: W. B. Saunders; 1992;796.
12. Warren JW, Tenney JH, Hoopes JM, et al. A prospective microbiologic study of bacteriuria in patients with chronic indwelling urethral catheters. *J Infect Dis.* 1982;146:719-723.
13. Warren JW. Catheter-associated urinary tract infections. *Infect Dis Clin North Am.* 1987;1:823-855.
14. Wong ES, Hooton TM. *Guidelines for prevention of catheter-associated urinary tract infections.* US Department of Health and Human Services, Public Health Service, Atlanta, GA: Centers for Disease Control and Prevention; 1981.

Cholera in a 3-Year-Old Child in Bangladesh

EMILY RHINEHART

CLINICAL PRESENTATION

Kochel is a 3-year-old boy who lives with his parents and four siblings in a medium-size coastal city in Bangladesh. His family, of modest means, has a two-bedroom apartment. Although there is electricity and running water in their home, none of the utilities are reliable.

Early one morning Kochel awakened his mother when he began to vomit. Within two hours he began to complain of abdominal cramps and diarrhea. His stool was very watery, with small flecks of mucus (commonly described as rice-water stool), and had a slightly fishy odor.[1] Through the morning Kochel had more frequent episodes of watery diarrhea.

Kochel's mother took him to the local clinic, where they frequently see children with diarrhea. The clinic nurse and a physician obtained the history of Kochel's recent onset of diarrhea from his mother. They also obtained a sample of his stool for gross examination. Kochel's symptoms, especially his vomiting, mild abdominal pain, frequency of diarrhea and lack of fever, along with the distinctive odor and character of his stool, led them to a clinical diagnosis of cholera.[2]

The clinic staff was aware that many of the cases of diarrhea that they treat are caused by *Vibrio cholerae*. Although laboratory tests such as microscopic examination of the stool and stool cultures are available, clinical diagnosis is usually relied on in areas like Bangladesh, where cholera is endemic.

Once this presumptive diagnosis was made, the staff knew that assessment of the patient's dehydration, electrolyte balance, and serum glucose level was critical. The administration of fluids containing glucose and electrolytes must occur promptly, since rapid fluid loss in severe cases of diarrhea can lead to shock and death.[1,2,3] The clinic nurse and physician assessed Kochel's fluid status by taking his vital signs, examining his skin and mucus membranes, and calculating the amount of fluid loss based on his mother's description of the frequency and volume of his diarrhea and vomiting. Kochel's pulse was moderately rapid (110 beats/minute) and his blood pressure was low (88/58). His respirations were normal at 22, and he had no fever. His oral mucous membrane and tongue looked dry and his skin had poor turgor. Kochel was also irritable and restless. Their impression was that Kochel was moderately dehydrated.[4,5] A blood sample was obtained for serum glucose and electrolyte determination, and oral fluid replacement was begun.

Kochel and his mother remained in the clinic, where the mother was given oral rehydration fluid to administer to Kochel over the next several hours. After calculating the amount of fluid replacement necessary based on the assessment, the nurse instructed her to have Kochel drink 250 ml (8 oz) of fluid every hour (about 60 ml every 15 minutes) for rehydration.[4,5] Although Kochel's diarrhea continued, his vomiting stopped and he was able to drink sufficient amounts of fluid. Kochel was also begun on oral antibiotic treatment with tetracycline. His mother was given antibiotics for his four siblings as well.[5]

After several hours, Kochel was sent home with his mother, who was given two more packets of oral rehydration mixture to mix with boiled water. She was instructed to give Kochel 100-200 ml of fluid each time he had a diarrhea stool.[5] She was told to bring Kochel back to the clinic in the morning. If Kochel had not been able to take the oral fluid in adequate amounts, the doctor in the clinic would have sent him to the local hospital for intravenous fluid replacement. However, since his illness was of a short duration when he came to the clinic and he was able to take oral fluids, intravenous fluids were unnecessary.[2,3]

Kochel's diarrhea continued but was less frequent through the night and during the next several days. He visited the clinic each day for 3 days to allow the nurses and physicians to follow his course of illness and make sure he was taking adequate oral fluids. His mother was given two oral rehydration packets at each visit. Within a week, Kochel was feeling much better and had no more diarrhea.

HOST-ENVIRONMENT INTERACTION
The host

Cholera is an acute infection of the small intestine caused by *V. cholerae*. The bacteria that cause cholera are usually ingested in contaminated water or food.[2,3,4]

Cholera is found throughout the world and affects persons of all ages. However, in endemic areas such as the Indian subcontinent and Asia, many adults who are repeatedly exposed to cholera develop immunity; and, small children, who have not been previously exposed to the organism, are at greatest risk for infection. When the organism reaches previously uninfected populations, adults are at highest risk for infection.[2,4] Breastfeeding provides some protection to infants and very young children by delaying or preventing their contact with food and water that may contain the microorganism. Recurrences of infection are rare, suggesting that immunity is acquired and maintained after infection.[1,2,4]

Not all persons exposed to *V. cholerae* become infected or ill. Host defenses such as gastric acidity and gut motility can interfere with or prevent the toxin from reaching the small intestine. After infection, natural immunity develops, as evidenced by circulating antibodies and lower incidence in adults in endemic areas.[2]

Some cases of cholera are mild, resulting primarily in diarrhea and other gastrointestinal symptoms. Virtually all persons recover from these infections if treatment is begun promptly and continued until symptoms are gone. However, severe infections, in which patients have voluminous diarrhea, can be rapidly fatal. This is due to the rapid loss of water and electrolytes which leads to hypovolemia, acidosis, and potassium depletion. Children, especially infants, can become severely dehydrated much more rapidly as they are especially susceptible to hypokalemia and hypoglycemia.[2,4]

Physical assessment is very important in determining the degree and severity of dehydration. The patient with moderate dehydration will complain of thirst and have a slight decrease in skin turgor and an increase in pulse rate. The blood pressure usually remains normal. However, if fluid loss continues without replacement and more severe dehydration occurs, weakness, lethargy, severe thirst, a very rapid, thready pulse rate and a drop in blood pressure occur. In severe cases the sensorium is affected, and the stuporous patient may eventually become comatose.[2,4]

The microbiologic environment

V. cholerae are short, curved aerobic gramnegative bacilli with polar flagella. Many serogroups of vibrios may cause diarrhea in humans. The two main pathogens are *V. cholerae* and *V. parahemolyticus*. *V. cholerae* serotype 01 has been associated with epidemics. *V. parahemolyticus* invades tissue of the colon and causes diarrhea. *V. cholerae*, the organism causing Kochel's illness, is not an invasive organism. It secretes an exotoxin that affects the intestinal mucosa in the small intestine by impairing normal absorption of sodium chloride. This leads to excessive water and electrolyte secretion that causes the watery diarrhea.[2,4]

Cholera organisms can survive for about 5 days in fresh water. Survival is prolonged in brackish water, among aquatic plants, and in decaying organic matter. Survival of the organism in food or on fomites is generally shorter.[2]

Cholera is transmitted by the oral-fecal route through ingestion of food or water contaminated with feces. The incubation period is 24 to 48 hours, after which there is an abrupt onset of diarrhea and often vomiting. Humans can be asymptomatic carriers of *V. cholerae* for extended periods.[1,3,4] Excrement from both acute and asymptomatic carriers may contaminate clean water supplies if sanitary sewer systems do not exist or are inadequate. Old or overburdened systems may leak into the clean water supplies.

Laboratory diagnosis of cholera is made by obtaining a stool specimen and plating it on thiosulfate citrate bile salts sucrose (TCBS) agar, a selective media. The *V. cholerae* ferments the sucrose, and the colony appears yellow. The organism is then identified by using biochemicals and type-specific antibodies.[5] Most hospitals and clinic laboratories in the United States are not prepared to culture *V. cholerae*, so specimens for *V. cholerae* are likely to be sent to a reference laboratory, such as a state health department. In nations such as Bangladesh, where the disease is prevalent or there is an epidemic, physicians rely on the clinical findings rather than culture or other laboratory methods to make the diagnosis.

The physical environment

In nations with reliable, adequate sewage systems, sewage is treated to eliminate pathogenic organisms such as *V. cholerae*. Water supplies are treated by filtration and chlorination to minimize microbiologic contamination. Routine testing of water supplies is performed to detect coliform bacteria, which is evidence of contamination.[7]

Where treatment of sewage and provision of safe drinking water is unreliable or nonexistent, risk of infection may be high.[6] Sewer systems may be open drains that carry raw sewage to a river or large body of water. This type of system may allow sewage to contaminate the groundwater and water supplies. Even closed systems that contain the sewage may be old or poorly maintained, allowing leakage into groundwater or other clean water supplies such as reservoirs. If there is no system to treat and test water, people may drink contaminated water and become infected. Ingestion of enteric pathogens such as *V. cholerae* can also occur via consumption of fish, especially shellfish, from contaminated water when the fish are eaten raw or inadequately cooked.[6]

In Kochel's medium-sized city, the sewage system is old and overburdened. Much sewage flows in open drains and contaminates the groundwater. When the system is overburdened, raw, untreated sewage flows into the Bay of Bengal, which contaminates the fishing areas close to shore.

The social environment

Cholera occurs most often in areas with unsanitary living conditions and high population density. When utility services are not available on a regular basis, or are not reliable, those who depend on the services are at risk for infection.[1,2,6]

Kochel's family has no control over the quality of the general water supply. They must rely on the local government to maintain sanitation and supply of safe drinking water.

Bottled water is unavailable or very expensive. Kochel's family's simple diet consists primarily of fresh fruits, rice, vegetables, and fish. Fruits and vegetables may be contaminated during preparation if rinsed with contaminated water and eaten raw or undercooked. Fish should also be well cooked, especially if caught in potentially contaminated water. In some cultures, raw fish is part of the regular diet. Kochel may have become infected with *V. cholerae* from ingesting contaminated food or drinking water or bathing, playing, or swimming in contaminated water.[1]

PREVENTION AND CONTROL

Prevention of cholera depends on adequate sewage treatment and availability of safe drinking water.[1,2,5,6] When the infrastructure that provides these safeguards is well developed, cholera is limited to isolated instances, and threats of epidemics mainly exist in times of social disruption or natural disasters when drinking water may become contaminated from overflowing sewer systems.[6,7] When the infrastructure and economic conditions necessary to ensure a clean, safe water supply which, in turn, depends on a reliable sewer system are inadequate, risk of enteric disease may be significant. The cost to develop and maintain these services is significant. The World Health Organization (WHO) has produced guidelines for cost effective preservation of safe drinking water and management of sewer systems.[7]

Vaccines against cholera are available but have not produced long-lasting immunity and do not prevent shedding of the organisms from carriers who are asymptomatic. Efforts continue to develop a more effective oral vaccine.[1-5]

Cholera is one of three internationally notifiable diseases. It does not occur frequently in the United States or western Europe but did occur in large epidemics in South America in the early 1990s.[5,6] Public health authorities can play an important role in recognizing clusters and epidemics of diarrheal illnesses by collecting reports of individual cases, analyzing the data, and disseminating findings to local medical personnel or health clinics.[5,6] The health system can also provide valuable educational materials to citizens, including instructions for boiling drinking water and eating only foods that have been thoroughly cooked and carefully prepared.

In areas like Bangladesh, where cholera is endemic, public health officials frequently publish information about cholera and other diarrheal diseases. The information explains how diarrheal illnesses are transmitted, as well as recommendations for preparation of food and water to prevent infection. The recommendations suggest boiling any water that may be used for drinking, cooking, or rinsing fruits or vegetables and avoiding consumption of raw fish. Recommendations emphasize that fish should be well cooked. Public health officials also emphasize basic hygiene, especially handwashing after use of the toilet.

The nurse at the clinic discussed these recommendations with Kochel's mother. She was reminded to wash her own hands thoroughly and often when she was caring for Kochel, especially after helping him use the toilet or washing him. The nurse reminded her that she was at risk for ingesting the cholera bacteria herself or could contaminate food she prepared for others in the family.

Treatment of an individual with cholera consists of fluid replacement, which is simple, inexpensive, and generally effective. In a child like Kochel with moderate dehydration, oral rehydration is the first intervention.[1,3,4] Intravenous rehydration may be necessary in cases of severe dehydration. In Bangladesh, WHO oral rehydration fluid packets are available and were provided to Kochel. Each packet contains glucose, sodium chloride, potassium, and sodium bicarbonate and is mixed with a liter of water. The fluid is administered to the patient in amounts based on body weight and estimated fluid loss. Physical signs and symptoms are monitored. Once fluid balance is restored, oral rehydration must continue if diarrhea and fluid loss persist.

Antibiotics can also be used in the treatment of cholera. Administration of tetracycline or doxycycline may decrease the symptoms, required treatment, and duration of the illness as well as the number of organisms excreted by an infected host.[3-5] Where risk to household contacts is high, these persons should receive prophylactic antibiotics.[3,4]

Staff who work in hospitals or clinics where patients with cholera are cared for must reduce the risk of nosocomial transmission. The staff should wash hands after caring for each patient to protect themselves and other patients from person-to-person transmission of organisms. Gowns and gloves are often used in the United States when contact with feces is anticipated during care of a patient with infectious diarrhea. In other nations these supplies may not be affordable or available. In either case, reliance on good handwashing is critical.

SUMMARY TABLE 25.   Cholera in a 3-year-old child in Bangladesh

Host-environment model	Case presentation	Factors that influence infectious process	Prevention and control
Host factors	3-year-old boy	Some immunity after repeated exposure Young children without prior exposure highly susceptible	Vaccine not effective
Microbiologic factors	*Vibrio cholera*	Diarrhea producing exotoxin Organisms survive in fresh and brackish water	Rehydrate
Physical environment	Inadequate utilities	Lack of sewage treatment and safe drinking water	Control and treat sewage and drinking water Provide bottled water for drinking and cooking Ingest only fully cooked foods
Social environment	Social or political instability or poverty	Breast-feeding may delay contact with contaminated food or water Compromised utility construction or maintenance	Encourage breast feeding where appropriate Educate about preparing food and water for ingestion Support public health interventions

SUMMARY

Cholera is an acute infection of the small intestine that manifests as a diarrheal illness. It is caused by *V. cholerae*. The organisms are transmitted to persons via the fecal-oral route through ingestion of contaminated water or food. Cholera occurs in geographic areas where sewage treatment and safe drinking water are inadequate. Infections present singly, in clusters or in widespread epidemics. Although cholera can be a mild gastrointestinal infection, it frequently causes profuse watery diarrhea leading to severe dehydration. Symptoms can occur rapidly, and death may ensue if treatment is not begun promptly. The very young are at greatest risk for the most severe outcomes.

The primary treatment is rehydration. Oral rehydration is used in mild to moderate cases when the person can tolerate oral fluids. Intravenous fluids are used only in persons who are severely dehydrated. Oral antibiotics such as tetracycline or doxycycline may decrease the symptoms and shorten the duration of the illness.

Prevention is best achieved through management of sewage and provision of safe drinking water. Cases of cholera must be reported to health authorities so that preventive measures can be implemented.

REFERENCES

1. Black RE. Cholera. In Maxcy KF, Rosenau MJ, Last JM, eds. *Public Health and Preventive Medicine*. East Norwalk, CT: Appleton & Lange; 1992.
2. Greenough WB III. *Vibrio cholerae*. In Mandel GL, Douglas RG, Bennett JE, eds. *Principles and Practice of Infectious Diseases*, 3rd ed. New York, NY: Churchill Livingstone; 1990.
3. Keusch, GT, Bennish M. Cholera. In Feigin R, Cherry J, eds. *Textbook of Pediatric Infectious Diseases*. Philadelphia, PA: W. B. Saunders; 1992.
4. Pierce NV. Cholera. In Warren K, Mahmoud AAF, eds. *Tropical and Geographic Medicine*. New York, NY: McGraw Hill; 1984.
5. Swerdlow D, Ries A. Cholera in the Americas. *JAMA*. 1992;267(11):1495-1499.
6. Tauxe R, Blake P. Epidemic cholera in Latin America. *JAMA*. 1992;267(11):1388-1390.
7. World Health Organization: *Guidelines for Drinking Water Quality*. Geneva: WHO, 1984.

Human Immunodeficiency Virus in a Female Who Injects Drugs

M A R I E C . T S I V I T I S

CLINICAL PRESENTATION

Susan Forbes is a 26-year-old woman from Brooklyn who lives in a fourth-floor walk-up apartment with her two children, aged 4 years and 28 months. She is enrolled in a computer training program, which she began after successful completion of a drug treatment program 3 months ago. Ms. Forbes was a cocaine-injecting addict for approximately 1 year before the birth of her first child. For the past 5 years she has not injected drugs, but she occasionally smokes crack cocaine and drinks alcohol two or three evenings each week.

Ms. Forbes shares her apartment with a male friend, John Hart, also a former injecting drug user (IDU). She has recently suspected that Mr. Hart has returned to his former drug habits. Because of his multiple-substance abuse problems, she has tried to discontinue their regular sexual relationship. This is difficult for her because they continue to live together and share the same bed. Sometimes when they are together smoking crack cocaine and drinking alcohol, she feels the temptation to resume her injecting drug use, but so far she has avoided this. Ms. Forbes is also concerned about Mr. Hart's poor influence on her children, but he often helps her when she is feeling ill and sometimes takes care of the children for an hour or two so she can go to the grocery store. She has not yet had the courage to ask Mr. Hart to move out of the apartment, and when they

talk about his drug use, he gets angry and yells at her and the children.

For the past 2 weeks, Ms. Forbes has had abdominal pain. She attributed this to increasing stress from her child care responsibilities, her troubled relationship with Mr. Hart, and difficulties keeping up with schoolwork. One evening a neighbor took Ms. Forbes to the local hospital emergency department (ED) when she was unable to walk to her class 10 blocks away. The ED physician examined her carefully, noting the abdominal pain and a fever. The physician diagnosed probable pelvic inflammatory disease (PID) and because of her severe pain recommended admission to the hospital for intravenous (IV) antibiotics. Ms. Forbes was distressed but agreed to be admitted to the hospital. Mr. Hart was watching the children at home, but Ms. Forbes did not want to leave the children with him while she was hospitalized. After several telephone calls she was able to make arrangements for her neighbor to return to the apartment and take the children to their grandmother's home.

Three days after the initiation of IV antibiotics, Ms. Forbes felt better and requested to be discharged from the hospital. The physician told her she had culture-confirmed gonorrhea, genital warts, and cervical dysplasia. He discussed the usual course of therapy for gonococcal PID and noted that Ms. Forbes might also have an infection with chlamydia. He prescribed antibiotics effective against both organisms and told Ms. Forbes that since she was feeling better, she could continue the antibiotics in an oral form for 10 days following her discharge from the hospital.

The physician also suggested that Ms. Forbes be tested for human immunodeficiency virus (HIV) before she left the hospital. Ms. Forbes was startled at the suggestion, indicating that she had not been injecting drugs for years and felt fine. She added that she had never shared needles with sick people. However, after further discussion, Ms. Forbes agreed that her injection of drugs in the 1980s, relations with other IV drug users during that time, and occasional exchange of sex for drugs when she was low on money, might have placed her at risk for infection. Consequently, she agreed to have an HIV test. The nurse provided pretest counseling. She discussed the consequences of a positive test result for Ms. Forbes, her children, and her sex partner(s). The nurse also told her that several drugs were available that could help people who were newly diagnosed as HIV infected. Some of these drugs, taken early in the course of HIV infection, appear to delay the onset of more serious illness and enable the infected person to continue with a normal life for some time. Ms. Forbes signed the consent form, and the test was performed.

Ms. Forbes was discharged from the hospital that afternoon and continued taking oral antibiotics to complete her treatment. She returned to the clinic 2 weeks later, where she was advised that her PID was resolving but that her HIV antibody test was positive. Ms. Forbes was devastated. The nurse and physician again explained the implications of a positive HIV antibody test. After the discussion the physician referred Ms. Forbes to the AIDS treatment center.

At the treatment center, she was screened for several infections, including tuberculosis and syphilis. Her children were also examined and

screened for antibodies to HIV, since both were born after the time of their mother's highest risk of infection, and both were old enough to have cleared maternal antibody. Both of Susan's children were HIV negative. These results were consistent with information that 15% to 40% of children born to infected mothers are infected in the perinatal period.[12]

The staff at the AIDS treatment center referred Ms. Forbes to a women's HIV/AIDS support group. There she was able to express her fears, process her grief, begin to cope with some profound issues, and make choices. She learned about stress management, life planning, resources and benefits, and treatment options, and she received peer group reinforcement and support during the continuing difficulties in her complex life.

HOST-ENVIRONMENT INTERACTION
The host

All humans and some primates are susceptible to infection with HIV. Because HIV is transmitted through blood and some other body fluids, such as semen and vaginal secretions, certain behaviors place some people at significant risk for acquiring the virus. It is well established that HIV is transmitted through sexual activities, blood exchange, birth, and breastfeeding. Sharing of drug paraphernalia among IDUs is associated with a particularly high risk of HIV exposure. This practice is more common in some geographic areas than others.

The presence of HIV infection in needle-sharing or sexual partners of an individual places him or her at risk for exposure to HIV. Although no conclusive evidence indicates a genetic predisposition for HIV infection,[6] genetic factors may contribute to the speed of onset and severity of HIV-related immunodeficiency.[17] The mechanisms of immune damage and the rapidity of onset and progression are highly variable. Factors that may accelerate the rate of progression of HIV infection include preexisting health status, (nutrition and general health) presence of other chronic or acute conditions such as lung or metabolic disease, and recurrent or persistent infections. Chronic abuse of alcohol, injected or noninjected drugs, and tobacco may also accelerate the course of the disease. In particular, coinfections and superinfections with other viruses, bacteria, and parasites, as well as symptomatic Kaposi's sarcoma, may accelerate progression (box).[11,15]

In the first 2 to 4 weeks of HIV infection, symptoms often include an acute flulike syndrome and swollen lymph nodes. These symptoms may be overlooked or may be perceived as of little consequence. This is particularly likely in people who have other pressing social, economic, or health concerns such as homelessness, drug addiction, or lack of access to medical care.

Antibodies against HIV can usually be detected within 3 to 12 weeks after infection, but unless the individual is tested, he or she may not be aware of the infection. Following resolution of the initial mild syndrome, no overt evidence of HIV infection may be apparent for many months or years (average is 9 years). The first evidence of infection may be symptoms of a secondary opportunistic infection or malignancy. These conditions are a consequence of advanced cellular immunosuppression and are used as markers to

---

indicate that the disease has progressed sufficiently to be classified as acquired immunodeficiency syndrome (AIDS). This classification is used for surveillance and reporting to public health agencies and the Centers for Disease Control and Prevention (CDC).[4] Both men and women may acquire a variety of opportunistic infections as HIV infection progresses. However, women have a disproportionate number of epithelial malignancies and are unlikely to have Kaposi's sarcoma.[7] Women are also more likely to have *Pneumocystis* pneumonia and develop reproductive tract complications.

Progression from HIV infection to serious disease and finally AIDS may occur more slowly in younger adults, who may have a relatively stronger cell-mediated immune system and enhanced CD4 lymphocytes.[17] Early presentation of AIDS may be in the form of persistent generalized lymphadenopathy, recurrent or chronic infections, such as bacterial pneumonia, nonhealing ulcers and wounds, oral thrush and other forms of candidiasis, recurrent or persistent mucocutaneous herpes simplex infection, bacteremia with endocarditis, vaginitis or salpingitis (PID), and tuberculosis (pulmonary with or without extrapulmonary involvement). These infections may be more severe as a result of the deterioration of the immune system.

Other manifestations of altered cellular immunity include premalignant or malignant conditions (i.e., cervical dysplasia and carcinoma, Kaposi's sarcoma, primary lymphoma of the brain, and certain non-Hodgkin's lymphomas). In addition, superficial fungal infections of the skin or nails may develop, as well as varicella-zoster, or shingles, which may be dermatomal or multidermatomal in distribution. Deterioration of immune function is usually irreversible and ultimately leads to infections with opportunistic agents such as *Pneumocystis carinii*, *Cryptococcus neoformans*, *Toxoplasma gondii*, mycobacteria, and cytomeg-

---

SOME AGENTS OF COINFECTION WITH HIV

Viral: cytomegalovirus, herpes simplex virus, human T-lymphotropic virus 1, Epstein-Barr virus, human papilloma virus
Bacterial: mycoplasma, spirochetes, gonococci
Parasitic: cryptosporidia, amoebae, blood parasitemia

alovirus.[15] Other late manifestations include neuropathies, encephalopathy, severe weight loss (slim disease), and organ failure (e.g., renal failure). Eventually, one or more infections or malignancies lead to death.

Studies have suggested that IDUs may have a faster progression of disease symptoms than HIV-positive persons who are not IDUs.[9,11] This hypothesis remains controversial.

The risk of transmission of HIV through sexual contact is enhanced by conditions that disrupt the mucosa or epithelium, such as genital ulcer disease, gonorrhea, syphilis, chancroid, and possibly genital warts and other lesions.[5,11,14] Many IDUs who have these lesion producing STD's do not seek treatment and unknowingly place themselves at greater risk of acquiring HIV through infected sexual partners.

Ms. Forbes was unaware of her exposure to and primary infection with gonococcus and did not seek medical care. Her infection progressed to involve the upper reproductive tract. She was also unaware of her genital warts, another STD that disrupts the reproductive mucosa. Her history of contact with multiple sex partners during her days of drug injection probably contributed to her exposures to a variety of STDs.

The proportion of newly reported cases of AIDS in IDUs is rapidly increasing. The CDC reports that of the 334,344 adult cases of AIDS reported through September 1993, 80,713 (24%) were attributable to injecting drug use, and drug injection was a major risk behavior in an additional 32,892 (10%) patients who reported multiple modes of exposure.[1] Of the 40,702 women with AIDS reported to the CDC through September 1993, 49% had personal history of drug injection.[6] Another 20% did not inject drugs themselves but were the sexual partners of men who were IDUs. Thus, for 69% of the women with AIDS in the United States by September 1993, injecting drug use was a contributing factor. Of the remaining women, 17% acquired their infection from men who were HIV positive but did not inject drugs, 6% through infected blood products, and for 8% the route of transmission was classified as undetermined, other, or under investigation. In addition, although half the women with AIDS reported injecting drug use, they could have acquired HIV either via this route or through sexual contact.

The microbiologic environment

HIV is a ribonucleic acid (RNA) retrovirus. An important characteristic of these viruses is the enzyme reverse transcriptase, which transcribes viral RNA into DNA which can integrate into the host cell's DNA. HIV invades and destroys cells, particularly those in the immune system and the nervous system, which have the CD4 protein on their surface. The CD4 lymphocyte, also known as the T-helper cell, is especially affected because of the relative number of CD4 sites on its surface. As the CD4 lymphocyte population is depleted, cellular immunity deteriorates. The period between time of infection to onset of serious clinical disease varies widely. The diagnosis of an AIDS-defining illness may require 2 to 10 years, with a mean of 9 years. Antiviral therapies attack several phases of viral replication. Nucleoside analogs, such as zidovudine, the first and most widely used anti-HIV drug, interrupt assembly of the virus.

The physical environment

Air, water, and food play no role in the transmission of HIV. Fomites (inanimate objects), such as drug injection equipment, can transmit HIV only if it becomes contaminated with HIV-containing body substances and delivers the virus through the skin to mucous membranes or to nonintact skin.[8] Needle sharing has been widespread among injecting drug users in certain communities. Even if this sharing were not anonymous,[3,8,9] the advantage of knowing the identity of one's needle-sharing partners is negated by the long incubation period of HIV, which makes it virtually impossible to distinguish an HIV-infected partner from one who is uninfected.

Specific environmental settings, such as correctional facilities, drug rehabilitation centers, and "shooting galleries" where drugs and injection equipment are shared, provide ample opportunities for the transmission of blood-borne agents such as HIV. The furtive nature of the injection drug use, the relative anonymity of equipment-sharing partners, the lack of access to clean injection equipment, and the unsafe sexual practices that may accompany substance abuse all contribute to transmission.[8,9,12,13]

The social environment

Living conditions of many, although not all, IDUs are marginal. Crowding, unsanitary conditions, and social instability may be common features of daily life. Housing, financial, and legal problems complicate the IDU's life, sometimes making the simplest of infection prevention measures nearly impossible to implement. The perceived ease and glamour of a lucrative career in street drug trafficking may attract young people who see it as a way to overcome the economic and educational disadvantages. In addition, the numbing or physical comfort of highs from drug use may be especially appealing to someone whose daily existence is harsh or unrewarding.

Sexual activity, as evidenced by the high prevalence of teenage pregnancy, may have early onset in impoverished, urban communities with limited or no access to family planning and health services.[2] Adherence to one's cultural norms is motivated by the needs for acceptance and belonging that are particularly strong in adolescence. Ethnic and social traditions that accept or promote early sexual activity or pregnancy may increase the risks of HIV transmission (e.g., a woman's first child before age 17, a man's first sexual encounter before age 14) (see Chapter 4).

Discrimination exists against many persons infected with HIV. Social support may erode during the frequent health crises of the HIV-infected. Persons who are part of the IDU's nondrug using social network may abandon or distance themselves if either drug use or HIV infection is perceived as a lost cause. The nursing, medical, and dental care of the infected IDU may also be affected by the biases of health care providers who have little understanding of HIV and the drug use culture and sometimes little interest in learning about it.

Compliance with preventive strategies, related to both sexual and drug use behaviors, is often complicated by lack of social support systems in the community.[9,14] Although IDUs fear HIV and contagion, the lack of a nondrug using supportive network or the resources to comply with recommendations make it difficult to suspend risky behaviors. The cycle of drug use may include periods of recovery followed by relapses into use and addictive behaviors.

The editor of the *American Journal of Public Health* stated several years ago that "the United States is faced with three plagues: AIDS, drug abuse, and poverty . . . and the greatest of these is poverty."[18] Ms. Forbes' situation is but one example of how intertwined these three issues are for society in the United States and throughout the world. The global HIV epidemic poses a tremendous challenge to all members of society and particularly to health care providers. This is perhaps most pronounced in members of the drug-using community and their sexual partners. A multidisciplinary, comprehensive effort is essential to the control of this infectious disease, and must include education to prevent the spread of HIV and facilities and resources for the diagnosis and treatment of HIV-infected individuals.

PREVENTION AND CONTROL

In addition to the prevention and control strategies proposed for the containment of HIV (e.g., safer sex practices), multiple strategies are needed to support behavior changes of the IDU. Education, comprehensive drug treatment, and rehabilitation services are essential to break the cycle of drug addiction and high-risk behavior. However, until the IDU is able to stop using drugs, prevention depends on the disinfection of needles, syringes, and other paraphernalia or the provision of clean or sterile supplies. Needle exchange programs, although politically controversial, have reduced the transmission of HIV and other bloodborne viruses and bacteria.[9] Disinfection of needles, syringes, and other contaminated IDU paraphernalia with bleach solutions has also been tested.[9,16] Usually, the recommended technique includes precleaning, and at least two flushes with a solution of high concentration or undiluted household bleach, followed by several flushes of tap or clean water. This procedure may be ineffective if inadequately performed, consequently, injecting drug users must be trained and motivated to perform the techniques reliably and consistently.

Chemotherapy may delay progression of immune deficiency, prevent opportunistic infections, and temporarily control the disabling effects of chronic infections. For example, in a patient with early diagnosis of HIV infection, *Pneumocystis carinii* prophylaxis can prevent most recurrences; suppressive therapy for infections such as toxoplasmosis of the central nervous system will prevent overwhelming infection; and symptomatic treatment can reduce the severity of chronic diarrhea of intestinal protozoan infections. Treatment may be difficult when the infecting strain of HIV has developed resistance to antiviral agents. Despite careful monitoring, some resistance to antimicrobial agents has developed (cytomegalovirus resistant to acyclovir, herpes simplex virus resistant to acyclovir, *Mycobacterium tuberculosis* resistant to isoniazid and other antimycobacterial drugs). The hope for the future is the development of an effective vaccine against HIV.

SUMMARY

Ms. Forbes's acute episode of PID resolved, and for the next several months she was relatively symptom free. She continued to be monitored by the AIDS care team to detect problems promptly and to provide appropriate treatments. Her cervical dysplasia was confirmed as benign but she remained under close observation for the next 2 years, until her death.

Ms. Forbes's family was initially frightened and angered by the news that she was HIV infected and likely to become progressively more ill over time. The family could not cope with this information, and except for her grandmother, they remained unsupportive throughout the remainder of her life. After her diagnosis, Ms. Forbes joined a women's support group for recovering IDUs with children. There she was able to discuss her anger, frustration, and guilt and share fears about her own and her children's future. Mr. Hart continued to live with Ms. Forbes and agreed to be tested for HIV soon after her diagnosis was made. He was also found to be HIV infected and sought medical attention at the same clinic where Ms. Forbes received care. He occasionally attended the support groups provided by the hospital for HIV-infected men but was unwilling to give up his injecting drug use completely, stating that he needed an occasional fix to cope with his impending death. As he also became progressively more ill, he and Ms. Forbes did the best they could to provide care for one another. Ms. Forbes's children moved permanently to their grandmother's home, and she became their legal guardian. In this environment they were provided some stability in their daily lives.

Twenty-eight months after her initial diagnosis of HIV infection, Susan was admitted to the hospital with *Pneumocystis carinii* pneumonia and died within 48 hours. At this time she weighed less than 100 lb and had all the signs of wasting syndrome. Mr. Hart was admitted

SUMMARY TABLE 26.   Human immunodeficiency virus in a female who injects drugs

Host-environment model	Case presentation	Factors that influence infectious process	Prevention and control
Host factors	26-year-old woman History of injecting drug use and risky sexual behaviors Sexually transmitted disease	Genital ulcer disease facilitates transmission Frequency and volume of exposure to HIV may increase risk Impaired immunity from other medical conditions increases risk	Vaccine not available Provide adequate nutrition Control chronic diseases to maintain immune status
Microbiologic factors	Human immunodeficiency virus (HIV)	Injection of HIV-contaminated material Sexual transmission	Give antiretroviral agents to delay progression Prophylaxy and treat opportunistic infections
Physical environment	High-incidence urban community	Blood-contaminated parenteral drug use paraphernalia, including blood-soiled items with indirect host contact (cooker, cotton)	Disinfect shared drug use paraphernalia Recognize/remove from "risky" settings to prevent relapses into risky behaviors
Social environment	Injecting drug use Inadequate psychosocial and/or financial support by significant others and by community Unprotected sex	Access to barrier protection (e.g., condoms) Drug treatment programs Clean drug use equipment Culturally appropriate educational programs Increased incidence of risky sexual practices when under the influence of drugs or when incentives to take risk exist (physical force, exchange of sex for drugs or money)	Educate to reduce or prevent exposure (e.g., drug use prevention and rehabilitation, safer sex and needle use programs) Develop and implement appropriate programs, including role-playing exercises, risk-specific and gender-specific support groups

to the same hospital 2 weeks later and died shortly thereafter.

HIV infection has become one of the most significant public health issues of this century. It has raised many associated social and policy issues such as discrimination and bias (see Chapter 10). All humans and some primates are susceptible to the infection. The disease is transmitted through sexual activities, blood exchange, birth, and breastfeeding. The proportion of new cases of AIDS in IDUs is increasing rapidly. More than half of women with AIDS have a history of injecting drugs.

REFERENCES

1. Centers for Disease Control and Prevention. *HIV/ AIDS surveillance reports*. Atlanta, GA: October 1993.
2. Centers for Disease Control and Prevention. Pregnancy and birth rates: United States, 1990. *MMWR*. 1993;42:733-737.
3. Centers for Disease Control and Prevention. Impact of new legislation on needle and syringe purchase and possession—Connecticut, 1992. *MMWR*. 1993;42:145-148.
4. Centers for Disease Control and Prevention. 1993 revised classification for HIV infection and expanded case definition for AIDS among adolescents and adults. *MMWR*. 1992:41(RR-17):1-19.
5. Centers for Disease Control. Condoms for the prevention of sexually transmitted diseases. *MMWR*. 1988; 37:133-137.
6. Diaz T, Buehler JW, Castro KG, Ward JW. AIDS trends among Hispanics in the United States. *Am J Public Health*. 1993;83:504-509.
7. Fineberg SA, Schinella R. Human immunodeficiency virus infection in women: report of 102 cases. *Mod Pathol*. 1990;3:575.
8. Grund JP, Kaplan CD, Adriaans NF. Needle-sharing in the Netherlands: an ethnographic analysis. *Am J Public Health*. 1991;81:1602-1607.
9. Joseph SC. *Dragon within the Gates: The Once and Future AIDS Epidemic*. New York, NY: Carrol and Graf; 1992.
10. Lawrence J: Women and AIDS: an overview and specific disease manifestations. *AIDS Reader*. September/ October 1991.
11. Levy J. Transmission of HIV and factors influencing progression to AIDS. *Am J Med*. 1993;95:86-100.
12. National Institute for Drug Abuse. *Needle-Sharing among Intravenous Drug Abusers: National and International Perspectives*. U.S. Department of Health and Human Services, No. (ADM)89-1567, 1989.
13. Office of Technology Assessment. *The effectiveness of drug abuse treatment*. Washington, DC: U.S. Government Printing Office; 1990.
14. Roper WL, Peterson HB, Curran JW. Commentary: condoms and HIV/STD prevention—clarifying the message. *Am J Public Health*. 1993;83:501-503.
15. Sande MA, Volberding PA. *The Medical Management of AIDS*, 3rd ed. Philadelphia, PA: W. B. Saunders; 1992.
16. Valdeserri RO, Jones TS, West GR, Campbell CH, Thompson PI. Where injecting drug users receive HIV counselling and testing. *Public Health Rep*. 1993; 108:294-296.
17. Weiss RA. How does HIV cause AIDS? *Science*. 1993; 260:1273-1279.
18. Yankauer A: The deadliest plague. *Am J Public Health* 1989;79:821-822 (editorial).

SUGGESTED READINGS

Centers for Disease Control and Prevention. Technical guidance on HIV counseling. *MMWR*. 1993;42:11-17.

Centers for Disease Control and Prevention. Update: barrier protection against HIV infection and other sexually transmitted diseases. *MMWR*. 1993;42: 589-591.

Durham JD, Cohen FL. *The person with AIDS: nursing perspectives*, 2nd ed. New York, NY: Springer; 1992.

Flaskerud JH, Ungvarski PJ. *HIV/AIDS: A Guide to Nursing Care*, 2nd ed. Philadelphia, PA: W. B. Saunders, 1992.

Bone Marrow Transplant Patient with Cytomegalovirus Infection

BARBARA R. MOONEY

CLINICAL PRESENTATION

Sam Luff is a 30-year-old man who received an allogeneic bone marrow transplant (BMT) from his brother. He was diagnosed with multiple myeloma 1 year before his BMT and was treated with various chemotherapeutic agents, which induced a short-lived remission. He was referred for BMT after his relapse. Mr. Luff was in excellent health before his diagnosis of multiple myeloma. He lives in a three-bedroom single-family home in a small suburban community with his wife and two young children. He is the owner of a small construction company; his wife has been helping him to manage the business since his illness. He is well supported by his extended family and the community.

Two weeks prior to his BMT, Mr. Luff was serologically screened for a number of infectious agents, including cytomegalovirus (CMV). CMV serology was positive, indicating prior infection. It is unclear when or how he acquired his infection, whether in early childhood, from blood transfusions, from his wife (who is also seropositive), or from his small children.

Mr. Luff was admitted for BMT to a high-efficiency particulate air (HEPA) filtered private patient room on the BMT unit. After his BMT he contracted an oral yeast infection, which was treated with local therapy, and had a febrile episode, which was treated with systemic antibiotics for 7 days. He suffered significant psychologic depression during his long hospitalization. A bronchoalveolar lavage performed on posttransplant day 28 was negative for CMV. Mr. Luff was discharged on posttransplant day 32 on systemic antibiotics for slightly decreased breath sounds with occasional crackles in the left lower lobe.

After discharge, Mr. Luff was visited daily by a home care IV therapy nurse and was seen in the BMT clinic twice a week. Two weeks after his discharge he began to feel run down but did not tell his doctors because he did not want to be hospitalized again. Ten days later he began having shortness of breath, increasing fatigue, and decreased appetite. At his next clinic appointment 2 days later, Mr. Luff was immediately readmitted to the BMT unit. His chest x-ray film showed diffuse infiltrates, and the bronchoalveolar lavage was positive for CMV. The physician ordered antiviral therapy for CMV pneumonia. Mr. Luff's respiratory status rapidly deteriorated, and he was transferred to the critical care unit for intubation. Despite intensive supportive treatment, he continued to deteriorate and died 2 days after readmission.

HOST-ENVIRONMENT INTERACTION
The host

The competence of the host's immune system is the most important determinant of the advent and outcome of symptomatic CMV disease. The most serious CMV infections occur in persons who are severely immunosuppressed, either from the disease or from immunotherapy. CMV is one of the most important and frequent causes of infection in transplant patients, developing in many of these patients.[2,3,6] The risk of nosocomial infection is highest during the 3 weeks following the transplant, during which time host defenses are severely suppressed. As the bone marrow engrafts and reconstitutes its hematologic components, the risk of infection decreases but does not disappear.[6] Radiotherapy can delay the marrow recovery, and procedures, such as intravenous therapy, that override the host's physical barriers may contribute to infection risk.

Many immunosuppressed persons are at risk for CMV infections such as pneumonia, retinitis, and hepatitis. Primary CMV infection in transplant recipients normally presents with onset of acute symptoms 40 to 60 days after infection. Recurrent infections generally occur more than 60 days after transplant and have a slower onset of symptoms. Mortality in transplant recipients with CMV pneumonia has been reported to be as high as 90%.[5] It also appears that CMV disease in immunocompromised patients may predispose the patient to other opportunistic infections and contribute to graft-versus-host disease.[2]

The microbiologic environment

CMV is a member of the virus family *Herpesviridae* and is also known as human herpesvirus 5. A deoxyribonucleic acid (DNA) virus, CMV is very similar in form and structure to herpes simplex virus and varicella-zoster virus. Virus particles reproduce in the human fibroblast; the viral envelope is derived from the nuclear membrane of the host cell.

Humans are the only known hosts for CMV. During active infection the virus is shed into urine, saliva, genital secretions, and breast milk. Transmission can occur when these virus-containing body substances come into direct contact with mucous membranes of a susceptible host. Transmission can also be accomplished through blood transfusions and organ or tissue transplants from an infected donor. Some 40% to 90% of people are infected by the time they are adults, usually in early childhood by contact with respiratory secretions.[4]

As with all types of herpesviruses, initial infection may be followed by latency and periodic recurrences of symptoms. Symptoms of initial infection with CMV can range from none to severe disease and death. Outcome is dependent on the status of the host's immune system. Adults with normal immune systems most often have inapparent infections, although mononucleosis-like symptoms may occur; CMV is the major cause of transfusion-acquired mononucleosis syndrome.[4] The incubation period for CMV has not been clearly defined, but it may be weeks to months. Recurrences range from asymptomatic viral shedding to serious systemic infections that are most often associated with immune system compromise.

Diagnosis may be based on clinical evidence of active infection in conjunction with (1) recovery of virus from tissue culture of body excretions or organs, (2) a rise in antibody titers, (3) specific rapid diagnostic tests, or (4) microscopic examination of specimens from an infected organ. A combination of these methods is more reliable than any single method. The appearance of CMV's large intranuclear inclusions and presence of early CMV antigen in bronchoalveolar lavage specimens may be diagnostic for CMV pneumonia when accompanied by clinical signs and symptoms of respiratory disease in an immune compromised person. Periodic bronchoalveolar lavages may be performed in an attempt to recognize early viral replication in transplant patients. In addition, periodic cultures of the buffy coat of white cells in the patient's blood may also reveal early viral replication.

The physical environment

The physical environment contributes little to the natural history of CMV infection in transplant patients. Theoretically, the virus is excreted into the environment in body substances and can be transmitted from person or object to another person. Though fomites may be soiled with secretions containing CMV, they have never been shown to be a significant factor in CMV transmission. The environmental sources of greatest consequence are the transplanted tissues or organs or blood transfusions containing CMV.[3]

CMV has a worldwide distribution and varies by geographic location. CMV infection does not appear to occur seasonally.

The social environment

CMV infection risk varies by socioeconomic status. Infection during childhood is widespread in geographic areas and countries with low socioeconomic levels, sometimes affecting 100% of the population as opposed to 40% in areas with better economic and social conditions. In the United States, seroprevalence is highest in lower income groups. Sexual contact is the most common route of transmission in adults. As with other sexually transmitted diseases, risk of infection increases with numbers of sexual partners.

Since most transplant patients who develop CMV infections are seropositive before transplantation, the social environment plays little role in this population. However, risk of infection can theoretically be influenced by the degree of health care provider compliance with infection control precautions during the preparation of transplant tissues, blood transfusions, invasive procedures, and maintenance of the environment. Inadequate technique during any of these processes may increase risk to the patient for exogenous acquisition of CMV infection.

PREVENTION AND CONTROL

Prevention and control efforts in seronegative transplant recipients must be directed toward preventing initial infection. In contrast, management of seropositive patients is limited to treatment of active viral replication to reduce severity of recurrences.

A number of interventions may be helpful in preventing CMV infection in the seronegative transplant recipient. Use of seronegative donors may provide the most protection; however, it is not always possible to avoid CMV positive donors when donors are few and tissue compatibility is difficult to achieve. Blood products from seronegative donors should also be used. If this is not possible, blood products should be treated to decrease the risk of CMV transmission, such as by removal of white blood cells. If a seronegative recipient receives an organ, tissue, or untreated blood products from a seropositive donor, prophylactic treatment with antiviral agents such as ganciclovir or CMV-specific immune globulin may help to avoid serious CMV disease. CMV vaccines have been tried with limited success.[5]

In the hospital, routine infection control practices, such as handwashing and use of barriers, should be used to reduce the risk of cross-infection from other patients or from health care workers who may be shedding CMV. The patient's family members may also be a source of transmission. If feasible, individuals with signs or symptoms of any illness should avoid direct contact with the immunocompromised patient. Transmission from an infected sexual partner may be prevented by consistent use of condoms. Handwashing before and after contact with children and family members may also interrupt transmission to the seronegative transplant recipient. With good preventive care, the risk of acquiring CMV or developing severe CMV disease during maximal immune suppression can be decreased.

Suppression of recurrent episodes of CMV in the seropositive transplant recipient is a challenge. The extreme suppression of the immune system necessary to avoid rejection of an organ or tissue results in CMV viral replication in approximately one half of seropositive patients. A number of these patients then progress to serious disease. Studies designed to suppress replication of herpesviruses, including CMV, during periods of extreme immune suppression by use of prophylactic antiviral agents such as acyclovir, ganciclovir, and immune globulins are in progress. However, there is risk that the organism will become resistant to those agents. Because of these problems, efforts are directed at early recognition of viral replication in the seropositive transplant recipient so that early treatment can be initiated.

Prevention and control in health care settings have included consideration of the risk to pregnant health care workers. In the past, pregnant health care workers were not assigned to seropositive or apparently actively infected patients. Some facilities screened all women health care workers of childbearing age for CMV antibody before assigning patients. It is now recognized that only 1 in 10 patients who shed CMV have symptoms recognized as evidence of CMV. Although one study suggested that there may be some risk to the pregnant health care worker of acquiring CMV in pediatric units where there is a high level of viral shedding, subsequent studies have shown little difference in incidence of CMV between pediatric, oncology, and hemodialysis nurses and persons in the general community.[1,4] Direct contact with body substances containing the virus is required for transmission; therefore, infection control practices that encourage handwashing and use of gloves during contact with body substances such as urine are adequate to avert transmission. However, to be effective, these interventions must be consistently used with *all* patients rather than just for patients perceived as likely to be shedding CMV. Reassignment of select staff in order to avoid contact with known CMV-positive patients is ineffective and will provide a false sense of security for the health care worker.

Mr. Luff had nonspecific symptoms 2 weeks after his discharge that may have indicated that CMV viral replication was occurring. His reluctance to be rehospitalized may have increased his chances of serious illness by delaying earlier intervention. Since CMV recurrence before posttransplant day 60 is uncommon, recurrence may have been unexpected and diagnosis delayed.

During Mr. Luff's brief final hospitalization, nurses and other health care providers consistently used routine infection control interventions and reminded family members to follow the same infection control precautions. No care providers were reassigned, and apparently no CMV was transmitted.

SUMMARY

It is estimated that 40% to 90% of adults have been infected with CMV.[4] Though most infections in healthy individuals do not produce symptoms, severe and often fatal CMV infection is a frequent and well-recognized consequence of immunosuppression in transplant recipients.

Efforts to prevent CMV infection and recurrence in persons receiving transplanted organs have had only limited success. Current efforts are being directed at developing new antiviral treatments to prevent initial infection for the CMV seronegative patient receiving seropositive organs or tissues and to suppress recurrent infection in seropositive patients. A CMV vaccine and monoclonal CMV antibodies, to prevent both initial and recurrent infections, are being developed. Research is also in process to develop immune system stimulators that may decrease the length and severity of immune system compromise in transplant recipients without encouraging organ rejec-

SUMMARY TABLE 27.   Bone marrow transplant patient with cytomegalovirus infection

Host-environment model	Case presentation	Factors that influence infectious process	Prevention and control
Host factors	30-year-old man Multiple myeloma Allogeneic bone marrow transplant	Universal susceptibility CMV positive by testing before transplant Immune suppression due to treatment	No vaccine available Vaccine under development
Microbiologic factors	Cytomegalovirus (CMV, human herpesvirus 5)	Mucous membrane contact with secretions or excretions (particularly urine) containing CMV Long incubation period Latency and periodic viral shedding	Use prophylactic treatment with antiviral agents during periods of induced immunosuppression (variably susceptible to antiviral agents)
Physical environment	Plays little role in infection	No apparent seasonality	Handle secretions and excretions using barrier precautions
Social environment	Risk related to socioeconomic level	Childhood spread due to crowding and decreased hygiene Sexual transmission in adults	Teach good hygiene and use of barriers Use condoms to prevent sexual spread

tion. Hopefully, CMV disease will become a rare and easily managed complication of organ and tissue transplantation with the success of these efforts.

REFERENCES

1. Adler SP, et al. Molecular epidemiology of cytomegalovirus in a nursery: lack of evidence for nosocomial transmission. *J Pediatr.* 1986;108:117-123.
2. Hibberd PL, Rubin RH. Infection in transplant recipients. In Bennett JV, Brachman PS, eds. *Hospital infections,* 2nd ed. Boston, MA: Little, Brown; 1992; 899-921.
3. Ho M. Cytomegalovirus. In Mandell GL, Douglas RG Jr, Bennett JE, eds. *Principles and Practice of Infectious Diseases,* 3rd ed. New York, NY: Churchill Livingstone; 1990;1159-1172.
4. Pomeroy C, Wengland JA. Cytomegalovirus: epidemiology and infection control. *Am J Infect Cont.* 1987; 15:107-119.
5. Smith CF. Cytomegalovirus pneumonia state of the art. *Chest.* 1989;95(March suppl):192S-197Sm.
6. Wey SB. Nosocomial infection in the compromised host. In Wenzel RP, ed. *Prevention and Control of Nosocomial Infections,* 2nd ed. Baltimore, MD: Williams & Wilkins; 1993;923-957.

SUGGESTED READINGS

Bale JF Jr, et al. The epidemiology of cytomegalovirus infection among patients with burns. *Infect Control Hosp Epidemiol.* 1990;11:17-22.
Pass RF, et al. Increased rate of cytomegalovirus infection among day care center workers. *Pediatr Infect Dis J.* 1990;9:465-470.
Rossier E, Miller H. Prospective study of the incidence of cytomegalovirus infection in renal allograft recipients, Ottawa, 1982-89. *Can Dis Wkly Rep.* 1990;16:231-233.
Sokol DM, Demmler GJ, Buffone GJ. Rapid epidemiologic analysis of cytomegalovirus by using polymerase chain reaction amplification of the L-S junction region. *J Clin Microbiol.* 1992;30:839-44.

Presumptive Pneumococcal Pneumonia in an Elderly Woman

PATRICIA A. TABLOSKI

GAIL A. HARKNESS

CLINICAL PRESENTATION

Lydia Maxwell is an 84-year-old woman who lives independently in a senior citizen housing project. She has a small apartment and manages well with the assistance of her son, who visits her regularly three or four times a week. Mrs. Maxwell eats one meal a day in a communal dining room and attends many social activities sponsored by the housing project. There are approximately 300 other residents in the building, and 50 to 75 residents typically congregate for social events. Mrs. Maxwell suffered a stroke (cerebrovascular accident, CVA) 9 years ago and has a left hemiparesis. She has lost several inches of height to osteoporosis and has decreased vital capacity because of vertebral shortening. Mrs. Maxwell avoids physician visits and does not believe in immunizations. She refuses the influenza vaccine each year based on her belief that she is allergic to eggs because she suffers diarrhea when she drinks eggnog.

Until 1 week ago, Mrs. Maxwell was alert, oriented, continent, and able to enjoy social activities with her friends and family. Her only medication is a diuretic, which she takes daily to control her blood pressure. However, one week ago her son noticed that Mrs. Maxwell was increasingly lethargic, spent more time in bed, and had occasional urinary incontinence. Her appetite also markedly decreased. Her son noted that most of the food

he brought to his mother on Monday afternoon remained in the refrigerator on Friday morning. Mrs. Maxwell was not coughing and offered no complaints of pain or shortness of breath but stated that she felt very weak. Her son took her to see the physician, who, after careful physical examination, diagnosed pneumonia probably caused by *Streptococcus pneumoniae* (the pneumococcus). Mrs. Maxwell was unable to produce sputum for culture and Gram stain. The physician ordered a chest radiograph and complete blood count (CBC) and prescribed amoxicillin. She requested that Mrs. Maxwell or her son call in 2 days to give her a progress report. Mrs. Maxwell was feeling stronger and regaining her appetite 2 days later. Within a week she was much better and at 10 days after her initial examination, the physician believed the pneumonia had resolved.

HOST-ENVIRONMENT INTERACTION
The host

The major host factor associated with community-acquired pneumonia is advanced age. Contributing factors include smoking; alcohol abuse; chronic lung disease; recent history of viral upper respiratory tract infection; neurologic disease, which may contribute to microaspiration of secretions of the oropharynx; and sedating and dehydrating medications.[1] Healthy elderly persons with diagnosed lung disease may have diminished mucociliary clearance, decline in cell-mediated immunity as evidenced by a diminished response to challenge antigens, and decline in neutrophil function such as that resulting from diabetes.[7]

The estimated incidence of pneumococcal pneumonia in the United States is 68 to 260 cases per 100,000 people per year, or between 150,000 and 570,000 cases per year.[2] A serious complication is the development of bacteremia in 20% to 25% of those infected. About 5% of cases of complicated pneumonia are fatal. Community-acquired pneumonia in the United States is the most common infectious cause of death and is the fifth overall leading cause of death in the elderly (3.3 million cases of diagnosed pneumonia and 24.1 deaths per 100,000 population).

Humans are the reservoir of *S. pneumoniae.* The organism is a common resident of the human upper respiratory tract and has been isolated from up to 70% of some healthy adults. Pneumonia follows aspiration of the organism into the lungs. Pneumococcal pneumonia is endemic in the United States. The incubation period is usually 1 to 3 days. Infants, the elderly, and individuals with underlying medical problems are at particular risk. Risk to individuals older than 40 years is three to four times that of younger adults. In elderly persons, pneumonia sometimes goes undiagnosed because the symptoms may be subtle. The typical symptoms of pneumonia in the young, which include fever, chills, cough, sputum production, and pleuritic chest pain, are often decreased or absent in the elderly. Mrs. Maxwell's symptoms were very mild.

Interpretation of laboratory findings of patients with significant illness who have impaired pharyngeal clearance mechanisms may be complicated by pharyngeal colonization with gram-negative rods, which may contaminate sputum samples collected for microscopic examination and culture. These organisms often are not responsible for the lower respiratory infection and may obscure the real pathogens, which may be present in extremely low numbers and go unnoticed in the Gram stain or culture.[3]

Multiple pathologies or the simultaneous presence of pathology in several organ systems may interact with the normal changes of aging to produce an atypical presentation of disease. Symptoms of pneumonia in the elderly are falls, decreased oral intake, changes in mental status and level of orientation, and lethargy.[5] As in Mrs. Maxwell's case, decreased appetite may develop. Elderly persons who are relatively isolated from others and live alone are at particular risk of advanced illness because no one may be present to notice early changes in their general function.

The microbiologic environment

S. pneumoniae is a gram-positive, lancet-shaped coccoid bacterium that usually occurs in pairs. The complex polysaccharides that make up the organism's capsule are antigenic and can be used to classify strains of the organism by their reaction with specific antibodies (serotype). There are 84 known serotypes; 23 account for 90% of infections.[2] The pneumococcal vaccine now available protects against these 23 serotypes. Encapsulated organisms resist phagocytosis by white blood cells. The organism invades and multiplies in the alveolar spaces of the lungs. Several toxins produced by *S. pneumoniae* appear to be linked to an abrupt onset of symptoms and a fulminant clinical course in some people.

S. pneumoniae is common in the upper respiratory tract and is transmitted person to person via droplets. Contact with articles recently contaminated with secretions may also transmit the organism. Coughs and sneezes can spray millions of droplets containing organisms into the air to be inhaled by others nearby.

The physical environment

Several environmental factors are associated with the transmission of *S. pneumoniae* in the elderly. Outbreaks usually occur in the colder months of the year, especially during and immediately after influenza outbreaks. The organism is spread by contaminated droplets of oral and nasal secretions via coughs, sneezes, or contaminants on hands. This is especially a problem when people congregate indoors for extended periods, as may be the case in housing for elderly persons. Many older persons, including Mrs. Maxwell, maintain their homes at temperatures in the middle to upper 70s, which may dry the air and the oropharynx, and contribute to the risk of respiratory infection.

The social environment

Congregate housing, assistance from family and paid helpers, communal eating, church attendance, shopping in crowds, volunteering at a nursing home or day-care center, and other group activities that many older persons enjoy may place them at risk for exposure and infection. Many elderly persons would be unable to live independently without these supports. However, crowded environments where persons are in frequent close contact support the transmission of microorganisms. During outbreaks of influenza and upper respiratory infection, older persons at risk should avoid contact with others who are obviously infected and pay extra attention to obtaining adequate nutrition and rest. It is probably impossible and undesirable for Mrs. Maxwell to insulate herself completely from exposure to infection because of the negative psychologic consequences of social isolation; however, discretion in selecting activities may reduce her infection risk.

PREVENTION AND CONTROL

Prevention and control strategies should support the host's defenses. The value of the influenza vaccine has been well documented and is recommended for all older persons. Influenza vaccine reduces influenza-related morbidity and mortality by 70% to 90% among vaccinated individuals.[6] Most deaths in the elderly related to influenza are the result of secondary pneumonias (often *S. pneumoniae*) or progression of the influenza to primary viral pneumonia. During an average year, 10,000 to 20,000 excess deaths attributable to *S. pneumoniae* may occur during influenza epidemics.[6]

Pneumococcal vaccination is recommended for the elderly, persons at high risk (e.g., those having had a splenectomy), and those who have had a bacterial pneumonia. The vaccine should be given before extreme old age as the immune response and the resulting vaccine effectiveness decreases with advanced age or post-splenectomy.[4] Many factors affect vaccine acceptance. As in Mrs. Maxwell's case, some older people refuse the vaccine for inappropriate reasons, and some primary care providers fail to offer the vaccine or provide education regarding its effectiveness.

Other preventive strategies include careful attention to nutritional and fluid intake; avoidance of smoking, alcohol, and sedating drugs; and avoidance of crowded places during outbreaks of influenza and upper respiratory infections. Frequent handwashing and careful disposal or disinfection of items contaminated with discharges from the respiratory tract are important control measures. Older persons and their families should be instructed to seek early medical attention for subtle changes that may signal the onset of pneumonia in the elderly. For those at risk and living alone in isolated areas, a telephone monitoring system can alert others to the onset of illness. Although 75% of older persons with pneumococcal pneumonia can be treated as outpatients, some require hospitalization and administration of intravenous antibiotics.

Treatment considerations for community-acquired pneumonia include severity of the illness, presence of underlying disorders, community supports available to the patient, reliability of the caregivers, and the motivation and compliance of the patient. Sputum may be difficult to obtain from an older person. Chest radiographs may be of poor quality because of poor inspiratory efforts. A CBC may fail to show the typical left shift (i.e., presence of young forms of neutrophils) seen in younger patients responding to bacterial infection. Diagnosis is often based on a physical examination, which notes wheezes and crackles in the lungs and perhaps dullness on percussion. Appropriate antimicrobials for the community-residing elderly include amoxicillin, trimethoprim-sulfamethoxazole, oral cefuroxime and erythromycin. Lack of response to initial treatment within 48 hours should prompt a more aggressive diagnostic effort, including induced sputum and blood cultures. Hospitalization may be required to support hydration, oxygenation, correction of metabolic disturbances, nutrition, and monitoring for complications such as secondary infections and exacerbations of chronic illnesses.

SUMMARY

Pneumococcal pneumonia in community-residing elderly persons is a serious illness. It often goes unrecognized because of its atypical or subtle presentation. This may result in excess morbidity and mortality. The mode of transmission is primarily by droplets of secretions from the oropharnyx. Preventive strategies include annual immunization against influenza; one-time administration of pneumococcal vaccine; avoidance of smoking, alcohol, and sedating drugs; and maintenance of adequate nutrition and hydration. Older persons and their families should seek early treatment for the elder's falls, confusion, and loss of appetite. Those living alone should be monitored regularly for changes in function, especially in winter. Treatment should begin

SUMMARY TABLE 28.   Presumptive pneumococcal pneumonia in an elderly woman

Host-environment model	Case presentation	Factors that influence infectious process	Prevention and control
Host factors	Elderly woman	Neurologic insult Dehydrating medication Lack of vaccine	Accept influenza and pneumococcal vaccine
Microbiologic factors	*Streptococcus pneumoniae*	Contaminated droplets in crowded areas	Administer antibiotics
Physical environment	Congregate housing; high temperatures and dry air in apartment	Frequent contact with others Dry mucous membranes	Practice frequent handwashing Avoid infected persons Avoid over-heated, dry air
Social environment	Frequent interaction with many people Crowded environments	Frequent touching, kissing, proximity when coughing and sneezing	Avoid crowds and infected persons during outbreaks

early and include antimicrobial therapy and general supportive measures including hydration, appropriate nutrition, respiratory support and evaluation for complications. Care should be monitored to ensure efficacy of treatment.

REFERENCES

1. Keroack MA. The clinical challenge of pneumonia in the elderly. *Geriatric Focus on Infectious Diseases.* 1992; 1;3:6.
2. Mufson MA. *Streptococcus pneumoniae.* In Mandell G, Douglas RG, Bennett JE, eds. *Principles and Practice of Infectious Diseases,* 3rd ed. New York, NY: Churchill Livingstone; 1990.
3. Ristuccia P. Microbiologic aspects of infection in the compromised host. *Nurs clin North Am.* 1985;20;1: 171-179.
4. Roughmann KR, Tabloski PA, Bentley DW, Schiffman GS. Immune response of elderly adults to pneumococcus: variations by age, sex and functional impairment. *J Gerontol.* 1987;42;3:265-270.
5. Rowe J, Minaker J. Geriatric medicine. In Finch CE, Schneider EL, eds. *Handbook of the Biology of Aging.* New York, NY: Van Nostrand Reinhold; 1987; 932-960.
6. Ruben FL. Prevention and control of influenza. *Am Int Med.* 1987;82,6a;31-35.
7. Weart CW. Outpatient management of lower respiratory tract infection. *Clin Rev.* 1992;2;1:73-77.

SUGGESTED READINGS

Fraser D. Patient assessment: infection in the elderly. *Journal of Gerontological Nursing,* 1993;19;7:5-11.

Johannsen JM. Chronic obstructive pulmonary disease: current comprehensive care for emphysema and bronchitis. *The Nurse Practitioner* 1994;19;1:59-67.

Kind AC, Williams DN. Management guidelines for streptococcal pharyngitis. *Hospital Medicine,* 1994;30;3: 19-23.

Koster F. Respiratory tract infections. In Barker LR, Burton JR, Zieve PD, eds. *Principles of Ambulatory Medicine,* ed 3, Philadelphia; Williams & Wilkin; 1991.

Lange-Alberts ME, Shott S. Nutritional intake: use of touch and verbal curing. *Journal of Gerontological Nursing,* 1994;20;2:36-40.

Lorensen M. Health and social support of elderly families in developed countries. *Journal of Gerontological Nursing,* 1992;18;6:25-32.

Melillo KD. Interpretation of laboratory values in older adults. *The Nurse Practitioner,* 1993;18;7:59-67.

Pascucci MA. Measuring incentives to health promotion in older adults: understanding neglected health promotion. *Journal of Gerontological Nursing,* 1992;18;3: 16-23.

Sack RB, Barker LR. Immunization to prevent infectious disease. In Barker LR, Burton JR, Zieve PD, eds. *Principles of Ambulatory Medicine,* 3rd ed. Philadelphia, PA: Williams & Wilkin; 1991.

Respiratory Syncytial Virus in a Special Care Nursery

DOROTHY J. THOMAS

CLINICAL PRESENTATION

On July 15, 1993, George Mills, a 2-month-old previously healthy boy, was admitted for evaluation of a choking spell. George was a vaginally delivered term infant who weighed 8 pounds at birth. He was sent home at 1 day of age and has developed normally. George lives at home with his parents and 2-year-old brother who attends a day-care center 3 days a week. On the day of admission, George's mother reported that he had choked and turned blue twice that morning while taking his formula. He also had been fussy and had felt warm for the 3 preceding days. A family history revealed that his brother was recovering from a mild cold.

George appeared to be well nourished, alert, and responsive when he was admitted. The nurse practitioner noted good air exchange, scattered bilateral crackles, some wheezing, and slightly increased respiratory rate. However, George was afebrile, and had a cardiac murmur on chest auscultation. George's nasal mucosa was slightly reddened. A small amount of clear discharge was present. His chest radiograph showed bilateral haziness, which was initially interpreted as evidence of possible aspiration pneumonia. Cardiac evaluation detected a moderate ventricular septal defect. Within 24 hours George developed a fever of 39.6° C (103.3° F) (rectal) and progressive respiratory symptoms. The nurse placed George in a private room and notified the physician of the change in his condition. A nasal washing was submitted to the laboratory at the time the fever was noted. It was positive for respiratory syncytial virus (RSV).

HOST-ENVIRONMENT INTERACTION
The host

RSV is found worldwide and is the single most important respiratory pathogen of infants and young children. It is the leading cause of pneumonia in infants. Most children have sustained at least one infection by age 2 years.[8,9,17,26] Most infants who have primary infection with RSV have some degree of symptomatic respiratory illness, with pneumonia and bronchiolitis representing the more severe manifestations (box). Reinfection is generally milder than primary infection and may be asymptomatic. Infection limited to the upper airways usually presents as a coldlike illness or otitis media. Upper airway involvement alone resolves in 4 to 8 days, usually without residual disease.[17] Lower tract involvement (bronchiolitis or pneumonia) may require 7 to 21 days for resolution.[16] Lower respiratory tract infection results in necrosis of the ciliated epithelial cells of the bronchi and alveoli, inflammation-producing edema, increased secretions, and mucous plugging of the small bronchioles. This mucous obstruction can result in air trapping and decreased gas exchange, leading to decreased ventilation, hypoxemia, and respiratory acidosis.[1,8,10,17,26]

Most children recover completely; however,

RANGE OF CLINICAL PRESENTATION OF RSV INFECTION IN INFANTS AND YOUNG CHILDREN

INITIAL PRESENTATION

Cough
Fever (low grade and intermittent)
Otitis media
Pharyngitis
Rhinitis
Diffuse wheezing
Rhonchi and rales
Irritability

INITIAL SYMPTOMS

Poor feeding
Difficulty swallowing
Tachypnea
Retractions
Dyspnea
Cyanosis

LATE SIGNS

Chest hyperextension
Lethargy
Apnea (may be a presenting sign in very
    young infant)
Hypoxemia

Compiled from references 1, 3, 7-9, 16, 26, 28.

severe clinical illness and mortality are associated with young age, underlying cardiopulmonary disease, and deficient immunologic function.[3,8,17,21,26] The young infant has anatomically smaller airways, so minimal inflammation and tissue necrosis can produce pulmonary obstruction. The developing lung may also be more susceptible to the cytopathic effects of the virus.[8,17] Infants and children with decreased pulmonary function also have a more difficult time compensating for decreased gas exchange and clearing mucous plugs.[3,21,35]

Antibody production does not always confer protection but does appear to reduce clinical symptoms. Reinfection occurs in older children and young adults and is a major factor in the spread of infection to the very young infant.[8,17,26] The level of maternally transferred antibody is an important determinant of infection in an exposed infant. If maternal titers are high, infants infected before 1 month of age are usually asymptomatic.[8,14,17,26] These asymptomatic infants may be a source of infection for other infants.

The microbiologic environment

RSV is a medium-sized, enveloped ribonucleic acid (RNA) virus in the family *Paramyxoviridae*.[8] Humans are the natural host for the virus, although clinical infection has been seen in nonhuman primates such as chimpanzees. Antibodies have been detected in domestic animals such as cows and dogs, but the significance of these infections for humans is unknown.[8,17,26,31] Two strains of RSV, A and B, have been identified.[8,17,33] There does not appear to be any clinical or epidemiologic difference between the two strains, and they circulate with equal frequency during an outbreak. Community outbreaks are most common in the winter months in cold climates, but lower levels of infection occur throughout the summer months.[7,34]

The incubation period can range from 2 to 8 days but is typically 4 to 6 days.[17] After inoculation of the virus through the mucous membranes of the nose and eyes, viral maturation and replication takes place in the epithelial cells of the respiratory system. The virus spreads throughout the respiratory system by cell-to-cell transfer and may involve the airways at all levels.[1,8,15,10,17,26] Virus is excreted heavily in respiratory secretions. Viral particles survive for up to 6 hours when deposited on environmental surfaces and for 30 minutes on cloth or paper.[18]

Viral antigens can be detected in nasal secretions by a number of assays available for rapid diagnosis of RSV infection.[8,9,15,17,24,33] Respiratory secretions are obtained by nasal washing or nasopharyngeal swab, and testing is performed by immunofluorescence or enzyme-linked immunoabsorbent assay (ELISA). Results from these assays can be available within a few hours in most circumstances. Since RSV is very labile, optimum test results may be obtained by holding the specimen at 4° C (39° F) and transporting to the laboratory within 2 to 4 hours of collection.[24,29] Viral culture may also be used as an adjunct to rapid testing. If viral culture is performed, the inoculation of secretions into viral media should be done within 4 hours of collection.[18,29] Some patients shed virus and thus remain infectious for extended periods. Repeated testing may be indicated for long-stay patients in hospital.

RSV is transmitted when droplets of respiratory secretions containing the virus are deposited on or transported to the mucous membranes of the eyes, nose, or mouth. Direct transmission may occur when hands contaminated with secretions come in contact with mucous membranes of the nose or eyes.[8,17,26]

The physical environment

Pediatric units present opportunities for transmission of many viral agents, including RSV.[14,32] The infant's or child's inability to assist with care requires more direct contact with personnel and increased potential for transmission. Lack of hygiene in children may lead to environmental contamination with secretions containing viral particles.[17,18,32] The infectiousness of RSV makes it an especially important nosocomial pathogen. Children admitted to pediatric units during RSV outbreaks are at substantial risk for acquiring nosocomial RSV infection.[1,9,14,18]

Hospital staff may play a major role in the nosocomial transmission of RSV infection, whether or not they are infected.[1,8] Caregivers' hands may be contaminated during direct patient care or by contact with virus-contaminated surfaces. Visitors may also transmit RSV, particularly if they participate in patient care. Visitors, staff, and patients all present the

healthcare setting with prevalence of infection representative of the community. Older infants and toddlers may transmit it through their social contacts with other children and a tendency to put things in their mouths.

Given the time of year and presence of a congenital heart defect, respiratory infection was not initially suspected. Therefore, George was admitted to a 24-bed medical-surgical nursery unit consisting of four six-bed rooms for infants. One room was designated for chronically ill, ventilator-dependent infants. Family participation in care was encouraged in this unit. Each multiple-bed room had an attached private room for parent teaching and sibling visits.

Open units enable health care personnel to readily observe and monitor the children. However, these units may present risk of microorganism transmission if sinks are not placed at convenient locations for handwashing between patients and if spacing between beds is inadequate.[14,18,32] The lack of physical barriers may increase the socialization between visitors and patients and the risk that an infected adult or older child will have contact with an infant.

The social environment

Parents of children with RSV may have great anxiety regarding the child's illness and prognosis.[19,28] Education can help them to deal with their concerns, to find ways to be part of the child's care, and to reduce the risk of transmission of RSV to themselves, other family members, or patients. Nosocomial transmission may also occur if staff are not fully educated about the risks or are not compliant with barrier precautions established by the hospital.

PREVENTION AND CONTROL

Prevention of infection is difficult because of lack of vaccine and the ease of transmission. Development of an effective vaccine presents several challenges.[16,17] The most severe disease is in the very young infant; therefore, a vaccine would have to be effective despite the infant's immature immune system and in the presence of maternal antibody. Since the infection is often asymptomatic, it is reasonable to advise parents of very young infants or infants at risk for complicated RSV to avoid unnecessary contact with the public or infected persons during winter cold and flu season.

Most infected children can be managed at home. If hospitalization is necessary, control of nosocomial transmission requires a comprehensive approach.* Control measures should include monitoring for community levels of infection, surveillance for nosocomial infections, and recognition that infection may occur in all seasons and affect adults and children of all ages. Hospital visitors should be limited, particularly young children and individuals with coldlike symptoms, when RSV is known to be in the community. RSV containment precautions should be used routinely to manage all suspect cases. Handwashing is essential after all contact with the patient and his or her environment. Although standard precautions[6] are routinely used in the unit, more rigorous precautions to prevent and control nosocomial transmission of RSV have been recommended including masks and eye protection during outbreaks.[2,13,14,18,22,32] The use of gown, gloves, and eye-nose protection has been shown to reduce the risk of nosocomial transmission in some reports.[22,23,28] Use of private rooms and/or cohort placement of patients infected with RSV has been recommended,[13] but most hospitals do not have sufficient private rooms for the number of potential RSV patients admitted, particularly during a community outbreak. Health care workers must be aware that placing the child in a private room will not protect the staff from the virus or eliminate hand transmission between patients.

---

*References 2, 8, 9, 12, 14, 17, 22, 23, 32.

Although the exact role of fomites in person-to-person transmission has not been evaluated, it is reasonable to have established procedures for the cleaning and disinfection of toys, high chairs, playpens, and other items between patients.[32]

Presumptive diagnosis of RSV may be made during community outbreaks or when the patient is managed in the home. However, viral studies to determine the etiology of infection should be done if hospitalization is required.[9,15] Identification of the virus guides assessment for potential complications, selection of antiviral therapy, and implementation of infection control measures, including cohorting of patients with the same viral infection. Community outbreaks of RSV occur during winter months in temperate climates. This is the season during which adenovirus, influenza, and other respiratory viruses are also prevalent.

When George developed fever and his respiratory symptoms worsened, his nurse placed him in one of the unit's private rooms. Mask and eye protection procedures were added to the standard universal precautions. When RSV infection was confirmed, the physicians of the other patients in the nursery were advised of their patients' possible exposure to RSV, and the patients were monitored carefully for signs and symptoms of infection over the next several days. At the time of this exposure, prophylaxis for RSV was under research and not available for general use. The presence of young infants with chronic cardiopulmonary conditions made the presence of RSV infection particularly risky.[3] No prophylaxis is available to prevent infection after exposure. However, RSV-specific immune globulin is being tested for use with high risk patients.[8,16] All patients who shared a room with George were maintained as a closed cohort for 7 days. Within 5 days, two exposed infants, one health care worker, and George's mother were symptomatic and confirmed to

SUMMARY TABLE 29.   Respiratory syncytial virus in a special care nursery

Host-environment model	Case presentation	Factors that influence infectious process	Prevention and control
Host factors	2-month-old boy Congenital heart defect	Age: young infant (smaller diameter of airway in young child more likely to cause symptoms)	No vaccine or prophylaxis available Test hospitalized children with respiratory infections to identify etiologic agent
Microbiologic factors	Respiratory syncytial virus (RSV)	Human is only host Transmission is by direct contact through large-droplet aerosols and inoculation of eye and nose by contaminated fingers Virus is excreted heavily in nasal secretions and can survive for several days in environment	Use ribavirin for children with underlying cardiopulmonary disease or immunodeficiency (RSV-specific immune globulin being tested for use in high risk patients)
Physical environment	Open nursery in an acute care facility	Open nursery may provide more opportunity for RSV transmission Parents and other visitors may touch or play with other patients Shared items, such as playpens, toys, high chairs, etc., may become sources for fomite transmission	Private room or cohort with other RSV-infected patients Maintain isolation procedures until patient is RSV negative Maintain precautions that control respiratory secretions Clean toys and other shared items between patients Clean all potentially contaminated surfaces Disinfect fomites

Continued.

SUMMARY TABLE 29. Respiratory syncytial virus — cont'd

Host-environment model	Case presentation	Factors that influence infectious process	Prevention and control
Social environment	Patient lives with his parents and an older sibling	Other children frequently serve as the source of infection for younger infants Adult health care providers and visitors may also play a role in transmission Social interactions between children in playroom settings may increase risk of transmission	Cohort infected infants and toddlers Restrict ill personnel from contact with high-risk patients and remove from duty when possible Limit visitors during peak seasons Restrict RSV-positive patients from playroom activities Limit at-risk patients' contact with crowds or other children with colds during community outbreaks

have RSV infection. The infants and George required only supportive therapy to resolve the infection. The health care worker was off duty for 10 days until she became RSV negative. George's mother was restricted to George's room while visiting.

Specific antiviral therapy with ribavirin may be indicated for some patients.* The American Academy of Pediatrics[9] has published guidelines for therapy, and George met these criteria based on his congenital heart defect, age, and degree of respiratory distress. Some evidence suggests that health care professionals in contact with the drug aerosol for extended periods absorb some of the drug,[7,27,28] and, although no adverse effects have been re-

ported, specific precautions for use of the drug have been proposed.[9,27] It is reasonable for health care workers, especially pregnant personnel, to be familiar with their facility's procedures for ribavirin administration and to obtain additional information if they do not feel comfortable with their knowledge of the drug. Guidelines for management of ribavirin therapy have been published.[4,5,11,27,30]

SUMMARY

RSV is a highly communicable virus that can produce significant morbidity and mortality in the high-risk pediatric patient. Nosocomial transmission can result in increased hospital stay and medical costs. George's infection was considered community acquired because his

*References 3, 9, 11, 17, 19, 20, 25.

symptoms developed not later than 24 hours after admission. The source of George's infection was most likely his older sibling, who could have been infected in the day-care center. Nurses implemented more stringent barrier precautions based on George's symptoms. Their prompt addition of personal protective barriers and transfer of George to a private room helped prevent additional nosocomial transmission of RSV. Nurses must consider the possibility of infection in family members and provide education, barriers, and/or visitor restrictions to reduce the risk of transmission from a family member to patients, staff, or other visitors. Health care providers must exclude themselves when they may have upper respiratory infections of their own.

REFERENCES

1. Adams DA, McFadden EA. Respiratory syncytial viral infection in infants: nursing implications. *Crit Care Nurs.* 1990;10(20):74-79.
2. Agah R, et al. Respiratory syncytial virus (RSV) infection rate in personnel caring for children with RSV infections. *Am J Dis Child.* 1987; 141:695-697.
3. Anderson LJ, Parker RA, Shrikas RL. Association between respiratory syncytial virus outbreaks and lower respiratory deaths in infants and young children. *J Infect Dis.* 1990;161:640-646.
4. Bradley JS, Connors JD, Compogiannis LS, Eiger LI. Exposure of health care workers to ribavirin during therapy for respiratory syncytial virus. *Antimicrob Agents Chemother.* 1990;34(4):668-669.
5. Centers for Disease Control. Assessing exposures of health care personnel to aerosols of ribavirin—California. *MMWR.* 1987;37(36):560-563.
6. Centers for Disease Control. Update: universal precautions for prevention of transmission of human immunodeficiency virus, hepatitis B virus, and other bloodborne pathogens in health care settings. *MMWR.* 1988;37(24):377-387.
7. Centers for Disease Control and Prevention. Current trends: respiratory syncytial virus outbreak activity—United States, 1992. *MMWR.* 1993;42:5-7.
8. Chanock RM, McIntosh K, Murphy BR, Parrott RH. Respiratory syncytial virus. In Evans AS ed. *Viral Infections of Humans: Epidemiology and Control,* 3rd ed. New York, NY: Plenum Medical Book Co., 1989: 525-544.
9. Committee on Infectious Diseases, American Academy of Pediatrics: Ribavirin therapy of respiratory syncytial virus. In *Report of the Committee on Infectious Disease,* 22nd ed. Evanston, IL: 1991;581-587.
10. Corey MA, Clore ER. Management of the infant with respiratory syncytial virus. *J Pediat Nurs.* 1991;6(2): 92-93.
11. Eggleston M. Clinical review of ribavirin. *Infect Control.* 1987;8(5):215-218.
12. Gala CL, et al. The use of eye-nose goggles to control nosocomial respiratory syncytial virus. *JAMA.* 1986; 256(19):2706-2708.
13. Garner JS, Simmons BP. Guidelines for isolation precautions in hospitals. *Infect Control.* 1993;4:245-325.
14. Goldman D. Transmission of infectious diseases in children. *Pediatr Rev.* 1992;13(8):283-292.
15. Goldwater PH, et al. A survey of nosocomial respiratory viral infections in a children's hospital: occult respiratory infection in patients admitted during an epidemic season, *Infect Control Hosp Epidemiol.* 1991;12:231-238.
16. Hall CB. Vaccines for respiratory syncytial virus: from ghosts to genetic genomes. *Semin Infect Dis.* 1991; 2(3):191-196.
17. Hall CB. Respiratory syncytial virus. In Feigen RD, Cherry JD, eds. *Textbook of Pediatric Infectious Diseases,* 3rd ed. Philadelphia, PA: W.B. Saunders, 1992;1633-1656.
18. Hall CB, Douglas RG Jr. Modes of transmission of respiratory syncytial virus. *J Pediatr.* 1981;99:100-103.
19. Harris J, Culp S, Nicolayson T, et al. Respiratory syncytial virus: a pediatric nursing plan of care. *J Pediatr Nurs.* 1992;7(2):128-132.
20. Jury DL. More on RSV and ribavirin. *Pediatr Nurs.* 1993;19(1):89-91.
21. Laufer DA, Edelson PJ. Respiratory syncytial virus infection and cardiopulmonary disease. *Pediatr Ann.* 1987;16(8):644-653.
22. Leclair JM, et al. Prevention of nosocomial respiratory syncytial virus infections through compliance with glove and gown isolation precautions. *N Engl J Med.* 1987;317:329-334.
23. Madge P, et al. Prospective controlled study of four infection control procedures to prevent nosocomial infection with respiratory syncytial virus. *Lancet.* 1992;340:1079-1083.
24. Michaels MG, et al. Respiratory syncytial virus: a comparison of diagnostic modalities. *Pediatr Infect Dis J.* 1992;11:613-616.
25. Miller H. Respiratory syncytial virus and the use of ribavirin. *Matern Child Nurs J.* 1992;17:238-241.
26. Murphy MD. Respiratory syncytial virus. In Donowitz L ed. *Hospital Acquired Infection in the Pediatric Patient.* Baltimore, MD: Williams & Wilkins; 1988;207-217.
27. National Institute for Occupational Safety and Health.

Hazard evaluation and technical assistance interim report, HETA 91-104, Cincinnati, 1991, The Institute.

28. Nederhand KC, Solon J, Sweet JI, Conner SC. Respiratory syncytial virus: a nursing perspective, *Pediatr Nurs.* 1989;15(4):342-345.

29. Rabalais GP, Stonth GG, Ladd KL, Cosh KM. Rapid diagnosis of respiratory viral infection by using a shell viral assay and monoclonal antibody pool. *J Clin Microbiol.* 1992;30:1505-1508.

30. Shinya I, Koren G. Exposure of pregnant women to ribavirin contaminated air: risk assessment and recommendations. *Pediatr Infect Dis J.* 1993;12:2-5.

31. Sinnott JT, Gilgrist LS, Ellis L. Respiratory syncytial virus. *Infect Control Hosp Epidemiol.* 1988;9(11):465-468.

32. Stover BH. Pediatric units. In Berg R, ed. *APIC Curriculum for Infection Control Practices.* Dubuque, IA: Kendall-Hunt; 1988(3):1189-1227.

33. Talis A, McIntosh K. Respiratory syncytial virus. In Isenberg HD, ed. *Microbiology Procedures Handbook.* Washington, DC: American Society for Microbiology; 1992(2):883-888.

34. Washburne JF, Becchirie JA, Jamison RM. Summertime respiratory syncytial virus infection: epidemiology and clinical manifestation *So Med J* 1992;85(6):579-583.

35. Wong DL. The child with respiratory dysfunction. In Wong DL, Whaley LF. *Essentials of Pediatric Nursing,* 4th ed. St Louis, MO: Mosby–Year Book; 1993:710-756.

SUGGESTED READINGS

1. Chernoff AE, Snydman DR: Viral infections in the intensive care unit. *New Horizons.* 1993; 1(2):279-301.

2. Krilov LR, Harkness SH: Inactivation of respiratory syncytial virus by detergents and disinfectants. *Pediatr Infect Dis J.* 1993; 12:582-4.

3. Prows CA, Shortridge L, Kenner C, Lemasters G: Nature and prevalence of ribavirin aerosol administration in U.S. pediatric hospitals. *Pediatr Nurs.* 1993; 8(6):370-75.

4. Rabalais GP, Stonth GG, Ladd KL, Cosh KM: Rapid diagnosis of respiratory viral infection by using a shell viral assay and monoclonal antibody pool. *J Clin Microbiol.* 1992; 30:1505-1508.

5. Tristram DA, Welliver RC: Respiratory syncytial virus vaccines: Can we improve on nature? *Pediatr Ann.* 1993; 22(12):715-18.

Pertussis in an Infant

BETH HEWITT STOVER

CLINICAL PRESENTATION

Beatrice Lindsey, a 7-week-old girl, is a 34-week gestation infant of a 16-year-old mother. Both live with Beatrice's grandparents. Because of her low birth weight and respiratory distress shortly after birth, Beatrice was on assisted ventilation for 1 week and spent 3 weeks in the intensive care nursery. She improved and was sent home. Over the next 4 weeks she became congested during feedings. Her formula was changed from cow's milk to a soy-based formula, but there was no improvement. On March 14 she began vomiting formula shortly after feedings. She was admitted to the children's hospital on March 18 after a 1-week history of runny nose, coldlike symptoms, choking episodes during feedings, and vomiting after feedings. A protracted cough lasting almost 2 minutes and culminating with forceful spitting of formula through the nose and mouth was noted during the nursing admission assessment. Her mother had a cold at the time Beatrice was admitted. Beatrice's vital signs at time of hospitalization were: fever, 101° F (38.3° C); heart rate, 140; and respirations, 88 with subcostal retractions. Admission diagnosis was bronchiolitis. Respiratory syncytial virus (RSV) was the suspected agent. Her chest radiograph showed bilateral pulmonary infiltrates. A few crackles were heard on auscultation of the lungs.

Beatrice was admitted to a private room, and the nurses instituted precautions to prevent transmission of RSV. These precautions included use of gown and gloves by those having direct contact with her and gloves when having contact with items that may have been contaminated with respiratory secretions.[4] Nose and eye protection were not used. Beatrice's white blood count was 17,000, with a lymphocytosis of 75%. The RSV antigen test by enzyme-linked immunosorbent assay (ELISA) was negative on both March 18 and 20.

On the night of March 21, Beatrice's respiratory rate increased, respirations became more shallow, and she became agitated. The nurse noted thick nasopharyngeal secretions, protracted coughing, and frequent choking episodes. Pertussis (whooping cough) was suspected. The direct fluorescent antibody stain (DFA) for pertussis was positive. Five days later the nasopharyngeal culture had grown *Bordetella pertussis*. Oral erythromycin was prescribed, and Beatrice was placed on contact precautions to prevent droplet transmission of organisms. Health care workers were required to mask when in the room with her.[4] Because Beatrice's mother had coldlike symptoms, nasopharyngeal swabs were obtained from her for pertussis DFA and culture. Beatrice's mother was also infected with *B. pertussis*, and she also received oral erythromycin before Beatrice was discharged.

Sixteen health care workers were identified as having unprotected exposure to Beatrice's respiratory secretions. These staff were considered exposed to pertussis and provided with

14 days of erythromycin prophylaxis. No secondary cases were identified.

HOST-ENVIRONMENT INTERACTION
The host

Pertussis is an endemic disease of worldwide importance. Epidemic peaks occur in 3- to 4-year cycles. The annual incidence and mortality from pertussis before the introduction of vaccine was 150 cases and 6 deaths per 100,000 population.

In the prevaccine era, pertussis occurred primarily in children between ages 1 and 5 years. Since vaccination schedules now protect older children, the highest incidence of infection occurs in infants under 1 year of age.[5,13] Vaccine-induced and natural immunity are of limited duration. Most individuals lose their immunity before adulthood because immunity is no longer maintained by repeated exposure and vaccine is contraindicated in adults.[6,13] Consequently, pertussis in individuals over 15 years of age has increased in recent years,[5,9-12,14-20] and pertussis immunity may not be passed on to infants at birth.[13]

Humans are the only hosts for pertussis. The incidence of infection is greater in females than males. Adolescents and adults have become a major source of pertussis exposure to non-immunized and partially immunized infants and children.[11,14,15] Outbreaks of disease have been reported among high-school students, staff and residents of a facility for developmentally disabled persons, and hospitalized patients and their care providers.*

Pertussis is manifested in three stages: catarrhal, paroxysmal, and convalescent. The symptoms may continue for up to 8 weeks. Clinical symptoms are age specific. The disease is usually asymptomatic to very mild in adults; however, the very young infant may have severe complicated disease.[6,16]

---

*References 3, 8-10, 12, 17, 19, 20.

The age-specific manifestations are outlined below.

Infants
Catarrhal stage

Rhinorrhea, cough, and conjunctival injection develop and are occasionally accompanied by a low-grade fever. Nasopharyngeal secretions increase and become thick and tenacious. This stage lasts 7 to 10 days. Beatrice had runny nose, cough, and coldlike symptoms on admission.

Paroxysmal stage

Coughing episodes increase. Numerous forceful expiratory coughs may occur, followed by a sudden massive inspiratory effort, the classic "whoop." Beatrice's cough lasted almost 2 minutes and forced her to expel formula. The whoop may be absent in infants less than 6 months of age, as in Beatrice's case. Circumoral cyanosis, swelling around the eyes, and excessive salivation may occur. A mucous plug may be coughed up, and vomiting may follow the coughing paroxysm. Apnea may be a prominent feature in very young infants. This stage may have a duration of a few days to 3 to 4 weeks.

Convalescent stage

Paroxysms and vomiting decrease. However, coughing may persist for 3 to 4 weeks and in some patients up to several months.

Pneumonia is the most frequent complication of pertussis and is responsible for most pertussis-related deaths in children under 3 years of age. Seizures, coma, encephalopathy, and secondary infection (e.g., otitis media) may occur.

Older children, adolescents, and adults

Symptoms of pertussis in older children and adults vary and frequently are atypical. Mild upper respiratory infection may be an initial symptom and may be followed by a persistent cough. The whoop usually is absent, although the cough may be severe and protracted. The cough associated with pertussis in adolescents and young adults has been reported to extend beyond 3 months.[5] The infected adult may not be identified because most do not require medical evaluation or, if medical care is sought, pertussis may not be considered in the differential diagnosis of a cough. Often, as in Beatrice's case, pertussis in an adolescent or adult may be identified after pertussis in a susceptible infant has been diagnosed.

The microbiologic environment

B. pertussis is a fastidious small, nonmotile gram-negative pleomorphic rod. The organism enters the respiratory tract via inhalation of infected droplet nuclei. The organism attaches itself to epithelial cells of the trachea and proliferates, damages the respiratory mucosal surfaces, and disrupts mucociliary clearance. Leukocytosis associated with a significant lymphocytosis occurs in the infected individual. Chest radiographs may show infiltrates in the perihilar region. Antibodies against pertussis are produced, and lifelong immunity usually follows.

Nasopharyngeal secretions may be tested by direct fluorescence for presence of organisms. Culture of *B. pertussis* requires inoculation of nasopharyngeal mucus on Bordet-Gengou media or other selective media and incubation for up to 7 days. False-negative results may be obtained late in the course of disease or if the specimen is of poor quality. Of the several methods to test for pertussis, many are time-consuming, costly, require special equipment, or are under investigation. Current diagnostic methods for pertussis identification are neither sensitive nor specific.[3,6,13,18]

The physical environment

Transmission of *B. pertussis* requires direct exposure to an infected individual. Infectious droplets are expelled during coughing paroxysms. Susceptible individuals within close range of the patient (under 5 feet) inhale these particles, and the organism invades the respiratory tract. Once infected droplets have been inhaled, 6 to 20 days (average of 7) of incubation may elapse before symptoms appear.[13,16] Pertussis, when introduced into a susceptible population, will produce disease in 50% to 100% of susceptible persons. The incidence of pertussis has little seasonal variation.[6]

The social environment

Some parents have elected not to have their infants immunized because of reservations based on religious beliefs or reports of neurologic sequelae from pertussis immunization. Neurologic disorders associated with prior pertussis immunization and certain other neurologic conditions may contraindicate use of pertussis vaccine.[16] Since vaccine-induced *B. pertussis* immunity decreases with age, older children and adults are at increased risk for pertussis when it is introduced into such settings. Once pertussis is acquired, the infected individual can transmit it to susceptible persons.

Beatrice's medical history revealed that she had not received pertussis immunization and that Beatrice's mother attended a local high school, where several students had coldlike symptoms. During the day the infant stayed at a baby sitter's home. The nurse at the local health department was informed of these two pertussis cases and attempted to identify individuals who had been significantly exposed. The health department physician provided erythromycin prophylaxis for those exposed.

PREVENTION AND CONTROL

The incidence of pertussis in the United States has decreased since vaccine was introduced in the 1950s. A killed whole-cell pertussis vaccine combined with diphtheria and tetanus toxoid (DTP) has been used for immunization. An acellular pertussis vaccine (DTaP) recently received U.S. Food and Drug Administration (FDA) approval.[3,4] The standard immunization schedule includes three primary doses of whole-cell vaccine at 2-month intervals beginning between ages 6 weeks and 2 months, followed by a booster dose 6 to 12 months after the third dose (age 15 months). A fifth dose is given between ages 4 and 6 years. DTaP vaccine is recommended for the fourth and fifth vaccine doses for children who have previously received the whole-cell vaccine.[3,4] Pertussis immunization is not recommended for individuals over age 7 years because of age-related risk of complications.

Studies of pertussis outbreaks in Great Britain and the United States have clearly shown that reduction of incidence of pertussis is directly related to vaccine use. When vaccine use decreases, the incidence of pertussis increases in new susceptible cohorts of young children.[6] If pertussis is to be reduced worldwide, effective immunization programs must be maintained in the United States, and DTP and DTaP must be made available to infants and children globally.

Health care providers should maintain a high index of suspicion for pertussis in any infant or young child when an upper respiratory infection progresses to include a frequent, severe, and spasmodic cough followed by paroxysms and vomiting. Any young infant with rhinorrhea, lacrimation, conjunctival injection, apneic episodes, and a cough associated with feeding should be evaluated for pertussis. When *B. pertussis* is suspected, the affected child should be placed in a private room and contact precautions should be followed to prevent transmission by droplets until effective antimicrobial therapy has been administered for 5 to 7 days.[7,16]

The antibiotic of choice for treating pertussis is erythromycin estolate ester (EES). EES pen-etrates the respiratory tract and produces effective blood levels. It also eliminates *B. pertussis* organisms from the nasopharynx, shortening the duration of communicability and reducing the severity of symptoms if instituted early in the course of the infection. Trimethoprim-sulfamethoxazole is occasionally used as an alternate antimicrobial when EES is contraindicated; however, its efficacy has not been established.

Secondary cases of pertussis have been reported in hospitals; therefore, compliance with precautions and reporting of unprotected exposure are important. Although there have been no controlled trials of EES for prophylaxis in health care settings, staff who have had close contact with an infected child should be given chemoprophylaxis.[2,6,16,17] EES prophylaxis should also be administered to household contacts. Family members should be evaluated for illness and if symptomatic, restricted from visiting or given EES therapy and requested to stay in the room with the patient until at least 5 to 7 days of EES treatment has been completed. Household contacts under age 7 years who have not completed a full series and booster doses of pertussis immunization may be given a dose of vaccine.

SUMMARY

Pertussis is a communicable disease of worldwide importance. Pertussis is highly contagious to susceptible persons who are close to an infected individual with coughing paroxysms. Increased vaccine use has been associated with a general decline in disease and with a shift of the majority of reported cases in the United States from children aged 1 to 5 years to infants under 1 year of age. Today, undiagnosed infected adolescents and adults who have lost vaccine immunity may represent a major source of infection. This was the case with Beatrice. Her undiagnosed, pertussis-infected adolescent mother, who had

SUMMARY TABLE 30. Pertussis in an infant

Host-environment model	Case presentation	Factors that influence infectious process	Prevention and control
Host factors	7-week-old girl, previously healthy	Human is only host All nonimmune persons are susceptible	Immunize at recommended schedule Consider postexposure prophylaxis (oral erythromycin) for susceptible close contacts of infectious person
Microbiologic factors	*Bordetella pertussis*	Droplet aerosols during coughing paroxysms from infected individual Highly transmissible	Treat with erythromycin
Physical environment	Home of teenage mother and baby sitter	Close contact with infected persons	Place infant in private room on contact precautions to prevent droplet transmission, caregivers wear a mask
Social environment	16-year-old mother who attends local high school with others who have had "coldlike" symptoms	No prior immunization	Report case to health department Evaluate mother for evidence of pertussis Advise mother to inform health department of school friends with whom she has had recent contact or who have had similar illness

received a complete series of pertussis immunizations, was the likely source.

Whole-cell pertussis vaccine has been effective in preventing pertussis. Because of sporadic reports of vaccine complications, some parents have been reluctant to vaccinate their children. Criteria have been developed for deferral of pertussis immunization in infants having specific underlying neurologic conditions and those who have experienced specific adverse events following receipt of previous pertussis immunization. The new acellular pertussis vaccines are effective and FDA approved. Because adverse reactions are reported to be less with the acellular pertussis vaccines, it may be preferable to administer these as the 4th and 5th pertussis vaccine doses. Recently pertussis vaccine has been combined with *Haemophilus influenzae* type B vaccine. Additional research is needed before a pertussis vaccine which can provide long-term immunity and can be given to adolescents and adults will be available.

Diagnosis of pertussis is often based on clinical findings because laboratory techniques lack sensitivity and specificity. The U.S. Public Health Service has established a clinical case definition to identify cases and provide a marker in community outbreaks.[1,18] Prevention and control measures include use of specific precautions during care of infected individuals, EES treatment to limit duration of contagiousness and shorten the clinical course, EES prophylaxis of contacts, and completion of the vaccine series by young infants and children.

REFERENCES

1. Centers for Disease Control: Case definitions for public health surveillance, *MMWR.* 1990;39 (RR-13):26-27.
2. Centers for Disease Control: Diphtheria, tetanus and pertussis: recommendations for vaccine use and other preventive measures—recommendation of the Immunization Practices Advisory Committee. *MMWR.* 1991; 40(RR-10).
3. Centers for Disease Control: Pertussis surveillance—United States, 1989-1991. *MMWR.* 1992;41(SS-8):11-19.
4. Centers for Disease Control: Pertussis vaccination: acellular pertussis vaccine for reinforcing and booster use—supplementary ACIP statement. *MMWR.* 1992; 41(RR-1):1-10.
5. Centers for Disease Control and Prevention. Pertussis outbreaks—Massachusetts and Maryland, 1992. *MMWR.* 1993;42:197-200.
6. Feigin RD, Cherry JD. Pertussis. In Feigin RD, Cherry JD, eds. *Textbook of Pediatric Infectious Diseases,* 3rd ed. Philadelphia, PA: W. B. Saunders; 1992.
7. Garner JS, Simmons BP. Guidelines for isolation precautions in hospitals. *Infect Control.* 1983;4 (suppl):316-349.
8. Halsey NA, Welling MA, Lehman RM. Nosocomial pertussis: a failure of erythromycin treatment and prophylaxis. *Am J Dis Child.* 1984;134:521-522.
9. Hammond J, Alter SJ, Gilchrist M. Hospital infection containment for *Bordetella pertussis.* Abstract 930 in Program and abstracts of the twenty-third Interscience Conference on Antimicrobial Agents and Chemotherapy, Washington, D.C., American Society for Microbiology; 1984.
10. Lambert HJ. Epidemiology of a small pertussis outbreak in Keny County, Michigan, *Public Health Rep.* 1965;80:365-369.
11. Linnemann CC Jr, Nasenbery J. Pertussis in the adult, *Ann Rev Med.* 1977;28:179-185.
12. Linnemann CC Jr et al. Use of pertussis vaccine in an epidemic involving hospital staff. *Lancet.* 1975;2: 540-543.
13. Mandell GL, Douglas RG Jr, Bennett JE, eds. *Principles and Practice of Infectious Diseases,* 3rd ed. New York: NY: Churchill Livingstone; 1990.
14. Mortimer EA Jr: Pertussis and its prevention: a family affair. *J Infect Dis.* 1990;161:473-479.
15. Nelson JD. The changing epidemiology of pertussis in young infants: the role of adults as reservoirs in infection, *Am J Dis Child.* 1978;132:371-375.
16. Peter G, et al, eds. *Report of the Committee of Infectious Diseases,* 23rd ed. Elk Grove Village, IL: American Academy of Pediatrics; 1994.
17. Stakette RW, et al. Evidence for a high attack rate and efficacy of erythromycin prophylaxis in a pertussis outbreak in a facility for the developmentally disabled. *J Infect Dis.* 1988;157:434-440.
18. Strebel PM, et al. Pertussis in Missouri: evaluation of nasopharyngeal culture, direct fluorescent antibody testing, and clinical case definition in the diagnosis of pertussis. *Clin Infect Dis.* 1993;16:276-285.
19. Valenti WM, Pincus PH, Messner MK. Nosocomial pertussis: possible spread by a hospital visitor. *Am J Dis Child.* 1980;134:520-521.
20. Wassilak SGF, et al. Pertussis outbreak in a Colorado high school: use of a new ELISA. Abstract 725 in Program and abstracts of the twenty-third Interscience Conference on Antimicrobial Agents and Chemotherapy. Washington, DC: American Society for Microbiology; 1984.

SUGGESTED READINGS

Bass JW. Pertussis. In Donowitz LG, ed. *Hospital Acquired Infections in the Pediatric Patient.* Baltimore, MD: Williams & Wilkins; 1988.

Halperin SA, Bortolussi R, Wort AJ. Evaluation of culture, immunofluorescence and serology for the diagnosis of pertussis. *J Clin Microbiol.* 1989;27:752-757.

Marlow DR, Redding BA, eds. *Textbook of Pediatric Nursing,* 6th ed. Philadelphia, PA: W. B. Saunders; 1988.

Onorato IM, Wassulak SGF: Laboratory diagnosis of pertussis: the state of the art. *Pediatr Infect Dis J.* 1987; 6:145-151.

Occupationally Acquired Hepatitis B in a Health Care Worker

MARJORIE J. STENBERG

CLINICAL PRESENTATION

Ron Mest is the night charge nurse on the busy 12-bed medical intensive care unit (MICU) of a 350-bed city hospital. The unit admits seriously ill medical patients, occasional trauma patients, and some surgical patients when the surgical ICUs are full. Mr. Mest is 32 years old, has been a nurse for 10 years, and has worked in the MICU for 8 years. He lives in a nearby suburban area with his wife, who is also a nurse. She works part-time and cares for their two daughters, who are 5 and 7 years old.

Mr. Mest has become increasingly fatigued over the last 5 weeks. He finds himself exhausted midway through his shift. His appetite has decreased, resulting in an unplanned 8-pound weight loss. After one particularly strenuous night during which he had two episodes of vomiting and abdominal discomfort, he reported to the occupational health office on his way out of the hospital.

A physical examination revealed a fine rash on the chest, right upper quadrant tenderness, and faint icterus of the skin and sclera. His vital signs and complete blood count (CBC) were normal. His serum glutamic-oxaloacetic transaminase* (SGOT) was 500 IU/L (normal: 7 to 40 IU/L), and the serum glutamate pyruvate transaminase* (SGPT) was 900 IU/L

*AFT (aspartine aminotransferase) often used for SGOT and ALT (alanine aminotransferase) for SGPT.

(normal: 40 IU/L). The lactate dehydrogenase (LDH) was normal and the bilirubin 9.2 mg/dl (normal: 0.2 to 1.2 mg/dl). From these findings, the physician suspected that Mr. Mest had hepatitis B. Serologic tests were ordered for hepatitis A, B, and C viruses because a specific diagnosis cannot be made clinically, and the prophylaxis, control measures, and long-term patient management are specific for each.

Mr. Mest told the examining physician he did not know of any exposure to hepatitis A, which is contracted from virus-contaminated water or foods and transmitted by the fecal-oral route. He did recall two needle sticks and one blood exposure to his ungloved hands in the past 6 months but knew of no hepatitis B or jaundiced patients in the unit during that time. The physician noted that none of these exposures was documented in his occupational health record. When asked about this, Mr. Mest explained that it was too difficult to be seen quickly in the busy emergency room where exposures were handled. After work he usually rushed home to allow his wife to get to her job. He also said he thought this busy schedule contributed to his failure to be immunized against hepatitis B, even though the vaccine had been available at no cost for years to hospital employees whose work included contact with blood and body fluids.

Mr. Mest was sent off duty. During the next week he became progressively more jaundiced and remained on sick leave for 3 more weeks. His serologic tests were positive for hepatitis B surface antigen (HBsAg) and the immuno-globulin M (IgM) fraction of antibody to the hepatitis B core antigen (anti-HBc), indicating that his illness was attributable to hepatitis B. Hepatitis Be antigen (HBeAg) was negative. Individuals who are positive for HBeAg are highly infectious. Mr. Mest was also positive for the immunoglobulin G (IgG) fraction of antibody against hepatitis A, demonstrating previous infection and recovery. He was nega-tive for hepatitis C antibody. He was still jaundiced by the sixth week of his illness but felt better, and at 8 weeks he returned to nonpatient care light-duty assignments.

Three months after he first began to feel fatigued while working, Mr. Mest tested posi-tive for antibody against HBsAg. This test provided evidence that he had recovered from the disease. He was able to return to duty in the MICU and is immune to further infection from hepatitis B.

HOST-ENVIRONMENT INTERACTION
The host

Hepatitis B is a viral infection of the liver that occurs worldwide. Humans are the only reservoir. The infection has a slow, insidious onset after an incubation period ranging from 4 to 28 weeks. The earliest symptom may be a serum sickness–like illness with a maculo-papular rash, urticaria, arthralgias, and low-grade fever. This may last for several days to weeks before the appearance of jaundice. Sub-clinical infections are frequent, and although they present no symptoms, the liver enzymes are usually elevated. Mild infections do not produce jaundice but in more severe cases are preceded by headache, nausea, malaise, vom-iting, and loss of appetite. The appearance of jaundice and symptoms coincides with high levels of virus in the blood. These symptoms and the jaundice disappear as antibodies ap-pear in the blood. The duration and severity of the disease may be inoculum related and age related. Large-volume exposures (e.g., transfu-sions) and age over 40 years are associated with severe infection and increased mobidity and mortality.[7]

Symptoms typically resolve in 3 to 4 months. However, 5% to 10% of HBV infected adults will not resolve and will remain positive for surface antigen (HBsAg) indefinitely. These individuals may transmit hepatitis B to others through blood and body fluids that may have a high titer of virus. Of these carriers, 70% will develop chronic persistent hepatitis, 30% will have chronic active hepatitis, and 1% to 2% will later develop hepatocellular carcinoma.[7]

In the United States, 5% to 10% of the population has been infected with hepatitis B. This is an estimate extrapolated from the results of testing volunteer blood donors and others. Acute and chronic infection is more common in Africa, Asia, and the Caribbean than in the United States. There are estimated to be more than 70 million chronic carriers worldwide.[4,7] The incidence of infection among the U.S. born is highest in low socio-economic groups, injection drug users and their sexual partners, those who received transfusions in the era before serologic screen-ing of blood for HBV, multiply transfused dialysis patients, persons engaging in unpro-tected sex with multiple partners, prostitutes, institutionalized mentally retarded persons, and health care workers with blood contact.

Transmission of HBV in the health care setting results from exposure to the blood of infected persons. Susceptible persons are not all at equal risk, which varies according to the work setting, duration of occupation, and frequency of exposure to blood.[6] Features of the physical and social environment are sig-nificant.

The microbiologic environment

HBV is a small deoxyribonucleic acid (DNA) virus of the *Hepadnaviridae* family. Liver cells are the primary target of the virus, though limited evidence indicates that pancreatic infection may occur. The virus and excess viral outer coating material (HBsAg) are found in many body fluids, but the levels are highest in blood, semen, and saliva. Transmission via saliva is very rare; the primary routes of transmission are sexual contact, blood-to-blood contact such as occurs when needles are shared, and from an infected mother to the unborn child. Transfusion was an important mechanism of transmission before serologic screening of blood donors was possible. The risk from this source has decreased significantly but is not entirely eliminated.

Many viral components can be identified in the blood of infected persons, whether the infection is acute or chronic. These components include the whole virus or Dane particle, surface antigen, and antibody to the core segment (box). Surface antigen (HBsAg) is the envelope, or outside, of the virus. This antigen appears in the blood about 3 to 6 weeks after the onset of active infection. At the same time, a related antigen, HBeAg, may also be detected in the blood. Its persistance is associated with high infectivity of body fluids. This is followed in 2 to 3 weeks by the appearance of antibody to the core of the virus (anti-HBc); core antigen is found in the viral core and in liver cells and does not circulate independently. Core antibody persists, possibly for life, but the level decreases with time.

When a person recovers from HBV infection, the surface antigen disappears from the blood and is replaced by surface antibody (anti-HBs). Persons who have recovered from the disease have both anti-HBs and anti-HBc. Persons whose immunity is from vaccine will have only anti-HBs. Chronic infection is evidenced by persistence of HBsAg and failure to develop anti-HBs. To determine whether an infection is recent or long past, a test for the IgM fraction of the core antibody is performed. Since IgM lasts only about 6 months after infection, detection of the IgM fraction indicates recent infection. As IgM disappears, it is

---

HEPATITIS B ANTIGENS AND ANTIBODIES

ANTIGENS: PRESENT IN ACTIVE INFECTION

HBsAg	The viral particle of surface; indicates active infection or the carrier state
HBcAg	An antigen not in the blood and present only in liver cells; no serology tests done to measure this
HBeAg	Antigen associated with virulence; low infectivity if absent

ANTIBODIES: PRESENT IN CONVALESCENCE AND RECOVERY

Anti-HBs (HBsAb)	Indicates recovery from infection or antibody from the vaccine; immunity persists even though titer may drop below level of detection
Anti-HBc (HBcAb)	Indicates a person has had disease; only appears after infection
IgM	Core antibody fraction seen only in early infection; lasts about 6 months
IgG	Core antibody fraction that appears later in recovery, after IgM
Anti-HBe (HBeAb)	Appearance in recovery period indicates low infectivity

---

replaced by IgG fraction against core antibody. The course of the infection can be monitored using periodic assessments of these antigens and antibodies (Figure 31-1).

The physical environment

The risk to health care workers for developing HBV in the course of their employment is directly related to their occupational exposure to blood. Thus the physical environment plays a significant role in the transmission of this virus. Serologic screening during clinical trials of HBV vaccine detected the percentage of hospital employees in various areas of practice with serologic markers (antibodies and antigens) indicating past or present infection, and the frequency of patient and blood contact for

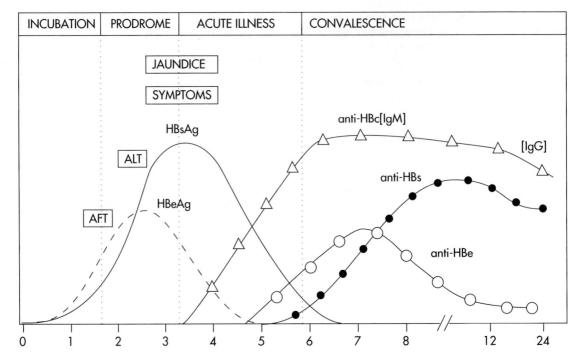

FIGURE 31-1. Course of acute hepatitis B with recovery. SGOT, AFT-aspartine aminotransferase. SGPT, ALT-alanine aminotransferase. HBsAG-surface antigen, HBeAG-e antigen, anti-HBc (HBcAb)-antibody to core, anti-HBs (HBsAb)-antibody to surface, anti-HBe (HBeAb)-antibody to the e antigen.

each of these categories (Table 31-1). Emergency room nurses who reported frequent exposure to both blood and patients, often in uncontrolled situations, showed the highest prevalence (30%) of HBV markers. The prevalence for other workers who reported much less patient contact but more frequent blood exposures were pathology (27%), blood bank (26%), and laboratory staff (24%). These same areas still carry the greatest risks for health care workers for blood and body fluid exposures. These findings are placed in context when compared to the prevalence of 5% in volunteer blood donors, who more closely reflect the experience of the general population than do many health care personnel.

The use of the HBV vaccine and universal precautions in health care settings has probably contributed to a reduction of the inci-dence of HBV infection in health care professionals. For those who work in high-risk areas and remain unvaccinated, the risk of HBV infection remains.

In 1982 Dienstag demonstrated that 17% of nurses in ICUs had HBV serologic markers.[1] ICU care providers continue to be at risk of exposure to HBV as they work with central venous pressure monitoring, arterial lines under pressure, and peripheral lines that require extensive manipulations. Surgical and trauma patients often have bleeding wounds. Occasionally dialysis is performed in these settings. Risk may be reduced by the use of barrier precautions and engineering controls such as safer needle devices or needleless systems. Although some nursing personnel may view HIV as their major bloodborne pathogen threat, the Centers for Disease Control and

TABLE 31-1. Blood and patient contact and the presence of hepatitis B serologic markers in various hospital employee groups*

Work setting (No. tested)	Exposure to patients	Exposure to blood	Percent positive for hepatitis B markers
ED nurses (30)	Frequent	Frequent	30
Pathology staff (26)	Frequent	Frequent	27
Blood bank personnel (39)	None	Frequent	26
Laboratory technicians (85)	None	Frequent	24
Intravenous team (68)	Frequent	Frequent	22
Surgical house officers (66)	Frequent	Frequent	17
Intensive care nurses (94)	Frequent	Occasional (MICU) to frequent (SICU)	10
Medical house officers (89)	Frequent	Occasional	8
General ward nurses (76)	Frequent	Occasional	5
Dietitians (19)	Occasional	None	5
Volunteer blood donors (462)	—	—	5

MICU, Medical intensive care unit; SICU, surgical intensive care unit.
*Adapted from Dienstag JL. Ryan DM. Occupational exposure to hepatitis B virus in hospital personnel: Infection or immunization? *Am J Epidemiol*. 1982;115:26-39. From Stenberg MJ. Hepatitis B and ED nurses: the disease, the risks, and the vaccine. *J Emerg Nurs*. 1983;9(3):125-128. Used with permission.

Prevention (CDC) reports that risk of HBV infection is much greater. Approximately 8000 HBV infections occur in health care workers every year and that 200 to 300 workers die yearly as a result of occupationally acquired HBV infections. [7,10]

Exposure for most occupational groups in health care occurs from percutaneous needle sticks or injuries caused by sharps contaminated with the blood of infected patients; mucocutaneous exposures result in far fewer infections. The risk of transmission of HBV from a needle stick with blood from a patient with acute or chronic HBV infection is 10% to 30%. [10] This reflects the very high titers of virus in the blood of HBV-infected patients, estimated to be 10^6 to 10^{11}/ml. The high level of underreporting of exposures seriously complicates their management and prophylaxis. Mr. Mest's case is an example of how failure to report can result in serious infection. If his needle sticks had been appropriately managed, he would have been started on the vaccine at the time of his first injury, which may have prevented his illness.

While it is clear that most nosocomial transmission of HBV is from patients to health care workers, transmission to patients from infected dentists, surgeons, respiratory therapists, and operating room personnel has been documented. [8] However, this is a rare occurrence related to the level of antigenemia in the infected health care worker and the potential for blood-to-blood contact during care. Invasive procedures such as those involving blind suturing (e.g., vaginal hysterectomy) may injure the provider. These injuries may result in such transmission. Routine nursing care by an infected individual provides few if any opportunities for blood-to-blood contact and is unlikely to pose a threat to patients. [11]

The social environment

Mr. Mest's behavior contributed to his risk of infection. He allowed a hectic schedule of work and child care to contribute to his risk of

HBV infection by interfering with his timely reporting of needle sticks and immunization. Since the protocol for follow-up after blood exposure at Mr. Mest's hospital included identifying and testing the patient source of the blood, Mr. Mest's failure to report his needle stick also prevented identification of the patient source and that patient's HBV status. The lack of investigation had implications for the patient's health and that of others close to the patient.

Mr. Mest's infection may have had a considerable effect on his own family. His wife should have been evaluated for hepatitis B immune globulin (HBIG) immediately after Mr. Mest's diagnosis and tested to determine whether she was infected. If not infected, she should have received vaccine. The Mests would have been advised to use condoms for intercourse until she had completed the vaccine series and demonstrated antibody. Although some evidence suggests that small children in the home may be infected through mucous membrane contact with such common items as toothbrushes, this mode of transmission probably occurs infrequently when sanitation is adequate and parents are aware of the mechanisms of transmission of the disease. Mr. Mest's children should have been vaccinated according to the Centers for Disease Control and Prevention (CDC), Advisory Committee on Immunization Practices (ACIP), and American Academy of Pediatrics (AAP) recommendations (see Chapter 5).[6]

Risk of HBV infection is associated with sexual activity initiated at a young age, low socioeconomic status, lack of access to health care, intravenous drug use, and sex with injection drug users. Country-specific prevalence of markers of past infection range from less than 20% in western Europe, Australia, New Zealand, and the United States to 20% to 60% in eastern Europe, Japan, and Russia and more than 60% in southeast Asia, Africa, and China. The local political environment, as reflected in policy development and resource commitment to public health and medical care, contributes to a population's risk for acquiring HBV (see Chapter 10). The high cost of HBV vaccine has hindered public health intervention in all but the most affluent circumstances.

PREVENTION AND CONTROL

Safe and effective vaccines have made the prevention of HBV technically possible. A serum-derived vaccine was introduced in 1981, and although its safety was proved, at that time many health care workers feared the vaccine was contaminated with the agent that might ultimately prove to be responsible for the newly recognized (1981) AIDS. In health care settings where the vaccine was offered free to staff, only 24% of those eligible were vaccinated.[9] In private facilities where the vaccine cost was more than $100 to employees, acceptance was even lower.

Genetically engineered vaccines became available in 1987 and have replaced the serum-derived vaccine. The U.S. Occupational Safety and Health Administration (OSHA) has mandated that all employers must provide vaccine free to workers at risk[10] (see Chapter 6). To prevent perinatal transmission of HBV, prenatal and perinatal care should include HBsAg testing and administration of hyperimmune globulin (HBIG) and the first of three doses of the vaccine to babies born to infected or chronic carrier mothers.[4] Universal immunization consistent with recent CDC, ACIP, and AAP recommendations may minimize the need for prenatal and perinatal screening.

Prevention of exposures to blood and body fluids in health care settings is based on education, universal precautions, engineering controls, use of personal protective equipment, and careful postexposure management. Education about prevention of HBV, including the importance of the vaccine and its availability without charge, must be provided to new

SUMMARY TABLE 31.   Occupationally acquired hepatitis B in a health care worker

Host-environment model	Case presentation	Factors that influence infectious process	Prevention and control
Host factors	32-year-old MICU nurse	Health care workers at medium to high risk of infection Nurse not immunized and did not report exposures	Give hepatitis B vaccine for prevention Report exposures Give HBIG for post-exposure management if unprotected
Microbiologic factors	Hepatitis B virus	Blood of infected patients or carriers has very high titer of virus Needle sticks transmit HBV Patients often asymptomatic	Antiviral therapy not available Treat asymptomatically
Physical environment	ICUs present risk for HBV	ICU care often includes complex vascular devices with: exposure to blood, bleeding problems, drainage, and frequent needle use	Universal precautions; use of safety devices in patient care (needleless systems)
Social environment	Virus may be transmitted to family	Sexual activity IV drug use Health care workers at occupational risk	Prevent infection in wife: use safer sexual practices, vaccine Children at low risk but should also receive vaccine

employees who may be at risk at the time of employment. In addition, employers must provide annual continuing education and a plan for postexposure management.

Standard infection control precautions and techniques must be integrated by health care providers into all patient care and other procedures. These systems provide mandated barrier precautions to protect health care workers from body substances that may transmit bloodborne pathogens. Personal protective equipment cannot prevent such injuries as needle sticks, but gloves can decrease the amount of blood introduced into the wound by a such an injury.[2] Engineering controls such as safe needle disposal containers located in area of sharps use can help reduce needle stick injuries if sharps are placed immediately in containers without recapping. All employers must continuously evaluate and consider purchasing equipment that eliminates the use of needles or other sharps.[3,10]

Careful evaluation and management of exposure to blood or body fluids can prevent HBV in persons sustaining percutaneous or extensive mucous membrane exposures. The most important element in such a program is education of health care workers about the importance of reporting exposures immediately. It is estimated that a considerable number of sharps injuries and needle sticks are not reported, especially in areas with potential for frequent accidents, such as the operating room.[5] When the exposed person is unvaccinated, reporting provides the opportunity to test the source and give vaccine and high anti-HBs titer immune globulin at once. The immune globulin will provide passive antibody until vaccine-stimulated antibody is formed or presence of antibody is confirmed. HBIG contains 1:100,000 units of anti-HBs. If this is not available, immune globulin containing 1:1000 units of anti-HBs may be useful. Had Mr. Mest reported his needle sticks at the time they occurred, his disease probably could have been prevented.

SUMMARY

The incidence of HBV is increasing in the United States, especially among young people. In spite of this increase and the potential for serious outcomes, less than 10% of the 22 million people at high risk for HBV have been vaccinated.[4] The morbidity and mortality associated with cirrhosis, chronic infection, and hepatocellular carcinoma can be substantially reduced by proper control measures. Vaccination of persons at risk and incorporation of the vaccine into effective childhood immunization programs could eliminate the disease.

REFERENCES

1. Dienstag JL, Ryan DM. Occupational exposure to hepatitis B virus in hospital personnel: Infection or immunization? *Am J Epidemiol* 1982;115:26-39.
2. Gerberding JL, et al. Risk of exposure to surgical patients' blood during surgery at San Francisco General Hospital. *N Engl J Med* 1990;322:1788-1796.
3. Jagger J, et al. Rates of needlestick injury caused by various devices in a university hospital. *N Engl J Med* 1988;319:284-288.
4. Katkov WN, Dienstag JL. Prevention and therapy of viral hepatitis. *Semin Liver Dis.* 1991;11(2):165-174.
5. Lynch P, White MC. Perioperative blood contact and exposures: a comparison of incident reports and focused studies. *Am J Infect Control* 1993;21:357-363.
6. Polder JA, Tablan OC, Williams WW. Personnel health services. In Bennett JV, Brachman PS, eds. *Hospital Infections,* 2nd ed. Boston, MA: Little, Brown; 1992.
7. Robinson WS. Hepatitis B virus and hepatitis delta virus. In Mandell GL, Douglas RG, Bennett JE, eds. *Principles and Practice of Infectious Diseases,* 3rd ed. New York, NY: Churchill Livingstone; 1990.
8. Sheretz RJ, Marasok RD, Streed SA. Infection control aspects of employee health. In Wenzel RP, ed. *Prevention and Control of Nosocomial Infections,* 2nd ed. Baltimore, MD: Williams & Wilkins; 1993.
9. Stenberg MJ. Hepatitis B and ED nurses: the disease, the risks, and the vaccine. *J Emerg Nurs.* 1983;9(3):125-128.
10. U.S. Department of Labor, Occupational Safety, and Health Administration: Occupational exposure to bloodborne pathogens, final rule. *Federal Register.* December 6, 1991; 56:64004-64182.
11. Valenti W. Selected viruses of nosocomial importance. In Bennett JV, Brachman PS, eds. *Hospital Infections,* 2nd ed. Boston, MA: Little, Brown; 1992.

SUGGESTED READINGS

Doebbeling BN, Wenzel RP: Nosocomial viral hepatitis. In Mandell GL, Douglas RG, Bennett JE, eds. *Principles and Practice of Infectious Diseases,* 3rd ed. New York, NY: Churchill Livingstone; 1990.

Fedson DS. Immunizations for health-care workers and patients in hospitals. In Wenzel RP, ed. *Prevention and Control of Nosocomial Infections,* 2nd ed. Baltimore, MD: Williams & Wilkins; 1993.

Lau JYN, Alexander GJM, Alberti A. Viral hepatitis. *Gut.* 1991;(suppl) S47-S62, September.

Margolis HS, Alter MJ, Adler, SC. Hepatitis B: evolving epidemiology and implications for control. *Semin Liver Dis.* 1991;11(2):84-92.

Marks JF. Viral hepatitis: unscrambling the alphabet. *Nursing 93,* 1993;23:34-41.

Tuberculosis Transmission in a Pediatric Hospital

BETH HEWITT STOVER

CLINICAL PRESENTATION*

Case I

Adam Jones, a 14-month-old boy from eastern Kentucky, was admitted to Children's Hospital in March 1990 for evaluation of failure to thrive, fever, and cervical lymphadenopathy. He was born at 25 weeks' gestation and weighed 750 g (1 lb, 10 oz). He required assisted ventilation for 3 weeks and developed chronic lung disease. Adam had a grade IV intraventricular hemorrhage, which required placement of a ventriculoperitoneal shunt. He was discharged home after a 3½ month hospitalization.

At admission, Adam's weight was 3.64 kg (8 lb), and he appeared severely malnourished. A chest radiograph revealed left upper lobe consolidation superimposed on chronic lung disease; no cavity was present. Adam was given 2 weeks of intravenous (IV) antibiotics, but he continued to have febrile episodes, and his chest radiographs did not show improvement.

On the 15th hospital day, his physicians added *Mycobacterium tuberculosis* (MTB) to the differential diagnosis. Tuberculosis (TB) control precautions were not instituted, since hospital policy at that time did not require that airborne disease precautions be used to manage tuberculosis-infected pediatric patients. A tuberculin (purified protein derivative, PPD) skin test was administered by his nurse. At 48

hours induration was 15 mm. Acid-fast organisms were noted on a direct stain of a suctioned sputum specimen and lymph node aspirate. MTB was recovered from cultures of urine, lymph node, sputum, and bone marrow.

Contact tracing identified Adam's father as having active pulmonary TB. He was present at Adam's admission but when diagnosed was asked to stay home and not resume visiting until after he had received 3 to 4 weeks of antituberculosis treatment. Despite the request, the father insisted on visiting again after only 1 week of therapy. To accommodate the father's wish to visit his son, Adam was transferred from a standard private room to a negative-pressure isolation room. The father was permitted to visit but was instructed to wear a mask at all times, as were staff when the father was present.

Adam needed frequent suctioning and chest physiotherapy. Before the diagnosis of MTB was made on the 15th hospital day, staff did not mask during those procedures. All exposed health care workers who had provided care to Adam were offered the PPD skin test; 50 of 61 exposed personnel were tested 12 weeks after exposure. Two nurses and one medical student, all of whom had negative tests within the previous 12 months, were PPD positive (>10 mm induration). One nurse was exposed on the evening of Adam's admission, and the other cared for Adam for four 12-hour work shifts before the diagnosis was made and treatment started. The medical student was

---

*These two cases are reprinted, in part, with permission from the editor of *The Lancet*.[13]

exposed repeatedly during 15 working days. Transmission from the father to the first nurse and the medical student could not be ruled out. The second nurse was never exposed to the father. These three staff had no other known contact with TB.[13]

Case II

Joseph Morgan, a 5-month-old boy, was admitted to the same hospital for persistent left upper lobe pneumonia, fever, and weight loss. A direct stain of a gastric aspirate showed acid-fast organisms. MTB was cultured from both gastric aspirate and cerebrospinal fluid (CSF). Both of Joseph's parents were PPD nonreactive and had normal chest radiographs.

Because Joseph had a prominent cough and because MTB transmission from a child to health care workers appeared to have occurred several months previously, staff who cared for Joseph were offered PPD skin tests. Of 33 exposed health care providers, 28 were tested within 8 weeks and again 12 weeks after exposure. One nurse had a 10 mm induration PPD skin test 7 weeks after her first exposure. She had cared for Joseph during five 12-hour work shifts, two of which occurred before he began treatment. This nurse had a negative PPD skin test 3 months previously and no other contact with TB in the preceding 12 months.[13] Airborne disease precautions were not implemented, since transmission of MTB from an infant had not been thought likely.[16]

HOST-ENVIRONMENT INTERACTION
The host

Infection caused by MTB is a major global health problem. At least 3 million deaths associated with MTB are estimated to have occurred worldwide in 1990.[1] Homeless persons (see Clinical Study 7), residents of chronic care facilities, persons with human immuno-deficiency disease (HIV) and acquired immu-nodeficiency syndrome (AIDS), and those with other diseases that compromise the immune system are also at risk for MTB-associated morbidity and mortality.

Although the incidence of active MTB infection is lowest in infants and children, those younger than 5 years of age are at highest risk of disease following infection and are at greatest risk for death from MTB.[14]

Infants are especially susceptible to infection, and malnourished infants and children such as Adam are at risk for developing serious disease from MTB. Adolescent and pregnant women are also at increased risk for infection after exposure. Measles and influenza may lower an individual's resistance to tuberculosis.[11,14] Incidence of MTB infection is high in many countries. MTB has been a particularly serious health problem for Native Americans and Alaskan Inuits.

Children usually acquire MTB from an infected member of the household. However, scattered reports cite children such as Joseph who have acquired MTB from other contacts. Infected children are rarely reported to transmit MTB to others.[12,14,16] Epidemiologists and others have believed that the sputum of infants and children contained fewer tubercle bacilli than that of adults and that children were not likely to produce sputum during coughing episodes.[4,8,13] For this reason, airborne disease precautions have not been routinely used to manage infants and young children with pulmonary MTB.[9,13]

Clinical manifestations of MTB vary by site of infection and host susceptibility. Asymptomatic infection occurs in most cases. Asymptomatic infection is identified by a skin reaction (induration) when PPD, a preparation of MTB proteins, is injected intradermally. Symptoms of active infection in infants and children may include any of the following: weight loss, fever, anorexia, cough, wheezing, dyspnea, lethargy, and night sweats. Hilar, mediastinal, and cervical lymphadenopathy is most common in infants and children. Hilar adenopathy may be accompanied by atelectasis. One or more lung segments may be affected. Segmental lesions are seen most frequently in infants. Pleural effusion may be seen in children over age 2 years. Calcified lesions and cavitation are less often seen in children than adults. Progressive primary pulmonary MTB occurs occasionally.

Approximately 20% of MTB in infants and children is extrapulmonary. Miliary MTB can occur in children, especially infants, through lymphohematogenous spread of the tubercle bacilli, as occurred with Adam. Tuberculous meningitis occurs most frequently in children under age 6 years. Joseph had evidence of tuberculous meningitis. Cutaneous, skeletal, and renal MTB, and superficial lymph node scrofula (tuberculous cervical lymphadenitis) also occurs in children. Neonatal MTB infection may produce symptoms in the second or third week of life.[14]

The microbiologic environment

MTB is one of the mycobacteria that infect humans. Other mycobacteria species that cause disease include *avium, africanum,* and *bovis.*[7] Primates, dogs, cats, and other mammals having contact with humans can become infected with MTB; however, humans are the major reservoir. MTB is an aerobic, nonmotile, non-spore-forming pleomorphic, weakly gram-positive rod 1 to 5 μm long. The cell wall is composed of lipids of high molecular weight, which retain stain despite an acid rinse—thus the designation acid-fast bacilli (AFB). Although the organism replicates every 15 to 24 hours, visible colony growth on solid media may take 3 to 6 weeks.

Sputum frequently is difficult to obtain from infants and children unless bronchoscopy or lung aspiration is performed. Gastric aspirates collected from these patients before arising may yield AFB. Older children and adolescents may be able to expectorate sputum with the use of a nebulized aerosol treatment. Spinal fluid, an early-morning urine specimen, and bone marrow and tissue biopsy of infected body fluids may yield AFB in patients with extrapulmonary TB. Rapid recovery and diagnosis can be achieved with the use of deoxyribonucleic acid (DNA) probes and radiometric culture (Bactec) techniques.

Mycobacteria replicate slowly, therefore antimicrobial therapy must be administered for many months. Mutations can occur during therapy which confers antimicrobial resistance. Therapy must include multiple antimicrobials to insure that an active agent is included. Premature discontinuation of drugs or prescription of the wrong or too few antimicrobials has resulted in the emergence of strains of MTB that are resistant to multiple antimicrobials (multi-drug resistance tuberculosis or MDRTB). Antimicrobial sensitivity testing should be performed routinely, since the frequency of drug resistance is increasing.

The primary mode of transmission of MTB is via the air.[3,5] Infectious droplet nuclei form when liquid droplets of respiratory secretions from an infected individual are expelled by coughing, sneezing, or talking. The liquid evaporates and the droplet nuclei may remain suspended in air for long periods. When the nuclei containing MTB are inhaled, the organisms multiply within the new host's bronchioles. Transmission may also occur as a result of inoculation into a superficial skin lesion. Transmission has also occurred transplacentally and during delivery. Nosocomial transmission via contact with heavily contaminated objects has infrequently been reported[14] (see Clinical Study 7).

The physical environment

The physical environment plays an important role in the transmission of MTB. Since infectious droplet nuclei can remain suspended in the air for long periods and since the organism can remain viable, the air plays an important role in transmission of MTB. In the hospital setting, nonprotected contact with MTB-infected patients and medical treatments have been implicated in nosocomial transmission.[8,10,13,14] In Adam's case, it was speculated that chest physiotherapy and suctioning procedures may have aerosolized infectious droplet nuclei and exposed staff. Staff may have inhaled infectious droplet nuclei during these cough-stimulating procedures.[3]

Seasonal occurrence of MTB has been observed among children in the Northern Hemisphere.[7,14] It is speculated that close contact with infected household members during winter months in closed settings with limited air exchanges increases exposure. Hospitals where rooms did not achieve proper negative air pressure and exhaust without recirculation have been implicated in MTB transmission.[8] Patients not suspected of having MTB have disseminated tubercle bacilli in the surrounding environment with subsequent transmission to others. Initially neither Adam nor Joseph was suspected of having MTB.

The social environment

MTB infection is associated with overcrowded and poor living conditions and undernutrition. Adam was malnourished secondary to severe developmental delay, oropharyngeal discoordination, and gastroesophageal reflux. The family received minimal support to help them deal with these medical issues. Visits from the traveling nurses were infrequent and the family's compliance with prescribed care was inconsistent.

No one in Joseph's family was identified as being infected with *Mycobacterium tuberculosis*, and no source of MTB was ever identified. Identification of exposed persons may be difficult or impossible among highly mobile groups. As more individuals and families become homeless and travel from one shelter to another and from city to city, transmission risk increases (see Clinical Study 7). Prison

inmates, injecting drug users, alcoholics, and elderly persons who live in poor conditions are at risk for MTB exposure. Many of these individuals do not have easy access to preventive health care or medical care during illness. Some of these individuals may be exposed, acquire MTB infections, or develop active disease, but because of poor access to medical care will not seek medical attention promptly and will have undiagnosed disease for many weeks or months. Lack of compliance with preventive therapy and treatment may be related to the individual's inability to understand the disease process and need for continued therapy. These conditions are conducive to the spread of MTB.

PREVENTION AND CONTROL

Social improvements such as education of those at high risk and public health TB control programs are vital for the prevention and control of MTB.[3,5] Children and other individuals at risk should receive adequate nutrition to maintain immunity and lessen the likelihood of active disease. While the patient is in the hospital, nurses and dietitians should teach family members the importance of medication compliance and proper nutrition. Improved living conditions, including decreased crowding and adequate ventilation, decrease the opportunity for TB transmission. Early identification and treatment of newly infected individuals (recent TB skin test converters) are effective measures to prevent emergence of active disease. Public health nurses participate in education, case finding, screening, contact follow-up, and medication administration in the national initiative to prevent and control MTB.

Employer-based PPD skin-testing programs may identify individuals exposed to an unrecognized case of active disease when the prevalence of infection is high. MTB testing programs may be useful in hospitals, home health agencies, physicians' offices, extended care facilities, shelters for homeless persons, and licensed day-care facilities. Annual TB testing in childhood is recommended for those at high risk for MTB infection.[12] The Mantoux PPD skin test is the preferred method for screening individuals for MTB. The PPD must be placed intradermally, not subcutaneously. The test should be interpreted on the basis of the diameter of induration measured in millimeters. The person interpreting the PPD should do so with eyes closed while palpating the site in order to detect the induration before measuring.

Preventive therapy with isoniazid (INH) is recommended for new PPD skin test converters whose infection is not active and persons having close contact with persons newly diagnosed with MTB.[5] Persons in certain high-risk groups, regardless of age, should be considered for INH preventive therapy.[5] Additionally, in the absence of known high-risk factors, persons in high-incidence groups under 35 years of age with PPD skin conversion of 10 mm or greater are candidates for preventive therapy. When a reactive skin test is observed, a chest radiograph should be obtained. If there is no evidence of pulmonary disease, INH chemotherapy should be initiated.

Children who are contacts of persons with active tuberculosis are candidates for tuberculosis prophylaxis even if the child's skin test is negative and the child has no evidence of active disease. This is especially important for immunocompromised children and all children under the age of 4 years who are household contacts of a person with active tuberculosis.[12] Children with a reaction of greater than or equal to 5 mm of induration are considered to have a positive skin test if they 1) are close contacts of individuals with tuberculosis, 2) have a chest radiograph consistent with a healed tuberculous lesion, or 3) have HIV infection. Those children who have reactions of greater than or equal to 10 mm induration are considered positive when 1) age is less than 4 years, 2) a medical risk factor is present (e.g., diabetes, chronic renal failure, malnutrition, Hodgkin's disease or lymphoma), 3) when the child's parent is from an area of the world where tuberculosis is prevalent or 4) they are frequently exposed to adults at high risk for tuberculosis. Children age 4 years or older who have 15 mm of induration or greater are considered positive regardless of whether they have any identified risk factor.

For children, the American Academy of Pediatrics (AAP) recommends 9 months of daily INH therapy. When compliance is low, twice-weekly directly observed therapy (DOT) can begin after 1 month of daily therapy. When drug-resistant MTB is suspected, preventive therapy should be carefully selected and may include more than one agent.[4]

Uncomplicated active pulmonary disease in children is usually treated with INH, rifampin, and pyrazinamide for 2 months, followed by INH and rifampin for 4 months. When drug resistance is likely, ethambutol or streptomycin should be added to the treatment regimen.[12,14] A 9- to 12-month regimen is recommended for severe disseminated disease in children. Because both Adam and Joseph had disseminated (pulmonary and extrapulmonary) MTB, each received multidrug therapy for 12 months.

To prevent transmission of MTB in health care settings, the latest recommendations of the Centers for Disease Control and Prevention (CDC) should be followed.[2] For many years, infants and young children such as Adam and Joseph were not thought to be contagious.[9,14] When a child has MTB, usually an adult household contact is the source. The infected adult source may be a parent day-care provider, visitor, or teacher.[10,14]

Occasionally, as in Joseph's case, the individual with active disease may not be identified. Unless a household contact is known to have active MTB, this disease may not be considered in the initial differential diagnosis. In these situations, as in both Adam's and Joseph's cases, the patient may be hospitalized without MTB precautions. Adam's father was the source for his infection and could not be ruled out as the source for transmission to two health care workers, although he was asked to mask at all times during his visits. In 1981 at Birmingham (England) Children's Hospital, a 3-year-old was hospitalized and found to have a spinal tumor caused by MTB.[10] The child's mother later was identified as having cavitary pulmonary MTB. She was the source of an outbreak of MTB that infected 36 patients, visitors, and staff. As with Adam and Joseph, this case illustrated the need for a high index of suspicion for MTB and prompt use of controlled airflow for management of the pediatric patient and respiratory precautions for health care providers.

Precautions for airborne-spread organisms should be continued until there is clinical improvement, cough has decreased, and the number of organisms on AFB smears is decreasing or absent.[3] When drug-resistant organisms are suspected, precautions should be continued until AFB smear of sputum is free of organisms on 3 successive days. When MTB is confirmed, the degree of contagiousness in the pediatric patient and any infected family member or visitor should be determined.

Restricting an infected family member from visiting until he or she is determined to be noncontagious may or may not be possible. Adam's father was requested not to visit until he had completed 3 to 4 weeks of antituberculous therapy and his symptoms had resolved; however he did not comply with the request. In this case, the hospital staff tried to accommodate the father while protecting staff and other patients from exposure. It is appropriate to appeal to the county or state public health officer for assistance with management of patients, visitors, or anyone else obstructing appropriate management of tuberculosis.

Communicability is believed to be greatest in patients with a productive cough, pulmonary cavitary disease, and AFB seen in sputum or gastric aspirate smears. Length of infectiousness varies. The CDC notes that noninfectiousness can be established when a patient is receiving effective chemotherapy and the sputum collected on 3 consecutive days is free of tubercle bacilli on AFB smear.[3]

The CDC guidelines for control of MTB in health care settings recommend ultraviolet light irradiation and high-efficiency ventilation for patient care rooms, areas such as endoscopy suites, and emergency departments.[2,3] Use of respirators is recommended for providers of direct care and those participating in bronchoscopy and other cough-inducing procedures. Contaminated environmental surfaces, medical instruments, and equipment should receive appropriate disinfection or sterilization as usual. Proposed revisions to the guidelines from the CDC recommend and an interim rule from the Occupational Safety and Health Administration mandates that high efficiency particulate air (HEPA) respirators be worn to protect health care personnel who care directly for individuals with suspected or confirmed MTB.[2,16] This requirement is controversial.

Health care providers should report a diagnosis of MTB infection to the county health department. The health department can assist by testing and evaluating household members and other contacts in an effort to identify the source or secondary cases of MTB. This is how Adam's father was found to be infected. Case finding, treatment for persons found to have active disease, and treatment of asymptomatic or inactive infection (PPD skin test converters) are important MTB prevention and control measures.

Patient compliance with therapy is imperative for effective treatment of MTB. Individuals must be given understandable instructions and explanations. Follow-up should include careful monitoring. When compliance with therapy cannot be ensured, patients should be required to take their medications in the presence of a health care provider. If the family does not administer medication to a child with active MTB, or if the infected adult with active disease refuses to comply with directly observed therapy, temporary hospitalization may be necessary to ensure appropriate treatment.

Education is a necessary component of prevention and control of MTB. Persons at high risk for exposure or infection should be instructed about symptoms of MTB and the need for prompt medical attention if symptoms develop or if they are exposed to active, potentially communicable infection. Persons with active disease should be taught about communicability and be informed of and encouraged to practice measures to reduce the

SUMMARY TABLE 32. Tuberculosis transmission in a pediatric hospital

Host-environment model	Case presentation	Factors that influence infectious process	Prevention and control
Host factors	Case I: 14-month-old boy; malnourished Case II: 5-month-old boy	All humans are susceptible Chronic lung disease Young age Prematurity Failure to thrive	Support nutrition
Microbiologic factors	*Mycobacterium tuberculosis* (MTB)	Airborne transmission by airborne droplet nuclei Increased prevalence of resistant strains	Treat with antitubercular therapy
Physical environment	Case I: household source for MTB Case II: source not identified	Contact with susceptible hosts MTB diagnosis in both situations was not considered during initial medical evaluations, thereby increasing numbers and frequency of exposure	Use private room with negative air pressure and no recirculation of the air (exhausted outdoors) Use gown if contamination of clothing is likely; gloves if extrapulmonary and lesion drainage Use mask when in room with patient, using current recommended mask/respirator
Social environment	Case I: cared for in home by mother; father found to have active pulmonary MTB	Case I: close household contact with source of MTB	Revise patient care policy for MTB in infants/children Educate health care workers to:

Continued.

SUMMARY TABLE 32.   Tuberculosis — cont'd

Host-environment model	Case presentation	Factors that influence infectious process	Prevention and control
	Case II: cared for in home by mother No source identified through contact tracing by county health department	Case II: none identified	1. Suspect MTB in pediatric patients with symptoms such as weight loss; fever; lymphadenopathy of hilar, mediastinal, cervical, or other lymph nodes; pulmonary involvement of lung segment or lobe with atelectasis; consolidation or pleural effusion 2. Understand potential risk for MTB transmission in the pediatric setting 3. Use airborne disease precautions and protect staff having contact 4. Report cases to local county health department so contacts can be (a) screened, (b) started on appropriate therapy, and (c) educated and monitored for compliance with treatment regimens (d) directly observed taking medication if necessary

numbers of bacilli expectorated into the air. These measures include use of masks, tissues for covering the nose and mouth during coughing episodes and sneezing, controlled airflow, and minimizing sharing of air during the infectious period. Strong emphasis should be placed on the need to complete therapy. Nurses caring for these patients in hospital and public health clinics can actively participate in the education process.

SUMMARY

MTB is a communicable disease that has been recognized for centuries. Improvements in social conditions and nutrition dramatically decreased morbidity, mortality, and incidence. Since the mid-1980s, the incidence of MTB infection has increased.[6,8,11,14,15] The increase can be attributed to recent immigration from countries having high prevalence of infection; crowded living conditions; homelessness; an aging population, including many individuals exposed and initially infected in the preantibiotic era; exposed HIV-infected individuals; and the emergence of drug-resistant MTB.[1] The U.S. Public Health Service has launched an initiative to eliminate MTB by the year 2010.[1] Cooperation from public health authorities, researchers, and health care providers will be necessary if that goal is to be accomplished. The infected individual must be cooperative and compliant with the antimicrobial therapy regimen if the emergence of resistant organisms, severe morbidity, and further transmission of disease is to be avoided. Research is needed to evaluate the efficacy of currently recommended control measures and develop antimicrobials that can effectively treat strains of MTB that are resistant to drugs currently available.

REFERENCES

1. Centers for Disease Control. Center for Prevention Services, Division of Tuberculosis Control: *USA* (narrative text), Atlanta GA: April 1990.
2. Centers for Disease Control and Prevention: *Draft Guidelines for Preventing the Transmission of Tuberculosis in Healthcare Facilities*, 2nd ed. *Federal Register*. 1993;58:52810-52854.
3. Centers for Disease Control: Guidelines for preventing the transmission of tuberculosis in health care settings, with special focus on HIV-related issues. *MMWR*. 1990;39 (RR-17): 1-29.
4. Centers for Disease Control: Management of persons exposed to multi drug-resistant tuberculosis, *MMWR*. 1992;41(RR-11):38-45.
5. Centers for Disease Control: Screening for tuberculosis and tuberculosis infection in high-risk populations and the use of preventive therapy for tuberculosis infection in the United States. *MMWR*. 1990;39;(RR-8): 1-12.
6. Centers for Disease Control: Tuberculosis morbidity in the United States—1992. *MMWR*. 1991;42:696, 697, 703, 704.
7. Des Prez RM, Heim CR. Mycobacterium tuberculosis. In Mandell GL, Douglas RG Jr, Bennett JE eds. *Principles and Practice of Infectious Diseases*, 3rd ed. New York, NY: Churchill Livingstone; 1990.
8. Edlin BR, Tokars JI, Grieco MH, et al. An outbreak of multi-drug resistant tuberculosis among hospitalized patients with the acquired immunodeficiency syndrome. *N Engl J Med*. 1992;326:1514-1521.
9. Garner JS, Simmons BP. Guidelines for isolation precautions in hospitals. *Infect Control*. 1983;4(suppl): 316-349.
10. George RH, et al. An outbreak of tuberculosis in a children's hospital. *J Hosp Infect*. 1987;8:129-142.
11. Inselman LS. Tuberculosis in children: an unsettling forecast. *Contemp Pediatr*. 1990;(10):110-130.
12. Peter G, et al eds. *Report of the Committee on Infectious Diseases*, 23rd ed. Elk Grove Village, IL: American Academy of Pediatrics; 1994.
13. Rabalais G, Adams G, Stover B. PPD skin test conversion in health care workers after exposure to *Mycobacterium tuberculosis* infection in infants. *Lancet*. 1991;338:826.
14. Smith MHD, Starke JR, Marquis JR. Tuberculosis and opportunistic mycobacterial infections. In Feigin RD, Cherry JD eds. *Textbook of Pediatric Infectious Diseases*, 3rd ed. Philadelphia, PA: W. B. Saunders; 1992.
15. Snider DE, Dooley SW. Nosocomial tuberculosis in the AIDS era with an emphasis on multi drug-resistant disease. *Heart Lung*. 1993;22:365-369.
16. Wallgren A. On contagiousness of childhood tuberculosis. *Acta Pediatr Scand*. 1937;22:229-234.

SUGGESTED READINGS

Marlow DR, Redding BA. *Textbook of Pediatric Nursing*, 6th ed. Philadelphia, PA: W. B. Saunders; 1988.
Nemir RL, Krasinski K. Tuberculosis in children and adolescents in the 1980s. *Pediatr Infect Dis J*. 1988; 7:375-379.
Smith MHD. Tuberculosis in children and adolescents. *Clin Chest Med*. 1989;10:381-395.
Snider D. Pregnancy and tuberculosis. *Chest*. 1984; 86(suppl 3):105-135.
Starke JR. Modern approach to the diagnosis and treatment of tuberculosis in children. *Pediatr Clin North Am*. 1988;35:441-464.

Legionnaires' Disease: Possible Acquisition on a Cruise Ship

TERESA C. HORAN

CLINICAL PRESENTATION

On August 6 Elliot Peale, a 74-year-old man, sought treatment for acute respiratory distress in the emergency department (ED) of University Hospital. His symptoms were dyspnea, fever (39° C, 102.2° F), cough, pleuritic chest pain, and diarrhea. His initial chest x-ray film revealed diffuse, patchy, multisegmental pneumonia involving several lobes. An expectorated sputum specimen was collected for Gram stain and culture. He was admitted to the medical intensive care unit and antibiotic therapy was begun with cefotaxime.

Mr. Peale's personal history revealed that he is an insulin-dependent diabetic, has chronic obstructive pulmonary disease (COPD), and is on medication for hypertension. He has smoked for more than 30 years and regularly consumes moderate amounts of alcohol. Mr. Peale and 49 other members of his independent senior living community had just returned from a two-week vacation in the Caribbean aboard a cruise ship.

Mixed bacterial flora was seen on the Gram stain of the sputum collected on August 6. The culture revealed no definitive pathogen. By August 8, Mr. Peale's condition had worsened. A chest film showed increased density and spreading of infiltrates, and he required increased ventilatory support. Suspecting atypical pneumonia, his physician ordered the collection of a respiratory specimen by deep suction. It was submitted to the lab for direct fluorescent antibody (DFA) test for *Legionella* and specifically cultured for *Legionella*. Erythromycin was added to Mr. Peale's antibiotic regimen.

On August 9 the results of the DFA test were reported positive for *Legionella*. Treatment with erythromycin was continued and the cefotaxime was discontinued. On August 12 *Legionella pneumophila* serogroup 1 was isolated from the respiratory secretion specimen obtained on August 8. By August 20, Mr. Peale's condition had stabilized and he was discharged four days later.

HOST-ENVIRONMENT INTERACTION

The host

Multisystem illness with pneumonia caused by *Legionella* is called Legionnaires' disease. It is one of the two principal respiratory syndromes of legionellosis. The other is a self-limited influenza-like illness without pneumonia called Pontiac fever. The characteristics of the two infections are compared in Table 33-1.[2] Erythromycin is the antibiotic treatment of choice. Both diseases are transmitted by breathing aerosols containing *Legionella* organisms. Legionnaires' disease acquired its name as a result of an outbreak affecting a large group of American Legion members who were attending a convention in Philadelphia in 1976.[8]

Skin and soft tissue infections due to *Legionella* have also been reported such as among

TABLE 33-1. Characteristics of respiratory diseases caused by *Legionella*

Characteristics	Diseases	
	Pneumonia	Pontiac fever*
Incubation period	2–10 days	36 hours
Attack rate	<5%	95%
Mortality	5%–30%	0%
Seasonality	Year-round with cases more common in summer/fall	—
Persons predominantly affected	Middle-aged to elderly persons with underlying medical conditions (cigarette smoking, immunosuppression, chronic cardiovascular or pulmonary conditions, diabetes mellitus, malignancy, alcohol addiction)	Working-age adults without underlying medical conditions
Onset/recovery	Variable/gradual	Sudden/48 hours
Fever/headache	>39° C/common	Low grade/common
Other symptoms	Cough, dyspnea, diarrhea, delirium, pleuritic chest pain	Flu-like symptoms
Chest radiograph	Segmented, multilobar	Negative

Adapted from Barbaree JM: Perspectives on the ecology and control of *Legionella.* In International Symposium on Water-Related Health Issues, November 1986, American Water Resources Association.

*Several species of *Legionella,* including *L. pneumophila, L. feeleii, L. micdadei,* and *L. anisa,* have been implicated as causative agents but have not been isolated from a patient with Pontiac fever.

patients undergoing bone marrow, cardiac, and renal transplants.[1,3,11,13,16]

Whether a person acquires legionellosis after exposure to a contaminated water source depends on several factors, including the type and intensity of exposure and the general health of the exposed individual. Persons with the highest risk of disease are those suffering from severe immunosuppression or chronic underlying illnesses (e.g., hematologic malignancy or end-stage renal disease). Persons at moderately increased risk are those with diabetes mellitus, chronic obstructive pulmonary disease (COPD), or nonhematologic malignancy, those who smoke cigarettes, and the elderly. However, nosocomial Legionnaires' disease has also been reported among pediatric patients.[4]

As in Mr. Peale's case, Legionnaires' disease is indistinguishable from pneumonia that has other causes. Men are affected two to three times as often as women, although this may be related to differences in prevalences of underlying conditions or likelihood of exposure to contaminated aerosols.

Microbiologic environment

Of the 30 species of *Legionella*, 18 have been associated with disease in humans. Although there are 48 serogroups, most human infections are caused by *L. pneumophila* serogroups 1 and 6 and *L. micdadei*. These ubiquitous aquatic organisms are small gram-negative rods with fastidious nutrient requirements. They are also intracellular organisms that parasitize human mononuclear phagocytes, that is, monocytes and alveolar macrophages.

Several laboratory tests identify *Legionella:* culture isolation or visualization using immunofluorescent microscopy [e.g., direct fluorescent antibody (DFA)] of respiratory secretions or tissue, and, for *L. pneumophila* serogroup 1, antigen detection in urine by radioimmunoassay or antibody detection at ≥1:128 in paired acute and convalescent serum samples by the indirect immunofluorescent antibody (IFA) test.

These tests complement one another, and none is 100% sensitive. Therefore, even if one or more of them is negative, legionellosis cannot be ruled out. Because culture isolation is the most specific test, growth of legionellae is considered significant. It usually takes 2 to 7 days for visible colonies to appear on specially prepared nutrient agar (buffered charcoal yeast extract agar with added α-ketoglutarate) incubated at 35° C (95° F).

Exposure occurs when respirable droplets (1 to 5 μm) of contaminated water are inhaled by humans. Although the infectious dose for *L. pneumophila* is not known, available data suggest that one colony-forming unit of bacteria in 50 L of air can successfully infect a susceptible host.

L. pneumophila accounts for more than 80% of the 250 to 400 confirmed cases of legionellosis reported annually to the Centers for Disease Control and Prevention (CDC). The true incidence of legionellosis is probably much higher than that reported via CDC's passive surveillance system, since diagnostic tests for legionellae are not routinely performed on patients with pneumonia. The risk of hospital-acquired legionellosis is not the same at all hospitals and the proportion of nosocomial pneumonia attributed to *Legionella* species has been reported to range from none to 30%.[10,11,15]

The physical environment

Although *Legionella* organisms have been found in most naturally occurring wet environments (e.g., lakes, rivers, wet soil), these sources have not been linked with human disease. Some man-made water environments, such as cooling towers of hospitals, hotels, and businesses, evaporative condensers, shower heads, and faucets can become colonized with *Legionella* and serve as reservoirs from which the organisms are disseminated.[5,7-9] Several physical factors that enhance colonization are warm temperature (25° to 42° C, 77° to 108° F), stagnation, scale, and sediment. Warm recirculated water with abundant organic and inorganic material and microorganisms, such as that found in water cooling systems, provides an ideal habitat for growth. The presence in water systems of other microflora, especially protozoa, is another factor that can promote colonization of *Legionella*. Legionellae can infect and multiply in amoebae and ciliated protozoa, as they do when they infect human mononuclear phagocytes. The intracellular environment of protozoa can support the nutritional needs of *Legionella* when the surrounding water cannot. Consequently, protozoa can be a reservoir of legionellae in unfiltered potable water.

Air-conditioning intake vents and windows can pull in drift from cooling towers contaminated with *Legionella*, which are inhaled by persons inside. Outdoors, contaminated aerosols have been inspired and caused disease in persons located as far as 200 m (218 yards) from the tower. In one investigation, persons as distant as 3.2 km (2 miles) may have been exposed. Air-conditioning systems that do not use water evaporation, such as most residential units, do not transmit disease.

Other devices that have been associated with legionellosis include showers, respiratory therapy equipment contaminated with tap water, whirlpools, and decorative fountains. In Canada, blind water fittings (i.e., shock absorbers that reduce noise in pipes) in a hospital plumbing system were found to be reservoirs of *L. pneumophila*.[14] In Louisiana, a large community outbreak of Legionnaires' disease was traced to an ultrasonic misting machine used in a grocery store vegetable case.[12] The ramifications of this outbreak are extensive, since the misting machine is similar in design to ultrasonic humidifiers used in homes. Person-to-person transmission of legionellosis and transmission via food, inhalation of dust (e.g., from a construction site), or aspiration of secretions has not been established.

The social environment

There has been at least one outbreak of *Legionella pneumonia* associated with a cruise ship.[6] In such a setting with air-conditioned cabins, recreation areas, and dining rooms where persons congregate, *Legionella*-contaminated aerosols may be inhaled. Another possible source of Mr. Peale's exposure was the shower head in his cabin. Mr. Peale's long history of smoking, diabetes, and COPD would increase his risk of acquiring infection if legionellae were present.

PREVENTION AND CONTROL

Mr. Peale's single case of Legionnaires' disease would be insufficient evidence to implicate the cruise ship as the source of infection. That link requires an epidemiologic investigation, which would not be undertaken unless an increase in cases were noted by public health officials. Health care providers (private physicians, laboratorians, or in the case of a hospital, the infection control staff) are responsible for reporting Legionnaires' disease to the health department. For example, if other residents of Mr. Peale's seniors' community who had also

---

*The amount of free residual chlorine (FRC) varies in a hyperchlorination procedure with the type of device being decontaminated. For example, for emergency decontamination of a water cooling tower during an outbreak, an FRC level of 50 ppm (50 mg/L) is necessary. However, if a hot water system is the source, an FRC level of ≥ 1 ppm at tap outlets running continuously would be required.[17]

made the cruise had gotten Legionnaires' disease and been reported, it is likely that the health department would have noted an increase and initiated a study.

The ill residents and other cruise patrons would then be interviewed to identify exposures among infected persons. In the case of the cruise ship, perhaps a link could be found with congregating in certain areas supplied with conditioned air or exposure to a common water source. Next, case-control or cross-sectional studies would be done to test hypotheses relating common exposures to disease. Laboratory studies (e.g., subtype matching) of patient isolates, water, and implicated devices (e.g., the cooling tower of the cruise ship) would then be done to establish an epidemiologic link between human disease and a specific source. Simply identifying legionellae from an aerosol-producing device does not necessarily implicate it as the source of disease, since the organisms are found in many aquatic environments. Finally, environmental studies may be conducted to determine whether the aerosols contain viable organisms in droplets of respirable size.

Once a source has been identified, it must be decontaminated. The procedures used depend on the type of device and establishment in which contamination is found. Contaminated cooling towers and evaporative condensers should be drained, mechanically cleaned with a dispersant (e.g., automatic dishwasher detergent), and hyperchlorinated.* For a contaminated water system, the entire system must be flushed with water that has been either superheated (>65° C, 150° F) or hyperchlorinated. Further, because scale or sediment in contaminated hot-water storage tanks, water heaters, faucets, and shower heads can harbor organisms and protect them from the biocidal effects of chlorine and heat, they must be drained and mechanically cleaned or replaced.

A routine maintenance program must follow the above principles to decrease the

SUMMARY TABLE 33. Legionnaires' disease: possible acquisition on a cruise ship

Host-environment model	Case presentation	Factors that influence infectious process	Prevention and control
Host factors	74-year-old man with chronic obstructive pulmonary disease, diabetes mellitus, and hypertension	Smoking, old age, male gender, immunosuppression, chronic cardiovascular or pulmonary conditions	Vaccine not available
Microbiologic factors	*Legionella pneumophila*	Inhalation of 1 CFU/50 L contaminated aerosol	Treat with erythromycin
Physical environment	Possible sources are contaminated aerosols from air-conditioning cooling tower or water system of the cruise ship	Warm recirculated water loaded with organic and inorganic material and microbes. Predominance of cases in summer and fall. Not person-to-person spread	Outbreak control: For cooling tower, drain, mechanically clean, and hyperchlorinate system. For water system, flush pipes and hyperchlorinate or superheat water. Maintenance: For cooling tower, clean regularly and use biocide; for water system, prevent stagnation and obstruction of water in pipes; maintain water temperatures above 50° C (122° F) or continuously infuse chlorine; alternatively, hyperchlorinate or superheat water intermittently
Social environment	Long history of smoking and drinking alcohol; possible exposure in air-conditioned areas or from contaminated water on the cruise ship	Lack of compliance with maintaining clean water in cooling tower	Develop and implement protocol for maintaining uncontaminated water in cooling towers, plumbing, etc. Monitor compliance

chance that *Legionella* will recontaminate the system. Regular cleaning and use of chlorine or other biocides is recommended for cooling tower maintenance. Constant free residual chlorine levels of 1 to 2 mg/L or a temperature of >50° C (122° F) at the tap may be adequate for water system maintenance. Alternatively, systems may be periodically hyperchlorinated or superheated. Unfortunately, corrosion of plumbing fixtures and the possibility of scalded skin are the main disadvantages of these approaches.

Surveillance for new cases should continue for 6 to 12 months after an outbreak to assess the success of intervention. Concurrently, the source should be monitored for the presence of *Legionella* and maintenance procedures altered if necessary.

There is no evidence to support routine bacteriologic culturing of man-made aquatic environments as a means of preventing outbreaks of legionellosis. Instead, biocide use and regular draining and cleaning of cooling towers and evaporative condensers has been recommended to keep legionellae from reaching high concentration levels. Two new methods—ultraviolet light and ozone—are being evaluated as alternatives to chlorine and heat. Another preventive approach would be vaccination of susceptible persons. To date, two preparations have been successfully tested in animals but not yet in humans. Since person-to-person transmission of Legionnaires' disease has not been reported, barrier precautions beyond normal asepsis and standard precautions in hospital or nursing home settings are not necessary.

SUMMARY

Legionnaires' disease most commonly affects older adults with underlying medical problems, especially those that contribute to immunosuppression or restricted cardiopulmonary function. The mode of transmission is inhalation by susceptible persons of aerosolized droplets containing viable *Legionella* bacteria. The incubation period ranges from 2 to 10 days, and clinical presentation is indistinguishable from those of other pneumonias. Attack rates are usually <5%, but mortality rates can be much higher (up to 30%).

Legionella are found in nearly all natural wet environments and in many man-made ones, notably water cooling towers and evaporative condensers of hospitals, hotels, and businesses. Water delivery systems in hospitals have also been implicated in outbreaks of legionellosis.

Prevention and control strategies are aimed at eliminating delivery of contaminated water to persons susceptible to infection and decreasing the number of viable organisms in the water. These include drainage, mechanical cleaning, and use of biocides (e.g., chlorine) or heat. Vaccines to the infection have been tested in animals but not yet in humans.

REFERENCES

1. Ampel NM, Wing EJ. *Legionella* infection in transplant patients. *Semin Respir Infect.* 1990;5:30-57.
2. Barbaree JM. Perspectives on the ecology and control of *Legionella*. In Tate CL. Jr., editor: *International Symposium on Water-Related Health Issues.* American Water Resources Association, Atlanta, 1986;51-55.
3. Benz-Lemoine E, et al. Nosocomial Legionnaires' disease in a bone marrow transplant unit. *Bone Marrow Transplant.* 1991;7:61-63.
4. Brady MT. Nosocomial Legionnaires' disease in a children's hospital. *J Pediatr.* 1989;115:46-50.
5. Breiman RF, et al. Association of shower use with Legionnaires' disease: possible role of amoebae. *JAMA.* 1990;263:2924-2926.
6. Centers for Disease Control and Prevention: Outbreak of pneumonia associated with a cruise ship, 1994, *MMWR* 43(28).
7. Dondero TJ, et al. An outbreak of Legionnaires' disease associated with a contaminated air-conditioning cooling tower. *N Engl J Med.* 1980;302:365-370.
8. Fraser DW, et al. Legionnaires' disease: description of an epidemic of pneumonia. *N Engl J Med.* 1977;297:1189-1197.
9. Garbe PL, et al. Nosocomial Legionnaires' disease: epidemiologic demonstration of cooling towers as a source. *JAMA.* 1985;254:521-524.
10. Johnson JT, Best MG, Goetz N. Nosocomial legionel-

losis in surgical patients with head and neck cancer: implications for epidemiological reservoir and mode of transmission. *Lancet.* 1985;2:298-300.

11. Kugler JW, et al. Nosocomial Legionnaires' disease: occurrence in recipients of bone marrow transplants. *Am J Med.* 1983;74:281-288.

12. Mahoney FJ, et al. Communitywide outbreak of Legionnaires' disease associated with a grocery store mist machine. *J Infect Dis.* 1992;165:736-739.

13. Matulonis U, Rosenfeld CS, Shadduck RK. Prevention of *Legionella* infections in a bone marrow transplant unit: multifaceted approach to decontamination of a water system. *Infect Control Hosp Epidemiol.* 1993; 14:571-575.

14. Memish ZA, et al. Plumbing system shock absorbers as a source of *Legionella pneumophila. Am J Infect Control.* 1992;20:305-309.

15. Muder RR, et al. Nosocomial Legionnaires' disease uncovered in a prospective pneumonia study: implications for underdiagnosis. *JAMA.* 1983;249:3184-3188.

16. Schwebke JR, Hackman R, Bowden R. Pneumonia due to *Legionella micdadei* in bone marrow transplant recipients. *Rev Infect Dis.* 1990;12:824-828.

17. Wisconsin Department of Health and Social Services. Control of *Legionella* in cooling towers: summary guidelines. Madison, WI: Wisconsin Division of Health; 1987.

SUGGESTED READINGS

Ampel NM, Wing EJ. Legionellosis in the compromised host. In Rubin RH, Young LS, eds. *Clinical Approach to Infection in the Compromised Host.* New York, NY: Plenum Medical Book Co.; 1988.

Breiman RF, Fraser DW. Legionellosis. In Maxcy KF, Rosenau MJ, Last JM, eds. *Public Health and Preventive Medicine,* 13th ed. East Norwalk, CT: Appleton & Lange; 1992.

Edelstein PH. The laboratory diagnosis of Legionnaires' disease. *Semin Respir Infect.* 1987;2:235-241.

Hoge CW, Breiman RF. Advances in the epidemiology and control of *Legionella* infections. *Epidemiol Rev.* 1991;13:329-339.

Rodgers FG, Pasculle W. *Legionella.* In Balows A, et al, eds. *Manual of Clinical Microbiology,* 5th ed. Washington, DC: American Society for Microbiology; 1991.

Centers for Disease Control and Prevention. "Draft guideline for prevention of nosocomial pneumonia," 59 *Federal Register* 22 (2 Feb 1994), 4980-5022.

Group B Streptococcal Disease in an Infant

LORRAINE M. HARKAVY

CLINICAL PRESENTATION

Darcelle Johnson, a married 19-year-old gravida 2, para 1 woman went to the hospital's labor and delivery unit at about 40 weeks gestation in early labor with membranes that had ruptured 6 hours before. Her prenatal care had been limited but she appeared to be in good health. Effacement and dilatation progressed smoothly, and 18 hours after her membranes ruptured, she delivered a 3290-g (7 lb, 4 oz) girl by spontaneous vaginal delivery under epidural anesthesia. The infant's Apgar scores were 8 and 9 at 1 and 5 minutes. At 15 minutes after birth, the delivery room nurse observed the infant having respiratory distress and a dusky color. She called the neonatologist to examine the baby.

The neonatologist observed retractions, grunting, cyanosis on oxygen, poor tone and movement, and poor skin perfusion. She estimated the neonate's gestational age to be 36 weeks. She obtained a cord arterial blood pH which was 7.16 (normal >7.25). A chest x-ray was ordered; the radiologist interpreted it as normal. A Gram stain of gastric contents revealed polymorphonuclear leukocytes and gram-positive cocci in pairs and chains. The baby's arterial blood gas showed the P_{CO_2} to be 67 (normal 31-47) and the P_{O_2} to be 50 (normal 42-58). The infant was too sick to have a lumbar puncture.

The infant was treated with mechanical ventilation plus oxygen. Penicillin and gentamicin were started after blood and tracheal cultures were obtained. By 8 hours, the baby required 100% inspired oxygen with peak end expiratory ventilator pressures of 43/5 cm of water, ventilation rates of 90 breaths per minute, muscle paralysis with pancuronium, and blood pressure support with dopamine. Treatment with extracorporeal membrane oxygenation was deferred because of intraventricular hemorrhage. The baby died at age 49 hours in spite of continued antimicrobial therapy, intravenous gamma globulin, and blood pressure support with dobutamine, and tolazoline. The mother was febrile postpartum and was treated with ampicillin and gentamicin. Admission blood cultures from the baby, reported after death, were positive for *Streptococcus agalactiae*, a species of group B streptococcus (GBS). Maternal cultures were not obtained.

HOST-ENVIRONMENT INTERACTION
The host

GBS disease is a major cause of neonatal morbidity and mortality worldwide. Indeed, GBS is the most common cause of neonatal sepsis in the United States, resulting in more than 2000 infant deaths annually.[14] Infant sepsis is associated with 20% to 30% mortality.[5]

In the neonate, GBS disease occurs as two distinct syndromes, classified as early onset (EOS) or late onset (LOS) disease. EOS, often acquired perinatally, is characterized by septicemia, pneumonia, and a low incidence of meningitis (about 5% to 10%). The major clinical manifestations are tachypnea, respiratory distress, cardiovascular instability (hypotension, poor perfusion, acidosis), and cyanosis persisting despite administration of oxygen. Radiographs are rarely diagnostic and may mimic that found in hyaline membrane disease, aspiration pneumonia, or mild wet lung with transient tachypnea.

LOS occurs most often after 1 week of age and sometimes as late as 5 months of age. It often attacks otherwise apparently healthy infants and manifests as meningitis more than 90% of the time. In addition to meningitis, GBS infections have been reported to include sepsis; pneumonia; cerebritis; conjunctivitis; disseminated intravascular coagulation; empyema; endocarditis; otitis media; skin, scalp, and soft tissue lesions; ventriculitis; osteomyelitis; lung abscess; ethmoiditis; and subdural effusion.

As with Ms. Johnson's baby, the prognosis of infants with GBS disease can be poor. EOS sepsis is associated with a mortality of 13% to 37%.[3] Absent a positive blood culture, mortality from clinical infection (positive tracheal aspirate or surface cultures) is below 5%. Half of the survivors of septic shock may develop periventricular leukomalacia (necrosis of white matter) of the brain. Among the 5% to 10% who develop meningitis, about one-fifth exhibit major neurologic morbidity, such as mental retardation, uncontrolled seizures, blindness, abnormal head size, quadriparesis, diabetes insipidus, or mild mental retardation. Another fifth develop less incapacitating sequelae, including unilateral deafness, borderline retardation, monoparesis, controlled seizures, and language delay. The likelihood of detecting neurologic deficit increases with the child's age at follow-up.

Endogenous risk factors in infant and mother for this disease include prematurity, prolonged rupture of the membranes, chorioamnionitis (often unrecognized), and heavy maternal colonization with GBS at the time of delivery. The latter may be manifest as multiple colonized anatomic sites of the mother, persistence of maternal colonization throughout pregnancy, and heavy or rapid growth on maternal cultures. Many cases of GBS disease occur in term or near-term infants with membranes ruptured for less than 24 hours. Katz and Bowes[10] maintain that as many as 50% of infections occur despite intact fetal membranes at the time of presentation. The exact mechanism of transmission of GBS from mother to infant has not been determined. The GBS may reach the fetus through hematogenous spread, through direct penetration of the amniotic membranes, ascension of the organism through the open cervix, or in the birth canal.

Invasive infection in the infant appears to be related to several immunologic deficiencies. Maternal antibodies to GBS of all types cross the placenta, and the level of maternal antibodies correlates with the outcome. Mothers with culture-negative or colonized babies have significantly higher titers than do mothers of infected babies.[1] Unfortunately, only 15% to 40% of women have detectable antibodies, and only 12% have levels considered protective.[5]

Deficiencies in the complement system, decreased mobility of polymorphonuclear cells (PMNs), decreased ingestion of bacteria by PMNs, and early and rapid depletion of PMNs after invasion of mucous membranes by GBS may play a role in infants' susceptibility to GBS. Prevalence of GBS colonization is so highly variable that intervention strategies should not be based on demographics alone. This variation may reflect the inconsistent sensitivity of the methods of detecting colonization as much as true variation in colonization. Carriage in the same woman may be detected at some times but not others. For example, serial cultures in pregnant women have identified an overall 19% prevalence of colonization during pregnancy, but only half are positive in all three trimesters.[11] Prevalence of colonization is the same (about 8%) in each trimester. Antibiotics can only temporarily eliminate colonization, since the woman's vagina may be recolonized from her intestinal tract or her sexual partner. The mother is rarely ill from GBS before delivery, although GBS can cause asymptomatic bacteriuria or urinary tract infections. She may develop chorioamnionitis, especially after premature or prolonged rupture of the membranes. Emptying the uterus is often curative. Cesarean delivery increases the risk of uterine infection, which manifests as endometritis, by providing devitalized tissue as nutrient for the bacteria.

The microbiologic environment

Streptococci are identified using Lancefield groups. There are over a dozen groups (A-V). Group B is represented by *Streptococcus agalactiae,* which belongs to the family *Streptococcaceae* and the genus *Streptococcus.* This organism can grow under aerobic and anaerobic conditions (facultative) and is found in the genitourinary and gastrointestinal tracts of humans. GBS is a gram-positive diplococcus that can grow on a variety of growth media. Some media containing antibiotics can enhance detection of GBS by limiting growth of other organisms. GBS sometimes causes β-hemolysis of red blood cells.

The five major types of GBS associated with perinatal infections are categorized by other cell wall carbohydrates (S substance) and the presence or absence of a protein. The serotype designations are types Ia, Ib, Ic, II, and III. Although neonatal infections have been caused by all serotypes of GBS, group III is the most common in both maternal carriers and septic infants, especially those with meningitis.

The physical environment

The physical environment played a relatively minor role in the transmission of GBS in Ms. Johnson's case since the infection was transmitted from Ms. Johnson to her baby. Organisms producing EOS disease are usually acquired from the mother during labor or delivery. Multiple vaginal examinations during labor and transvaginal intrauterine electrodes or catheters can increase the incidence of congenital sepsis, including that due to GBS. Our understanding of the epidemiology of LOS disease is very limited. Only half of the infants who develop LOS disease have a mother with the same GBS. The source of infection in the other 50% is unknown.

While not significant in this case, the hospital environment can be a source of GBS. Clusters and outbreaks have occurred in nurseries.[5] Environmental factors that appear to play a role in transmission of organisms include the placement of newborns in large open wards with no barriers between babies, overcrowding resulting in close contact of susceptible hosts, and understaffing that may result in uneven application of important infection control measures such as hand washing and barrier precautions. Outbreaks of GBS disease linked to an infected caretaker have not been described; however, LOS disease does occur in chronically hospitalized newborns even without a history of GBS colonization. Presumably, the infants acquired the organism from an adult's hands.[1]

The social environment

An infant's risk of GBS infection has been associated with the social environment of the mother. Age, parity, socioeconomic status, geographic location, and ethnic origin all have been associated with colonization of pregnant women. The prevalence of GBS is greatest in women who are in their teens, are sexually active, and use intrauterine contraceptive devices. GBS colonization is also greatest during the first half of the menstrual cycle.[2] African-Americans and Hispanics of Caribbean origin may also have a higher prevalence independent of age, sexual activity and contraception.[6] Women who have had fewer than three pregnancies, are of low socioeconomic status, and have a high frequency of sexual intercourse with more sexual partners are more likely to be carriers.

Pregnancy and marital status have no independent effect on GBS colonization rates.

PREVENTION AND CONTROL

Chemoprophylaxis has been very effective in preventing both maternal endometritis and neonatal infection. The preferred approach is to identify women who are carriers of GBS and administer a penicillin (usually ampicillin) during labor and delivery.[8] GBS may be identified during pregnancy on cervical or vaginal cultures if appropriate media are used. Combined rectal and cervical swabs may identify twice as many carriers of GBS.[4] The timing of cultures for optimal benefit to the baby is unknown, but culture early in the third trimester and when needed intrapartum has been found to reduce neonatal infection when followed by antimicrobial therapy. Failure to eliminate all neonatal infection was a consequence of deliveries before 32 weeks, failure to use intrapartum prophylaxis, or maternal sepsis at hospital admission. Hospitalized women at high risk, for example those with premature rupture of membranes or in preterm labor, may be screened with one of several rapid assays for GBS antigen. The sensitivity for GBS detection of these methods ranges from 4% to 88%.[15] Heavy colonization is detected in 63% to 100% of cases. Delivery by cesarean section increases the need for chemoprophylaxis to prevent endometritis.

A review and analysis of 19 different screening and treatment strategies for the management of group B streptococcus in obstetrics suggested that the greatest cost-benefit would be obtained by universal treatment, treatment based on risk factors, treatment based on preterm delivery, or 36 week culture status.[13]

Management of the infants born to mothers who have had prophylaxis remains controversial. Asymptomatic or not, the infant may be placed in a special nursery room and observed or be treated with antibiotics (a penicillin and an aminoglycoside) until cultures are normal. Symptomatic infants are usually presumed infected and treated.

High maternal antibody titers may protect the infant against GBS disease, since these antibodies cross the placenta. However, only 12% to 20% of women are immune.[5] The vast majority of mothers of infected infants lack levels of antibody considered protective. Vaccines against GBS are being developed. A type III polysaccharide vaccine administered to women 24 to 37 weeks pregnant induced a significant rise in antibody level in about two-thirds of the women.[4] Administration of intravenous immune globulin to the preterm newborn as prophylaxis against nosocomial infection of any type has no proven value. Even with high natural or induced maternal antibody titers, newborns can be infected during preterm delivery as a consequence of inadequate transfer of antibodies across the placenta or exposure to a large inoculum of bacteria.

Appropriate and accepted infection control measures, though not specific to the control of GBS, minimize transmission of GBS in the nursery.[9] These measures include scrupulous hand washing, rapid identification of infections that require additional precautions such as cohorting or nursery closure, and interventions to reduce the risk of infection and colonization of the infant. The latter includes triple-dye cord care, which can reduce colonization of the umbilical cord. Bathing the stabilized infant is appropriate. All maternal secretions should be cleansed from the infant using soap, water, and sponges. The infant's routine care should include cleaning of the perineum and buttocks in the same manner. Caregivers should wear gloves during the initial bath.

Rooming-in of well infants with their mothers and segregation of infected patients reduce exposure of infants to GBS and may minimize risk of cross-contamination by staff. Cohorting of infants and staff has been used to contain

SUMMARY TABLE 25. **Group B streptococcal disease in an infant**

Host-environment model	Case presentation	Factors that influence infectious process	Prevention and control
Host factors	Term newborn infant	Large inoculum Immature immune system	Maternal vaccine under development Obtain prenatal GBS culture to identify colonized mothers
Microbiologic factors	Group B streptococcus *Streptococcus agalactiae*	In utero and intrapartum contact Approximately 30% of women colonized prenatally Less commonly acquired in nursery or home	Use antimicrobial prophylaxis for colonized mother and/or infant
Physical environment	Delivery Nursery	Intimate contact with bacterium Internal monitoring devices	Eliminate bacterium from birth canal Practice scrupulous handwashing
Social environment	Mother presented in advanced labor without prenatal care	Infection established when presenting for care	Provide universal access to care Educate about preterm labor and premature rupture of membranes Counsel about future pregnancies

outbreaks, however, a recent report challenges the usefulness of cohorting.[7]

Patient management strategies for GBS should be outlined in nursery policies and should specify appropriate precautions including identification of susceptible hosts, discharge of patients if possible to minimize the population of susceptible hosts, and use of antimicrobial prophylaxis.

Up to 20% of culture-negative babies are colonized after admission to the nursery, presumably via unwashed hands.[12] Thus, handwashing and use of gloves may be critical to preventing transmission of GBS.

Supportive care and antibiotics are the primary treatment of GBS infection. Penicillin is the drug of choice for the infant.[1] Synergism of combined penicillin and aminoglycoside therapy can overcome the few (about 5%) strains of penicillin-tolerant GBS reported. Mechanical ventilation and cardiotropic agents (such as dobutamine and dopamine) may be required for support.

The antimicrobial of choice for the mother who develops GBS endometritis is penicillin, although broad-spectrum cephalosporins are often used until culture and sensitivity reports are available. Antibiotic therapy of the symptomatic mother may be changed from intravenous to oral after the symptoms subside.

Neonatal prophylaxis with a single dose of IM penicillin can significantly reduce the incidence of EOS GBS infection in healthy term newborns whose mothers are GBS carriers. Though universal prophylaxis without maternal screening is less expensive, it does not prevent disease acquired in utero or by preterm infants. Despite its apparent effectiveness, penicillin prophylaxis is not universally practiced.

SUMMARY

S. agalactiae was recognized as a cause of maternal and perinatal infection half a century ago. The incidence rose dramatically in the early 1970s. Since then there has been a fairly constant incidence of streptococcal sepsis in infants in the range of 2 to 4 per 1,000 live births. GBS is a common cause of chorioamnionitis and endometritis as well.

GBS causes both acute and chronic disease. EOS disease, which often results in sepsis, kills up to 30% of the babies affected. LOS disease may result in long-term sequelae requiring continuing medical care.

Disease is most often the result of infection from the mother's organisms. Because maternal colonization is usually silent, delivery may occur prematurely or the mother may be infected when admitted to the hospital. Prevention of neonatal infection is not always possible; therefore, newer interventions are under evaluation, including vaccines against GBS to be used during pregnancy and prophylactic antimicrobial therapy of the newborn.

When neonatal infection does occur, attention to hand washing, barrier techniques and other appropriate infection control measures appears to reduce the risk nosocomial transmission of GBS.

REFERENCES

1. Baker CJ, Kasper DL. Correlation of maternal antibody deficiency with susceptibility to neonatal group B streptococcal infection. *N Engl J Med.* 1976;294:753-756.

2. Baker CJ, Goroff DK, Alper S, et al. Vaginal colonization with group B streptococcus: a study in college women. *J Infec Dis.* 1977;135:392-397.
3. Baker CJ. Group B streptococcal infection in neonates. *Pediatr Rev.* 1979;1(1):5-15.
4. Baker CJ, Rench MA, Edwards MS, Carpenter RJ, et al. Immunization of pregnant women with a polysaccharide vaccine group B streptococcus. *N Engl J Med.* 1988; 319(18):1180-1185.
5. Baker CJ, Edwards MS. Streptococcal infections. In Remington JS, Klein JO, eds. *Infectious Diseases of the Fetus and Newborn Infant.* Philadelphia, PA: W.B. Saunders; 1990.
6. Committee on Infectious Diseases and Committee of Fetus and Newborn. Guidelines for prevention of group B streptococcal infection by chemoprophylaxis. *Pediatrics.* 1992;90(5):775-778.
7. Ehrenkranz NJ, Sanders CC, Eckert-Schollenberger D, Hufcut RM, et al. Lack of evidence of efficacy of co-horting nursing personnel in a neonatal intensive care unit to prevent contact spread of bacteria: an experimental study. *Pediatr Infect Dis J.* 1992;11(2):105-113.
8. Gotoff SP, Boyer KM. Prevention of group B streptococcal early onset sepsis. *Pediatr Infect Dis J.* 1989; 8(5):268-270.
9. Harkavy KL. Neonatal/infant care units. In Berg R, ed. *The APIC Curriculum for Infection Control Practice.* Dubuque, Iowa: Kendal Hunt 1988:3.
10. Katz V, Bowes WA. Perinatal group B streptococcal infections across intact amniotic membranes. *J Reprod Med.* 1988;33(5):445-449.
11. Lewin EB, Amstey MS. Natural history of group B streptococcus colonization and its therapy during pregnancy. *Am J Obstet Gynecol.* 1981;139:512.
12. Paredes A, Wong P, Mason EO, et al. Nosocomial transmission of group B streptococci in a newborn nursery. *Pediatrics.* 1977;59(5):679-682.
13. Rouse DJ, Goldenberg RL, Cliver SP, et al. Strategies for the prevention of early-onset neonatal group B streptococcal sepsis: A decision analysis. Obstetrics & Gynecology April, 1994, 83(4), 483-494.
14. Strickland DM, Yeomans ER, Hankins GDV. Cost-effectiveness of intrapartum screening and treatment for maternal group B streptococci colonization. *Am J Obstet Gynecol.* 1990;163:4-8.
15. Yancey MK, Armer T, Clark P, Duff P. Assessment of rapid identification tests for genital carriage of group B streptococci. *Obstet Gynecol.* 1992;80(6):1038-1047.

SUGGESTED READINGS

Apgar BS, Green LA. Preventing group B streptococcal sepsis in the newborn. *Am Fam Physician.* 1994; 49(2):315-318.

Coleman RT, Scherer DM, Maniscalo WM. Prevention of neonatal group B streptococcal infections: advances in maternal vaccine development. *Obstet Gynecol.* 1992; 80:301-309.

Dillon HC, Khare S, Gray BM. Group B streptococcal carriage and disease: A 6-year prospective study. *J Pediatr.* 1987 110(1):31-36.

Edwards MS, et al. Long-term sequelae of group B streptococcal meningitis in infants. *J Pediatr.* 1985; 106(5):717-722.

Gibbs RS, et al. Consensus: Perinatal prophylaxis for group B streptococcal infection. *Pediatr Infect Dis J.* 1992;11(3):179-183.

Klein JO, Marcy SM, Bacterial infections. In Remington JS, Klein JO, eds. *Infectious Diseases of the Fetus and Newborn Infant.* Philadelphia, PA: W.B. Saunders; 1990.

Platt WM, Gilson KGJ. Group B streptococcal disease in the perinatal period. *Am Fam Physician.* 1994;49(2): 434-442.

Pyati SP, Pildes, MD, Jacobs NM, et al. Penicillin in infants weighing 2 kg or less with early-onset group B streptococcal disease. *N Engl J Med.* 1983;308(23):1383-1389.

Weisman LE, Stoll BJ, Cruss DF, et al. Early-onset group B streptococcal sepsis: a current assessment. *J Pediatr.* 1992;121:428-433.

Schoolteacher with Malaria

MARTHA LONG

CLINICAL PRESENTATION

Melissa Rivers is a 36-year-old schoolteacher who lives in Seattle. She enjoys traveling to exotic places on her summer vacations and recently took a 3-week trip to Kenya, where she planned to see Nairobi and Mombasa and go on safari to the game parks. Unexpectedly, 2 days after she arrived, she was invited to visit one of the rural villages located on a small lake. She stayed there for 3 days and then continued the rest of her trip.

Ms. Rivers had been given mefloquine to take prophylactically to prevent malaria, but she had forgotten to start it until the day before the trip. She had also taken other prophylactic medications, including vaccine for yellow fever and immune globulin to prevent hepatitis A. In Seattle she returned to school right away, was very busy, and did not continue to take the mefloquine for the additional 4 weeks recommended after leaving an area endemic for malaria.

Approximately 2 weeks after her trip, Ms. Rivers developed fever, chills, myalgia, headaches, and fatigue. She had no other symptoms, such as chest or abdominal pain or arthralgia, and no history of any underlying disease or allergies. Thinking she was still tired from her trip and had acquired a viral illness, Ms. Rivers self-medicated with acetaminophen for 5 days and continued to work. When her chills and fever did not subside, she sought medical treatment.

Initially, her physician also thought Ms. Rivers had a severe viral infection. She was lethargic and dehydrated. It was only when she described the persistent, periodic shaking chills occurring at approximately 48-hour intervals that the physician suspected another cause for the illness and began a systematic work-up. As part of the history, he asked Ms. Rivers about her activities during the past month. She described her trip to Africa. The physician inquired about food and water intake, daily activities, and mosquitoes. Ms. Rivers said she had been very careful about eating only cooked food and bottled or treated water and had not gone swimming, but that during her stay in the rural village, she was practically "eaten alive" by the mosquitoes. The physician considered malaria a possibility, since her symptoms were consistent with the illness and she had recently been to an endemic area. He ordered a series of blood tests, requesting that the laboratory technologist perform a manual (not automated) differential white blood count as part of a routine complete blood count (CBC), including a smear to look for malarial organisms. The smear was positive for *Plasmodium falciparum*, and Ms. Rivers was diagnosed with malaria. She was treated with oral quinine and tetracycline for 7 days. After treatment, Ms. Rivers made a full recovery.

HOST-ENVIRONMENT INTERACTION
The host

Malaria is one of the most important infectious diseases in the world. Its effect on the social and economic development of many societies is significant. It is estimated that approximately 100 million cases occur annually in Africa alone, with 1 million deaths attributable to malaria each year.[7] Susceptibility is universal. Adults from highly endemic areas such as Africa may exhibit tolerance because of continual exposure to the infectious agent occurring over many years. One species of malaria, *P. vivax*, rarely affects black Africans, theoretically because the *P. vivax*-specific receptors are not present on the erythrocyte. Another species, *P. falciparum*, achieves only low blood levels in persons with sickle cell trait. Most deaths in the world are from *P. falciparum.*[7]

Malaria infection usually presents with high fever, chills, and rigors. The initial stage of malaria is easily mistaken for a viral illness and may produce nonspecific symptoms such as headaches, myalgia, fatigue, and malaise several days before onset of the high fever, chills, and rigor. Some individuals complain of localized symptoms, such as abdominal pain, chest pain, and arthralgia. Malaria is well known for imitating other diseases, which frequently results in delayed diagnosis. The typical paroxysm of malaria is a violent rigor that lasts for a few minutes to an hour and is followed by a rapidly rising fever that approaches 40° to 41.1° C (104° to 106° F), usually lasting 3 to 8 hours.[5]

There is no vaccine to prevent malaria, but work to develop one has recently been promising.

The microbiologic environment

Malaria is an obligate intracellular protozoan in the genus *Plasmodium*. There are four species: *P. falciparum, P. vivax, P. malariae,* and *P. ovale*. Infection with *P. falciparum* is the most common. In endemic areas, infection with one or more species may occur.

Humans and mosquitoes are the only important reservoirs of *Plasmodium*. In fact, the mosquito is the definitive host and the human the intermediate host. The female *Anopheles*

mosquito is the vector responsible for almost all transmission to humans. After a mosquito feeds on a human already infected with the protozoan and whose blood contains the sexual stages of the parasite (gametocytes), a complicated sequence of events takes place. Within the mosquito, male and female gametes unite, forming a cyst in which thousands of sporozoites develop. The sporozoites mature, and those that reach the salivary glands may be injected into and infect a human when the mosquito takes a blood meal, typically at dusk or early evening. Once infected, the mosquito remains infected and able to transmit the disease.

After inoculation into the human, the sporozoites rapidly enter the liver hepatocytes. There they develop into exoerythrocytic or hepatic schizonts which rupture, releasing thousands of merozoites that invade erythrocytes. The infected erythrocyte evolves into an erythrocytic schizont. The schizont ruptures, releasing merozoites that invade more erythrocytes. Some of these develop into gametocytes that infect mosquitoes; others of the erythrocytes repeat the cycle by developing into erythrocytic schizonts (Figure B).

The cycle of amplification, rupture, and reinvasion leads to ever-increasing levels of the parasite in the bloodstream and produces the pathologic and clinical manifestations of malaria. No clinical manifestations appear until 10 to 14 days after the bite of an infected mosquito, when the first infected erythrocytes rupture.

In addition to transmission by the mosquito, malaria may rarely be transmitted by transfusion of merozoite containing blood or blood products, through sharing of contaminated needles, or transplacentally.

Diagnosis is established by demonstration of the parasite in the red blood cell. Species identification is based on the appearance of infected erythrocytes and the morphology of the erythrocytic and extraerythrocytic for MS in blood smears. Several microscopic evalua-

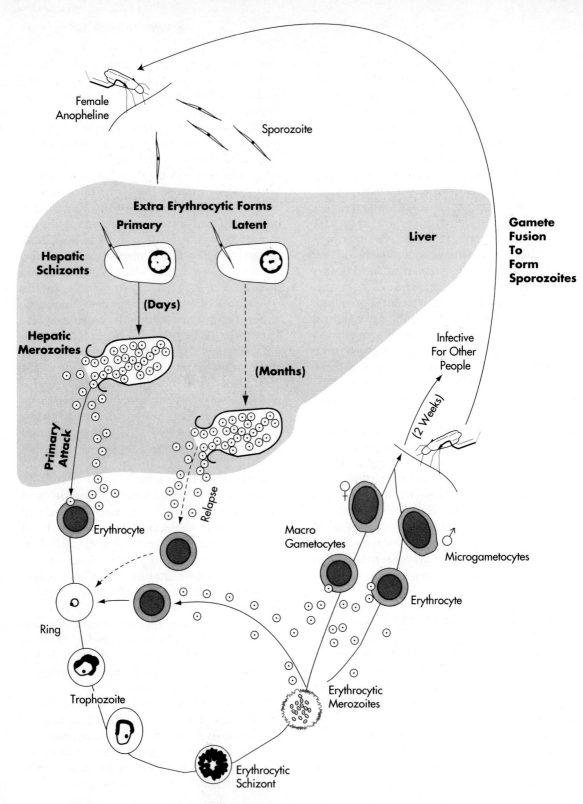

FIGURE 35-1. The life cycle of plasmadia in humans. Adapted from Wyler D: *Plasmodium* Species. In Mandell GL, Douglas RG, Bennett, JE, eds. *Principles and Practice of Infectious Diseases*, 3rd ed. New York, NY: John Wiley & Sons; 1990:2057.

tions may be necessary, since levels of parasitemia vary as the life cycle of the agent progresses or as a consequence of treatment. It is important to identify the infecting species because treatment is species specific. *P. falciparum* produces greater morbidity and mortality. *P. vivax* and *P. ovale* produce the risk of relapse of the disease because of delayed maturity within the liver.

The physical environment

Several environmental factors are associated with transmission of malaria. The vector of malaria is the *Anopheles* mosquito. There are approximately 60 species of this insect throughout the world. The disease is usually associated with travel to or living in the tropics and subtropics. In Ms. Rivers's case, the exposure during her African trip was the source of her infection.

In the United States, malaria was once transmitted in many geographic areas. Although malaria was eradicated from the United States during the 1950s,[7] the *Anopheles* mosquito persists. About 1,200 cases of malaria are reported in the U.S. annually.[4] Cases reported in the United States are primarily in individuals who acquired the disease in endemic areas, such as those entering the country for the first time (e.g., migrant workers) and those who have traveled to high-prevalence areas. A very small number of cases in the United States are the result of direct transmission involving an indigenous mosquito.[4] Transmission in the United States has also occurred through blood transfusions from infected individuals.[6]

The largest U.S. outbreak since 1952 involved 30 people in San Diego County in 1988.[1] Recent cases reported from Florida and southern California have been associated with infected migrant workers.[2] Factors in the physical environment that affect transmission of malaria are standing water and open sewers, which are sites of mosquito breeding. These conditions are found in all parts of the world. In areas of California and Florida where outbreaks occurred, sanitary facilities and housing were substandard.[4]

The actual amount of time spent outside does not seem to be associated with risk in tropical and subtropical climates if unscreened doors and windows are opened to aid air circulation. Proximity to a heavily infested area, such as a lake, increases the chance of infection.

Seasonal factors influence the occasional transmission in the United States. People tend to spend more time outside in mosquito-infested areas in warm weather. In the tropics and subtropics, where warm weather is the norm, no seasonal factors affect transmission.

The social environment

Economic development has made funds for control efforts available in many tropical countries and resulted in decreased incidence of malaria. Unfortunately, malaria remains prevalent in areas with less socioeconomic development. Since its eradication from the United States in the 1950s, cases of imported malaria have coincided with military activity in endemic regions such as the Pacific region in World War II and Vietnam.[6] More frequent travel of Americans to endemic areas and of persons from endemic areas to the United States has increased disease incidence in U.S. inhabitants. Transmission by mosquito can occur from persons from endemic areas to persons who have never traveled to an endemic area. Transmission may be aided when those infected have limited access to medical care, which provides an ongoing, undiagnosed source of mosquito infection, or when living conditions include proximity to standing water sources of mosquitoes.

U.S. citizens who travel to endemic areas and contract malaria often do so because of prophylaxis failure which is the consequence of administration of an ineffective drug, or noncompliance with the prophylactic regimen.

SUMMARY TABLE 35.   Schoolteacher with malaria

Host-environment model	Case presentation	Factors that influence infectious process	Prevention and control
Host factors	36-year-old healthy woman	No reliable immunity	No vaccine Provide prophylactic antimalarial medications
Microbiologic factors	*Plasmodium falciparum*	Bite by mosquito carrying organism Many antigenic forms	
Physical environment	Bite from infected *Anopheles* mosquito	Standing water Lack of proper clothing/insecticide	Eliminate standing water; eliminate mosquitoes and their larvae Wear protective clothing; use insecticide Use screens or mosquito nets
Social environment	Travel to endemic area of world	Limited access to medical care No organized mosquito abatement program	Increase access to medical care Improve organized mosquito abatement Educate traveler to take chemoprophylaxis at appropriate time

PREVENTION AND CONTROL

Prevention and control strategies are aimed at decreasing exposure to the *Anopheles* mosquito. Removal of standing water and open sewers eliminates breeding grounds for mosquitoes. When water cannot be removed, mosquito larvae may be eliminated through the use of larvicides and/or larvivorous fish.

In endemic areas, living quarters should be well screened and mosquito nets used between dusk and dawn. It may be useful to spray living and sleeping areas nightly with an insecticide containing pyrethrum.

Persons who travel to endemic areas should be instructed to cover their arms and legs with clothing when going out in the evening. Insect repellent that contains DEET (diethyltoluamide) should be applied to exposed skin surfaces.

Chemoprophylaxis is recommended for travelers to endemic areas, including children and pregnant women, who expect exposure to mosquitoes. The specific chemoprophylaxis used depends on the area of travel because resistance of *Plasmodium* to some prophylactic agents has been reported in many areas of the world. Travelers should be instructed to begin the medication 1 week before arriving in the endemic or high-risk area and continue chemoprophylaxis for at least 4 to 5 weeks after leaving the endemic area even if they feel well.

Prevention of transfusion-associated malaria requires proper screening of blood donors. Asymptomatic persons who have traveled to an endemic area but received no antimalarial drugs may donate blood 6 months after their return. Asymptomatic persons who have taken chemoprophylaxis, have had the disease, have immigrated, or are visiting from endemic areas may donate blood 3 years after the drugs are discontinued or after departure from the endemic area.[3,6]

Prevention of congenital malaria requires careful education and chemoprophylaxis of pregnant travelers to endemic areas. Although chemoprophylaxis is not contraindicated in pregnant women, they should consider the need for travel to such areas.

Injection drug abuse–associated malaria may be prevented by programs aimed at eliminating drug use.

Ms. Rivers took appropriate medications and used good sense in taking some precautions when she was in an area where malaria was endemic. However, she failed to follow the anti-malarial prophylaxis regimen prescribed for her. Fortunately, she recovered fully.

SUMMARY

Malaria is a disease of importance worldwide. Persons at risk of the disease are primarily travelers to and inhabitants of endemic areas. The mode of transmission is through the bite of an infected *Anopheles* mosquito. The incubation period is usually 12 to 14 days or longer. Factors associated with disease transmission include outdoor activity during the evening hours in endemic areas and inadequate skin protection.

Prevention and control strategies are aimed at decreasing the mosquito population and at the education of travelers regarding proper chemoprophylaxis and clothing to be worn outdoors during the evening hours.

REFERENCES

1. Centers for Disease Control: Transmission of *Plasmodium vivax* malaria, San Diego County, California, 1988 and 1989. *MMWR.* 1990;39:91-94.
2. Centers for Disease Control: Mosquito-transmitted malaria—California and Florida, 1990. *MMWR.* 1991; 40:106-108.
3. Johnson LW. Preventive therapy for malaria. *Am Fam Physician.* 1991;44:471-478.
4. Lederberg J, Shope RE, Oaks Jr SC, eds. *Emerging Infections: Microbial Threats to Health in the United States.* Washington, DC: Institute of Medicine, National Academy Press, 1992;29.
5. Shulman ST, Phair JP, Sommers HM eds. *The Biologic and Clinical Basis of Infectious Disease.* Philadelphia, PA: W. B. Saunders, 1992.
6. Wyler, D: *Plasmodium* species. In Mandell GL, Douglas RG, Bennett, JE, eds. *Principles and Practice of Infectious Diseases,* 3rd ed. New York, NY: John Wiley & Sons; 1990.
7. Zucker JR, Campbell CC. Malaria: principles of prevention and treatment. *Infect Dis Clin North Am.* 1993; 7(3):547-567.

SUGGESTED READINGS

Centers for Disease Control and Prevention: Recommendations for the prevention of malaria among travelers. *MMWR.* 1990;39:1-10.

Chin W, Coatney GR. Parasitic infections: malaria (Part 3). In Last JM, ed. *Public Health and Preventive Medicine.* New York, NY: Appleton-Century-Crofts; 1980.

Hoffman SL. Diagnosis, treatment and prevention of Malaria. *Med Clin North Am.* 1992;76:1327-1355.

Wiest PM, Opal SM, Romulo RL, Olds GR. Malaria in travelers in Rhode Island: a review of 26 cases. *Am J Med.* 1991;91:30-35.

Winters RA, Murray HW. Malaria—the mime revisited: fifteen more years of experience at New York City Teaching Hospital. *Am J Med.* 1992;93:243-246.

Selected Organizations With Guidelines for Infection Prevention and Control

American Association of Critical Care Nurses
101 Columbia
Aliso Viejo, CA 92656
714-362-2400

American Association of Occupational Health Nurses
50 Lenox Pointe
Atlanta, GA 30324
404-262-1162

American College of Nurse Midwives
1522 K St. NW, Suite 1000
Washington DC 20005
202-289-0171

American Nephrology Nurses Association
North Woodbury Rd., Box 56
Pitman, NJ 08071
609-589-2187

American Society for Microbiology
1325 Massachusetts Ave NW
Washington DC 20005-4171
202-737-3600

Association of Operating Room Nurses
10170 East Mississippi Ave.
Denver, CO 80231
303-755-6300

Association for Professionals in Infection Control and Epidemiology
1016 16th St. NW
Washington DC 20036
202-296-2742
(Note: In addition to their own guidelines, APIC has published a Resource List for Standards and Guidelines, 1993, which lists guidelines from numerous other agencies)

Centers for Disease Control and Prevention
Hospital Infections Program
1600 Clifton Rd.
Atlanta, GA 30333
404-639-1550

Intravenous Nurses Society
Two Brighton St.
Belmont, MA 02178
617-489-5205

Joint Commission on the Accreditation of Healthcare Organizations
One Renaissance Blvd.
Oakbrook, IL 60181
708-916-5600

Occupational Health and Safety Administration
Department of Labor
200 Constitution Ave. NW
Washington DC 20210
202-513-7075

Oncology Nursing Society
501 Holiday Rd.
Pittsburgh, PA 15220
412-921-7373

Society for Hospital Epidemiology of America
875 Kings Highway, Suite 200
West Deptford, NJ 08096
609-853-0411

US Environmental Protection Agency
Office of Solid Waste
401 M St. SW
Washington DC 20460
800-858-7377

US Food and Drug Administration
Centers for Devices and Radiological Health
8757 Georgia Ave.
Silver Spring, MD 29010

Glossary

This is a list of selected terms frequently encountered in discussions of infections and their control. It should be used as a supplement to a medical dictionary and clinical and microbiology texts.

---

acid-fast bacilli (AFB) bacteria, including mycobacteria, that are not de-colorized by acid-alcohol after staining with specific dye

acute sera sera obtained during the acute phase of an illness. "Paired sera" consist of one specimen obtained during the acute phase of infection and one obtained during the convalescent phase, by which time antibody to a causal microorganism would have developed. Presence of microorganism-specific antibodies in the convalescent sera which are absent in the acute sera suggests the microorganism was the etiologic agent of disease

agar dried mucilaginous derivative of seaweed that is used as the solidifying agent in bacteriological culture media because it resists decomposition by bacterial enzymes

airborne suspended on air currents. See "droplet nuclei"

allergy acquired hypersensitivity to a substance that results in the release of histamine and manifests as eczema, hives, hayfever, asthma, or other pathological manifestation of immune response

anamnestic response rapid immune response including antibody titer rise following repeat exposure to an antigen. Occasionally referred to as secondary immune response

anaphylaxis immediate, transient, sometimes severe, allergic reaction characterized by contraction of smooth muscle and dilation of capillaries. Involves IgE antibodies, mast cells, and basophils

antibiotic antimicrobial derived from mold or bacteria that inhibits growth of other organisms

antibody a protein usually developed in response to an antigen which facilitates the inactivation or disposal of the substance or microorganism carrying the antigen

antigen a substance recognized by the body as "foreign" that induces the immune response

antigenic drift minor mutations resulting in alteration of the antigens of a virus. Typical of influenzae

antigenic shift major alteration in the antigenic composition of a viral strain

antimicrobial chemical compound that destroys or prevents development of microorganisms

antisepsis prevention of infection by eliminating or preventing growth of infectious microorganisms

antiseptic chemical compound applied to skin or tissue to prevent growth of infectious microorganisms

asepsis a condition free from potentially pathogenic microorganisms

aseptic technique methods used during patient care, including surgery, to prevent microbial contamination. Sterile technique

autoantibody antibody occurring in response to antigenic components of the host's own tissues

auxotyping diagnostic tests that distinguish strains of bacteria (e.g., *Neisseria gonorrhoea*) according to their requirements for specific substances

Bacillus stearothermophilus a spore-forming bacterium that is highly resistant to heat and used to confirm the appropriate function of steam sterilizers

Bacillus subtilis a spore-forming bacterium that is used to confirm the appropriate function of ethylene oxide and dry heat sterilizers

bacteremia bacteria in the blood

bacteriocins heterogeneous group of substances produced by select bacteria that have a lethal effect on other bacteria

bacteriophage typing the subspecies classification of bacteria according to their susceptibility to infection by viruses which do not uniformly infect all strains of the species

bacteriocidal capable of destroying bacteria

bacteriostatic capable of inhibiting growth and reproduction of bacteria but not causing their destruction

basophil a granular leukocyte with an irregularly shaped nucleus and cytoplasm that contains coarse granules which stain blue with basic dyes

beta-lactamase an enzyme produced by some bacteria that splits the beta-lactam ring of penicillin and other beta-lactam compounds, destroying their antibacterial activity

binary fission asexual reproduction in which the cell divides into two identical daughter cells

bioavailability the rate and extent to which a drug or metabolite enters the circulation and reaches the site of action

biological indicator encapsulated live spores used to monitor sterilization (e.g., *B. stearothermophilus* for steam sterilizers, *B. subtilis* for ethylene oxide sterilizers)

biotyping characterization of microorganisms according to their physiologic characteristics

body substance isolation (BSI) system of infection precautions intended to prevent bidirectional transmission of microorganisms among patients and caregivers based on the premise that blood, body fluids, non-intact skin, and mucous membranes of every patient may contain infectious microorganisms or are susceptible to the introduction of microorganisms

capsule an outer covering of variable composition of some bacteria that can confer increased resistance to environmental degrada-

tion such as that imposed by a host's immune response

cell culture growth of cells in the laboratory for experimental or diagnostic purposes

chemical indicator chemical agent that indicates, usually by color change, presence of conditions necessary to achieve sterilization

cleaning the physical removal of organic material. The first step in disinfection or sterilization that enhances the effectiveness of the subsequent disinfection or sterilization processes

coagulase positive/negative refers to the ability of a microorganism (usually staphylococci) to produce an enzyme that will coagulate citrated plasma

coliform any gram-negative, lactose fermentative, rod-shaped bacteria that resembles *Escherichia coli*

colonization reproduction of microorganisms at a site in the absence of clinical signs of infection, tissue invasion, or significant immune response

colony-forming unit (CFU) single or aggregate of microorganisms capable of producing a visible colony on culture media. Colonies representing CFUs are counted to quantitate organisms in clinical specimens

commensal the species in a symbiotic relationship that derives benefit without harming the host. Commensal microorganisms may produce clinically significant infection if the host's immune capabilities are compromised or they are introduced to another host site

complement protein components of the immune system that react in series as part of the immune response and facilitate chemotaxis and phagocytosis of immune system cells and destruction of microorganisms

contaminants chemical, organic, or infectious material on normally sterile or clean sites

contamination the introduction of impurity such as potentially infectious microorganisms

convalescent sera serum obtained during the convalescent phase of an illness and tested for presence of pathogen-specific antibody as evidence that the specific pathogen was the cause of recent infection

cyst a phase in the life cycle of some parasites during which they are enclosed in a protective wall

cytokine non-antibody proteins that mediate activity of cells of the immune system

decontamination process of rendering a person, object or area free from contaminants such as infectious microorganisms

disease a definite morbid process having characteristic symptoms

disinfection elimination of vegetative forms of potentially infectious microorganisms from inanimate objects

DNA (deoxyribonucleic acid) the molecule which, by its configuration of nucleic acids, determines biologic functions and hereditary identity. Considered to be the autoreproducing component of chromosomes and of many viruses, and the repository of hereditary characteristics and genetic information. The complex proteins are arranged as two long chains that twist around each other to form a double helix joined by bonds between the complementary components

DNA probe diagnostic technology that provides rapid detection or identification of microorganisms by identification of microorganism-specific sequences of nucleic acids in DNA or RNA

droplets particles of moisture generated by coughing, sneezing, laughing, or procedures such as suctioning, sputum induction, or bronchoscopy which may contain infectious microorganisms but do not remain suspended in air and normally travel a distance less than three feet

droplet nuclei the airborne residual of evaporated droplets usually less than five microns in size and capable of reaching the alveoli if inhaled

ecology the study of interrelationships among living organisms and their environments

ELISA (enzyme-linked immunosorbent assay) a rapid enzyme immunoassay method used to identify the etiologic agent of infection in which either an antibody or an antigen is linked to an enzyme. The resulting complex retains both immunologic and enzymatic ac-tivity and participates in antigen-specific reactions that allow identification of the antigen by means of detection of enzymatic activity of the antigen-antibody complex

endemic a disease or condition that is continuously present in a population

endogenous originating within a host

endotoxin gram-negative bacterial cell wall constituent capable of initiating shock in the host who is infected or exposed to the cell wall components, such as across a dialysis membrane

enteric inhabiting the gastrointestinal tract

enterotoxin a toxin specific for the cells of the intestinal mucosa

enzyme a protein that catalyzes chemical reactions

eosinophil a granular leukocyte having cytoplasm that contains coarse, round granules which are readily stained by eosin

epidemic attacking many people in any region at the same time. Widely diffused and rapidly spreading

epidemiology the quantitative study of health events in populations and the factors that determine the frequency and distribution of those events

epitope site of antibody attachment on an antigen

exogenous originating or produced outside the host

exotoxin poisonous substance formed within and released by a microorganism (usually gram-positive bacteria)

facultative able to live under either aerobic or anaerobic conditions

fiberoptic an optical system of flexible bundles of glass or plastic fibers that convey an image

flagella organelles of locomotion that appear as projections from certain microorganisms

fluorescent antibody/antigen testing laboratory method that allows visual identification of antigens that consists of antibody or antigen attached to a fluorescent molecule and allowed to react with an antigen or antibody to be identified by visualization under fluorescent light. Fluorescent antibody/antigen techniques permit rapid diagnosis of various kinds of infection

fomite an object that is not in itself harmful but is able to harbor pathogenic microorganisms and thus may serve as an agent of transmission of infection

genotype the genetic constitution of an individual

genus a taxonomic category that is a subdivision of the family or tribe and is divided into species

hematogenous derived from or transported by blood. Often refers to transportation of infectious agents from one body site to another via the blood

HEPA filter high-efficiency particulate air filter capable of capturing from the air particles larger than three microns

herd immunity protection from an infectious disease provided to susceptible members of a group by immunity of other members of the same group who do not transmit an infectious agent

hypersensitivity an exaggerated immune system response to stimuli; allergy

incubation period the time in the development of infectious disease between the entrance of the pathogen and the appearance of clinical symptoms

infection invasion and multiplication of microorganisms in body tissues, resulting in local cellular injury due to competitive metabolism, toxins, intracellular replication, or immune response

immune globulins a family of proteins that are capable of binding antigens. Five major classes exist in adults:

IgA: 10-15% relative amount present in human serum. IgA is the principal immunoglobulin in exocrine secretions such as milk, respiratory secretions and tears

IgD: less than .1% in human serum. The exact function of IgD is not known but it appears to play a role in activating complement

IgE: less than .01% in human serum. IgE is produced in the respiratory tract and associated with allergic reactions and response to parasitic infections. Its specific immune function is unknown

IgG: 80% in human serum. IgG is the principal immunoglobulin of sustained immunity which is also capable of crossing the placental barrier

IgM: 5-10% in human serum. IgM is the first immunoglobulin to be generated in immune responses

immune response the cell mediated and humoral immune reactions to antigens which preserve the integrity of the host from infectious organisms and other degradative environmental agents

immunocompromised a state of defective or failed immune response

immunoelectrophoresis a method of distinguishing proteins and other materials (e.g., antigens) on the basis of their electrophoretic mobility and antigenic specificities (i.e., reaction with specific antibodies)

immunoglobulin another term for immune globulin; antibody

in vitro performed or occurring outside of the living individual

in vivo performed or occurring on or in a living individual

incidence the number of new events, such as new cases of diseases, occurring in a defined population during the specified time individuals were at risk

india ink a dye used to stain fluid which is then examined under a microscope for the presence of microorganisms. *Cryptococcus neoformans* in spinal fluid exhibits a characteristic, clear halo indicating the presence of a capsule when stained with india ink

inflammatory response a process consisting of histologic and cytologic reactions that occur in the affected blood vessels and adjacent tissue in response to stimulation such as injury or infection and is manifested as rubor (redness), dolor (pain), calor (heat production), and tumor (swelling)

interferon a class of glycoproteins that function as antiviral agents

KOH (potassium hydroxide) preparation treatment of specimen or skin scraping with potassium hydroxide to dissolve host tissue remnants and reveal fungal hyphae

latency a state in which disease is present but not

manifest. Some conditions have a long latent period from the time of initial infection to the appearance of disease, or symptomatic episodes separated by asymptomatic periods

latex agglutination laboratory procedure for identifying antigen or antibody in a specimen by reaction with complementary antigen or antibody to which visible molecules of latex have been bound

leukopenia abnormally low number (<5000/cu mm) of white blood cells (leukocytes) in blood

lymphocyte mononuclear, non-granular leukocyte formed in lymphatic tissue, normally constituting 22-28% of the total leukocytes in the circulating blood. B and T lymphocytes are important components of the immune system

lymphokine substance released by sensitized lymphocytes on contact with specific antigens that stimulates activity of macrophages and monocytes

lysis lethal disruption of cell

lysozome intracellular vacuole containing enzymes that break down certain proteins and carbohydrates

macrophage a mononuclear, phagocytic cell from the bone marrow widely distributed throughout the body

minimum inhibitory concentration (MIC) the lowest concentration of antimicrobial agent that will inhibit bacterial growth

monoclonal antibody antigen-specific antibody produced by a single clone of cells

neutrophil mature granulocytic white blood cell normally representing 54-65% of circulating white cells

normal flora microorganisms usually inhabiting the surfaces and spaces of larger organisms, generally without adverse effect

nosocomial infection infection developed or initiated during stay or work in a health care facility and not present or incubating at the time of admission

pandemic widespread epidemic distributed throughout a region or continent or globally

parasite an organism dependent on a living host for nutrients

pathogen microorganism capable of causing disease

pathogenicity the ability to produce disease

phagocytosis the process of ingestion and digestion of bacteria, cells, tissue, or foreign particles by single cells of the immune system or unicellular organisms

phenotype the combined manifested characteristics of an organism that distinguish it from other organisms

pili short, hair-like organelles that protrude from bacterial cells and facilitate attachment and conjugation

plasmid extrachromosomal genetic material in bacteria not essential to the cell's function that may be transmitted by conjugation. Resistance capabilities are often transferred among bacteria of the same or different species on plasmids

polymicrobic involving several species of microorganisms

polymorphonuclear leukocytes (PMNs) phagocytic leukocytes with variably shaped nuclei

prevalence the number or proportion of individuals in a population who have a specific characteristic, condition, or disease at a specific point in time

prions infectious agents more primative than viruses which appear to consist only of protein and lack nucleic acid. Includes agents of Scrapie and Creutzfeldt-Jakob disease

pyocin bacteriocin produced by strains of *Pseudomonas* that can be used to type other microorganisms according to their relative susceptibility

reservoir place where a microorganism maintains its presence and from which it may be transmitted

restriction endonuclease typing laboratory technique used to determine genetic relatedness in which enzymes (endonucleases) cut viral DNA at unique and specific sites and fragments are separated by electrophoresis according to their molecular weights and charge and visualized radiographically

reverse transcriptase an enzyme in retroviruses that catalyzes the production of DNA from a viral RNA template

ribosome an internal cell structure that is the site of protein synthesis

RNA (ribonucleic acid) a nucleic acid macromolecule constructed on a DNA template which, in turn, provides the template for amino acid assembly into proteins. The basic determinant of biologic function and hereditary identity in some viruses

saprophyte an organism that grows on dead organic matter

sensitivity ability of a laboratory test to correctly identify all true positive cases of a condition

septicemia systemic disease caused by the presence of microorganisms and/or their toxic products in the circulating blood

serologic diagnosis diagnosis based on the detection of specific antibody or other constituents of serum

serotyping identification of organisms based on their antigenic composition as detected by specific antibody

source the immediate location from which a microorganism is transmitted to a host

species a taxonomic level subordinate to genus

specificity ability of a laboratory test to correctly identify all true negative cases of a condition

spore the living but dormant stage of the life cycle of some bacteria, fungi, and other organisms. Spores are usually relatively resistant to environmental extremes and less metabolically active than other forms

sterile free of all life forms including spores

sterilization destruction of all life forms including spores

strain a homogeneous population of organisms descendant from a common ancestor or, in microbiology, isolate

superinfection infection that occurs as a complication of a previous infection and is caused by a different microorganism

surveillance systematic observation intended to detect the occurrence and distribution of disease or other events in a population

synergism combined action of two or more agents, structures, or processes that produces a result greater than that of each acting separately

teratogenic causing congenital malformations or disturbed fetal development

toxin a poison produced by pathogenic bacteria or other organisms which is toxic for other living organisms. A toxin is distinguished from a simple chemical poison by its high molecular weight and antigenicity

toxoid a toxin that has been treated to destroy its toxic properties but which retains its ability to stimulate the production of antitoxin antibodies and, thereby, produce active immunity

transcriptase enzyme that catalyzes production of RNA from a DNA template. The first stage of protein production that is followed by the assembly of amino acids into proteins based upon the sequence of ribonucleic acids (translation)

translocation transposition of two segments between nonhomologous chromosomes as a result of abnormal breakage

transposon a segment of DNA that can excise itself from a chromosome or plasmid and migrate to and integrate into another plasmid or chromosome

universal precautions infection prevention strategies implemented during patient care regardless of the patient diagnosis. These strategies include use of barriers such as gloves, cover clothing, and facial protection to prevent the health care provider's direct contact with blood or other substances which may contain bloodborne pathogens

vector an organism such as a tick, bloodsucking fly, or mite capable of transmitting infectious agents among hosts

vehicle an inanimate substance such as food, dust, or instrument, within or upon which infectious agents may be delivered to a susceptible host; fomite

virion viral particle consisting of the central core (nucleoid) containing DNA or RNA surrounded by a protein coat and often other structures. The virion is structurally complete and able to infect cells; virus

virulence the disease-evoking capability of an organism in a given host

Index